KININS IV
Part A

ADVANCES IN EXPERIMENTAL MEDICINE AND BIOLOGY

Recent Volumes in this Series

A Continuation Order Plan in available for this series. A continuation order will bring delivery of each new volume immediately upon publication. Volumes are billed only upon actual shipment. For further information please contact the publisher.

KININS IV
Part A

Edited by
Lowell M. Greenbaum
Medical College of Georgia
Augusta, Georgia

and
Harry S. Margolius
Medical University of South Carolina
Charleston, South Carolina

PLENUM PRESS • NEW YORK AND LONDON

Library of Congress Cataloging in Publication Data

International Kinin Congress (4th: 1984: Savannah, Ga.)
  Kinins IV.

  (Advances in experimental medicine and biology; v. 198)
  "Proceedings of the Fourth International Kinin Congress, held October 21-25, 1984, in
Savannah, Georgia"—T.p. verso.
  Includes bibliographies and index.
  1. Kinins—Congresses. 2. Kallikrein—Congresses. I. Greenbaum, Lowell M. II.
Margolius, Harry S. III. Title. IV. Title: Kinins 4. V. Series. [DNLM: 1. Kinins—
congresses. W1 AD559 v.198/QU 68 I593 1984k]
QP552.K5I54 1984   599′.019′24   86-9403
ISBN-13: 978-1-4684-5145-0   e-ISBN-13: 978-1-4684-5143-6
DOI: 10.1007/978-1-4684-5143-6

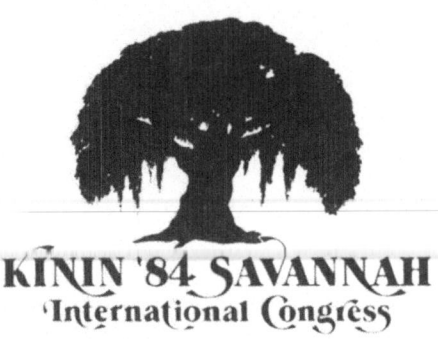

KININ '84 SAVANNAH
International Congress

Proceedings of the Fourth International Kinin Congress,
held October 21-25, 1984, in Savannah, Georgia

PREFACE

    Scientists from 25 countries came together at the Hyatt Regency
Hotel on October 21-25, 1984, for the 4th International Kinin Congress
in the beautiful city of Savannah, Georgia. Many of the delegates
enjoyed southern hospitality for the first time. The friendly city with
its streets lined with the Live Oak Tree (symbol of the Congress), the
balmy weather, and the excellent facilities of the hotel set the stage
for scientific events and exchange that proved so successful. The organization of the meeting was the result of many hours, days and weeks of
effort by many, including from Augusta Drs. James H. Sutherland, John
Catravas, William Davis, Jr., and Hiroshi Okamoto; and from Charleston,
SC, Julie Chao, Ronald Mayfield and Donald Miller. Special thanks go
to Ms. Cher Cornett of the Department of Medical Illustration at the
Medical College of Georgia for her talent in the design of the logo, as
well as the graphics of the program and abstracts. We are indeed
indebted to Dr. Paul Brucker, Director of the Division of Health Communications at the Medical College of Georgia, for his considerable aid in
spending time with us to arrange the programming format and continuity.
Ms. Sandra Usry provided very excellent and devoted secretarial help for
several years while the Congress was in the making. Thanks also to the
secretarial staff of the Department of Pharmacology at MCG, including
Rosiland Simmons and Jennie Doby for their expert assistance during the
meeting. We also wish to thank the many sponsors (NIH, Johnson &
Johnson, Bayer AG and Bayer AG/Miles, KabiVitrum AB, American Heart
Association, Medical College of Georgia Research Institute, Rich's
Travel, Bayer Yakhuin, Ltd., Bristol-Myers Co., Drug Science Foundation
of S.C., Sanwa Kagaku Ltd., Upjohn Co., Hoffmann-La Roche, Inc.,
Boehringer Ingelheim, Ltd., Burroughs Wellcome Co., Ciba Geigy Pharma-
ceutical, E. R. Squibb & Sons, Inc., Fujimoto Pharmaceutical Co., Ltd.,
Am. Cyanamid Co., G. D. Searle, E. I. DuPont de Nemours & Co.).

    During the early planning of the Congress, we learned of the death
of one of the world's great pharmacologists and discoverer of bradykinin, Professor Mauricio Rocha e Silva of Brazil. Professor Rocha e
Silva not only coined the name for bradykinin but was a staunch advocate
in his own special way for research all over the world to elucidate the
importance of kinins and kallikreins in health and in disease. It is
more than fitting that the 4th International Congress of Kinins was
dedicated to his memory and efforts. We were most fortunate that his
collaborator in the discovery of bradykinin and a great scientist in his
own right, Dr. Wilson Beraldo of Belo Horizonte, attended the Congress.
All of us were moved by his sincere tribute, as well as the tribute of
Dr. Mauricio Rocha e Silva, Jr., to Professor Rocha e Silva's contributions to science and society. Since the close of the Congress we
learned of the deaths of three pioneers in kinin research, Dr. John
Pisano (suddenly) of the NIH, Dr. Ulla Hamburg of Finland and Dr. Marion
Webster, formerly of the NIH. Each of these have left lasting impres-

sions on us because of their pioneering contributions, their strength of purpose in kinin research and their love of aiding others in our discipline. We will miss them. We are privileged that these volumes contain the last scientific communications of Drs. Pisano and Hamburg.

"Kinin '84 Savannah" had a number of "firsts". It was the first Kinin Congress to encompass four full days. It was the first Congress to institute "Frontier Lecturers" which provided us with information about areas of research which may be vital to our growth but with which we may not be familiar at this time. We are all indebted to the superb lecturers which included Dr. Hans Fritz (FRG), Dr. Robert Colman (USA), Dr. S. Nakanishi (Japan), Dr. John Shine (Australia), Dr. Allen Cuthbert (England) and Dr. T. Hokfelt (Sweden). This was the first Congress to utilize the concept of formal "Poster Discussions" so that all investigators had a chance to comment on their efforts in addition to the 200 posters on display. We are indebted to the discussion leaders who made the 14 sessions so meaningful. It was the first of the Kinin Congresses to have "competing" oral sessions and we wish to thank the Chairman and Co-chairman of these sessions, as well as the delegates themselves, for the excellence of the 80 oral presentations. This was the first international meeting at which the T-kinin - T-kininogen sysem was introduced, as well as several components of the kallikrein-kinin system in brain including kinins and kininases. The long sought-after antagonist to bradykinin as well as the isolation and characterization of the genes expressing kininogen synthesis was described. It was the first of our meetings to pay tribute to our pioneers in kinin research and we again salute the recipients, Drs. Melville Schachter (Canada), Ervin Erdös (USA), Wilson Beraldo (Brazil), Hector Croxatto (Chile), Tomoji Suzuki-(Japan), and Gert Haberland (FRG). It was the first meeting at which six young investigators from five countries were nominated as KabiVitrum Scholars and given special travel awards.

Our social times together also left some unforgettable memories. All of us will remember the warm friendship and the beauty of the evening and as we glided down the Savannah River on the riverboat to shuck oysters under the torchlight and accompanied by the southern jazz music of Fort Jackson. We were truly a "Kinin Family." The satellite meeting in Hilton Head and the visitations to Charleston and Augusta provided additional opportunities for interactions and friendships.

The 4th International Kinin Congress was a stimulating experience for us and we hope the pages of these volumes will keep the spirit and science of Kinin '84 Savannah alive for many years to come.

Lowell M. Greenbaum, Ph.D
President, IKC
Augusta, Georgia

Harry S. Margolius, Ph.D, M.D.
Vice President, IKC
Charleston, South Carolina

CONTENTS - PART A

TISSUE KININOGENASES

KININOGENS

CONTENTS - PART B

BLOOD CLOTTING FACTORS AND THE KALLIKREIN-KININ SYSTEM

NEW METHODS AND MECHANISMS IN STUDIES ON THE
KALLIKREIN-KININ SYSTEM

THE VARIED LOCALIZATION AND FUNCTIONAL SIGNIFICANCE OF KALLIKREIN-LIKE

ENZYMES IN SALIVARY GLANDS, PANCREAS, COLON, SEX GLANDS AND SPERMATOZOA,

INCLUDING EVIDENCE FOR THE PRESENCE OF NERVE GROWTH FACTOR (NGF) IN BULL

SPERM ACROSOME[1]

M. Schachter, M. W. Peret, The Late C. Moriwaki,
G. D. Wheeler, R. W. Matthews, J. G. Mehta and T. Labedz

Department of Physiology, University of Alberta
Edmonton, Alberta T6G 2H7

INTRODUCTION

There has been considerable recent progress in the cellular and sub-cellular localization of kallikreins (or kininogenases) and related serine proteases.[1-8] In this report, we review briefly our localization studies - some published and some new observations. These include studies on the salivary glands and colon of various mammals, the sex glands of the guinea pig, and the spermatozoa of boar, bull and man. In addition, we report our observations on the presence of Nerve Growth Factor (NGF) in bull sperm.

We describe and discuss the diverse subcellular localization of kallikreins in different tissues and emphasize the probable multiplicity of functions of these and related serine proteases which probably have a common molecular ancestry.

METHODS

Pure boar acrosin was provided by the late Professor C. Moriwaki. It gave only a single precipitation band in immunodiffusion tests with our antisera. Nerve growth factor, NGF (from mouse submandibular gland), and its specific antiserum were obtained from Collaborative Research Laboratories, Inc. (Mass., USA). This antiserum also gave single precipitation bands with pure mouse NGF or with mouse submandibular gland extracts.

Boar and bull semen were obtained from commercial sperm banks in the fresh state or frozen in liquid nitrogen. Fresh human semen was

---

[1]This communication duplicates in part, and extends our publication in Kinins III, Advances in Experimental Medicine and Biology, Vol. 156A, pp. 377-386, eds. H. Fritz et al., Plenum Press, New York, 1983. Due to printer's error, the legends to the figures were incorrect in the previous publication. Some of these figures are, therefore, correctly republished here.

obtained at our Hospital Infertility Clinic from healthy donors. Smears
of seminal fluid were made 1-2 hours after collection or after the thawing
of frozen samples. The fresh semen was diluted twice with phosphate-
buffered saline at pH 7.5; thawed boar or bull semen was diluted with the
commercial buffer provided. Smears were dried at room temperature or at
36ºC.

Immunocytochemical staining and related procedures were carried out
as previously described.[5-9]

RESULTS

Kininogenase (Kallikrein) in Salivary Glands

Cat   The kininogenase in the cat submandibular gland (also parotid
and sublingual) was localized by fluorescence immune staining and by the
immunoperoxidase method, using both light and electron microscopy (see
Methods). All our recent results are in accord with our previous
suggestion that this enzyme is located in small apical secretory granules
in the duct cells.[9-11] Although the secretion of the enzyme is effected
primarily by stimulation of the sympathetic nerve, its synthesis or storage
requires the integrity of the parasympathetic innervation. Thus, whereas
the kallikrein concentration of the gland, the apical duct granules, and
the specific immune staining are all greatly reduced after several days
of duct obstruction or after degenerative section of the parasympathetic
nerve, they are all unaffected by sympathetic denervation and subsequent
degeneration of these fibres.[11-12]

Figure 1 shows conventional electron micrographs of the submandibular
glands (from the same cat) with and without depletion of kallikrein, the
former after duct obstruction for several days. Note the almost complete
absence of apical duct granules in the obstructed (and kallikrein depleted)
gland. Figure 2 is an electron micrograph showing immune staining for cat
salivary kallikrein. The specific immune staining is in the apical
granules of a striated duct. The granules are less deformed by the methods
of fixation used for conventional than for immunoelectron microscopy.

Man and Dog   We have found, as have others,[13] that the salivary
glands of both man and dog contain relatively small amounts of kallikrein
compared to rat, cat and guinea-pig. Nonetheless, we obtained definitive
evidence of an apical ductal localization of kallikrein in the submandibular gland of dog and man using the immunoperoxidase method.[6]

Guinea-Pig   Submandibular gland kallikrein of the guinea-pig is
also localized by immunocytochemistry in the apical regions of the duct
cells.[5-6] Figure 3 shows such light microscopic results, as well as an
ordinary electron micrograph showing the small apical granules in the
guinea-pig's ducts, granules similar to those of the cat in Figure 1.

Kininogenases (Kallikrein and Kallikrein-Like Enzymes) in Pancreas

Yasuda and Coons[14] confirmed by immunofluorescence technique the
already presumed localization of amylase, chymotrypsin and trypsin in the
acinar cells of the pig pancreas. Since then, the same result has been
obtained by immunocytochemical techniques for kallikrein in the pancreas
of the rat[1] and pig.[15] My colleagues and I (unpublished) have confirmed these results and in the pancreas of the cat and dog as well.

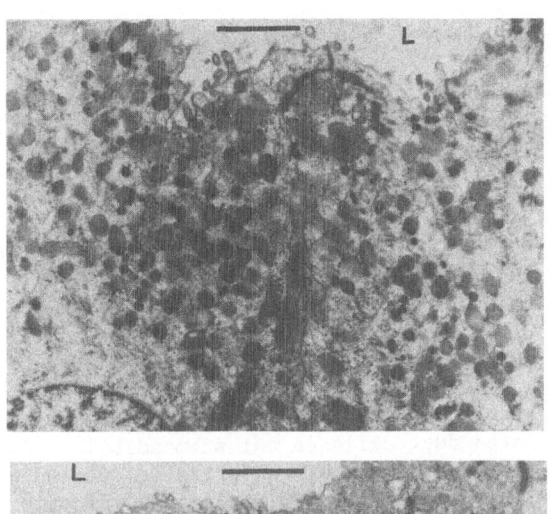

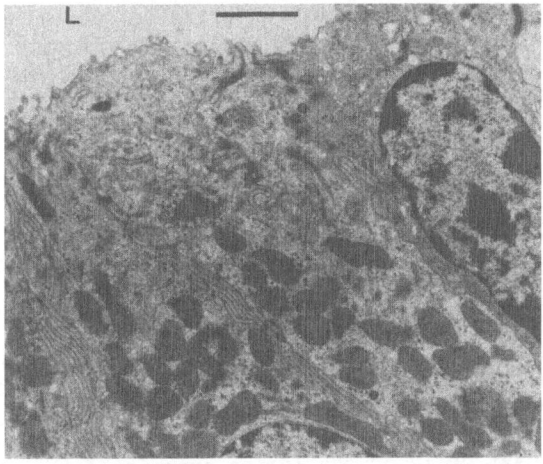

Figure 1. Electron micrograph of apical duct granules of cat submandibular gland in upper panel. Lower panel is a similar area in
contralateral gland depleted of granules (and of kallikrein)
after 3 days of duct ligation; the granules are absent and
mitochondria are more prominent. L, lumen.[11]

     Further, similar methods have detected a discrete localization of
kallikrein in beta cells of the islets of human pancreas, as well as in
acinar cells.[16] In a similar way, "trypsin-like activity" has been
demonstrated in isolated pancreas islet cells.[17] It is presumed that
such localized islet cell proteases are involved in insulin processing.
Further studies are required for the confirmation and precise identification of these proteases in the endocrine pancreas.

Kininogenase (Kallikrein, etc.) in Colon

     We have recently localized colon kallikrein in the goblet cells of
man, cat and rat by a variety of immunocytochemical techniques. No
evidence of this kallikrein was found in cells other than the goblet or
mucous cells of this organ.[7] Figure 4 illustrates our result of the
specific localization of kallikrein in goblet cells of the glandularis
mucosa of the cat colon using the immunoperoxidase method and antibody to
pure salivary gland kallikrein.

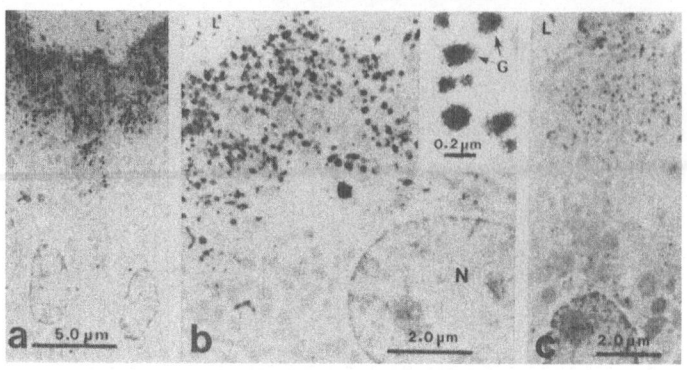

Figure 2. Immunoperoxidase localization of kallikrein in apical granules of striated duct cells in cat submandibular gland. (a) Low power electron micrograph of striated duct showing luminal particles. L, lumen. (b) Higher magnification than a, showing immunostained apical granules lining lumen above unstained mitochondria and nucleus (N). Inset: Highest magnification showing characteristic irregular, "studded" appearance of granules (G) due to PAP immune aggregates. (c) Control section of duct cell. Apical granules show only faint nonspecific stain. L, lumen. Original magnifications: (a) x925; (b) x2345; inset, x17,625; (c) x1980.[8]

These interesting results on kallikrein localization in mucous and goblet cells await confirmation by others using related techniques. We await such studies with interest in view of the many pitfalls in immunocytochemistry. However, a serine protease of the "group-specific protease", or GSP type, has been localized in intestinal goblet cells and also in atypical mast cells of the lamina propria of the small intestine using immunofluorescence techniques.[18] Also, using histochemical techniques, kallikrein-like activity has been demonstrated in mast cells of the lamina propria and submucosa of salivary glands and colon of different mammals.[19-21] My colleagues and I have also detected kallikrein-like enzymes histochemically in the lamina propria and submucosa of the colon and other parts of the gastrointestinal tract (unpublished).

Kininogenase (CGK) in the Coagulating and Prostate Glands of the Guinea-Pig

The first evidence of a kallikrein-like enzyme in reproductive organs was presented for the accessory sex glands of the guinea-pig by Schachter and his colleagues in 1961.[3-4,22-24] This potent kininogenase (the term was introduced at this time for this enzyme) was found in large amounts in the guinea-pig's coagulating gland and in lower concentrations in the prostate. Several other mammals examined, including man, however, did not appear to have it in their accessory sex glands as measured by the ability of extracts to release kinin in vitro and in vivo. This enzyme was later designated as CGK (Coagulating Gland Kininogenase) by Moriwaki and Schachter,[25] and it was found to release either bradykinin or kallidin, more likely the latter.[26] It was shown by immunocytochemistry to be present in most, if not all, cells lining the crypts of the coagulating gland[5] and is thought to be present in the soluble fraction of homogenates rather than in specific organelles.[27] We have shown (unpublished), using the immunoperoxidase technique, that CGK is also located in cells lining the lumen of the prostate gland. We conclude, therefore, that although the concentration of CGK are lower in the prostate than in the coagulating gland of the guinea-pig, the enzyme is

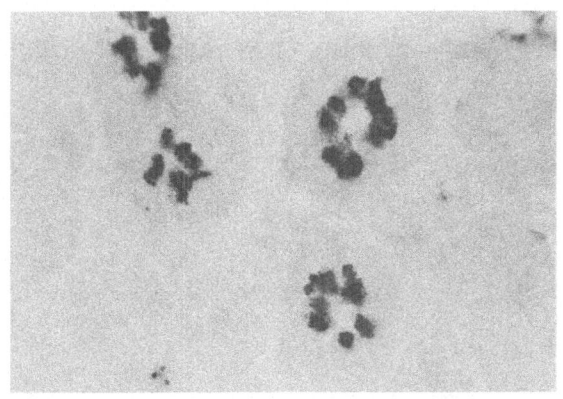

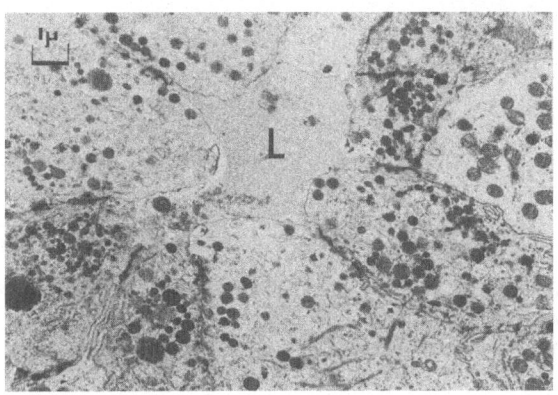

Figure 3. Guinea-pig submandibular gland. Upper panel: Light microscopic immunoperoxidase stained section showing localization of kallikrein in apical region of duct cells only. Original magnification x160.[6] Lower panel: Electron micrograph showing small apical granules in striated ducts. These granules correspond in position to areas of specific immune staining for kallikrein seen in upper panel (Shnitka, Peret and Schachter, unpublished).

also present in the prostate itself, where it is not due to contamination during its dissection from the adjacent coagulating gland. We have also confirmed the observations of Harper et al.[28] that, whereas the prostate gland has high concentrations of Nerve Growth Factor, the coagulating gland has little or none (Barton, et al., unpublished).

Antibody to guinea-pig CGK cross-reacted in the "Eliza" test with submandibular gland kallikrein with 2-5% of its specific activity with its own antigen. It failed to cross-react, however, even at high concentrations, with acrosin from bull, boar and man. The latter, however, cross-reacted strongly with one another.

Acrosin in Spermatozoa of Bull, Boar and Man, and Immunocytochemical Evidence for Nerve Growth Factor (NGF) in Bull Spermatozoa

A trypsin-like acrosomal kininogenase named acrosin has been isolated from sperm in recent years.[29-31] Previous immunocytochemical work has indicated that acrosin is present in the head region or acrosome of various mammals, e.g., in the bull,[32] ram,[33] and in man and other mammals.[27] Our work confirms and extends these observations as follows.

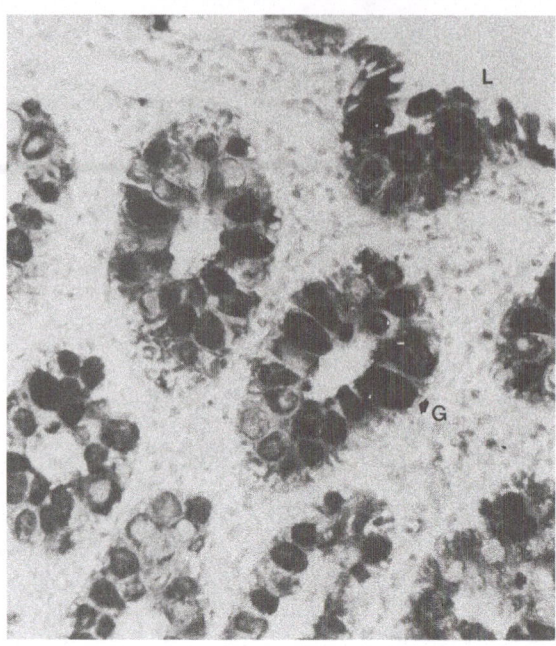

Figure 4. Localization of kallikrein in goblet cells of cat colon by
immunoperoxidase technique. G, goblet cell; L, lumen.
Original magnification x64.[7]

1. Acrosin localizes in the head region of spermatozoa from boar, bull
    and man with immunofluorescence and peroxidase techniques using anti-
    body to boar acrosin (Figure 5).

2. Antibody to boar acrosin cross-reacts strongly in different immuno-
    logical tests with acrosin from bull and man but does not with the
    guinea-pig sex gland kininogenase (CGK).

3. Bull spermatozoa also contain NGF. They react immunocytochemically
    with antibody raised to NGF prepared from mouse submandibular gland.
    The reaction with NGF antibody in the head of bull spermatozoa
    resembles that to acrosin (Figure 5). Whether the NGF thus de-
    tected in bull spermatozoa is produced there or transported, or simply
    adsorbed from the bull seminal fluid[34] remains uncertain for the
    present. Further experiments are necessary.

DISCUSSION

    Our results and those of others presented here confirm and extend
the ubiquity of closely related serine proteases in different organs and
in a wide variety of tissues and cells. We also confirm their chemical
similarities by our observations on the relative immunological cross-
reactivity between the kininogenases in the guinea-pig's coagulating and
salivary glands, by the high cross-reactivity between the kallikreins of
salivary gland, pancreas and colon in the cat, and between the acrosins
of spermatozoa of boar, bull and man. The enzymes classified as
kallikreins, kininogenases and many other serine proteases, so diverse in
their distribution and subcellular localizations, are now known from

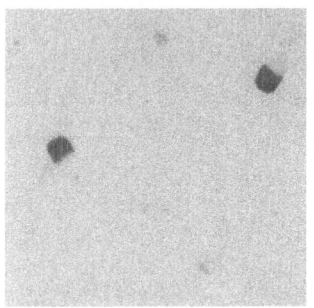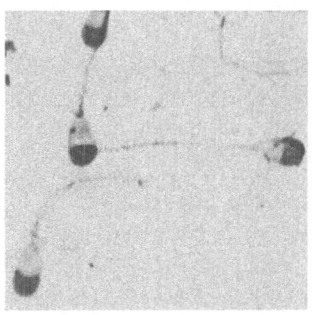

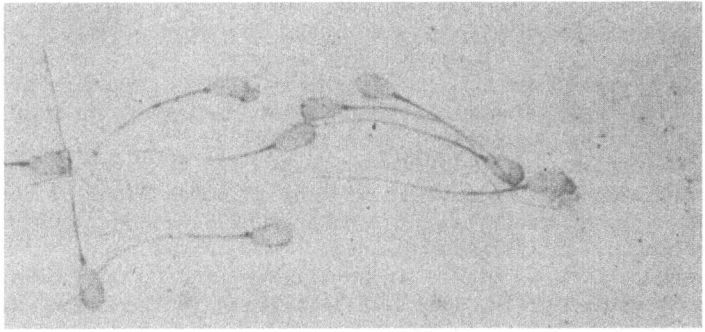

Figure 5. Localization of acrosin in head region of boar sperm (upper left) and NGF in head region of bull sperm. Lower panel shows control boar sperm without specific immune serum (similar negative controls are obtained with bull sperm).

chemical analyses to have extensive shared amino acid sequences, suggesting a common ancient ancestry for these enzymes.[3-4,35-39] Also, the γ subunit of NGF and the EGF-binding protein are closely related to the kallikrein-like esteroproteases.[40]

In the view of the above, we conclude: The serine proteases which are so similar in chemical structure and in their catalytic mechanisms that they are considered by some to have arisen from a common ancestral molecule, are, nonetheless, most diverse in their respective functions. Their relevant property is the proteolytic specificity whereby they exert their bioregulatory actions. The presence of their inhibitors in many mammalian cells and secretions and wide distribution of the latter in nature, reflect the ubiquitousness and probably the significance of the enzymes themselves.[3-4]

ACKNOWLEDGEMENTS

We are indebted to Drs. R. Peter Beck and Joe Scott of our Obstetrics Department and Infertility Clinic for making human sperm available to us. This work was supported by the Medical Research Council of Canada, the Alberta Heart Foundation, and the Alberta Heritage Foundation for Medical Research.

REFERENCES

1. T. B. Ørstavik, K. Nustad, and P. Brandtzaeg, Origin of kallikrein in rat and human exocrine glands and kidney, Clin. Sci., 57: 2395, (1979).

2. T. B. Ørstavik, K. Nustad, and P. Brandtzaeg, Localization of blandular kallikreins in rat and man, in: Enzymatic Release of Vasoactive Peptides ed. by F. Gross and G. Vogel, Raven Press, New York, pp. 137-149, (1980).

3. M. Schachter, Kallikrein localization and its significance, in: Enzymatic Release of Vasoactive Peptides ed. by F. Gross and G. Vogel, Raven Press, New York, pp. 151-160, (1980a).

4. M. Schachter, Kallikreins (kininogenases) - a group of serine proteases with bioregulatory actions, Pharmacol. Rev., 31:1, (1980b).

5. M. Schachter, B. Maranda, and C. Moriwaki, Localization of kallikrein in the coagulating and submandibular glands of the guinea-pig, J. Histochem. Cytochem., 26:318, (1978).

6. M. Schachter, M. W. Peret, C. Moriwaki, and J. A. A. Rodrigues, Localization of kallikrein in submandibular bland of cat, guinea-pig, dog and man by the immunoperoxidase method, J. Histochem. Cytochem., 28:1295, (1980).

7. M. Schachter, M. W. Peret, A. G. Billing, and G. D. Wheeler, Immunolocalization of the protease kallikrein in the colon, J. Histochem. Cytochem., 31:1255, (1983a).

8. M. Schachter, G. D. Wheeler, R. W. Matthews, M. W. Peret, and C. Moriwaki, Ultrastructural immunolocalization of kallikrein in apical granules of striated duct cells of cat submandibular gland, J. Histochem. Cytochem., 31:345, (1983b).

9. B. Maranda, J. A. A. Rodrigues, M. Schachter, T. K. Shnitka, and J. Weinberg, Studies on kallikrein in the duct systems of the salivary glands of the cat, J. Physiol., 276:321, (1978).

10. S. Barton, E. J. Sanders, M. Schachter, and M. Uddin, Autonomic nerve stimulation, kallikrein content and acinar cell granules of the cat's submandibular gland, J. Physiol., 251:363, (1975).

11. M. Schachter, S. Barton, M. Uddin, E. Karpinski, and E. J. Sanders, Effects of nerve stimulation, denervation, and duct ligation, on kallikrein content and duct cell granules of the cat's submandibular gland, Experientia, 33:746, (1977).

12. S. Beilenson, M. Schachter, and H. Smaje, Secretion of kallikrein and its role in vasodilatation in the submaxillary gland, J. Physiol., 199:303, (1968).

13. E. K. Frey, H. Kraut, and E. Werle, Das Kallikrein-Kinin System and Seine Inhibitoren, Enke, Stuttgart, (1968).

14. K. Yasuda and A. H. Coons, Localization by immunofluorescence of amylase, trypsinogen and chymotrypsinogen in the acinar cells of the pig pancreas, J. Histochem. Cytochem., 14:303, (1965).

15. T. Dietl, J. Kruck, and H. Fritz, Localization of kallikrein in procine pancreas and submandibular gland as revealed by the direct immunofluorescence technique, Hoppe Seyler's Z. Physiol. Chem., 359:499, (1978).

16. G. S. Pinkus, M. Maier, D. C. Seldin, O. Ole-Moiyoi, K. F. Austen, and J. C. Spragg, Immunohistochemical localization of glandular kallikrein in the endocrine and exocrine human pancreas, J. Histochem. Cytochem., 31:1279, (1983).

17. A. Dorn, G. Koch, H. Zuhlke, B. Arlt, D. Lorenz, and M. Ziegler, The immunochemical investigation of trypsin and trypsin-like activity in the small intestine, pancreas and isolated Langerhans islets, Acta Histochem., 63:26, (1978).

18. R. G. Woodbury, G. M. Gruzenski, and D. Lagunoff, Immunofluorescent localization of a serine protease in rat small intestine, Proc. Natl. Acad. Sci., U.S.A., 75:2785, (1978).

19. J. R. Garrett, J. D. Harrison, A. Kidd, K. Kyriacou, and R. E. Smith, Kallikrein-like activity in human salivary glands and colon, including mast cells, J. Physiol., 334:78P, (1982a).

20. J. R. Garrett, R. E. Smith, A. Kidd, K. Kyriacou, and R. J. Grabske, Kallikrein-like activity in salivary glands using a new tripeptide substrate, including preliminary secretory studies and observations on mast cells, Histochem. J., 14:967, (1982b).

21. J. R. Garrett, A. Kidd, K. Kyriacou, and R. E. Smith, New observations on the localization of kallikrein-like activity in human salivary parenchymal and mast cells by enzyme histochemistry, Histochem. J., 16:789, (1984).

22. K. D. Bhoola, R. May May Yi, J. Morley, and M. Schachter, Kinin-releasing enzyme in the accessory sex glands of the guinea-pig, J. Physiol., 159:34-35P, (1961).

23. K. D. Bhoola, R. May May Yi, J. Morley, and M. Schachter, Release of kinin by an enzyme in the accessory sex glands of the guinea-pig, J. Physiol., 162:269, (1962).

24. M. Schachter, Kinins of various origins, Ann. N. Y. Acad. Sci., 104:108, (1963).

25. C. Moriwaki and M. Schachter, Kininogenase of the guinea-pig's coagulating gland and the release of bradykinin, J. Physiol., 219:341, (1971).

26. K. Kizuki, C. Moriwaki, and H. Moriya, Kinin-converting factor in the dog pseudoglobulin fraction from heated plasma and kinin liberation from dog kininogen by guinea-pig coagulating gland kallikrein (CGK), Chem. Pharm. Bull. (Japan), 28:42, (1980).

27. S. Barton, J. Wimalasema, and M. Schachter, Subcellular location of the kininogenase in the coagulating gland of the guinea-pig, Biochem. Pharmacol., 22:1121, (1973).

28. G. P. Harper, Y. A. Barde, G. Burnstock, J. R. Carstairs, M. E. Dennison, K. Suda, and C. A. Vernon, Guinea-pig prostate is a rich source of nerve growth factor, Nature (London), 279:160, (1979).

29. H. Fritz, W. D. Schleuming, H. Schiessler, W. B. Schill, V. Wendt, and G. Winkler, Boar, bull and human sperm acrosin - isolation, properties and biological aspects, in: Proteases and Biological Control, ed. by E. Reich, D. B. Rifkin and E. Shaw, Cold Spring Harbor Laboratory, pp. 715-735, (1975).

30. L. J. D. Zaneveld, K. L. Polakoski, and G. F. B. Schumachen, The proteolytic enzyme systems of mammalian genital tract secretions and spermatozoa, in: Proteases and Biological Control, ed. by E. Reich, D. B. Rifkin and E. Shaw, Cold Spring Harbor Laboratory, pp. 683-714, (1975).

31. W. Muller-Esterl, S. Kupfer, and H. Fritz, Purification and properties of boar acrosin, Hoppe Seyler's Z. Physiol. Chem., 361:1811, (1980).

32. D. L. Garner, M. P. Easton, M. A. Munson, and M. A. Boane, Immunofluorescent localization of bovine acrosin, J. Exp. Zool., 191:127, (1975).

33. D. B. Morton, The occurrence and function of proteolytic enzymes in the reproductive tract of mammals, in: Proteases in Mammalian Cells and Tissues, ed. by A. J. Barrett, North Holland Publ. Co., Amsterdam, pp. 445-500, (1977).

34. G. P. Harper and H. Thoenen, The distribution of nerve growth factor in the male sex organs, J. Neurochem., 34:893, (1980).

35. R. M. Stroud, A family of protein-cutting proteins, Sci. Amer., 231: 74, (1974).

36. F. Fiedler, W. Shret, C. Godec, C. Hirschauer, C. Kutzbach, G. Schmidt-Kastner, and H. Tschesche, The primary structure of pig pancreatic kallikrein B., in: Kininogenase 4, ed. by G. L. Haberland, J. W. Rogen, and T. Suzuki, Schattauer, Stuttgart-New York, pp. 7-14, (1977).

37. H. Fritz, F. Fiedler, T. Dietl, M. Warwas, E. Truscheit, G. Kolb, G. Mair, and H. Tschesche, On the relationship between porcine, pancreatic, submandibular, and urinary kallikreins, in: Kininogenases 4, ed. by G. L. Haberland, J. W. Rogen, and T. Suzuki, Schattauer, Stuttgart-New York, pp. 15-28, (1977).

38. H. Neurath and K. A. Walsh, The role of proteases in physiological regulation: an overview, Fed. Eur. Biochem. Soc. Symp., 47:1, (1978).

39. F. Fiedler, Enzymology of glandular kallikreins, in: Bradykinin, kallidin and Kallikrein, ed. by E. G. Erdos, Springer-Verlag, Berlin, pp. 103-161, (1979).

40. M. A. Bothwell, W. H. Wilson, and E. M. Shooter, The relationship between glandular kallikrein and growth factor-processing pro-teases of mouse submaxillary gland, J. Biol. Chem., 254:7287, (1979).

KININOGENASE FROM RAT VASCULAR TISSUE

Hector Nolly,* A. Guillermo Scicli, Gloria Scicli, M. Cristina
Lama,* Ana M. Guercio,* and Oscar A. Carretero

Hypertension Research Division, Henry Ford Hospital, Detroit
Michigan 48202, *Department of Pathology, School of Medicine
Universidad Nacional de Cuyo, Mendoza, Argentina

SUMMARY

A kininogenase resembling glandular kallikrein ws partially purified
from vascular tissue and characterized. Saline perfused rat tail arteries
and veins were homogenized in 0.25 M sucrose containing 10 mM Tris-HCl (pH
7.4). The homogenate was centrifuged at 105,000 x g for 60 min and a vascular kininogenase was purified from the supernatant by chromatofocusing,
affinity chromatography on immobilized antibodies against rat urinary kallikrein, and gel filtration on Sephadex G-100. The inhibitory effects of
antibodies against rat urinary kallikrein were tested using equivalent kinin-
forming concentrations of rat urinary kallikrein and vascular kininogenase.
Kininogenase activities of both enzymes were similarly inhibited by urinary
kallikrein antibodies. Aprotinin (1,000 KIU) completely inhibited vascular
kininogenase activity while soybean trypsin inhibitor (100 µg) did not modify
its kinin-forming activity. Vascular kininogenase and rat urinary kallikrein
had the same elution volume when chromatographed on a Sephadex G-100 column
and had similar mobilities in 10% polyacrylamide gel electrophoresis. Kinins
released by vascular kininogenase were identified as bradykinin by reverse-
phase high performance liquid chromatography. Rat vascular kininogenase
appears to be similar to glandular kallikrein. Kinins released locally
by vascular kininogenase may contribute to the regulation of vascular tone.

INTRODUCTION

Kallikrein is known to be produced by the kidney, salivary glands,
pancreas, and other tissues[1] and also immunoreactive glandular kallikrein
is present in plasma.[2] It has been proposed that glandular kallikrein may
play a role in the regulation of blood flow to organs containing kallikrein
thereby indirectly participating in blood pressure regulation.[1] We have
previously reported the presence of both neutral and acid proteases in rat
mesenteric arteries capable of forming kinins.[3,4]

In our continuing investigation of kininogenase enzymes in vascular
tissue, we have determined that a kinin-forming enzyme different from plasma
kallikrein is also present in tail arteries and veins of the rat. This
enzyme was partially purified and characterized.

11

MATERIALS AND METHODS

Reagents

The following materials were obtained from commercial sources: molecular weight markers, polybuffer anion exchanger (PBE 94) and polybuffer 74 (Pharmacia Fine Chemicals); captopril (Squibb); polyacrylamide (Eastman Kodak); all other reagents used were analytical grade. Aprotinin was a kind gift from G. Haberland (A. G. Bayer, W. Germany).

Preparation of Tissue Extracts

One hundred male and female Sprague-Dawley rats (400-500 g) of both sexes were used. After sacrificing the animal by decapitation, the ventral artery and veins of the tail were exposed proximally through small incisions and catheterized with polyethylene tubing.[5] The tail was perfused through the artery with a buffered saline solution (pH 7.4) for 10-20 minutes at a flow rate of 1.0 ml/min until the effluent collected from the veins appeared visually free of blood. Subsequently, the vessels were removed, cleaned of any adherent fat and connective tissue and placed in Petri dishes containing a saline solution. The tail vascular bed was washed by renewing the saline solution several times. Then, the vessels were cut into 1-2 mm rings and kept frozen at -70°C.

For these experiments 4,200 mg of pooled tail vessels were used. The vessels were frozen and thawed four times. The tissue was suspended in three volumes of 0.25 M sucrose (pH 7.0) and homogenized on ice for four 15 second intervals with a polytron homogenizer. The homogenate was centrifuged at 1,000 g for 10 minutes to eliminate debris. The supernatant was further centrifuged at 105,000 g for 60 minutes in a L-5 Beckman ultracentrifuge. This supernatant was dialyzed overnight at 4°C against 0.01 M Tris-HCl buffer (pH 7.0) for further purification.

Chromatofocusing on Polybuffer Anion Exchanger 94 (PBE 94)

The supernatant of the vascular extract was applied to a polybuffer exchanger 94 column (20 x 1 cm) equilibrated with 0.025 M imidazole-HCl buffer (pH 7.4). A pH gradient between 7.0 and 4.0 was obtained by using polybuffer adjusted to pH 4.0. Proteins still bound to the gel after pH 4.0 were eluted with 0.01 M acetate buffer, pH 3.5, 1 M NaCl. During acid elution, the pH was rapidly neutralized by collecting on equal volumes of 2 M Tris-HCl, pH 8.5. The fractions obtained after the sodium acetate elution were pooled in three major fractions of 10 ml each. The fractions were dialyzed against distilled water, concentrated by evaporating under a nitrogen stream at 37°C, and frozen at -70°C until assayed for kininogenase activity.

Affinity Chromatography on Immobilized Kallikrein Antibody

The gamma globulin fraction of the rabbit antiserum against rat kallikrein was purified by precipitation with 40% ammonium sulfate. The kallikrein antibodies of this fraction were further purified by absorption to, and elution from a rat glandular kallikrein CH-sepharose column. For this, glandular kallikrein was purified from rat submandibular gland by chromatography on DEAE-Sephadex adsorption, elution from a aprotinin-sepharose gel, isoelectric focusing and gel filtration on HPLC using a TSK-250 column. One µg of the purified enzyme released 1.1 µg of kinin per minute when incubated with semi-purified dog kininogen.[6] On 12% slab polyacrylamide gel electrophoresis, purified kallikrein (20 µg) showed a 1major and a minor band both of which had kininogenase activity. One mg of purified rat submandibular gland kallikrein was covalently bound to activated CH-sepharose

(Pharmacia) as indicated by the manufacturer.

The kallikrein CH-sepharose gel was equilibrated with 0.1 M TRIS-HC1, 0.5 M sodium chloride, pH 8.0, and mixed with the anti-kallikrein antibodies for 2 hours at room temperature and then overnight at 4°C. After washing the gel to eliminate unbound material, the antikallikrein antibodies were eluted with 0.1 M acetic acid, pH 2.9. Purified kallikrein antibodies were coupled to activated CH-sepharose (Pharmacia) as suggested by the manufacturer. The antikallikrein-sepharose gel was equilibrated with 0.1 M sodium phosphate buffer, pH 7.4. The fraction containing kininogenase after chromatofocusing activity was dissolved in phosphate buffer and mixed with the antikallikrein-sepharose gel for 2 hours at room temperature followed by 24 hours at 4°C. Non-bound proteins were separated by successive washings first with 0.1 M sodium pyhosphate buffer (pH 7.4), and then with 0.1 M sodium phosphate buffer (pH 6.0) containing 1 M NaCl. The kininogenase activity was eluted with 0.1 M acetate buffer (pH 3.5) containing 1 M NaCl. Fractions of 3 ml were collected in equal volumes of 2 M Tris, pH 8.5. The samples were then dialyzed against distilled water, concentrated under a nitrogen stream, and frozen at -70°C until assayed for ininogenase activity.

Gel Filtration on Sephadex G-100 and Molecular Weight Determination

2 ml of the concentrated solution from the immunoaffinity chromatography step were applied to a Sephadex G-100 column (50 x 1 cm) equilibrated with 0.1 M phosphate buffer, pH 7.4. The column was eluted at a flow rate of 20 ml/hr. Fractions of 4 ml were collected, dialyzed against distilled water, and frozen at -70°C until assayed. Standards used for molecular weight determination were ovalbumin, chymotrypsinogen, and ribonuclease.

Discontinuous Polyacrylamide Gel Electrophoresis

Disc gel electrophoresis was performed in 10% polyacrylamide gels as described by Nustad and Pierce.[7] Each gel was cut into 2 mm slices and each slice was homogenized in the presence of 1 ml of 0.1 M sodium phosphate buffer (pH 7.4), centrifuged at 4,000 x g for 20 min., and the supernatant saved for ininogenase assay.

High Performance Liquid Chromatography of Kinins

Identification of kinins liberated during kininogenase assay was carried out by comparing the elution volume of kinins generated by the vascular homogenate with that of synthetic bradykinin and lys-bradykinin during reverse-phase high performance liquid chromatography (HPLC). Each kinin solution was injected into a C_{18} Bondapack column equilibrated with 10% acetonitrile in 0.05 M triethyl ammonium formate (TEAF), pH 4.4, and eluted with a linear gradient (10% to 20% acetonitrile in 0.05 M triethyl ammonium formate, TEAF, pH 4.4) with a flow rate of 1 ml/min.

Kininogenase Assay

Kinin-generating activity in tissue extracts and fractions were determined by incubation with partially purified dog kininogen by a method identical to that previously described,[6] except that the buffer was altered by the addition of captopril (10 µg/ml). Kinins were measured by RIA.[6]

Inhibition Studies

The effect of soybean trypsin inhibitor (SBTI) and aprotinin on vascular kininogenase activity was examined. SBTI was dissolved in 0.1 M Tris-HC1 (5,000 µg/ml) and aprotinin was diluted with 0.1 M Tris-HC1 (50,000 KIE/ml).

The vascular kininogenase was preincubated with 20 μl of the aforementioned inhibitors for 60 minutes at 37°C. The final concentrations of inhibitors was 100 μg of SBTI and 1,000 KIE of aprotinin per ml of sample. The mixture was then incubated with kininogen for assay of kininogenase as described. The gamma globulin fraction of the rabbit antiserum against rat urinary kallikrein was diluted in 0.1M Tris-HCl buffer (pH 7.4) to a final concentration of 20 mg/ml and an aliquot containing 10 μg proteins was added to the samples of vascualr kininogenase or urinary kallikrein and preincubated for 60 minutes at 37°C. As control, nonimmunized rabbit serum was used in the same concentration. After the preincubation period, the mixture was incubated with kininogen for assay of kininogenase activity.

Protein Determination

Protein determination was done by the method of Bradford[8] using bovine serum albumin as the standard. Protein concentration in column effluents was measured at 280 nm (A_{280}).

RESULTS

The results of the partial purification of rat vascular kininogenase are summarized in Table 1. Chromatofocusing resulted in a two-fold increase in the specific activity but total activity also increased after this step. With immunoaffinity the specific activity increased up to 68-fold. After gel filtration a 78-fold purification with 95% recovery was obtained.

On gel filtration on Sephadex G-100, vascular kininogenase and purified rat urinary kallikrein eluted similarly both in a single peak (Fig. 1). Kininogenase activity of both vascular and urinary kallikrein was inhibited by incubation with kallikrein antibodies. The apparent molecular weight of vascular kininogenase as calculated from the elution volume on gel filtration column was 37,000 daltons.

Mobility on disc polyacrylamide gel electrophoresis of both vascular kininogenase and urinary kallikrein was similar (Fig. 2).

Identification of the reaction products by reverse phase HPLC showed that kinins generated by vascular kininogenase had the same elution volume as synthetic bradykinin.

Table 1. Purification of Vascular Kininogenase from Rat Tail Vessels

PURIFICATION STEP	TOTAL PROTEIN (mg)	TOTAL ACTIVITY (μg BK hr^{-1})	SPECIFIC ACTIVITY (μg BK $mg^{-1}hr^{-1}$)	PURIFICATION FACTOR
Supernatant 105,000 g	1.80	1.68	0.9	1
Chromatofocusing	1.08	2.12	2.0	2.1
Immunoaffinity	0.028	1.92	68.4	73.3
Gel Filtration	0.022	1.60	72.7	77.9

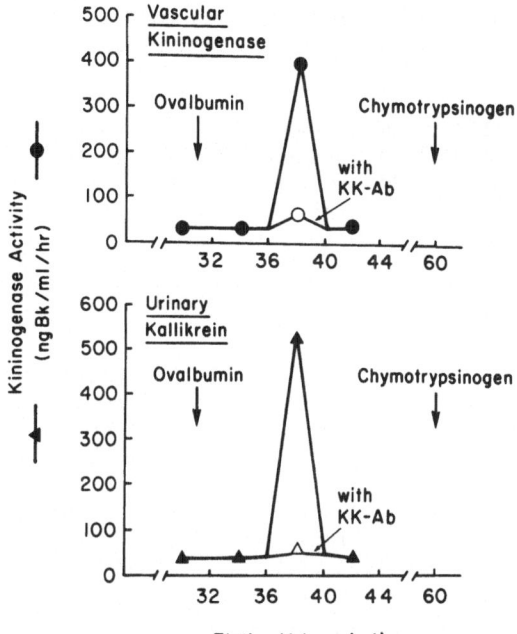

Fig. 1. Gel filtration of the purified vascular and urinary kininogenases
on Sephadex G-100. The column was eluted at a flow rate of 20
ml/hr. Fractions of 4 ml were collected. Open circles and triang-
les indicates inhibition of the kininogenase activity by kallikrein antibodies.

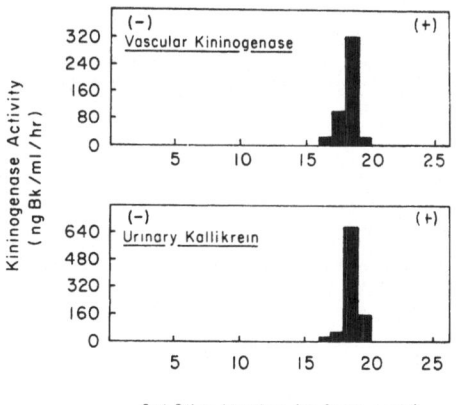

Fig. 2. Alkaline disc gel electrophoresis of the purified vascular kininogenase and of urinary kallikrein. Each slice (2 mm) was homogenized and centrifuged; the kininogenase activity was measured
in the supernatant.

The kininogenase activity of both vascular kininogenase and urinary kallikrein was completely inhibited by aprotinin, whereas it was resistant to soybean-trypsin inhibitor. In contrast, the kininogenase activity of trypsin and plasma was strongly inhibited by soybean-trypsin inhibitor (Table 2). Kininogenase activity of both enzymes was inhibited to the same extent by kallikrein antibodies. Nonimmunized rabbit serum had a negligible effect.

The different enzyme preparations were incubated for 60 minutes at 37°C, pH 8.5 with kallirkein antibody, nonimmunized-rabbit serum, aprotinin, or soybean-trypsin inhibitor, then the kininogenase activity was measured. The values represent the mean of at least three determinations. SBTI = soybean-trypsin inhibitor.

DISCUSSION

The present study demonstrates that a kinin-forming enzyme is present in tail arteries and veins of the rat. Vascular kininogenase was purified by a series of chromatographic steps with a very high yield. The property of the vascular kininogenase to bind strongly to immobilized kallikrein antiserum was used for its partial purification from vascular tissue. The combination of chromatofocusing, gel filtration and immunoaffinity chromatography resulted in a 70-fold purification. Due to the small amount of material available, the analytical techniques usually used to determine purity were not performed.

The unsensitivity of the vascular kininogenase to soybean-trypsin inhibitor readily distinguishes it from trypsin and plasma kallikrein. On the other hand, rat vascular kininogenase appears to be very similar to rat glandular kallikrein; both purified rat vascular kininogenase and urinary kallikrein had similar molecular weights, isoelectric points, electrophoretic mobilities, and inhibition profiles. The similar behavior of both enzymes when reacted with rabbit antiserum against rat urinary kallikrein strengthens the contention that they are very similar if not identical.

Table 1. Effect of Kallirkein Antibodies, Soybean-Trypsin Inhibitor and Aprotinin on Kinin-Generating Activity From Different Sources

Kininogenase Source	% Inhibition		
	Urinary KK-Ab	Aprotinin (1000 KIU/ml)	SBTI (100 µg/ml)
Vascular Tissue	82	96	5
Urine	91	95	4
Plasma	6	80	96
Trypsin	7	94	98

While the precise cellular localization of the vascular enzyme is still unknown, it could be speculated that the enzyme may play a role in regulating local vascular resistance and hence blood flow, either directly or through kinin release. If the enzyme is located in the endothelial lining it may participate in the regulation of phospholipase activity and local formation of arachidonic acid metabolites either directly or through kinin formation. If the enzyme is located in smooth msucle it may directly participate in regulation of vascular tone, and if located in the adventitia it could have a role in regulating vascular permeability.

In summary, a protease which resembles tissue kallirkein is present in vessels isolated from rat tails. This enzyme is present in an active form and is able to release kinins at physiological pHs. Kinin released locally by vascular kininogenase may contribute to the regulation of vascular tone.

ACKNOWLEDGEMENTS

The authors thank Mrs. Pat Piejak and Miss Susan Mastaler for typing the manuscript and Dr. Robert Murray for editing. This work was supported in part by NIH Grants HL 28982 and 15839.

REFERENCES

1. M. E. Webster, Kallikrein in glandular tissue, in: "handbook of Experimental Pharmacology, Bradykinin, Kallidin and Kallikrein," E. G. Erdos, ed., Springer, Berlin, Heidelberg, New York (1970).
2. S. F. Rabito, A. G. Scicli, and O. A. Carretero, Immunoreactive glandular kallikrein in plasma, in: "Enzymatic Release of Vasoactive Peptides," F. Gross and H. G. Vogel, eds., Raven Press, New York (1980).
3. H. L. Nolly, F. Bertini, and M. C. Lama, Kinin-forming enzymes in vascular tissue, Adv. Exp. Med. Biol., 156A:399-407 (1983).
4. H. Nolly and M. C. Lama, Vascular kallikrein: A kallikrein-like enzyme present in vascular tissue of the rat, Clin. Sci., 63:249s-251s (1968).
5. S. M. Friedman, B. Sustafson, D. Hamilton, and C. L. Friedman, Compartments of sodium in a small artery, Can. J. Physiol. Pharmacol., 46:673-679 (1968).
6. O. A. Carretero, N. B. Oza, A. Piwonska, T. Ocholik, and A. G. Scicli, Measurement of urinary kallikrein activity by kinin radioimmunoassay, Biochem. Pharmacol., 25:2265-2270 (1976).
7. K. Nustad and J. V. Pierce, Purification of rat urinary kallikrein and their specific antibody, Biochem., 13:2312-2319 (1974).
8. M. M. Bradford, A rapid and sensitive method for the quantitation of microgram quantities of protein utilizing the principle of protein-dye binding, Anal. Biochem., 72:248-254 (1976).

INTRACELLULAR AND INTERCELLULAR DISTRIBUTIONS OF ACID KININOGENASES IN

SPLEEN

Masako Watanabe and Keiko Yamafuji

Department of Food and Nutrition
Nakamura Gakuen College
Fukuoka, Japan

SUMMARY

Intracellular distributions of acid kininogenases were investigated
following the subcellular fractionation of bovine and rat spleens. Acid
kininogenases as well as other acid hydrolases were observed to be distributed in several fractons. Relatively high kinin forming activity was
found in two fractions which were considered to contain lysosomes from reticulum cells and from lymphocytes respectively. The latter fraction had
shown the higher sensitivity to thiol compound for its activation. These
findings led us to the separation of the free cells existing in spleen
each other. We adopted the techniques such as Ficoll-Isopaque centrifugation, plastic dish treatment and iron carbonyl treatment for this purpose.
Lymphocyte from rat thymus was also examined and proved to have acid kininogenase activity as well.

INTRODUCTION

We have been working on acid kininogenases of bovine spleen and have
reported on the partial purification and characterization[1] and on kinin
forming reactions.[2] Recently, we achieved the purification of the two
enzymes, one is thiol independent and the other is thiol sensitive, and now
undertaking structure studies. Throughout these works, were we not clear
to which cells among the several species of cells in spleen tissue the kinin
forming activity could be attributed. We are to report the intracellular
and intercellular distributions of acid kininogenases in spleen tissue in
this paper.

Subcellular fractionation was performed according to the procedure
described by Ragab et al.[3] Although this method was effective to prepare
lysosomes from rat liver, it failed to give single lysosomal fraction from
spleen. Acid kininogenases were detected in more than one fraction. According to the investigation of Bowers and de Duve,[4,5] lysosome from the
different member of the spleen cells has different set of acid hydrolases
and different density as the cause of complexity of the sedimentation patterns. In considering our results referring to their discussion, we came
to the conclusion that the lysosome which contain thiol independent kinin
forming enzyme belongs to reticulum cell and that which contain thiol dependent enzyme mainly belongs to lymphocyte. The lymphocytes were then

isolated from bovine and rat spleen and also from rat thymus and showed the acid kininogenase activity in all cases. Thus we could confirm the speculation made in elucidating the results of subcellular fractionation. The results concerning macrophage is still to be clarified.

MATERIALS AND METHODS

Bovine spleen and bovine blood were obtained at slaughter house. Bovine kininogen was prepared by the method described by Greenbaum and Hosoda.[6] Rat heated plasma[7] was used as the kininogen substrate in the case of examining the cells from rat tissues.

Ficoll and Isopaque (75% solution) were purchased from Pharmacia. Hanks and Eagle-MEM type 2 salt mixture were obtained from Nissui Co. Fatus calf serum (FCS) was the product of Gibco. Cytochrome C, p-nitrophenylphosphate and p-nitrophenyl-β-D-glucronide were the products of Sigma. Bovien hemoglobin was purchased from Wako. 2-mercaptoethanol and other chemicals in use were of highest quality available from Wako and Katayama Chemicals.

Subcellular Fractionation

About 20 pieces were cut from separate parts of bovine spleen and combined to make 60 g of starting material, or spleens removed from 10 rats were combined to make around 6 g of material. Spleen tissue was homogenized in two volumes of 0.2 M KCl with Waring blender in full speed for 20 sec. Resulting homogenate was centrifuged successively according to the procedure of Ragab et al.[3] as shown in Fig. 1. KUBOTA KR200FA centrifuge and RA3 roter (R_{max} = 108 mm) was used. The second density gradient centrifugation to get separation of lysosome and light lysosome was performed only in the case of rat. Pellet obtained in each step of centrifugation was suspended in 0.25 M sucrose and was subjected to freeze and thaw ten times. Freezing was performed in solid carbon-dioxide-acetone mixture and thaw was in 15° C water bath. The suspension thus lysed was then centrifuged at 6000 RPM for 20 min. The supernatant supplied the samples for protein determination and enzyme assays. Protein concentration was determined by Lowry's method.[8] Enzyme assays will be described in the last paragraph of this section.

Separation of the Cells

The procedures employed were mostly learned from the article by Harada et al.[9] The cells obtained by any of the following techniques were homogenized with Potter-Elvejem homogenizer in 0.34 M sucrose and lysed by freeze and thaw 5 to ten times prior to use for protein determination and for enzyme assay.

Cell suspension   The tissue was cut into frakes with scissors and picked with forceps in two volumes of Hanks solution. Thus obtained sludge was filtered through 80 mesh stainless shieve. Filtrate was then centrifuged at 1300 RPM for 7~10 min. Pellet was washed twice with MEM and suspended in appropriate amount of medium. This was called "Cell Suspension". If necessary, was lysed the contaminating erythrocyte with Tris-NH$_4$Cl buffer[11] to give "Red cell free cell suspension". Cell number was counted after May Gimsa or peroxidase staining.

Ficoll-Isopaque centrifugation   The experiments were undertaken following the instruction of Pharmacia text. Cell suspension was diluted to 3×10^6 cells/ml with Eagle-MEM medium shortly before use. 24 ml of this diluted suspension was layered on top of 15 ml of Ficoll-Isopaque solution which was the mixture of 24 volumes of 9% (w/v) Ficoll and 10 volumes of

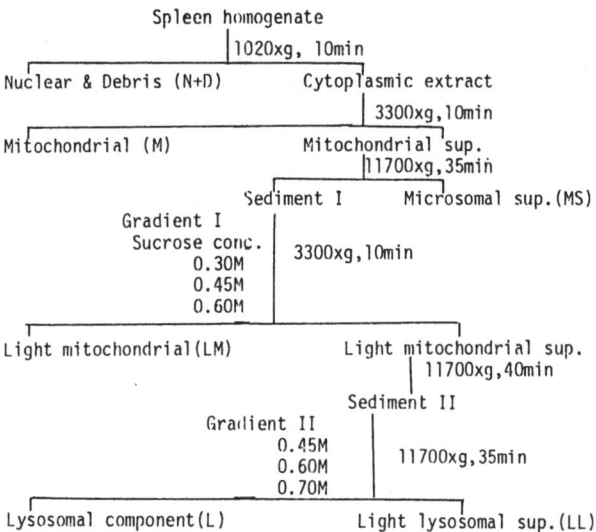

Fig. 1. Centrifugation scheme.

32.8% (w/v) Isopaque in each 50 ml siliconized glass centrifuge tube.
Centrifugation was performed at 20°C for 40 min at 1620 RPM (400 xg) with
KUBOTA KS-5000 centrifuge. White turbid layer appeared at the intermediate
phase was gently sucked and collected. Thus obtained lymphocyte fraction
was mixed with two volumes of medium and centrifuged at 1400 RPM for 10
min. Sedimented lymphocyte cells were washed two times and suspended in
appropriate amount of medium.

   Plastic dish treatment   The lymphocyte fraction from Ficoll-Isopaque centrifugation or red cell free cell suspension were subjected to
plastic dish treatment. The cell count of the starting suspension was
adjusted to 4 x 10^6 cells/ml with 10% (w/v) FCS-MEM. 5 ml of this suspension was applied on each plastic dish (Nipro 90 x 15 mm) and incubated at
37°C for 60 min. The suspension containing non-adherent cells was sucked
out from the dish. The dishes were rinsed three times with wormed medium.
The removed suspension and the washes were combined and centrifuged at 1300
RPM for 7 min. Sedimented cells were washed with MEM two times and suspended in minimum amount of the same medium. This fraction was designated
as "non adherent cell". The cells captured by the dish was detadhed with
ice cold 0.2% EDTA in Delbecco solution (PBS)[12] splashed from fine tipped
pipette. After standing at 2°C for 15 min, dishes were scrubbed with rubber
policeman and the suspension was sucked and collected. Then the dishes were
rinsed thoroughly with ice cold EDTA-PBS twice. The suspension and washes
were combined and centrifuged at 1300 RPM for 7 min. Pellet was washed
twice with MEM and finally suspended in the minimum amount of MEM. The
fraction thus obtained was designated as "Adherent cell".

   Iron carbonyl treatment   To 30 ml of cell suspension containing 3 x
10^8 cells add 15 ml of 5% iron carbonyl suspended homogeneously by means
of sonication in 5% Arabian gum dissolved in PBS. Incubation was carried
out at 37°C for 60 min with occasional stirring. Excess iron carbonyl and
the cells which were undertaking phagocytosis of iron carbonyl particles
were sedimented at the bottom of the flask. Supernatant was removed
without disturbing the precipitate with the aid of the magnet situated at
the bottom. Pellet obtained by the centrifugation of this supernatant was
washed twice with MEM. This fraction was further purified by Ficoll-Isopaque method.

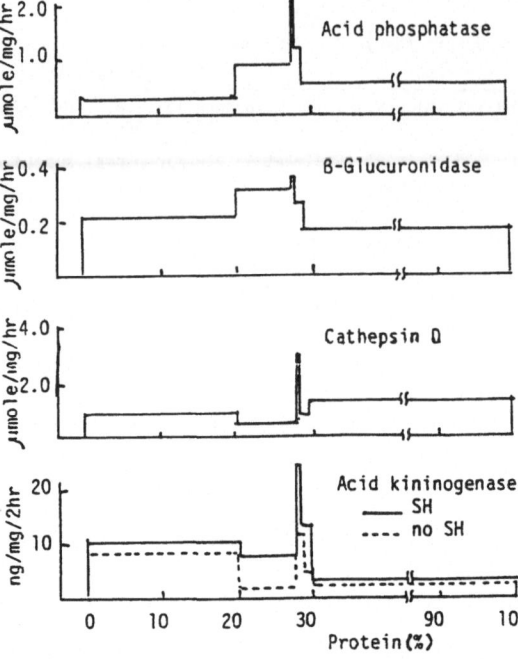

Fig. 2. Subcellular distribution of acid kininogenases and other acid
hydrolases in bovine spleen. Fraction were plotted in the order
of their isolation from left to right, N+D, M, LM, L and MS. Each
fraction is represented in the ordinate scale by its specific
activity. In the obscissa scale, each fractions represented by
its percentage of protein.

Enzyme Assay

Acid phosphatase was assayed by the rate of hydrolysis of p-nitrophenylphosphate at pH 5.2. The specific activity was expressed as μmoles
of p-nitrophenol produced by mg of protein in 1 hr. β-glucronidase was
measured by the hydrolysis of p-nitrophenyl-β-D-glucronide at pH 4.0.
The specific activity was expressed in the same manner as acid phosphatase.
Cathepsin D activity was estimated by the hydrolysis of 2% bovine hemoglobin
dissolved in 0.2 M acetic acid. Specific activity was respresented by
μmoles of tyrosin calculated from 280 reading of trichloroacetic acid supe.
Cytochrome C oxidase was measured as the decrease of reduced cytochrome C
read at 550 nm with time scanning. The rate constant was calculated.[13]
Acid kininogenase activity was measured by the assay on rat uterus contraction caused by produced kinin. Acetone powder of crude bovine bradykinin[6]
or heated rat plasma[7] was used as the substrate for each species. Incubation was carried out at 37°C for two hours in pH 4.4 acetate buffer with
and without addition of 0.2 M 2-mercaptoethanol. The specific activity was
represented as bradykinin equivalent produced by mg of protein.

RESULTS AND DISCUSSION

Subcellular fractions were obtained by the differential centrifugation
of which the scheme was shown in Fig. 1. The distribution patterns of acid
hydrolases in these fractions were shown in Fig. 2. High kinin forming
activity was found to be associated with light mitochondria or found in
lysosome itself. These kinin forming reaction and also the reaction by

Table 1. Distributions of the Acid Hydrolases and Cytochrome C Oxidase in the Subcellular Fractions of Rat Spleen

	N+D	M	LM	L	LL	MS
Protein (mg)	24.3±8.0	10.9±5.5	1.7±0.7	8.7±4.0	3.1±0.6	383.6±12.4
Specific activity						
Acid phosphatase (μmole/mg/hr)	7.6±2.0	13.0±0.30	13.4±4.6	11.5±3.1	13.6±4.6	4.0±1.2
ß-Glucronidase (μmole/mg/hr)	1.96±0.70	4.83±1.61	3.86±1.16	2.60±1.09	2.40±1.55	1.36±0.88
Cathepsin D (μmole/mg/hr)	1.87±0.56	4.56±1.23	12.2±10.3	3.49±1.14	12.4±5.7	1.18±0.41
Acid kininogenase (ng BK/mg/2hr) +SII	25.4±10.2	30.6±21.5	103.2±45.5	13.8±4.3	19.0±8.8	8.6±5.0
−SII	18.4±7.0	23.0±17.7	63.6±20.3	13.8±8.3	14.3±8.0	6.1±2.5
Cytochrome C oxidase (/sec/mg)	0.33±0.007	0.453±0.005	0.556±0.194	0.160±0.032	N.D.*	N.D.*

*Not detected   (n=4)

mitochondrial fraction were shown to be thiol sensitive. Relatively high but less thiol sensitive kinin formation was observed at nuclei and debris fraction. Other marker enzymes were also distributed in almost every fractions with different specific activity. ß-glucronidase which is characteristic of macrophage was shown to be concentrated largely in mitochondrial fraction. This fact suggested the possibility that the lysosomes of macrophage was sedimented with mitochondria. The results from the subcellular fractionation of rat spleen was summarized in Table 1. Ten rats were sacrificed at an experiment and mean values of four experiments (n=4) were shown in this table. In the case of rat, the second density gradient cen-

Table 2. Acid Kininogenase Activity in isolated Lymphocyte and Other Cells

		Cell number	Total protein (mg)		Specific activity (ngBK/mg)	Total activity (ng BK)
a						
Ficoll-Isopaque centrifugation	Cell suspension	6.5~6.9x10^8	~30	+SII	0.71	18.0
				−SII	2.22	57.5
	Lymphocyte fraction	1.1~3.7x10^7	~0.68	+SII	40.2	26.8
				−SII	19.7	13.1
(Plastic dish)	Non adherent cell	1.5~1.8x10^7	0.40~0.65	+SII	22.2	9.00
				−SII	12.2	4.96
	Adherent cell	0.82~2.0x10^6	~0.021	+SII	207	4.27
				−SII	209, ~0	4.30, ~0
b						
Plastic dish treatment	Before apply	1.4x10^8	0.657	+SII	7.71	5.07
				−SII	5.40	3.55
	Non adherent cell	1.7x10^7	0.0781	+SII	71.5	5.58
				−SII	70.0	5.47
	Adherent Cell	1.4x10^6	0.0145	+SII	272	3.94
				−SII	258	3.75
c						
Iron carbonyl treatment	Before treatment	3.0x10^8	———	+SII	0.71	——
				−SII	2.22	——
	After treatment	1.5x10^8	0.530	+SII	183	97.0
				−SII	151	79.8
(Ficoll -Isopaque)	Lymphocyte fraction	2.9x10^6	0.013	+SII	200	3.66
				−SII	214	3.92

trifugation step shown in Fig. 1 was carried out to give lysosome and light lysosomal supe. The assay of cytochrome C oxidase was performed to evaluate the reliability of the separation method and gave the satisfactory result, that is the localization of this enzyme in mitochondrial fraction. The results showed the similar tendency to bovine. High specific activity of kinin forming enzyme was found in light mitochondrial fraction. Relatively high activity was found in nuclei and debris fraction and mitochondrial fraction. Fairly large amount of acid kininogenases seemed to be contained in these two fractions considering their high protein concentration.

The distribution of lysosomal enzymes in all fractions in different rates reflect the fact that the lysosome originated in different cell differs in its density and the contents of enzymes. Bowers and de Duve described the phenomena in their studies of discrimination of the spleen cells as follows. Lysosome of reticulum cell has high density (1.30) as sediment with nuclei and debris. Next dense (1.19) lysosome is derived from macrophage and sediment with mitochondria. Lymphocyte release comparatively low density (1.15) lysosome which sediment concomitantly with light mitochondria. This lysosome and lighter lysosome may consist in lysosomal fraction. We concluded that thiol independent kininogenase come from lymphocyte and macrophage referring to their description.

Our next project was the separation of the different types of cells in spleen from each other. The cell population of "Red cell free cell suspension" was estimated to be 40~60% of small lymphocyte. 50~30% of large lymphocyte, 5% each of macrophage and granulocyte and no erythrocyte.

The results of the cell separation by three separate methods were summarized in Table 2. Table 2a shows the clel recovery and the acid kininogenase activity distribution after Ficoll-Isopaque centrifugation followed by plastic dish treatment. Isolated and purified lymphocyte proved to contain kinin forming enzyme which was partially active without addition of any activator and fully activated by the addition of thiol compound such as 2-mercaptoethanol. Application of this lymphocyte fraction to plastic dish resulted in large amount of non adherent cells composed of lymphocytes and small amount of adherent cells composed of macrophages and granulocytes. Adherent cell showed relatively high kinin forming activity per unit cell. This means that macrophage, though it is the minority in population, has high specific activity.

Table 2b shows the results from plastic dish treatment of red cell free cell suspension. This results are in good agreement with those in Table 2a. Effect of thiol compound was rather obscure in those assay where whole cell lysate was used as the enzyme sauce.

In Table 2c were shown the results of iron carbonyl treatment. "After treatment" means the fraction obtained from the supernatant and "Lymphocyte fraction" means that obtained by Ficoll-Isopaque centrifugation of "After treatment". The cell count certified the lymphocyte population to be more than 90% in this fraction. The specific activity was improved to some extent by this step but with poor cell recovery.

We have thus confirmed that lymphocyte is contributing to the acid kininogenase activity of spleen. We have not achieved the investigation as to the differentiation of subpopulation of lymphocyte yet. The only experiment along this line was the assay of acid kininogenase in the lymphocyte fraction from rat thymus. Thymuses were removed from 5 young rats. The cell suspension was prepared in the same manner as spleen. The results from the enzyme assay after plastic dish treatment are presented in Table 3. Adherent cell could not be detected in this case. Non adherent cell showed acid kininogenase activity which was improved by the addition of thiol

Table 3. Acid Kininogenase Activity in Lymphocyte from Rat Thymus

	Cell number	Total protein (mg)	Specific activity (ng BK/mg)		Total activity (ng BK)
Thymus cell suspension	2.10×10^8	1.157	+SH	69.0	79.8
			-SH	43.4	50.2
Non adherent cell	6.14×10^7	0.888	+SH	61.5	54.6
			-SH	30.4	27.0
Adherent cell	1.30×10^6	0.017	+SH	N.D.	
			-SH	N.D.	

compound. This finding made us suspect that T cell in spleen is contributing to the production of kinins which may be playing regulatory role in immune responses. Fujiwara reported that bradykinin effected supressively to the mitogen sensitivity of lymphocyte[14] and Okabe et al discussed the effect of kallikrein on cellular immune responses in vitro.[15]

The acid kininogenase from lymphocyte may possibly be the enzyme which has effect on cellular immune responses in vivo. Accumulation of the evidences in future is awaited.

REFERENCES

1. K. Yamafuji and M. Takeishi, Substrate specificities of acid kininogenases, Adv. Exp. Med. Biol., 120A:335 (1979).
2. Yamafuji, K. and M. Watanabe, Studies on the kinin formation by bovine spleen acid kininogenases, Adv. Exp. Med. Biol., 156A:409 (1983).
3. H. Ragab, C. Beck, C. Dillard, and A. L. Tappel, Preparation of rat liver lysosomes, Biochem. Biophys. Acta., 148:501 (1967).
4. W. E. Bowers and C. de Duve, Lysosomes in lymphoid tissue II. Intracellular distribution of acid hydrolases, J. Cell. Biol., 32:339 (1967).
5. W. E. Bowers and C. de Duve, Lysosomes in lymphoid tissue III. Influence of various treatments of the animals on the distributionof acid hydrolases, J. Cell. Biol., 32:349 (1967).
6. L. M. Greenbaum and T. Hosoda, Studies on the isolation of bradykininogen, Biochem. Pharmacol., 12:325 (1963).
7. S. Ohishi, Y. Uchida,, A. Ueno, and M. Katori, Bromelain, athiol protease from pineapple stem, depleltion high molecular weight kininogen by activation of hageman factor (Factor XII), Thrombosis Research, 14:665 (1979).
8. O. H. Lowry, N. J. Rosebrough, A. L. Farr, and R. J. Randall, Protein measurement with Folin phenol reagent, J. Biol. Chem., 193:263 (1951).
9. H. Harada, T. Kasahara, Y. Ito, and T. Kawai, Laboratory techniques for isolation, identification and removal of monocyte, Diagnostic Pathology (Rinsyo Byori in Japanese), Supplement: 87 (1981).
10. I. Ishikawa and G. Gimasoni, Isolation of Cathepsin D from human lymphocytes, Biochem. Biophys. Acta, 480:228 (1977).
11. T. Shiroishi, Preparation of lymph node. Protein, nucleic acid and enzyme, Supplement 24: Illustrated manual for animal experiment: 43, in Japanese (1981).
12. Y. Kagawa, Salt solutions, Biochemistry Data Book II: 924, Kagakudozin, in Japanese (1981).

13. Y. Orii, Purification and properties of bovine heart cytochrome oxydase. Protein, nucleic acid and enzyme, Supplement: Experiments in biological membrane II: 228, in Japanese (1974).

14. H. Fujiwara, Effects of chemical mediators (histamine, bradykinin, serotonin and acetylcholine) on lymphocyte activation by antigen or mitogen, Allergy, 31-1:29, in Japanese (1982).

15. T. Okabe, M. Hida, K. Takada, Y. Noose, M. Yamamoto, and Y. Kimura, Agents and action, Supplement 9:315 (1982).

LOCALIZATION OF KALLIKREINS IN THE HUMAN PAROTID GLAND AND IN THE HUMAN

KIDNEY: A COMPARATIVE STUDY OF IMMUNOHISTOCHEMISTRY AND ENZYME

HISTOCHEMISTRY

Kenjiro Kimura and Hiroshi Moriya*

The Second Department of Internal Medicine, Faculty of
Medicine, University of Toyko and
*Department of Biochemistry, Science University of Tokyo
Tokyo, Japan

SUMMARY

Kallikreins were localized in the human parotid gland and in the
human kidney from two different aspects of the enzyme: the enzyme antigenicity and the enzyme activity. In the human parotid gland, the
kallikrein antigenicity and the enzyme activity were identical in their
locations in the ductal cells. In the human kidney, however, the enzyme
activity was revealed in the proximal tubule without any corresponding
kallikrein antigenicity. Therefore, this activity may be due to esterases
other than kallikreins. The Kallikrein antigenicity was found to be
located in the basement membrane of tubules, in the interstitium as well
as in some granules of the proximal tubule. These results are compatible
with tissue kallikreins being formed in the ducts of the human parotid
gland and suggest that circulating tissue kallikreins in the plasma are
deposited in the human kidney.

INTRODUCTION

The histological localization of kallikreins in the various organs
has been investigated almost exclusively by immunohistochemical methods
using specific antibodies against kallikreins[1,2,3,4,5,6] However, as
these methods demonstrate only kallikrein antigenicity, no information
concerning the enzyme activity is obtainable. In order to obtain it, it
is necessary to apply enzyme histochemical methods, where synthetic substrates for kallikreins are used. The aim of the present work has been
to localize kallikreins in the human tissue by an immunohistochemical
method as well as by an enzyme histochemical method and to see if the
enzyme antigenicity and the enzyme activity revealed are identical in
their locations.[7,8]

MATERIALS AND METHODS

Normal human tissue was obtained as a part of specimens removed by surgery. Two parotid gland and nine kidneys were used in this work.

Frozen Sections

Blocks of tissue were frozen in isopentane cooled by dry ice. Four μm-thick frozen sections were cut in a cryostat.

Ethanol-Fixed, Paraffin Embedded Sections

Other tissue blocks from the same specimens were fixed overnight at 4°C in a mixture of 95 per cent ethanol and glacial acetic acid (99:1, v/v), dehydrated and embedded in paraffin. Four μm-thick sections were cut and placed on albumin-coated slide glasses.

Immunohistochemical Investigation

Ethanol-fixed sections were used. A rat antiserum against highly purified human urinary kallikrein was used as the primary antiserum in the immunoperoxidase staining, which was processed by using an unlabelled antibody peroxidase-antiperoxidase (PAP) method. This antiserum has been reported to be immunochemically monospecific by Miyaura and co-workers in 1981.[9]

Enzyme Histochemical Investigation

Frozen or ethanol-fixed sections were used. The incubation was carried out as described for rat kidneys.[10,11,12] Sections were incubated for 30 minutes at 37°C in the reaction medium containing Pro-Phe-Arg-Naphthylester 0.1 mg/ml as substrate and Fast Garnet GBC 0.6 mg/ml as coupler dissolved in 0.2 M tris HCL buffer, pH 6.8.

Some esterases other than kallikreins are also possible hydrolyzers of this substrate. Therefore, the enzyme activity revealed by this method was called kallikrein-like activity, because it may represent kallikrein as well as some other esterases if they are present in a sufficient amount for the demonstration.

RESULTS

The results were shown in Figure 1 and Figure 2.

The Human Parotid Gland (Figure 1)

The kallikrein antigenicity was demonstrated in the luminal side of the striated ducts and, to a lesser degree, in the same area of the excretory ducts. Outside of the parenchymal cells, it was also revealed in the interstitium surrounding these ducts. The kallikrein-like activity was revealed in the luminal side of the striated ducts as well as of the excretory ducts corresponding to the locations of the antigenicity. Some interstitial cells and white blood cells revealed the enzyme activity, too.

The Human Kidney (Figure 2)

The kallikrein antigenicity was demonstrated in the granules of some tubules. When compared to neighbouring PAS stained sections, these granules

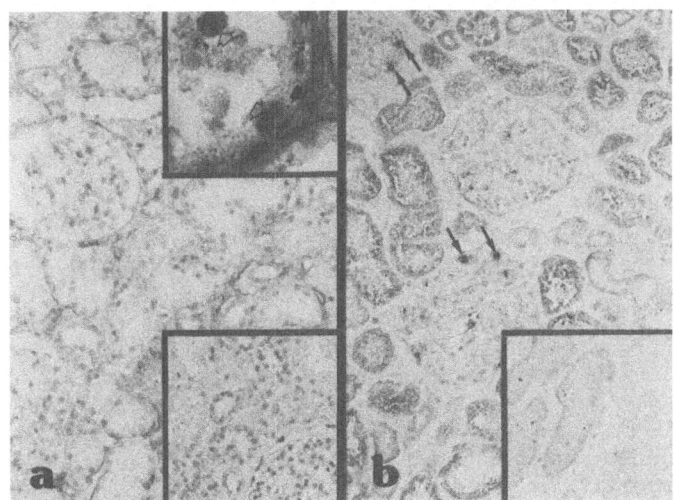

Figure 1. The human parotid gland. a. Kallikrein antigenicity. The
luminal side of the striated ducts (SD) and of the excretory
ducts (ED) is stained. The basement membrane of the ducts
(arrows) and the interstitium surrounding the ducts are also
stained. The insert: when the antiserum to which excessive
pure human kallikreins has been added in advance is used, any
staining is abolished (a control test) (x150).
b. Kallikrein-like activity. The enzyme activity is located
in the ducts (SD and ED) corresponding to the enzyme antigenicity. Some white blood cells and interstitial cells
(arrows) also show the enzyme activity. The insert: DFP inhibited the enzyme activity completely (x150).

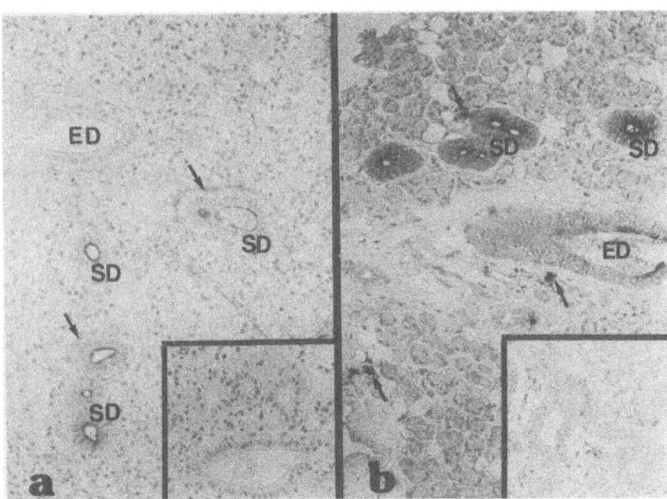

Figure 2. The human kidney. a. Kallikrein antigenicity is revealed in the
interstitium, in the basement membrane of tubules (filled arrows
in the upper insert) as well as in the cytoplasmic granules in
the proximal tubules (open arrows). The lower insert: the control test the same as that in Figure 1a. No staining is revealed (x150).   b. Kallikrein-like activity is located in the brush
border of the proximal tubules without any corresponding antigenicity. The insert: DFP inhibited the enzyme activity completely, including that in some white blood cells (arrows)
(x150).

were found to be located exclusively in cells from the proximal tubules. These granules were observed more frequently in the convoluted portions than in the straight portions and were suggested to be reabsorption granules (heterolysosomes). The kallikrein antigenicity was also revealed in the epithelial side of the basement membrane of all the tubules. Outside of the parenchymal cells, the interstitium revealed the antigenicity but to a slight degree.

The kallikrein-like activity was revealed in some tubules, which were proved to be the proximal tubule by comparing to neighbouring PAS-stained sections. Other tubular segments had no enzyme activity. Some interstitial cells and white blood cells also revealed the enzyme activity. Thus, no identification in the locations of the antigenicity and the enzyme activity was obtained in the human kidney.

As shown in the inserts of Figure 1a and Figure 2a, when the antiserum to which excessive pure human kallikreins had been added in advance was used, any immunostaining was abolished. Therefore, the staining revealed by the immunohistochemical method applied in the present work was specific to the human tissue kallikrein and represented the kallikrein antigenicity.

As shown in the inserts of Figure 1b and Figure 2b, di-isopropyl-fluorophosphate (DFP) inhibited all the kallikrein-like activity completely. Therefore, these enzyme activities were due to serine proteases to which kallikreins belong.

These results are summarized in Table 1. Identification in the locations of the kallikrein antigenicity and the kallikrein-like activity was obtained only in the straited ducts and in the excretory ducts of the parotid gland, which are surrounded by lines.

Table 1. Comparison of locations of kallikrein antigenicity and of kallikrein-like activity in the human parotid gland and in the human kidney

The Human Parotid Gland	Kallikrein Antigenicity	Kallikrein-like Activity
acinus	−	−
intercalated duct	−	−
striated duct	++	++
excretory duct	+	+
basement membrane of ducts	+	−
interstitium surrounding ducts	+	−
interstitial cells	−	+
The Human Kidney		
proximal tubule		
brush border	−	++
reabsorption granules	+	−
other tubular segment	−	−
interstitium	+	−
interstitial cell	−	+

DISCUSSION

In the parotid gland the kallikrein antigenicity and the kallikrein-like activity were identical in their locations in the striated ducts as well as in the excretory ducts. Thus it is concluded that kallikreins are present in an active form in these ducts. This is consistent with previous localization studies[1,3,5] and, moreover, with the concept of de novo synthesis of kallikreins in these ductal cells.[13] Therefore, the results also implied that the immunohistochemical and the enzyme histochemical methods used in the present work were suitable for the demonstration of kallikreins in the tissue.[7]

The same histochemical methods were applied in the human kidney. However, in contrast to the human parotid gland, no identification in locations of the antigenicity and the enzyme activity was obtained at any place. Thus the kallikrein-like activity revealed in the proximal tubule was regarded to be due to non-kallikrein esterases (serine proteases) because no corresponding antigenicity was present. Neither the antigenicity nor the enzyme activity was shown in any other tubular segments. Thus, in the renal parenchymal cells, active kallikreins were not demonstrated and this might imply that kallikreins are formed in too small amount to be demonstrated by the two histochemical methods applied in the present work. According to this assumption, Bonner et al.[14] demonstrated that kallikrein stores in the rat kidney were depleted markedly after the excretion of kallikreins from the isolated perfusion of the kidney and they regarded this due to an insufficient kallikrein synthesis in the kidney.

Out of the parenchymal cells, in the human parotid gland, the kallikrein antigenicity was demonstrated in the basement membrane of ducts as well as in the interstitium surrounding ducts. Recently, tissue kallikreins have been demonstrated in the plasma in the rat[15,16,17] as well as in the human.[18] They have been regarded to originate from the salivary glands and also from the pancreas and to be metabolized in the kidney.[16] Therefore, it is possible that the non-parenchymal kallikrein antigenicity revealed in the parotid gland are due to kallikreins secreted from the parenchymal cells, through the basement membrane of ducts, into the interstitium and then into the lymph or into the blood stream.

In the human kidney, the kallikrein antigenicity was revealed in re-absorption granules in the proximal tubule, in the tubular basement membrane and in the interstitium. This distribution is exactly the same as that of antibody fragment Fab (molecular weight: 50,000 daltons) injected into rats. Bariéty et al.[19,20] injected Fab in the rat and found it in the lysosomes in the proximal tubule, in the interstitium, in the basement membrane of all the tubules and in the basolateral membrane of tubular cell. Therefore, the kallikrein antigenicity found in the human kidney could be derived from tissue kallikreins in the plasma. The antigenicity in the reabsorption granules in the proximal tubule might be due to tissue kallikreins in the plasma passing across the glomerular capillary wall and reabsorbed from the tubular fluid. The antigenicity in the tubular basement membrane and in the interstitium might represent tissue kallikreins diffusing from interstitial capillaries and entering tubular cells across the tubular basement membrane. Then they might be excreted into urine. According to this assumption, Fink and Schleuning[21] demonstrated the pig pancreatic kallikrein infused into dogs could be excreted into urine and claimed that the renal transfer of endogenous tissue kallikrein from the blood into urine could contribute to the total amount of excreted urinary kallikrein.

The kallikrein antigenicities out of parenchymal cells in the human parotid gland and that in the human kidney had no corresponding enzyme activity. This could be explained by the presence of inactive kallikreins. It has been reported that tissue kallikreins in the plasma are present in an inactive form,[16] there are inhibitors of kallikreins in the plasma[22,23] and there are inactive kallikreins in the basolateral membrane of tubules.[24] These observations are consistent with the assumption of the presence of inactive kallikreins. However, a difference in sensitivity of the two methods has to be considered, as an immunohistochemical method, especially the PAP method applied in the present work, is much more sensitive for detection of enzymes than an enzyme histochemical method. Thus, even if active kallikreins are present in a concentration too small for recognition by the enzyme histochemical method, kallikreins still might be demonstrated by an immunohistochemical method.

Thus, in conclusion, the results of the present work are consistent with de novo synthesis of kallikrein in the parotid gland and favour the hypothesis that renal (urinary) kallikreins, at least partly, represent circulating tissue kallikreins originating from the salivary glands and from the pancreas.[21]

ACKNOWLEDGEMENTS

The authors would like to express their thanks to Dr. Poul Faarup, University Institute of Pathology, University of Copenhagen, Copenhagen, Denmark for his support and constructive criticism through the development of this study. This study was supported by a Danish National Scholarship, 1983 and the Danish Heart Association.

REFERENCES

1. T. B. Ørstavik, P. Brandtzaeg, K. Nustad, and K. M. Halvorsen, Cellular localization of kallikreins in rat submandibular and sublingual salivary glands, Acta Histochem., 54:183-192, (1975).
2. T. B. Ørstavik, K. Nustad, P. Brandtzaeg, and J. V. Pierce, Cellular origin of urinary kallikrein, J. Histochem. Cytochem., 24:1037-1039, (1976).
3. T. Dietl, J. Kruck, and H. Fritz, Localization of kallikrein as revealed by the indirect immunofluorescence technique, Hoppe-Seyler's Z. Physiol. Chem., 359:499-505, (1978).
4. J. A. V. Simson, S. S. Spicer, J. Chao, L. Grimm, and H. S. Margolius, Kallikrein localization in rodent salivary glands and kidney with immunoglobulin-enzyme bridge technique, J. Histochem. Cytochem., 27:1567-1576, (1979).
5. M. Schachter, M. W. Peret, C. Moriwaki, and J. A. A. Rodrigues, Localization of kallikrein in submandibular gland of cat, guinea pig, dog and man by the immunoperoxidase method, J. Histochem. Cytochem., 28:1295-1300, (1980).
6. G. S. Pinkus, O. Ole-Moiyoi, K. F. Austen, and J. Spragg, Antigenic separation of a nokinin-generating TAMe esterase from human urinary kallikrein and immunohistochemical comparison of their localization in the kidney, J. Histochem. Cytochem., 29:38-44, (1981).
7. K. Kimura, and H. Moriya, Enzyme- and immuno-histochemical localization of kallikrein. I. The human parotid gland, Histochemistry, 80:367-372, (1984).

8. K. Kimura, and H. Moriya, Enzyme- and immuno-histochemical localization of kallikrein. II. The human kidney, Histochemistry, 80:443-448, (1984).

9. S. Miyaura, Y. Matsuda, K. Yamaguchi, and H. Moriya, Detection and elimination of serum protein contaminants during the purification of human urinary kallikrein, Chem. Pharm. Bull., 29:855-860, (1981).

10. K. Kimura, M. Takagi, T. Igari, M. Ishii, T. Ikeda, T. Takeda, and S. Murao, Histochemical localization of kallikrein-like pro-phe-arg-naphthylester esterase activity in the rat kidney, Histochemistry, 75:91-98, (1982).

11. K. Kimura, Segmental localization of kallikrein-like pro-phe-arg-naphthylester esterase in the rat nephron, Acta Path. Microbiol. Scand. Sect. A, 91:35-42, (1983).

12. K. Kimura, Variations in kallikrein-like esterase activity in different segments of the rat nephron during salt-load and salt-depletion, Acta Path. Microbiol. Immunol. Scand. Sect. A, 91:43-51, (1983).

13. A. J. Mason, B. A. Evans, D. R. Cox, J. Shine, and R. I. Richards, Structure of mouse kallikrein gene family suggests a role in specific processing of biologically active peptides, Nature, 303: 300-307, (1983).

14. G. Bönner, U. Schwertschlag, M. Marin-Grez, and F. Gross, Effects of changes in perfusion pressure on renal and urinary kallikrein in the isolated perfusion rat kidney, Renal Physiol., 6:288-294, (1983).

15. D. Proud, S. Nakamura, F. A. Carone, P. L. Herring, M. Kawamura, T. Inagami, and J. J. Pisano, Kallikrein-kinin and renin-angiotensin systems in rat renal lymph, Kidney Int., 25:880-885, (1984).

16. W. J. Lawton, D. Proud, M. E. Frech, J. V. Pierce, H. R. Keiser, and J. J. Pisano, Characterization and origin of immunoreactive glandular kallikrein in rat plasma, J. Biochem. Pharmacol., 30: 1731-1737, (1981).

17. S. F. Rabito, A. G. Scicli, V. Kher, and O. A. Carretero, Immuno-reactive glandular kallikrein in rat plasma: a radioimmunoassay for its determination, Am. J. Physiol., 242:H602-H610, (1982).

18. E. Fink, T. Dietl, J. Seifert, and H. Fritz, Studies on the biological function of glandular kallikrein, in: Kinin II. Systemic pro-teases and cellular function, ed. by S. Fujii, H. Moriya, and T. Suzuki, Plenum Press, pp. 261-263, (1979).

19. J. Bariety, P. Druet, C. Sapin, M. Belair, and M. Paing, Study of the glomerular filtration barrier by detection of circulating anti-peroxidase antibodies and their fragments, in: Functional ultra-structure of the kidney, ed. by A. B. Maunsbach, T. S. Olsen, and E. I. Christensen, Academic Press, pp. 53-64, (1980).

20. J. Bariéty, P. Druet, F. Laliberté, M. Belair, M. Paing, and C. Sapin, Ultrastructural evidence by immunohistochemical techniques for a tubular reabsorption of endogenous albumin and certain cir-culating proteins in normal rat, in: Functional ultrastructure of the kidney, ed. by A. B. Maunsbach, T. S. Olsen, and E. I. Christensen, Academic Press, pp. 303-314, (1980).

21. E. Fink and M. Schleuning, Studies on the excretion of tissue kallikrein from blood into the urine, Hoppe-Seyler's Z. Physiol. Chem., 363:1331-1339, (1982).

22. Y. Hojima, M. Isobe, and H. Moriya, Kallikrein inhibitors in rat plasma, J. Biochem., 81:37-46, (1977).

23. R. Geiger, U. Stuckstedte, B. Clausnitzer, and H. Fritz, Progressive inhibition of human glandular (urinary) kallikrein by human serum and identification of the progressive antikallikrein as alpha 1-antitrypsin (alpha 1- protease inhibitor), Hoppe-Seyler's Z. Physiol. Chem., 362:317-325, (1981).

24. K. Yamada, and E. G. Erdös, Kallikrein and prekallikrein of the isolated basolateral membrane of rat kidney, Kidney Int., 22: 331-337, (1982).

STUDIES ON CARBOHYDRATE STRUCTURE AND IMMUNOLOGICAL PROPERTIES OF HUMAN URINARY KALLIKREINS

Hiroshi Moriya, Masahiko Ikekita and Kazuyuki Kizuki

Department of Biochemistry, Science University of Tokyo
Shinjuku-ku, Tokyo 162, Japan

SUMMARY

Some studies on carbohydrate structure and immunological properties of human urinary kallikreins purified from the human urine of healthy men (HUK) were investigated. A general technique for fractionating asparagine-linked oligosaccharides of HUK was applied. This involves serial chromatographies on concanavalin A-Sepharose 4B and other lectins bound Agarose. Asparagine-linked main oligosaccharides of both active and inactive types of HUK were mixture of tri- or tetra-antennary complex oligosaccharide having GlcNACβ1-4Manβ residue (bisecting GlcNAc) (type I-2), bi-antennary complex oligosaccharide having core Fucα1-6GlcNAc residue (type III-3), tri- or tetra-antennary complex oligosaccharides having Galβ1-4GlcNAcβ1-4 (Galβ1-4GlcNAcβ1-2)Manα-residue (type I-1-A-a) etc. Besides these structural studies, the method to probe the heterogenous profiles of HUK due to the different structures of carbohydrate chains bound, was devised without the complete purification of urinary kallikrein even with individual subject of not only active but also inactive forms of the kallikrein.

INTRODUCTION

Recently physiological and/or pathological meanings of varied carbohydrate structures bound to the glycohormones or glycoenzymes have been subjected to intense research by many investigators. Results have been shown, for instance, that half-life or clearance in blood of serum glycoproteins depends on their carbohydrate moiety. In addition, remarkable changes in the carbohydrate structures of certain glycoenzymes are induced by malignant tumor. Other important aspects of the role of the carbohydrate moieties had been previously shown, i.e., signals of immunological recognitions, cell aggregation phenomena, their stabilizing effect of certain high dimentional structures of glycoproteins and so on. In order to achieve a solution to the important physiological roles or pathological meanings of tissue kallikreins from these points of view, here the varied carbohydrate structures bound to kallikrein molecules forming (micro-) heterogenous molecules, were investigated.

MATERIALS AND METHODS

Materials

Human urinary, pancreatic and salivary kallikreins, monkey, dog and rat pancreatic kallikreins, and hog pancreatic submaxillary, renal and intestinal kallikreins were purified and prepared according to our previously described methods[1-3] with some modifications. Trypsin from hog pancreas and α-chymotrypsin from pancreas were purchased from Sigma Chemical Co., St. Louis, Mo., U.S.A. Hog pancreatic elastase I was prepared in our laboratory.[4] Other chemicals were of guaranteed reagent grade.

Methods

The vasodilator activity of kallikreins was determined by using anesthetized dogs with the method of Moriya et al.[5] and radioimmunoassay of HUK was done by the method of Morichi et al.[6]

Esterase and amidase assays of kallikreins and other proteases, double immunodiffusion, preprration of anti-HUK serum, sialidase treatment, isolation of oligosaccharides from HUK, radioactive labelling of oligosaccharides, fractionation of oligosaccharides, gel-permeation chromatography with immobilized lectins and treatment with glycosidases were done according to our previously described methods[7-8] with minor modifications.

Most other methods with kallikreins were done by our recently published methods.[9-12]

RESULTS AND DISCUSSIONS

Figure 1 shows the double immunodiffusion analysis of human kallikreins against rabbit anti-HUK serum. Our anti-HUK serum produced a single precipitin line of complete identity having no spurs with not only pure HUK but also crude HUK and any other human tissue kallikreins. This result means HUK which was employed to make anti-HUK serum as antigen was immunochemically complete pure. No cross-reaction occurred with pure hog pancreatic β-kallikrein A or B. We employed such the purest HUK through our structural studies on carbohydrate chains bound to HUK.

The summary of immunological cross-reactivation of various tissue kallikreins and other proteases is shown in Table 1. Rabbit anti-HUK serum also gave a single precipitin line of complete identity with monkey pancreatic kallikrein, but our anti-HUK serum was only specific for human tissue kallikreins including HUK derived from the urine of Bartter's snydrome patient.

The immunoelectrophoresis patterns of various human tissue kallikreins against the antisera to HUK showed the almost same immunoreactivity as in the case of double immunodiffusion analysis. However Bartter's HUK migrated slightly more slowly than normal HUK and human salivary kallikrein produced a very broad precipitin line against anti-HUK serum in our immunoelectrophoresis.[8] This observation means that Bartter's HUK was qualitatively somewhat different than normal HUK.

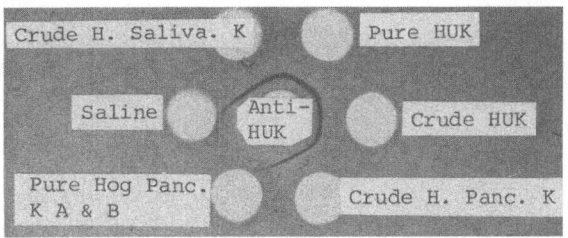

Figure 1. Immunological cross-reaction of various human tissue kallikreins against rabbit anti-HUK serum

Some of the structures of oligosaccharides bound to 2 major components of HUK had been previously proposed by us[7] in where structural studies had to be done with the purest material after complete purification. This matter makes difficulties to treat human urine, especially individual normal or patient urine. Therefore, here for the purpose of our clinical or pathological aspects, we have devised more convenient another way to probe the heterogenous profiles of urinaly kallikrein even with individual subject without complete purification. Figure 2 shows our schematic structures of carbohydrate chains for fractionating Asn-linked oligosaccharides by lectin-agarose affinity chromatographies which we devised. Con A (concanavalin A), E-PHA (erythroagglutinating phythohemagglutinin), WGA (wheat germ agglutinin), Lentil (letil lectin) and L-PHA (leucoagglutinating phytohemagglutinin) showed the different affinities of the

Table 1. Immunological Cross-Reactivities of Various Tissue Kallikreins and Other Proteases Against Rabbit Anti-HUK and Anti-Hog Pancreatic Kallikrein A and Anti-B Antibodies.

Antigens	Antibodies HUK	Hog Panc. K. A	Hog Panc. K. B
Hog Panc. K. A	−	+	+
Hog Panc. K. B	−	+	+
Hog Submaxillary K.	−	+	+
Hog Renal K.	−	+	+
Hog Intestinal K.	−	+	+
HUK	+	−	−
HUK (Bartter's Syndrome)	+	−	−
Human Panc. K.	+	−	−
Human Salivary K.	+	−	−
Monkey Panc. K.	+	−	−
Dog Panc. K.	−	−	−
Rat Panc. K.	−	−	−
Hog Panc. Trypsin	−	−	−
Hog Panc. Elastase I	−	−	−
Bovine Panc. α-Chymotrypsin	−	−	−

+: cross-reacted
−: not cross-reacted

varied N-Glycosidic carbohydrate structures by this method as shown on this figure. The kallikrein activities in each fraction were measured by both amidelytic and radioimmuno assays. And also the inactive (latent) kallikrein amount which can be only recognized as kallikrein activity after activation of trypsin treatment, were measured.

Figure 3 shows the possible proposed structures of carbohydrate chains bound to major 3 components of HUK suggested by our methods.

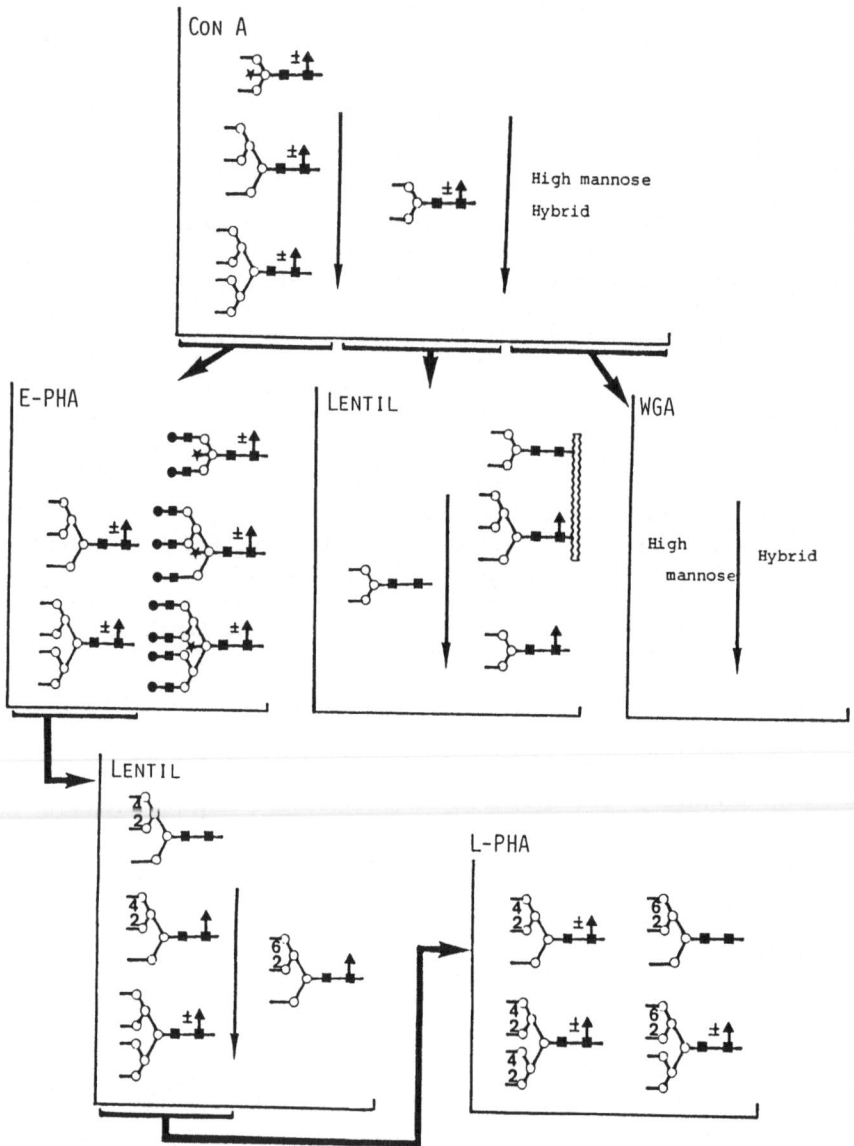

Figure 2.   Scheme for fractionating Asn-linked oligosaccharides by lectine-agarose affinity chromatographies.
Con A: Concanavalin A; E-PHA: Erythroagglutintting phytohemagglutinin; WGA: Wheat germ agglutinin; Lentil: Lentil lectin; L-PHA: Leucoagglutinating phytohemagglutinin.

●: Gal, ■:GlcNAc, O: Man,   *: GlcNAc (bisecting),
▲: Fuc, 2, 4 and 2, 6 show positions bound.

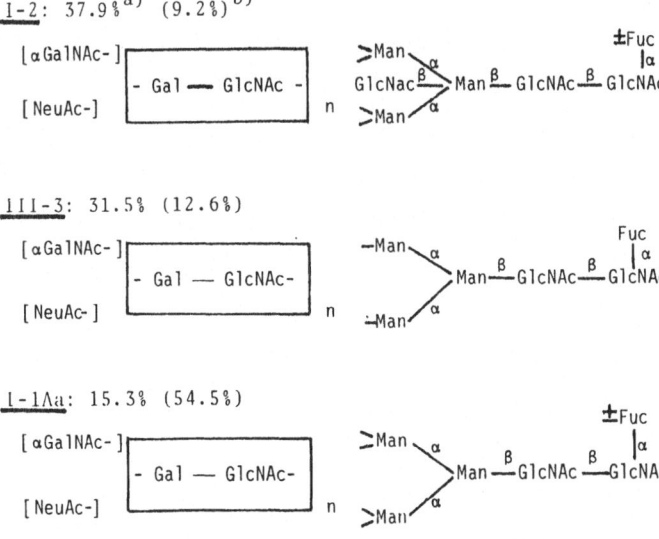

Figure 3. Proposed structures of I-2, III-3 and I-1-A-a Oligosaccharides from HUK

   n: the number of repeating βGal-βGlcNAc disaccharides or branches
   a: values represent the amounts of respective active type HUK present expressed as a percentage of the total active type HUK
   b: values in parentheses represent the amounts of respective inactive type HUK present expressed as a percentage of the total inactive HUK

There were 2 major components (types I-2 and III-3) obtained from the active and major 1 (types I-1-A-a) from the inactive kallikreins. These profiles of major components of not only active but also inactive kallikreins with normal subjects whichever individual or mixed big pool or urine, were usually observed approximately the same. On the contrary somewhat changes in these profiles due to the varied carbohydrate structures were seemed to be induced by certain pathological states, especially renal trouble and other clinical conditions which details are now under investigation. Thus the meanings of excreted changes of not only amount but also structural aspects of the fractionated heterogenous forms of urinary kallikrein due to the varied structures of carbohydrate moiety were considered to yield some important informations in the field of renal or other pathology or diagnosis. We are now making study of much more details and more samples of various urine, especially certain pathological states as well as the more detailed fundamental structural studies of carbohydrate moieties bound to human kallikreins. Our present observations with those can be expected very important to solve the problems of pathophysiological meanings of the tissue kallikreins.

ACKNOWLEDGEMENTS

    The authors would like to sincerely thank Professor T. Osawa, Faculty of Pharmaceutical Sciences, University of Tokyo, for his generous instructions in the carbohydrate analysis.

    This work was supported in part by grants from the Ministry of Education, Science and Culture, of Japan, the Japan Society for the Promotion of Science, the Takeda Science Foundation, the Suzuken Memorial Foundation and the Toray Science Foundation.

REFERENCES

1. H. Moriya, Y. Fukuoka, Y. Hojima, and C. Moriwaki, Measurement of the sugar contents and their effect on the electrophoretical behaviours of multiple forms of hog pancreatic kallikrein, Chem. Pharm. Bull., 26:3178-3185, (1978).

2. Y. Matsuda, K. Miyazaki, H. Moriya, Y. Fujimoto, and Y. Hojima, Studies on urinary kallikreins. I. Purification and characterization of human urinary kallikreins, J. Biochem., 80:671-679, (1976).

3. M. Ikekita, H. Moriya, S. Ozawa, and K. Kizuki, Studies on heterogenous components of hog pancreatic kallikrein - "Possible role of the neuraminic acid residues" -, Chem. Pharm. Bull., 29:545-553, (1981).

4. M. Ikekita, Y. Shiina, Y. Takemoto, K. Kizuki, and H. Moriya, An improved assay method for the elastinolytic activity of elastases with congo red-elastin, Yakugaku Zasshi, 103:1200-1205, (1983).

5. H. Moriya, H. Fukushima, K. Yamazaki, and C. Moriwaki, Biochemical studies on kallikreins and their related substances. II. An improved method of purification of hog pancreatic kallikreins, J. Biochem., 58:208-213, (1965).

6. S. Morichi, E. Sako, M. Tsukada, Y. Iga, S. Kitagawa, M. Nishida, K. Kizuki, M. Ikekita, and H. Moriya, Determination of active and inactive kallikrein in human urine by direct solid phase-radio-immunoassay, in preparation.

7. M. Ikekita, T. Tsuji, K. Yamamoto, T. Osawa, K. Kizuki, and Hm Moriya, The carbohydrate moiety of human urinary kallikrein, Chem. Pharm. Bull., 31:1052-1058, (1983).

8. M. Ikekita, K. Kizuki, and H. Moriya, Immunological relationships of the glandular kallikreins, Chem. Pharm. Bull., 31:2466-2472, (1983).

9. M. Ikekita, H. Moriya, K. Kizuki, and S. Ozawa, Measurement of carbohydrate contents in multiple forms of hog pancreatic kallikrein and their behavior on sodium dodecyl sulfate-polyacrylamide gel electrophoresis, Chem. Pharm. Bull., 28:1948-1950, (1980).

10. S. Miyaura, Y. Matsuda, K. Yamaguchi, and H. Moriya, Detection and elimination of serum protein contaminants during the purification of human urinary kallikrein, Chem. Pharm. Bull., 29:855-860, (1981).

11. H. Moriya, M. Ikekita, and K. Kizuki, Studies on heterogenous components of hog pancreatic kallikrein. II. Preliminary probe of the varied structures of carbohydrate chain of hog pancreatic kallikrein, Chem. Pharm. Bull., 29:1785-1788, (1981).

12. Y. Tamura, Y. Matsuda, K. Yamada, T. Takagi, T. Nishikawa, M. Watanabe, K. Mikami, H. Moriya, and A. Kumagai, Some aspects of urinary kallikrein in a patient with Bartter's syndrome, in: KININ. II. by S. Fujii, H. Moriya and T. Suzuki, eds., Plenum Publishing Co., Adv. Exptl. Med. Biol., 120B:515-524, (1979).

13. H. Moriya, M. Ikekita, and K. Kizuki, Some aspects of carbohydrate contents in glandular kallikrein, in: KININ III ed. by H. Fritz, N. Back, G. Dietze and G. L. Haberland, Plenum Publishing Co., Adv. Exptl. Med. Biol., 156A:309-316, (1983).

INITIAL OBSERVATIONS OF A KALLIKREIN-LIKE ENZYME ASSOCIATED WITH THE

PLASMA MEMBRANES OF RAT ADIPOCYTES

F. Mulholland, A. Ashford* and G.S. Bailey

Department of Chemistry, University of Essex, Colchester
UK *Biological Research Laboratories, May and Baker Ltd.
Dagenham, Essex, UK

SUMMARY

Homogenates of rat adipocytes and plasma membranes thereof were shown by radioimmunoassay to contain immunoreactive glandular kallikrein. On the basis of the hydrolysis of D-Val-Leu-Arg-p-nitroanilide, the kallikrein-like enzyme associated with the plasma membranes was found not to be stimulated by prior incubation with melittin or phospholipase A_2.

However, pre-incubation of the membrane preparation with trypsin did increase the activity of the enzyme. Furthermore, activation could also be achieved by incubating the plasma membranes with insulin at a dose that stimulated glucose uptake into intact adipocytes. On the other hand, incubation with insulin at a dose that did not increase glucose uptake into rat adipocytes was ineffective in activating the kallikrein-like enzyme.

INTRODUCTION

Over the last few years evidence has accumulated which indicates that the kallikrein-kinin system is able to control glucose uptake into responsive cells under certain conditions[1]. The ability of aprotinin to partially block the effects of insulin on glucose metabolism of skeletal muscle has been interpreted in terms of inhibition of a kallikrein-like molecule[2]. Furthermore, certain short-term intracellular effects of insulin on rat adipocytes appear to involve limited proteolytic action at the plasma membrane[3,4]. Thus, the present study was initiated to test for the presence of a kallikrein-like enzyme in rat adipocytes, and to investigate the factors responsible for its activation.

METHODS

The methodology adopted was largely that used by Nishimura and co-workers in their studies of activation of membrane-bound kallikrein in rat kidney[5]. Kallikrein activity was measured in terms of the hydrolysis of D-Val-Leu-Arg-pNA (S2266, Kabi) using the technique for turbid solutions. The unit of activity is nmole p-nitroaniline produced per minute. Immunoreactive kallikrein was measured by radioimmunoassay[6]. Protein concentration was measured by a modification of the Lowry procedure[7]. Adipocytes, isolated

by the method of Rodbell[8], were homogenized and DOC-treated, and were de-
salted by dialysis before RIA. Adipose plasma membranes were obtained as
described by Cushman and Wardzala[9]. Unless otherwise stated, pre-incubations of the membrane preparations were carried out at 37°C for 20 minutes
prior to starting the assay by addition of the substrate.

RESULTS AND DISCUSSION

The Existence of Immunoreactive Kallikrein in Adipose Cells and Adipocyte
Plasma Membranes

Radioimmunoassay of a DOC treated homogenate of rat adipocytes showed
it to contain an antigenic species that cross-reacted with antiserum to
kallikrein of rat submandibular gland (Figure 1).

The amount of immunoreactive kallikrein was estimated to be 0.69ug
kallikrein/mg protein. Similar results were found for a treated fraction
of adipocyte plasma membrane (Figure 2) where the amount of immunoreactive
kallikrein was found to be 1.1 ug kallikrein/mg protein. The kallikrein
measured by the RIA was not necessarily enzymically active. Thus kallikrein-
like activity was determined in terms of the hydrolysis of S2266.

The Effects of Phospholipase A_2, melittin and Triton X 100 on Plasma
Membranes

Pre-incubation of the plasma membranes with buffer alone or with
melittin (protein/peptide = 1/1 w/w) produced no measurable hydrolysis of
the substrate over a period of 60 minutes. A typical time-course for the
hydrolysis of S2266 by plasma membranes after prior incubation with
phospholilpase A_2 (protein/enzyme = 5.3/1 w/w) is shown in Figure 3. The
specific activities of the membrane preparation after various pre-incubations are shown in Table 1.

Table 1

Pre-incubation	Specific Activity v S2266 (units/mg protein)
+ phospholipase A_2	2.88
+ phospholipase A_2 + melittin	2.84
+ phospholipase A_2 + melittin + Triton X 100(1%)	2.87

Thus it would seem that the phospholipase A_2 had acted upon the plasma
membranes to activate or release an enzyme capable of hydrolyzing S2266.

However, as can be seen in Figure 3, even in the absence of plasma
membranes (blank), the phospholipase preparation produced significant
breakdown of the substrate. A commercial source of the phospholipase A_2,
isolated from Crotalus durissus terrificus (a rattlesnake venom), had been
used in the experiments. Such venoms are known to contain proteolytic
enzymes[10]. Thus it was considered possible that it was a proteolytic
contaminant rather than phospholipase A_2 itself that had been responsible
for the hydrolysis of the p-nitroanilide.

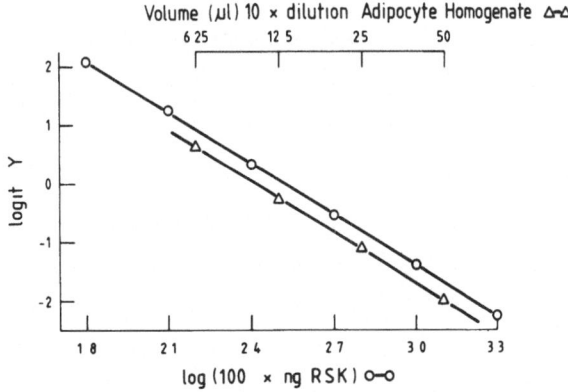

Figure 1. Cross-reactivity of rat adipocyte homogenate in RIA
for rat submandibular kallikrein.

To check that possibility, the experiments were repeated using that
preparation of phospholipase A_2 after incubation with phenylmethyl sulphonyl
fluoride. Under the conditions employed the potential inhibitor did not
reduce the ability of the preparation to act upon the plasma membranes.
However, no hydrolysis of S2266 occurred over 60 minutes following incubation of the membrane preparation with phospholipase A_2 isolated in our
laboratories from Naja naja siamensis (a cobra venom). Such Elapid venoms
are known to contain little or no proteolytic activity[10].

Thus, the kallikrein-like enzyme associated with the plasma membranes
of the rat adipocytes could not be activated by melittin or Triton X 100
or pure phospholipase A_2 and was distinct from the membrane-bound kallikrein
of rat kidney[5].

The ability of trypsin to stimulate the kallikrein-like activity of
the plasma membranes was then investigated.

The Effects of Trypsin on Plasma Membranes

Prior incubation of the membrane preparation with bovine trypsin,
followed by inhibition of the exogenous trypsin by excess Lima Bean Trypsin
Inhibitor, produced the results shown in Table 2.

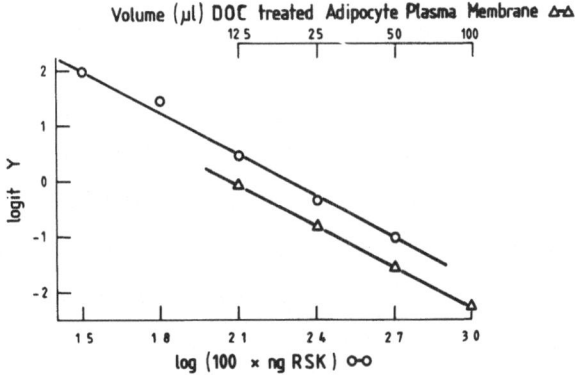

Figure 2. Cross-reactivity of adipocyte plasma membrane fraction
in RIA for rat submandibular kallikrein.

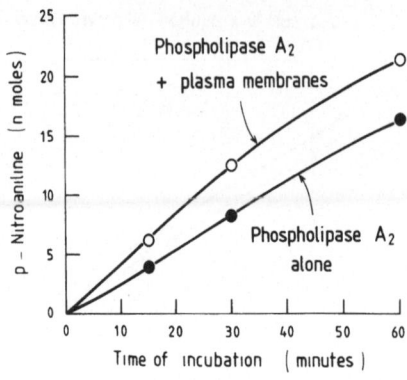

Figure 3. Time course of hydrolysis of S2266.

Table 2

Time of Pre-incubation (minutes)	Protein/Trypsin (w/w)	Specific Activity v S2266 (units/mg protein)
5	5.8/1	2.43
5	1.2/1	2.73
60	9.0/1	3.21
60	5.8/1	5.73
60	1.2/1	9.92

A time course of pre-incubations at a protein/trypsin ratio of 1.6/1 (w/w) is shown in Figure 4.

It can be seen that the level of activity of the plasma membranes increased with an increase in time of prior incubation and amount of trypsin added.

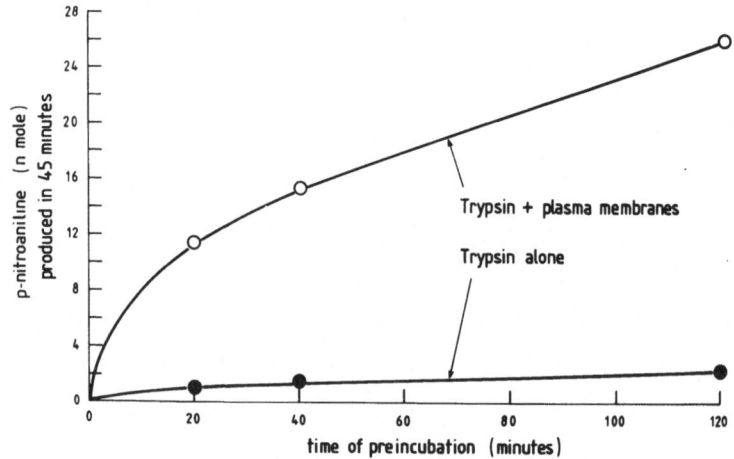

Figure 4. Effect of time of preincubation of trypsin and plasma membranes on activity towards S2266.

As it has been reported that trypsin can mimic certain actions of insulin on adipocytes[3], the ability of insulin to activate the plasma membranes was investigated.

The Effects of Insulin on Plasma Membranes

Two concentrations of insulin were chosen to be tested for the ability to activate the membrane preparation to hydrolyze the p-nitroanilide substrate. One amount of insulin (0.3 nM) was unable to stimulate glucose uptake into isolated adipocytes, whereas the other concentration (10 nM) was effective in that assay [data not shown]. Incubation of the plasma membranes with insulin (0.3 nM) prior to the addition of the substrate produced no subsequent detectable hydrolysis of S2266 over a period of 45 minutes. Some of the results of various pre-incubations using the higher level of insulin (10 nM) are shown in Table 3.

Table 3

Pre-incubation	Specific Activity v S2266 (units/mg/protein)
10 nM Insulin (30 mins) + buffer (60 mins) + LBTI (30 mins)	1.93
Buffer (30 mins) + Trypsin (60 mins) + LBTI (30 mins)	3.34
10 nM Insulin (30 mins) + Trypsin (60 mins) + LBTI (30 mins)	3.12

The protein/trypsin ratio was 3.81 (w/w).

LBTI = Lima Bean Trypsin Inhibitor.

It can be seen that incubation with insulin (10 nM) alone did produce activation of the membrane associated enzyme. However, the level of activity was not as great as that produced by trypsin activation. The combination of insulin and trypsin was not particularly effective.

In respect of earlier findings[1-4], it is interesting to speculate that the kallikrein-like enzyme found in the present study may well be involved in mediating the action of insulin on glucose uptake into rat adipocytes.

CONCLUSION

By means of radioimmunoassay and the measurement of the hydrolysis of a peptidyl p-nitroanilide, a glandular kallikrein-like enzyme has been found to be associated with the plasma membranes of rat adipocytes. The enzyme was not activated by preincubation with detergent, or melittin, or phospholipase. However, the activity was increased by prior incubation with trypsin. The ability of insulin to activate the kallikrein-like activity of the membrane preparation depended on its dose. An insulin dose that stimulated glucose uptake into intact rat adipocytes was also effective in increasing the activity of the membrane associated enzyme. A level of insulin that did not increase glucose uptake had no effect on the activity of the enzyme. Obviously, further work is necessary to test the possibility that the kallikrein-like enzyme is actually involved in the stimulation of glucose uptake by insulin.

REFERENCES

1. Wicklmayr, M., Brunnbauer, H. and Dietze, G.: The kallikrein-kinin-prostaglandin system. Involvement in the control of capillary blood flow and substrate metabolism in skeletal muscle tissue. Adv. Exp. Med. Biol. 156A: 625–638 (1983).

2. Dietze, G., Wicklmayr, M., Bottger, I. and Mayer, L.: Inhibition of insulin action on glucose uptake into skeletal muscle by a kallikrein-trypsin inhibitor. Hoppe-Seyler's Z. Physiol. Chem. 359: 1209–1215 (1978).

3. Seals, J.R. and Czech, M.P.: Evidence that insulin activates an intrinsic plasma membrane protease in generating a secondary chemical mediator. J. Biol. Chem. 255: 6529–6531 (1980).

4. Larner, J., Cheng, K., Schwartz, C., Dubler, R., Creacy, S., Kikuchi, K., Tamwa, S., Galasko, G., Pullin, C. and Katz, M.: Chemical mechanism of insulin action via proteolytic formation of mediator peptides. Mol. Cell. Biochem. 40: 155–161 (1981).

5. Nishimura, K., Ward, P. and Erdos, E.G.: Kallikrein and renin in the membrane fractions of the rat kidney. Hypertension 2: 538–545 (1980).

6. Proud, D., Bailey, G.S., Nustad, K. and Gautvik, K.M.: The immunological similarity of rat glandular kallikreins. Biochem. J. 167: 835–838 (1977).

7. Peterson, G.L.: A simplification of the protein assay method of Lowry et al. which is more generally applicable. Anal. Biochem. 83: 346–356 (1977).

8. Rodbell, M.: Effects of hormones on glucose metabolism and lipolysis. J. Biol. Chem. 239: 375–380 (1964).

9. Cushman, S.W. and Wardzala, L.J.: Potential mechanism of insulin action on glucose transport in the isolated rat adipose cell. J. Biol. Chem. 255: 4758–4762 (1980).

10. Tu, A.T.: Venoms. Chemistry and Molecular Biology, John Wiley, (1977).

BILE ACIDS AND THE INTESTINAL KALLIKREIN-KININ SYSTEM

I.J. Zeitlin, H.A.R. Al-Dhahir, S. Cook, A. Currie
and K. Donovan

Department of Physiology and Pharmacology, University of
Strathclyde, Glasgow, Scotland, U.K.

SUMMARY

1. We have measured concentrations of tissue kallikrein-like amidase
    (TKLA) in blood-free rat gastrointestinal tissue. TKLA was present
    in the gut wall from the stomach to the rectum with concentration
    peaks in the duodenum and caecum. When rats, fasted for 24 hr were
    compared with normally fed animals, the mean fasted TKLA levels rose
    significantly in the duodenum and proximal and distal colons and fell
    in the caecum. No other tissues showed concentration changes.

2. Sodium chenodeoxycholate and other bile acids have biological actions
    on the rat intestinal wall which are similar to those produced by the
    kallikrein-kinin system. We have previously reported that bile acids
    released TKLA from the rat colon wall. This TKLA was totally in-
    hibited by aprotinin.

3. We now report that intraluminal sodium chenodeoxycholate (30 mM) in-
    creases both colonic motility and colonic mucosal leakage. These
    increases are largely blocked by aprotinin.

4. The ability of intraluminal sodium taurochenodeoxycholate to increase
    vascular leakage in the rat stomach and colon was parallelled by its
    ability to release TKLA from these issues.

5. Our results are compatible with the mediation of these biological
    actions of the tested bile acids via activation of a serine proteinase,
    possibly tissue kallikrein.

INTRODUCTION

Eugene Werle, in 1960[1], reported the presence in mammalian intestinal
wall of a trypsin-activated hypotensive activity which was kallikrein-like.
The levels of this activity were much higher in the large than in the small
intestine. In rats the levels were unchanged by pancreatectomy, but were
increased by feeding such low bulk diets as egg, which produced the largest
changes, meat or fat. There has since been relatively little study of the
kallikrein-kinin system in the intestinal wall.

In 1965, Amundsen and Nustad[2], reported the presence of kinin-forming activity in the rabbit and rat intestine. In a series of papers from 1970 onwards, Zeitlin and co-workers reported the presence of a kallikrein-like kininogenase along the whole length of the rat gastrointestinal tract[3,4]. They showed that it occurred as a pre-active precursor[5], that it had a molecular weight of 33,000, which differed from that of rat plasma kallikrein[6] and that it had the inhibitor and substrate specificities of a tissue kallikrein[5,7].

Despite one dissenting voice[8], the presence of "tissue" kallikreins in rat gastrointestinal tract was confirmed by Moriwaki et al.[9] and Uchida et al.[10] who purified rat intestinal and stomach kallikreins respectively. These workers found in the small intestine two kallikreins with molecular weights 33,000 and 35,000 respectively[9] while in the stomach, a kallikrein with a molecular weight of 29,000 was found[10]. The kallikreins from both sources had the inhibitor and substrate specificities of a tissue kallikrein. Similarly the presence of a tissue kallikrein in human colonic mucosae, first indicated in 1973 by Zeitlin and Smith[11], was confirmed when human colonic kallikrein was purified by Zimmerman et al.[12].

Most recently, Schachter's group has used immunohistochemical techniques to localize tissue kallikrein in goblet cells of the colon[2] and small intestine, and in gastric mucous cells in rat, cat and man[13,14], while Miller et al.[15] have demonstrated a high rate of de novo immunoreactive tissue kallikrein synthesis in rat colonic tissue.

Although tissue kallikrein has been identified and localized in the gastrointestinal tract, nothing is yet known of the functional role, if any, of this "enterokallikrein". It is clearly of some value to determine whether any physiological or pathological states or maneuvres can alter gastrointestinal levels of kallikrein.

In the present study we have measured the concentration of tissue kallikrein-like amidase activity along the whole length of the rat gastrointestinal tract and describe results which indicate that biological actions of bile salts on the intestinal wall may be mediated by activation of a kallikrein-like enzyme.

METHODS

Total tissue kallikrein-like amidase (TKLA) was measured in gastrointestinal tissue, perfused free of blood, homogenized in distilled water (10 mg/g wet weight) and incubated under toluene (24 h, 22°C) to activate kallikreins. Amidase was assayed by incubating aqueous supernatant with H-D-Val.Leu.Arg.pNA. 2 HCl (S-2266, Kabi Ltd.) a glandular kallikrein-selective substrate, at pH 8.5.

Colonic motility was monitored in anaesthetized animals by inserting pairs of 3.5 mm balloons, rectally 4 cm and 6 cm into the proximally occluded colon. Pressure variations were detected using Statham pressure transducers. Motility was assessed as Motility Index determined as [Mean Wave Amplitude x Percent Motility].

Colonic vascular leakage was monitored following intravenous injection of I^{125}-labelled albumin, 30 min. prior to colonic perfusion. Colons were perfused for a 30 min. control period with Krebs solution alone and then for a further 30 min. with Krebs alone, or containing drugs. Perfusate was sampled at 5 min. intervals for I^{125}. Arterial blood was sampled at 15 min. intervals to determine the I^{125}-albumin clearance curve. Albumin leakage was expressed as perfusate counts percent of blood counts. An assessment of leakage during the whole 30 min period was determined as the area under the 30 min time-course curve.

Values are expressed as mean and standard error unless stated otherwise. Statistical differences between groups are determined using the Mann-Whitney U-test.

RESULTS

Intestinal Kallikrein Levels

In an earlier paper, we reported that although kallikrein-like kinin-forming activity was present along the whole rat gastrointestinal tract, dietary alterations produced concentration changes only in the duodenum, caecum and distal colon[16]. In the present study, we have likewise found TKLA in normally fed animals, along the whole gut, (Table 1), with activity peaks in the duodenum and in the caecum.

TABLE 1. Tissue kallikrein-like amidase (TKLA) in the gastrointestinal tracts of normally fed rats

Tissue	Number	TKLA Activity (n.Moles pNA Min $^{-1}$ g $^{-1}$ tissue)
Stomach	7	9.9 $\pm$ 0.95
Duodenum	7	128.9 $\pm$ 18.3
Jejunum	7	69.5 $\pm$ 8.2
Mid-ileum	7	93.4 $\pm$ 11.6
Terminal ileum	7	115.0 $\pm$ 14.2
Caecum	9	117.4 $\pm$ 5.4
Proximal colon	8	26.8 $\pm$ 2.2
Distal colon	8	26.0 $\pm$ 2.3
Rectum	7	23.2 $\pm$ 2.8

When rats were fasted for 24 h and given water ad libitum, statistically significant changes in mean TKLA were detected only in the duodenum (138.2 $\pm$ 13.1% of the mean fed value $p < 0.05$), caecum (68.2 $\pm$ 8.2%, $p < 0.01$) and proximal (170.5 $\pm$ 17.9%, $p < 0.05$) and distal (181.9 $\pm$ 21.5%), $p < 0.01$) colons. It is noteworthy that these changes were in the same directions as those in kinin-forming enzyme produced by feeding and fasting in our earlier study.

Effect of Bile Acids on Colonic Motility and Vascular Leakage

At the 1981 Kinin Symposium in Munich, we reported that bile acids released active kallikrein-like enzyme from rat colon both in vitro and in vivo[17]. In anesthetized animals, the enzymic activity was released into the lumen by intraluminal perfusion with 3.86 mM sodium chenodeoxycholate. The released enzyme was totally inhibited by aprotinin. Any biological actions of this bile acids which depend on kallikrein activation might therefore be expected to be inhibited by aprotinin.

The action of crystalline aprotinin (Trasylol (R)* was therefore examined on bile salt-induced colonic motility and mucosal vascular leakage in anaethetized rats. Pairs of small (3.5 mm) balloons were inserted rectally 4 cm and 6 cm into the proximally occluded colon to monitor motility. The colonic lumen was instilled for an initial 30 min with saline (2.5 ml) alone, followed by a second 30 min with saline alone or containing 30 mM

sodium chenodeoxycholate. This high concentration caused a large increase
(p < 0.01) in mean motility index at both 6 cm and 4 cm balloons (Table 2).
A further group of animals was pre-treated with a bolus intraarterial injection of 100,000 Units aprotinin per kg, 5 min prior to instillation,
followed by intraarterial infusion of 100,000 U aprotinin. Kg $^{-1}$ hr $^{-1}$.
In these animals, when 30 mM chenodeoxycholate was instilled in the presence
of 40,000 Units ml^{-1} aprotinin, the mean motility at both balloons was reduced by more than 94% of that in the absence of Trasylol (p   0.001,
Table 2).

TABLE 2. Changes in motility index induced during 30 min colonic
          intraluminal instillation of saline alone or containing
          drugs compared with a prior 30 min control instillation
          of saline alone (N in parentheses)

	Change in Motility Index at balloon:-	
	4 cm	6 cm
Saline	0 (5)	0 (5)
Bile (30 mM)	735 $\pm$ 96 (6)	306 $\pm$ 36 (9)
Bile & Trasylol	42 $\pm$ 23 (9)	19 $\pm$ 10 (9)

* Trasylol (R) is a registered trademark of Bayer A.G.

In a further study, colonic vascular leakage was determined in anesthetized rats during intraluminal colonic perfusion with Krebs solution
alone, or containing 30 mM sodium chenodeoxycholate. Krebs perfusion caused
little vascular leakage, neither during the first nor second 30 min (See
Figure 1, showing the percentage differences between areas under the time-
course curves for the first and second 30 min periods). Perfusion with
30 mM sodium chenodeoxycholate caused a large increase in mean leakage.
When animals were treated with aprotinin as described for the motility
studies, the mean increase in vascular leakage produced by the bile acid
was reduced by 71.4%.

This action of intraluminal bile acids on intestinal vascular leakage
is not consistent in every region of the rat gut. In further groups of
animals, gastric intraluminal perfusion with Krebs solution containing the
conjugated bile acid taurochenodeoxycholate caused no significant increase
in albumin leakage during the test period when measured as areas under the
time course curve (p < 0.05, n=5). Intraluminal perfusion of rat colons
with 30 mM sodium tauochenodeoxycholate induced a highly significant increase of 5442% (p < 0.05, n=5). However, this is not incompatible with
possible kallikrein involvement. Chopped rat stomach or colon (3 x mm
fragments) were incubated for 15 min in Krebs solution alone or containing
30 mM sodium taurochenodeoxycholate. No significant increase in release
into the incubate of active tissue kallikrein-like amidase was detected
from stomach in the presence of bile salt, however, a highly significant
increase of 47.3 $\pm$ 1.8% (p < 0.01, n=6) was detected from the colon. Thus,
rat colon showed both increased vascular leakage and TKLA activation in
the presence of tauochenodeoxycholate, while neither occurred in stomach.

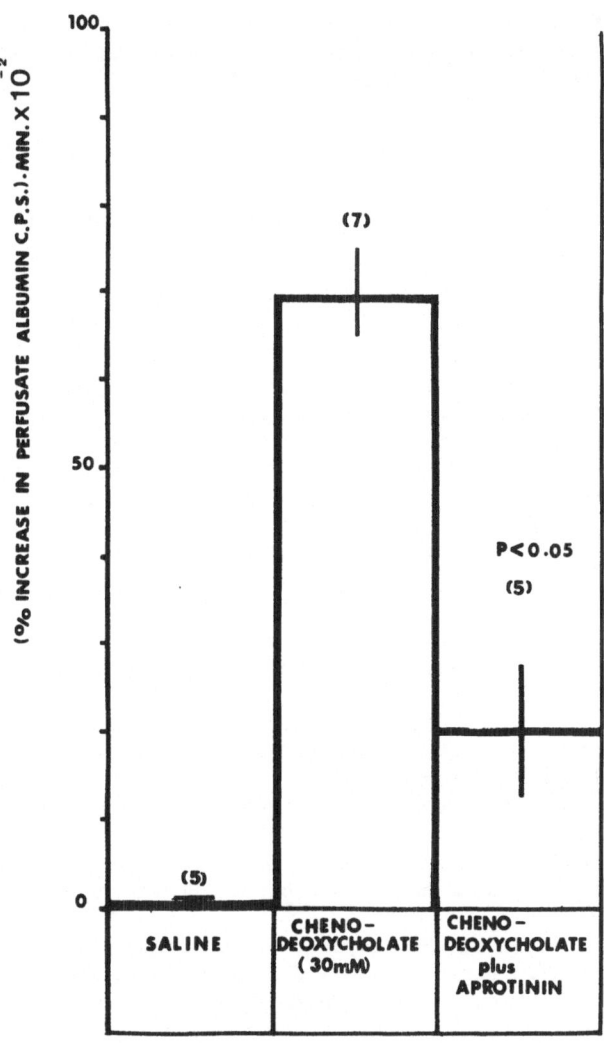

Figure 1. Vascular Leakage In Rat Colon:
Area Under Time – Course Drive
(Mean & S.E.)

DISCUSSION

We have found that tissue kallikrein-like activity is present along
the length of the gut wall of the rat. Several research groups have shown
that in rat and hamster gut the bile acids deoxycholate and chenodeoxycholate induce net water and electrolyte secretion and inhibit their absorption
[18,19]. These agents also increase mucosal permeability to large molecules
and stimulate colonic motility[20,21] and their biological properties are
parallelled to some extent by those of the kinin system. Kallikrein and
kinins both inhibit water and electrolyte absorption and induce net secretion of chloride[22,23], increase intestinal vascular permeability[24] and
stimulate rat colonic motility[25]. We have previously reported that bile
acids release active tissue kallikrein-like enzyme from rat intestinal
tissues[17,26] and that the colonic enzyme is totally inhibited by aprotinin
[17]. In the present study we have reported that the increases in both colonic
motility and vascular leakage induced by a high concentration of bile acid
are largely blocked by aprotinin. Furthermore, the actions of bile acid
on vascular leakage at two sites in the gut were parallelled by its ability

to release TKLA from the tissue at those sites. This provides circumstantial evidence that a serine proteinase, possibly tissue kallikrein, mediates these biological actions of the bile acids studied.

ACKNOWLEDGEMENTS

We are grateful to Professor G.L. Haberland of Bayer A.G. for a kind gift of Trasylol (R).

REFERENCES

1. Werle, E.: Kallikrein, kallidin and related substances. In: Polypeptides which affect smooth muscles and blood vessels. ed. by M. Schachter. Pergamon Press pp. 199–209 (1960).
2. Amundsen, E. and Nustad, K.: Kinin-forming and destroying activities of cell homogenates. J. Physiol. 179: 479–488 (1965).
3. Zeitlin, I.J.: Kinin-release associated with the gastrointestinal tract. Adv. Exp. Biol. Med. 8: 329–339 (1970).
4. Frankish, N.H. and Zeitlin, I.J.: The assay of tissue kallikrein in rat intestine. Br. J. Pharmac. 59: 517P (1977).
5. Zeitlin, I.J.: Pharmacological characterization of kinin-forming activity in rat intestinal tissue. Br. J. Pharmac. 42: 648–649P (1971).
6. Zeitlin, I.J., Singh, Y.N., Lembeck, F. and Theiler, M.: The molecular weights of plasma and intestinal kallikreins in rat. Arch. Pharmacol. 293: 159–161 (1976).
7. Zeitlin, I.J.: Rat intestinal kallikrein. Adv. Exp. Med. Biol. 21: 289–296 (1972).
8. Seki, T., Nakajima, T. and Erdös, E.G.: Colon kallikrein, its relation to the plasma enzyme. Biochem. Pharmacol. 21: 1227–1235 (1972).
9. Moriwaki, C., Fujimori, H., Toyono, Y. and Nagai, T.: Studies on kallikreins V. Purification and characterization of rat intestinal kallikrein. Chem. Pharm. Bull. 28: 3612–3620 (1980).
10. Uchida, K., Niirobe, M., Kato, H. and Fuji, S.: Purification and properties of rat stomach kallikrein. Biochim. Biophys. Acta. 614: 501–510 (1980).
11. Zeitlin, I.J., and Smith A.N.: Mobilization of tissue kallikrein in inflammatory disease of the colon. Gut. 14: 133–138 (1973).
12. Zimmerman, A., Geiger, R. and Kortmann, H.: Similarity between a kininogenase (kallikrein) from human large intestine and human urinary kallikrein. Hoppe Seyler's Z. Physiol. Chem. 360: 1767–1773 (1979).
13. Schachter, M., Peret, M.W., Billing, A.G. and Wheeler, G.D.: Immunolocalization of the protease kallikrein in the colon. J. Histochem. Cytochem. 31: 1255–1260 (1983).
14. Schachter, M., Wheeler, G.D. and Langridge, D.J.: Immunolocalization of kallikrein in goblet and mucous cells of the colon, small intestine and stomach. In this symposium.
15. Miller, D.H., Chao, J., Margolius, H.S.: Tissue kallikrein synthesis and its modification by testosterone or low dietary sodium. Biochem. J. 218: 37–43 (1984).
16. Frankish, N.H. and Zeitlin, I.J.: The effect of diet on tissue levels of kinin-forming enzyme in blood-free rat gastrointestinal tract. J. Physiol. 298: 361–370 (1980).
17. Al-Dhahir, H.A.R. and Zeitlin, I.J.: Bile salts activate glandular kallikrein-like activity in rat colon. Adv. Exp. Med. Biol. 156A: 463–467 (1983).

18. Forth, W., Rummel, W. and Glasner, H.: Zw resorptions-hemmenden
    Wirkung von Gallensauren. Arch. Pharmacol. 247: 382-383 (1964).
19. Gullikson, G.W., Cline, W.S., Lorenzsonn, V., Benz, L., Olsen, W.A.
    and Bass. P.: Effect of anionic surfactants on hamster small
    intestine membrane structure and function: relationship to surface
    activity. Gastroenterology. 73: 501-511 (1977).
20. Teichberg, S., McGarvey, E., Bayne, M.A. and Lifshitz, F.: Altered
    jejunal macromolecular barrier induced by α-dihydroxy deconjugated
    bile salts. Am. J. Physiol. 245: G122-G132 (1983).
21. Snape, W.J., Shiff, S. and Cohen, S.: Effect of deoxycholic acid on
    colonic motility in the rabbit. Am. J. Physiol. 238: G321-G325
    (1980).
22. Dennhardt, R. and Haberich, F.J.: Effect of kallikrein on the ab-
    sorption of water, electrolytes and hexoses in the intestine of
    rats. In: Kininogenases-Kallikrein. ed. by G.L. Haberland and
    J.W. Rohen. Schattauer pp. 81-82 (1972).
23. Cuthbert, A.W. and Margolius, H.S.: Kinins stimulate net chloride
    secretion by the rat colon. Br. J. Pharmac. 75: 587-598 (1982).
24. Fasth, S. and Hulten, L.: The effect of bradykinin on intestinal
    motility and blood flow. Acta. Chir. Scand. 139: 699-705 (1973).
25. Al-Dhahir, H.A.R. and Zeitlin, I.J.: The non-adrenergic non-choliner-
    gic (NANC) motility response in rat colon: Studies in possible
    transmitters. J. Physiol. 317: 93-94P (1981).

T-KININ AND T-KININOGEN – AN HISTORICAL OVERVIEW

Lowell M. Greenbaum
Department of Pharmacology, Medical College of Georgia
Augusta, Georgia 30912

It is well known that bradykinin liberation of trypsin from mammalian plasmas reflects the levels of high (HMW) and low molecular weight (LMW) kininogens of the plasma. Consequently the addition of trypsin to plasma is classically used to measure the total kininogen content of plasma of all species[1,2] by measuring the liberation of kinin. Kinin is generally measured by bioassay or by radioimmunoassay. It is important to understand that until 1983, when our laboratory on HPLC separation of kinins,[3] investigators could not differentiate clearly between bradykinin and its analogs by the bioassay or radioimmunoassay techniques. Many assumptions were made particularly in terms that HMW and LMW kininogens were the important proteins liberating kinins in all species. One piece of evidence that seemed to indicate that a third kininogen other than LMW or HMW was present in some fluids was the isolation of leukokininogen from human ascites fluid by Roffman and Greenbaum.[4] Leukokininogen was a poor substrate for kallikreins but did liberate a kinin (termed leukokinin by our laboratory) by either cathepsin D or trypsin. Hiroshi Okamoto joined our laboratory in 1982 and began a study on the relative concentration of leukokininogen compared to HMW and LMW kininogens in human, rabbit and rat plasmas. In order to obtain the total kininogen content, the classic concentration of 0.1 mg trypsin added to 1 ml of plasma was initially used. It was noted, however, that when rat plasma was treated with additional amounts of trypsin (up to 1.5 mg) there was a continuous and unexpected increase in released "kinin" especially from rat plasma.[5] The increase was almost 7 times the levels of total kininogen previously reported from rat plasma. As seen in Table 1, HMW kininogen (substrate releasing kinin from plasma by plasma kallikrein activated by glass powder) makes up a very small amount of the total kininogen content of the rat, rabbit and human plasmas when total kininogen is measured by release of kinin using large quantities of trypsin. We were very surprised by these findings and checked and rechecked for possible errors or misinterpretations of the data, as well as for contaminants of our trypsin preparations. However, the experiments were extremely reproduceable.[5] It was then decided to characterize the kinin generated by the high trypsin additions by column chromatography and by our new HPLC technique for separation of kinins. From these experiments, it was clear that a good part of the kinin generated was different from all known kinins and in January of 1983, we introduced the term "T-kinin" in the literature, to differentiate the kinin from bradykinin, Lys-bradykinin, and Met-lys-bradykinin, each of which was clearly differentiated from this new kinin by HPLC.[5] It followed

Table 1. Plasma Kininogen Levels in Normal Rats

Total[a]	T-kininogen[b] (ug kinin equiv./ml)	HMW+LMW-kininogen[c]	HMW-kininogen[d]
7.9±2.7 (100%)	5.7±1.0 (72%)	2.1±0.3 (27%)	1.1±0.1 (14%)

[a] Kinin liberated by trypsin.
[b] T-kinin liberated by trypsin.
[c] Bradykinin liberated by trypsin.
[d] Kinin liberated by glass powder.

Values are means ± S.D. of 5 rats.

then, that T-kinin must come from a substrate, "T-kininogen", rather than the well known HMW and LMW kininogens. Cathepsin D, an acid protease also released T-kinin from plasmas in a parallel manner as did trypsin[5] and thus we suspected that the third kininogen that we claimed existed and which we called leukokininogen in 1967[6] and was purified in 1979[4] was in probability T-kininogen. The confirmation that T-kinin generated by trypsin was in fact different than all known bradykinin analogs was published in 1983 following its isolation by Okamoto and Greenbaum[7] by procedures which included CM-cellulose, Biogel P-4 and reverse phase high-performance liquid chromatography. The final pure material which had a single N-terminal isoleucine was shown by amino acid analysis and sequence determination to have the structure of the undecapeptide ILE-SER-ARG-PRO-PRO-GLY-PHE-SER-PRO-PHE-ARG.[7] It is of interest that Bedi et al.[8] published the amino acid analysis of a "new peptide" isolated from acid protease treated rat plasma at the same time although no sequence had been determined. The discovery of T-kinin by our laboratory has several important meanings. First, it clearly demonstrated that HPLC technology makes possible the specific identification of kinins far beyond bioassay or radioimmunoassay ever could do. It is no longer satisfactory to assume that the kinin liberated by an inflammatory re-action is bradykinin or its classic analogs. A second meaning of the isolation of T-kinin and more recently T-kininogen[9] is that the "T-kinin – T-kininogen" system is a major system which may occupy an extremely important role in the inflammatory response.[10] The species which we have demonstrated to carry this system in blood and inflammatory fluids is the rat. Okamoto et al.[9] was first to show that two T-kininogens exist in rat plasma. Nakanishi has isolated the genes from rat liver for both these kininogens confirming this finding.[10] A major finding of the role of T-kininogen in inflammation has recently been discovered by Barlas et al.[11,12] who showed that T-kininogen dramatically increases 20 fold in plasma of Freund's adjuvant treated rats. This is in contrast to HMW and LMW kininogens which showed little or no change. In addition, the increase in T-kininogen paralleled the inflammatory condition of paw swelling. The anti-inflammatory agents indomethacin and dexamethasone, which reduced paw swelling, also reduced plasma T-kininogen levels in a parallel fashion. The dramatic increase in plasma T-kininogen in an inflammatory disease resembles, as discussed by Eisen,[13] an acute phase protein. This has been confirmed by Schreiber et al.[14] who isolated from rat the major ⍺-1 acute phase protein (MAP) whose sequence contains T-kinin. Thus T-kininogen and MAP of the rat appear to be one and the same. In addition to being an acute phase protein, Okamoto et al.[15] has shown that T-kininogen is a cysteine protease inhibitor; that it is an inhibitor of cathepsin B and papain. This confirms the work of Katunuma et al.[16] who showed that kininogens have properties of inhibiting certain thiol pro-teases. MAP was also shown to be a thiol protease inhibitor.[17] Muller Esterl showed that human plasma kininogens also are ⍺-cysteine pro-teinase inhibitors.[18]

T-kinin has been shown by our laboratory to have similar pharma-cological properties and potency as does bradykinin in that it contracts smooth muscle and lowers blood pressure.[19] The release of T-kinin from T-kininogen does not proceed by the action of kallikreins since T-kininogen unlike HMW and LMW-kininogen is resistant to kallikreins. A major question is whether T-kinin itself is released in inflammation. The question has been answered by the recent report from our laboratory that free T-kinin as well as bradykinin has now been shown to be present in plasma and fluids of rats injected with carageenin into a dorsal air pouch.[20] T-kinin is released by a neutral protease which is not kalli-krein. This exciting finding completes the concept that in some species such as the rat, that T-kinin - T-kininogen system is the major kinin releasing system. It also means that a specific T-kininogenase exists in bloos and on inflammatory fluids of the rat.

The variety of involvement of T-kininogen in the rat and perhaps in other species as far as inflammation is concerned is summarized in Figure 1.

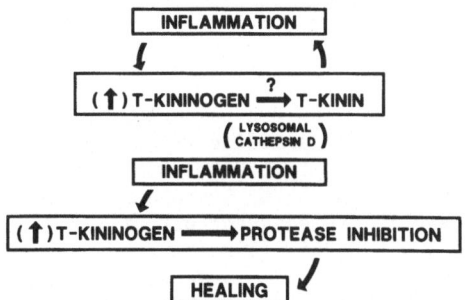

Figure 1. An inflammatory response in the rat results in the liver immediately synthesizing the major acute phase-protein T-kininogen. A neutral T-kininogenase catalyzes the release of T-kinin which produces the inflammatory response and causes the release of other mediators such as prostaglandins. T-kininogen also inhibits cysteine protease action (cathepsins) which could aid in the healing process.

In summary, T-kininogen is a unique protein that is rapidly synthesized in the liver in response to inflammation. It has three major properties:

1. An acute phase protein in the rat (MAP).
2. Thiol protease inhibitor.
3. The substrate from which T-kinin is released.

The speed of synthesis and the very large quantities seen in blood and liver indicates that it is a favored protein responding to signals for injury and inflammation. Its role in the rat must be considered of great significance. Its role in other species and in systems such as the CNS in the rat await clarification.

REFERENCES

1. C. B. Diniz, and I. F. Carvalho, A micromethod for determination of bradykinin under several conditions, Ann. N.Y. Acad. Sci., 104: 77-89, (1963).
2. Y. Uchida, and M. Katori, Differential assay method for high molecular weight and low molecular weight kininogens, Biochem. Pharmacol., 27:1463-1470, (1978).
3. T. K. Narayanan, and L. M. Greenbaum, Detection and quantitation of fluorescamine labeled bradykinin, its analogues and metabolites using high-performance liquid chromatography, J. Chromatogr., 306: 109-116, (1984).
4. S. Roffman, and L. M. Greenbaum, Properties of leukokininogen isolated from human neoplastic ascites, Biochem. Pharmacol., 28: 1043-1050, (1979).
5. H. Okamoto, and L. M. Greenbaum, Kininogen substrates for trypsin and cathepsin D in human, rabbit and rat plasma, Life Sci., 32:2007-2013, (1983).
6. L. M. Greenbaum, and K. S. Kim, The kinin-forming and kininase activities of rabbit polymorphonuclear leucocytes, Br. J. Pharm. and Chem., 29:238-247, (1967).
7. H. Okamoto, and L. M. Greenbaum, Isolation and structure of T-kinin, Biochem. Biophys. Res. Commun., 112:701-708, (1983).
8. G. S. Bedi, J. Balwierczak, and N. Back, A new vasopeptide formed by the action of a Murphy-Sturm lymphosarcoma acid protease on rat plasma kininogen, Biochem. Biophys. Res. Commun., 112:621-628, (1983).
9. H. Okamoto, and L. M. Greenbaum, Purification of the rat plasma T-kininogen, (This volume).
10. R. Kageyama, N. Kitamura, H. Okhuba, and S. Nakanishi, Primary structures of the mRNAs encoding the rat precurosrs for bradykinin and T-kinin, J. Biol. Chem., 260:12054-12059, (1985).
11. A. Barlas, H. Okamoto, and L. M. Greenbaum, T-kininogen - the major plasma kininogen in rat adjuvant arthritis, Biochem. Biophy. Res. Commun., 129:280-286, (1985).
12. A. Barlas, H. Okamoto, and L. M. Greenbaum, Increased plasma level of T-kininogen in rats treated with Freund's adjuvant, (This volume).
13. V. Eisen, New aspects of kinin formation, Trends in Pharm. Sciences, 69:190-191, (1985).

14. T. Cole, A. S. Inglis, C. M. Roxburgh, G. J. Howlett, and G. Schreiber, Major acute phase α_1-protein of the rat is homologous to bovine kininogen and contains the sequence for bradykinin: Its synthesis is regulated at the mRNA level, FEBS Lett., 182:57-61, (1985).

15. N. Itoh, F. Wakamori, H. Okamoto, and L. M. Greenbaum, T-kininogen as an acute phase reactant identical with thiol inhibitor in rat plasma, (This volume).

16. T. Sueyoshi, K. Enyoji, T. Shimada, H. Kato, S. Iwanaga, Y. Bando, E. Kominami, and N. Katunuma, A new function of kininogen as thiol-proteinase inhibitors: Inhibition of papain and cathepsins B,H and L by bovine, rat and human plasma kininogens, FEBS Lett., 182:193-195, (1985).

17. F. Esnard, and F. Gauthier, An acute phase reactant identical with α_1-acute phase globulin, J. B. Chem., 258:12443-12447, (1983).

18. W. Muller-Esterl, H. Fritz, W. Machleidt, A. Ritonja, J. Brzin, M. Kotnik, V. Turk, J. Kellarmann, and F. Lottspeich, Human plasma kininogens are identical with α_1-cystein proteinase inhibitors, FEBS Lett., 182:310-314, (1985).[1]

19. H. Okamoto, and L. M. Greenbaum, Pharmacological properties of T-kinin (Isoleucyl-Seryl-Bradykinin) from rat plasma, Biochem. Pharmacol., 32:2637-2638, (1983).

20. A. Barlas, K. Sugio, and L. M. Greenbaum, Release of T-kinin and bradykinin in carrageenin induced inflammation in the rat, FEBS Lett., 190:268-270, (1980).

INCREASED PLASMA LEVEL OF T-KININOGEN IN RATS TREATED WITH FREUND'S ADJUVANT

A. Barlas, H. Okamoto and L. M. Greenbaum

Department of Pharmacology and Toxicology
Medical College of Georgia
Augusta, GA 30912

SUMMARY

Studies have been carried out to clarify which component of plasma kininogen in rats increased in the inflammatory condition induced by an injection of Freund's complete adjuvant. Plasma T-kininogen, which was measured by assaying the amount of T-kinin liberated by trypsin treatment, remarkably increased in parallel with the severity of paw swelling following the intradermal injection of adjuvant into the rat hindpaw. Treatment with indomethacin or dexamethasone following an injection of adjuvant suppressed the increase in T-kininogen level as well as the development of paw swelling in rats. These results indicate that T-kininogen, the newly found precursor of T-kinin, is the main component of plasma kininogen which responds to the inflammatory stimulus in adjuvant arthritis.

INTRODUCTION

T-kinin (isoleucyl-seryl-bradykinin) was recently isolated from trypsin-treated rat plasma,[1,2] and the aminoacid sequence[3] and its pharmacological properties defined.[4]

T-kininogen has been discovered by our laboratory to be a major component of normal rat plasma kininogen making up some 70% of the total kininogen content.[5,6] The remainder is in the form of high molecular weight (HMW) and low molecular weight (LMW) kininogen. T-kininogen releases T-kinin when incubated with trypsin or cathepsin D,[2,3] while HMW- and LMW-kininogen release bradykinin when incubated with trypsin or kallikreins. HMW- and/or LMW-kininogens do not contain the Ile-Ser residues at the amino terminal position of bradykinin but contain a lysyl residue at this position. It has been reported in a variety of studies that experimentally-induced inflammation in the rat causes an elevation of plasma kininogen.[7-10] However, information is not known as to which of the kininogens is increased. In the current report, rats were subjected to an injection of complete Freund's adjuvant causing an inflammatory response and the kininogen profile of the plasma compared with that of control animals. Kininogen levels were also measured following the use of anti-inflammatory agents.

MATERIALS AND METHODS

Animals and Treatments

Male Sprague-Dawley rats, 6 weeks old, weighing 160-180 g, were used in all experiments. Freund's complete adjuvant was prepared buy suspending Mycobacterium in incomplete adjuvant (paraffin oil) at the concentration of 10 mg/ml and was intradermally injected into the rat left hind-paw (volume of 0.1 ml). Swelling of the injected paw was measured with a micrometer across a sagittal section as described by Newbould.[11] Five rats from each group were sacrificed to collect blood at days 1, 7, 14, 21, 28 and 42. To evaluate the effects of indomethacin (1.0 mg/kg) and dexamethasone (0.25 mg/kg), drugs were subcutaneously injected 30 min prior to the injection of adjuvant and thereafter at 24 hr intervals. As the control, normal rats received the same dosage of indomethacin or dexamethasone for the same period. Four rats of each group were sacrificed to collect the blood at day 3.

Collection of Plasma

Blood was collected from the abdominal aorta as described previously and centrifuged at 800 x g for 15 min at room temperature. Plasma was transferred to a plastic tube and kept at -70°C until used.

Assay of Plasma Kininogen Levels

Plasma kininogen levels were determined by assaying the total amount of kinin (Total kininogen), bradykinin (HMW kininogen plus LMW kininogen) and T-kinin (T-kininogen) released by treatment with an excess amount of trypsin as described previously.[2,3] Briefly, 100 μl of plasma was mixed with 900 μl of 0.03 N HCl and incubated for 15 min at 37°C to inactivate plasma kininases and aminopeptidases. Following the addition of 25 μl of 1 N NaOH, the sample was incubated with 250 μl of trypsin solution (5 mg/ml in 0.2 M Tris-HCl, pH 7.8) for 1 hr at 37°C. The reaction was terminated by heating in a boiling water bath for 10 min. Twenty μl of this sample was subjected to the RIA to determine the total amount of kinin (total kininogen). The remaining sample was mixed with an equal volume of 30% trifluoroacetic acid (TFA) following the centrifugation at 2,000 x g for 10 min. The supernatant was applied to an octadecyl-extraction column (1 x 2 cm), previously primed with 5 ml of methanol and 5 ml of 1% TFA. After washing the column with 1% TFA, kinins were eluted with 3 ml of 50% acetonitrile in 1% TFA. The eluate was evaporated and dissolved in 0.5 ml of distilled water. Kinins in the extract were separated by a reverse-phase HPLC as described previously.[12] Each fraction corresponding to bradykinin and T-kinin was evaporated followed by kinin immunoassay. HMW-plus LMW-kininogen level and T-kininogen level were calcualted as follows:

$$\text{Total amt of kinin} \times \frac{\text{Amt of kinin in bradykinin fraction}}{\text{Total amt of kinin eluted}} = \text{HMW \& LMW KGN}$$

$$\text{Total amt of kinin} \times \frac{\text{Amt of kinin in the T-kinin fraction}}{\text{Total amt of kinin eluted}} = \text{T-KGN}$$

HMW kininogen levels were determined separately by incubating the plasma with glass powder at pH 8.0 in the presence of o-phenanthroline, a kininase inhibitor.

62

Radioimmunoassay of Kinin

Kinins were assayed by RIA using an antiserum of rabbit for bradykinin-bovine serum albumin conjugate and ^{125}I-[Tyr^1]-kallidin according to the procedure described by Scicli et al.[13] Bradykinin and T-kinin exhibited an identical dose-response curve by weight in nanograms.

Assay of Plasma Protein

Protein was assayed by the method of Lowry et al.[14]

Materials

The following materials were obtained from commercial sources: trypsin (type XII, TPCK-treated from bovine pancreas, Sigma Corp.); Freund's incomplete adjuvant, Mycobacterium tuberculosis (Difco); bradykinin, [Tyr^1]-kallidin (Peninsula Corp); Na ^{125}I (carrier free, New England Nuclear); Octadecyl-extraction column, (J. T. Baker). T-kinin (Ile-Ser-bradykinin) was synthesized and supplied by courtesy of Dr. J. M. Stewart (Department of Biochemistry, University of Colorado Health Science Center).

RESULTS

Plasma total kininogen levels in complete adjuvant treated and control groups (incomplete-treated) increased within 24 hours after the injections (primary reaction) (Table 1). Total kininogen levels in the control group returned to normal after 14 days, while in the complete adjuvant-treated group, high levels of total kininogen were observed throughout the experimental period of 42 days. As also seen in Table 1, the increase in total kininogen is solely due to the increase in T-kininogen. HMW + LMW kininogen showed little change under these conditions.

A positive correlation was observed between the swelling of the injected paws and plasma T-kininogen levels in this experiment. Plasma protein concentration increased only 24 hours after the adjuvant injection, but not nearly to the extent of the kininogen increase. HMW-kininogen also increased, but it corresponded to merely less than 5% of the elevated kininogen (Table 2).

In order to determine if there is a relationship between the inflammation and plasma T-kininogen levels, two typical anti-inflammatory drugs, i.e., indomethacin and dexamethasone were administered to rats following the injection of adjuvant. As shown in Table 3, indomethacin and dexamethasone suppressed the development of paw swelling by 33 and 56%, respectively at day 3. Elevations of plasma T-kininogen levels were also suppressed by treatment with these drugs to a similar extent as the paw swelling. The administration of these drugs alone to normal rats did not change plasma kininogen levels.

DISCUSSION

Several investigators have measured kininogen levels as an indicator of the involvement of the kallikrein-kinin system in pathological states. In earlier reports, a number of investigators reported that injury or inflammation, such as caused by laparatomy, nephrectomy and an injection of acetic or croton oil, caused an elevation of serum kininogen level in rats.[7-10] However, it has never been clarified which component of plasma kininogen was actually altered. Our present studies confirmed that T-kininogen is a main component of plasma kininogen responded to the inflammatory

Table 1. Increases in Paw Thickness and Plasma T-Kininogen Levels of Rats Treated with Complete and Incomplete Freund's Adjuvant

Days after injection	KININOGENS LEVELS (μg kinin/ml)						PAW THICKNESS % INCREASE	
	TOTAL		HMW + LMW		T-KGN			
	Adj	Control	Adj	Control	Adj	Control	Adj	Control
0 (Normal)	6.03	6.03	1.21	1.21	4.82	4.82	0	0
1	31.67	26.33	1.46	1.35	30.21	24.98	46	39
7	119.60	19.42	2.99	1.39	116.61	16.43	80	21
14	57.08	11.03	2.74	1.31	54.34	9.72	56	15
21	59.17	9.87	2.48	1.40	56.69	8.47	61	17
28	28.97	9.43	1.42	1.35	27.55	8.08	53	16
42	30.03	8.98	2.87	1.47	27.16	7.11	54	12

Total kininogen, HMW + LMW kininogen and T-kininogen are indicated for the mean values of 5 rats at each day. Each value in paw thickness represents the mean of measurements in 5 rats converted to percent increase over the day zero.

Table 2. Plasma Protein Concentration and HMW-Kininogen Levels of Rats After the Injection of Freund's Complete Adjuvant

Days After Injection	Plasma Protein (mg/ml)	HMW-Kininogen (μg kinin equiv./ml)
0 (Normal)	52.9 ± 6.3	1.07 ± 0.08
1	65.8 ± 3.1	1.00 ± 0.14
7	59.4 ± 3.9	2.19 ± 0.36
14	58.7 ± 3.3	1.55 ± 0.29
21	53.7 ± 2.9	1.44 ± 0.13
28	52.8 ± 3.8	1.32 ± 0.17
42	49.2 ± 3.1	1.58 ± 0.14

HMW-kininogen levels are represented by the amount of kinin released with glass powder.

Table 3. Reduction of Plasma Kininogen Levels by Indomethacin and Dexamethasone of Rats Treated with Freund's Complete Adjuvant

	Kininogen Levels (µg kinin/ml)			% Inhibition of Paw Swelling	% Reduction of T-KGN Levels
	Total	HMW + LMW	T-KGN		
Normal	6.0 ± 1.2	1.21 ± 0.20	4.8 ± 1.0	–	–
Adjuvant	54.8 ± 6.8	1.41 ± 0.19	53.4 ± 6.9	–	–
Treated					
+ Indomethacin	36.0 ± 4.9	1.62 ± 0.10	34.4 ± 4.8*	33	35
+ Dexamethasone	24.1 ± 2.6	1.21 ± 0.25	22.9 ± 2.5**	56	58
Indomethacin Alone	5.5 ± 0.2	1.48 ± 0.30	4.0 ± 0.5	–	–
Dexamethasone Alone	5.8 ± 0.9	1.67 ± 0.51	4.1 ± 0.8	–	–

Plasma kininogen levels are measured on day 3 following the injection of Freund's complete adjuvant.

Indomethacin (1 mg/kg) and Dexamethasone (0.25 mg/kg) were subcutaneously injected once a day beginning at day zero.

* $p < 0.05$ as compared to adjuvant-treated group.
** $p < 0.001$ as compared to adjuvant-treated group.

condition. Since the levels of plasma T-kininogen closely correlated with the severity of inflammation and were suppressible by the administration of antiinflammatory drugs, it seems likely that this unique kinin precursor would be expected to contribute in some way in the process of inflammation or in tissue repair.

Cole et al. have reported that the major acute phase protein (MAP) of the rat is T-kininogen since it contains the sequence for T-kinin.[15] Thus T-kininogen is the major acute phase protein of the rat. It is also known to inhibit thiol proteinase.

Overall T-kininogen is an important protein which may be involved in the regulation of the inflammatory response.[16]

REFERENCES

1. H. Okamoto and L. M. Greenbaum, T-kinin generated by trypsin from rat plasma, Fedn. Proc., 42:1020 (1983).
2. H. Okamoto and L. M. Greenbaum, Kininogen substrates for trypsin and cathepsin D in human, rabbit and rat plasma, Life Sci., 32:2007-2013 (1983).
3. H. Okamoto and L. M. Greenbaum, Isolation and structure of T-kinin, Biochem. Biophys. Res. Commun., 112:701-708 (1983).
4. H. Okamoto and L. M. Greenbaum, Pharmacological properties of T-kinin (Isoleucyl-Seryl-Bradykinin) from rat plasma, Biochem. Pharmacol., 32:2637-2638 (1983).
5. L. M. Greenbaum, T. K. Narayanan, and H. Okamoto, Estimation of T-kininogen in rat plasma, Fedn. Proc., 43:437 (1984).
6. H. Okamoto, L. M. Greenbaum, and A. Barlas, Increased plasma levels of T-kininogen in rats with adjuvant arthritis, Fedn. Proc., 43:2150 (1984).
7. H. P. Zach and E. Werle, Changes in kininogen content of serum and some organs during injury and inflammation in rats, in: "Advances in Exp. Med. and Biol.," N. Back and F. Sicuteri, eds., Plenum Press, New York, 21:371-379 (1972).
8. D. R. Borges and A. H. Gordon, Kininogen and kininogenase synthesis by the liver of normal and injured rats, J. Pharm. Pharmac., 28:44-48 (1976).
9. C. G. Van Arman and G. W. Nuss, Plasma bradykininogen levels in adjuvant arthritis and carrageenin inflammation, J. Path., 99:245-250 (1969).
10. M. L. Reis, J. G. Leme, and L. S. Sudo, Plasma "kininogen" levels in rats with adjuvant arthritis, in: "Recent Progress on Kinins (Agents and Actions Supplements, 9:368-377)," H. Fritz, G. Dietze, F. Fiedler, and G. L. Harberland, Eds., Birkhauser Verlag, Basel-Boston-Stuttgart (1982).
11. B. B. Newbould, Chemotherapy of arthritis induced in rats by mycobacterial adjuvant, Brit. J. Pharmacol., 21:127-136 (1963).
12. T. K. Narayanan and L. M. Greenbaum, Detection and quantitation of fluorescamine-labeled bradykinin, its analogues and metabolites using high-performance liquid chromatography, J. Chromatogr., 306:109-116 (1984).
13. A. G. Scicli, T. Mindroiu, G. Scicli, and O. A. Carretero, Blood kinins, their concentration in normal subjects and patients with congenital deficiency in plasma prekallikreins and kininogen, J. Lab. Clin. Med., 100:81-93 (1982).
14. O. H. Lowry, N. J. Rosebrough, A. L. Farr, and R. J. Randall, Protein measurement with the folin phenol reagent, J. Biol. Chem., 193:265-275 (1951).

15. T. Cole, A. S. Inglis, C. M. Roxburgh, G. J. Howlett, and G. Schreiber, Major acute phase α_1-protein of the rat is homologous to bovine kininogen and contains the sequence for bradykinin: Its synthesis is regulated at the mRNA level, FEBS Lett., 182:57-61 (1985).
16. L. M. Greenbaum, T-kinin and T-kininogen, an historical overview (This Volume).

ISOLATION AND PROPERTIES OF TWO RAT PLASMA T-KININOGENS

Hiroshi Okamoto and Lowell M. Greenbaum

Department of Pharmacology and Toxicology, Medical College
of Georgia, Augusta, Georgia 30912

ABSTRACT

Two species of T-kininogen which release T-kinin (Ile-Ser-bradykinin) have been purified from plasma of rats treated with Freund's complete adjuvant. The molecular weight was estimated to be 69,000 for either T-kininogen I and II by SDS-polyacrylamide gel electrophoresis. Trypsin released one mole of T-kinin from one mole of either T-kininogen, but glandular kallikrein, including rat urinary and rat submandibular gland kallikreins and human urinary kallikrein, did not release any kinin from T-kininogens. Cathepsin D, which was purified from rat liver, released T-kinin from T-kininogens at pH 4.0. These results indicate that rat plasma contains two types of T-kininogen which differ from high molecular weight and low molecular weight kininogens.

INTRODUCTION

Plasma of vertebrates have been revealed to contain at least two distinct kininogens designated high molecular weight (HMW) and low molecular weight (LMW) kininogens which considerably differ in molecular weight and subceptibility to various kininogenases. Our recent studies have shown that rat plasma releases T-kinin (isoleucyl-seryl-bradykinin) in addition to bradykinin by trypsin treatment.[1,2] Since T-kinin does not contain lysyl-bradykinin structure, we have postulated a presence of new kininogen, T-kininogen, in rat plasma. Further a recent finding of our laboratory demonstrated that the increase in plasma kininogen levels of rats with adjuvant arthritis is exclusively due to the increased levels of T-kininogen, suggesting the importance of this kinin-precursor in the inflammatory condition.[3]

This study describes the purification procedures and some properties of T-kininogen from rats with adjuvant arthritis.

MATERIALS AND METHODS

Collection of plasma

Freund's complete adjuvant (5 mg Mycobacteria suspended in 1 ml of incomplete adjuvant) was injected intradermally into the left paws of 15 male Sprague-Dawley rats at the volume of 0.05 ml. Twenty four hr after the treatment, the citrated plasma was collected as described previously.[1]

Assay of kininogen

Kininogen in plasma or samples of each purification step was determined by assaying the amount of kinin released by trypsin as described previously.[1] Kinin was assayed by radioimmunoassay using rabbit anti-bradykinin serum and $125I$-[Try^1]-kallidin[4] according to the procedure described by Scicli et al.[5] T-kinin exhibited an identical dose-displacement curve with bradykinin in this system.

Identification of kinin

Kinins were identified by the elution profiles of kinin immuno-reactivity on the reverse-phase HPLC[6] and on CM-cellulose chromatography.[1]

Miscellaneous methods

Protein was assayed by the method of Lowry et al.[7] with bovine serum albumin as the standard. Disc-gel electrophoresis was carried out in 7.5% polyacrylamide gel as described by Davis.[8] SDS-polyacrylamide gel electrophoresis was done by the method of Weber and Osborn[9] using 5% gel.

Enzymes

Trypsin (TPCK-treated) was purchased from Sigma. Rat urinary kallikrein was purified by ammonium sulfate precipitation, DEAD-cellulose, Sephacryl S-200 and aprotinin-agarose chromatography. Human urinary kallikrein was purified as described by Geiger and Fritz.[10] Cathepsin D was purified from the lysosomal fraction of rat liver as described by Takahashi and Tang.[11] Rat submandibular gland kallikrein was kindly supplied by Dr. J. Chao, Department of Pharmacology, Medical University of South Carolina, USA.

RESULTS

Purification of rat plasma T-kininogen

T-kininogen was purified from rat plasma collected 1 day after the treatment of Freund's complete adjuvant. The following steps in the purification as summarized in Table 1.

One hundred ml of plasma was fractionated with solid ammonium sulfate and the precipitate between 20 and 60% saturation was collected. The precipitate was dissolved in distilled water and dialyzed against 50 mM sodium acetate, pH 6.3. The dialyzate was applied to a column of CM-Sephadex C-50 (1.5 x 40 cm), previously equilibrated with the dialysis buffer, and the pass-through fractions were collected. The pooled fraction was dialyzed against 20 mM Tris-HCl, pH 8.0, containing

Table 1. Purification of T-kininogen from adjuvant-treated rat plasma

	Protein (mg)	Kininogen (μg TK equiv.)	Kininogen/protein (μg TK equiv./mg)	Yield (%)
1. Plasma (100 ml)	7,050	4,302	0.61	100
2. $(NH_4)_2SO_4$ ppt. (20-60%)	4,575	2,894	0.63	67
3. CM-Sephadex C-50	3,059	3,197	0.91	74
4. DEAE-Sephadex A-50				
Peak I	325	1,133	3.48	26
Peak II	742	841	1.13	20
Peak I				
5. Sephacryl S-200	92	660	7.2	15
6. Hydroxylapatite	51	640	12.6	15
7. 2nd-DEAE-Sephadex	36	530	14.8	12
8. 2nd-Sephacryl S-200	19	343	18.2	8
Peak II				
5. 2nd-DEAE-Sephadex	200	459	2.3	11
6. Sephacryl S-200	35	376	10.7	9
7. Hydroxylapatite	20	359	18.2	8

0.1 M NaCl and then applied to a column of DEAE-Sephadex A-50 (1.8 x 40 cm), previously equilibrated with the dialysis buffer. The adsorbed protein was eluted with a linear gradient of NaCl concentration in 20 mM Tris-HCl, pH 8.0, between 0.1 M and 0.3 M with a total volume of 400 ml. Kininogen was eluted with two peaks designated as T-kininogen I and II. Each fraction was pooled and further purified as following procedures.

T-kininogen I fraction was dialyzed against distilled water followed by the lyophilization. The lyophilizate was dissolved in 20 mM Tris-HCl, pH 8.0, containing 0.1 M NaCl and applied to a column of Sephacryl S-200 (2.5 x 96 cm), previously equilibrated with the buffer. Kininogen was eluted with a single peak and the fractions were pooled and dialyzed against 10 mM sodium phosphate, pH 7.0. The dialyzate was applied to a column of hydroxylapatite (0.9 x 14 cm), previously equilibrated with the dialysis buffer. Kininogen was recovered in the non-adsorbed fractions. The fractions were pooled and rechromatographed on a column of DEAE-Sephadex A-50 with the same procedure was described above. The fractions containing kininogen were pooled and dialyzed against 20 mM Tris-HCl, pH 8.0, containing 0.1 M NaCl. The dialyzate was rechromatographed on Sephacryl S-200 column as described above. The final preparation of T-kininogen was stored at -60°C.

T-kininogen II fraction from the 1st DEAE-Sephadex A-50 column was rechromatographed on DEAE-Sephadex A-50 column followed by the chromatographies of Sephacryl S-200 and hydroxylapatite with the same procedures as described of T-kininogen I. T-kininogen II was also recovered in the non-adsorbed fractions of hydroxylapatite column. The fractions were pooled and stored at -60°C.

Homogeneity of T-kininogen preparations

The homogeneity of the resultant two kininogen preparations were assessed by gel electrophoresis. Disc-gel electrophoresis on 7.5% polyacrylamide gel revealed a single protein band for either T-kininogen I or II, but the mobilities were not identical. Each T-kininogen also showed a single band on SDS-polyacrylamide gel electrophoresis in the presence of mercaptoethanol, and the molecular weight was estimated as 69,000 for either T-kininogen.

Identification of kinin released from T-kininogen by trypsin

Kinin liberated from purified T-kininogen was identified by reverse-phase HPLC. In either kininogen, kinin immunoreactivity was eluted with a retention time corresponding to T-kinin and any immunoreactivity was not detected in the fraction corresponding to bradykinin. Therefore, the specific activity of purified T-kininogen I or II (18.2 µg T-kinin equivalent/mg protein) corresponds to 14.8 µmol T-kinin/mg T-kininogen. Based on the molecular weight of T-kininogen (69,000), one mg T-kininogen is calculated as 14.5 µmol which is in sufficient agreement with the specific activity of purified T-kininogen, indicating that one mol of T-kininogen I or II contains one mol of T-kinin.

Kinin liberation by various proteinases

Kinin liberation from purified T-kininogen was examined with glandular kallikreins and cathepsin D (Table 2). One µg of trypsin caused a complete liberation of T-kinin from 20 µg of T-kininogen I or II, but rat and human urinary kallikreins and rat submandibular gland kallikrein did not liberate any kinin from T-kininogen. Cathepsin D caused a complete liberation of kinin at the amount of 2 µg from T-kininogen at pH 4.0. The

Table 2. Kinin liberation from T-kininogen I and II by kinin-forming proteinases

Proteinase	T-kininogen	Kinin released (%)	Kinin*
Trypsin	I	100	T-kinin
(1 µg)	II	100	T-kinin
RUK[a]	I	1.1	Nd
(1 µg)	II	1.2	Nd
HUK[b]	I	0.8	Nd
(1 µg)	II	0.9	Nd
RSK[c]	I	4.5	Nd
(1 µg)	II	2.3	Nd
Cathepsin D	I	71.1	T-kinin
(1 µg)	II	70.0	T-kinin
(2 µg)	I	100	Nd
	II	100	Nd

T-kininogen (20 µg of I and II) were incubated in 0.1 M Tris-HCl, pH 8.0, with trypsin and kallikreins for 1 hr at 37°C. Cathepsin D was incubated with T-kininogen in 0.1 M citrate buffer, pH 4.0, for 1 hr at 37°C. 100% kinin liberation was equivalent to 0.29 nmol T-kinin.

[a] Rat urinary kallikrein

[b] Human urinary kallikrein

[c] Rat submandibular gland kallikrein

*Kinin was identified by HPLC and CM-cellulose chromatography.

Nd = not determined.

kinin liberation by cathepsin D was maximum at pH 4.5 in either kininogen, and the addition of pepstatin in the incubation mixture caused a complete inhibition of kinin liberation (data not shown). The kinin was identified as T-kinin by either method of HPLC or CM-cellulose chromatography.

DISCUSSION

Two species of T-kininogen was purified from adjuvant-treated rat plasma. Since both kininogens released only T-kinin by the action of trypsin and had a same molecular weight of 69,000 as judged by SDS-polyacrylamide gel electrophoresis, it is concluded that two species of T-kininogen with charge heterogeneity, which is probably due to a minor difference in the aminoacid composition, is present in rat plasma. In a separate experiment, two fractions releasing T-kinin by trypsin were also obtained from normal rat plasma by DEAE-Sephadex A-50 chromatography (data not shown), indicating that two T-kininogens are not specific for adjuvant-treated rats.

Rat plasma had been reported to contain two species of kininogens, i.e., HMW and LMW kininogens. Jacobsen showed the presence of two types of kininogen in rat plasma which differed in the susceptibility for kallikrein.[12] Bedi et al.[13] and Sakamoto et al.[14] have reported the purification of LMW kininogen with the molecular weight of 72,000 from rat plasma, and they described a low susceptibility of rat LMW kininogen for releasing kinin by glandular kallikreins. In the present study, we demonstrated that purified T-kininogen is entirely resistant to the action of glandular kallikreins, suggesting that T-kininogen is not LMW kininogen of rat. It may be concluded that rat plasma contains two species of T-kininogen and a LMW or related kininogen.

Cathepsin D released T-kinin from T-kininogen at the acidic pH. Lysosomal proteinases including cathepsin D have been implicated in the inflammatory process. Since plasma T-kininogen levels are closely correlated to the severity of inflammation,[3] a high concentration of T-kininogen seems tobe reached to the inflammed tissue and subsequently T-kinin will be released by the action of cathepsin D or other proteinases. T-kinin has been identified in plasma and inflammed fluids of the rat.[15]

ACKNOWLEDGEMENTS

Authors wish to thank Mrs. J. Jones for her technical assistance. This work was supported by NIH grant HL-32183.

REFERENCES

1. H. Okamoto, and L. M. Greenbaum, Kininogen substrate for trypsin and cathepsin D in human, rabbit and rat plasma, Life Sci., 32, 2007, (1983).
2. H. Okamoto, and L. M. Greenbaum, Isolation and structure of T-kinin, Biochem. Biophys. Res. Commun., 112, 701, (1983).
3. A. Barlas, H. Okamoto, and L. M. Greenbaum, T-kininogen - the major plasma kininogen in rat adjuvant arthritis, Biochem. Biophys. Res. Commun., 129, 280-286, (1985).
4. C. E. Odya, Y. L. Goodfriend, J. M. Stewart, and C. Pena, Aspects of bradykinin radioimmunoassay, J. Immunol. Methods, 19, 243, (1978).

5. A. G. Scicli, T. Mindroin, G. Scicli, and O. A. Carretero, Blood kinins, their concentration in normal subjects and in patients with congenital deficiency in plasma prekallikrein and kininogens, J. Lab. Clin. Med., 100, 81, (1982).

6. T. K. Narayanan, and L. M. Greenbaum, Detection and quantitation of fluorescamine-labeled bradykinin, its analogues and metabolites using high-performance liquid chromatography, J. Chromatogr., 306, 109, (1984).

7. O. H. Lowry, N. J. Rosenbrough, A. Farr, and R. J. Randall, Protein measurement with the Folin phenol reagent, J. Biol. Chem., 193, 265, (1951).

8. R. J. Davis, Disc electrophoresis - II. Method and application to human serum proteins, Ann. N.Y. Acad. Sci., 121, 404, (1964).

9. K. Weber, and M. Osborn, The reliability of molecular weight determination by dodecyl sulfate-polyacrylamide gel electrophoresis, J. Biol. Chem., 244, 4406, (1969).

10. T. Geiger, and H. Fritz, Human urinary kallikrein, Methods Enzymol., 80, 466, (1981).

11. T. Takahashi, and J. Tang, Cathepsin D from porcine and bovine spleen, Methods Enzymol., 80, 565, (1981).

12. S. Jacobsen, Substrates for plasma kinin-forming enzymes in rat and guinea pig plasma, Brit. J. Pharmacol., 28, 64, (1966).

13. G. S. Bedi, J. Balwierczak, and N. Back, Rodent kinin-forming enzyme system - I, Purification and characterization of plasma kininogen, Biochem. Pharmac., 32, 2061, (1983).

14. W. Sakamoto, K. Yoshikawa, S. Uehara, O. Nishikaze, and H. Honda, Purification and characterization of rat low molecular weight kininogen, J. Biochem., 96, 81, (1984).

15. A. Barlas, K. Sugio, and L. M. Greenbaum, Release of T-kinin and bradykinin in carrageenin induced inflammation in the rat, FEBS Lett., 190, 268-270, (1985).

CHARACTERIZATION OF KININOGEN DEFICIENCY OF BROWN NORWAY RAT MUTANT

KATHOLIEK STRAIN

Sachiko Oh-ishi[1], Izumi Hayashi[1], Takekazu Ino[1], Hisao Kato[2],
Sadaaki Iwanaga[2], and Takeshi Nakano[3]

[1]Department of Pharmacology, School of Pharmaceutical
Sciences, Kitasato University, Tokyo 108, [2]Department of
Biology, Faculty of Science, Kyushu University, Fukuoka 812
and [3]Department of Experimental Animal Sciences, School of
Medicine, Kitasato University, Sagamihara 228, Japan

SUMMARY

A deficiency in the plasma kallikrein-kinin system of Brown Norway
rat mutant Katholiek strain (B/N-Ka), first reported by Damas et al. was
further characterized. The prolonged activated partial thromboplastin
time (APTT) of B/N-Ka rat plasma was corrected by an addition of rat HMW-
kininogen, indicating B/N-Ka rat is deficient in HMW kininogen.

The study of kinin-release of plasmas of the three strains of rat
(B/N-Ka, B/N Ki and SD) by several kininogenases expressed that B/N-Ka rat
is deficient in LMW kininogen, in addition to HMW kininogen deficiency.

The plasmas of the three strains of rat were gel-filtered through
Sephacryl S-200 gel and profiles of kinin-release of the fractions were
examined by several kininogenases. The result demonstrated that normal
rat plasma contains three kinds of kininogen (HMW and LMW kininogens, and
T-kininogen), and B/N-Ka plasma contains only T-kininogen.

B/N-Ka rat plasma demonstrated T-kininogen antigen but no HMW kininogen by the study of immunodiffusion using their antisera raised in rabbits.

INTRODUCTION

A strain of rat, Brown Norway Mai pfd f (B/N) was originated at The
Wistar Institute, USA and has been kept at National Institutes of Health,
Bethesda. Recently, Marks et al. reported that Brown Norway rats kept
at NIH are normal in the plasma kallikgrein-kinin system.[1] The B/N rats
brought to Japan are also normal, in that the plasma releases a similar
amount of kinin to that of Sprague-Dawley rats (SD) by kaolin activation.
But B/N rat in Katholiek University, Belgium, was reported to be abnormal
in the kallikrein-kinin system.[2] We have confirmed the result of Damas et
al., and tentatively named the mutant strain in Katholiek University B/N
Katholiek and normal strain B/N Kitasoto, respectively.[3] Prolonged APTT
and characteristics of the plasma kallikrein-kinin system of B/N-Ka rat
have been previously reported.[3-5] In this paper, further characterization

of the deficiency of B/N-Ka rat will be described, in comparison with
normal strains of rat, such as B/N-Ki and SD, on the standpoint of the
kinin-release by various kininogenases, and the antigenic survey for
kininogens by using antisera raised in rabbits.

MATERIALS AND METHODS

Animals   Brown Norway Kitasato (B/N-Ki) and Brown Norway Katholiek (B/N-
Ka) rats were kept as previously described.[3]   Sprague-Dawley (SD) rats
(7-9 weeks old male and 5 weeks old female), and guinea pigs (male, 300-
400 g) were purchased from Shizuoka Experimental Animal Center (Hamamatsu).
Plasmas were prepared as previously reported.[3]

Gel chromatography   Four ml each of citrated plasma from three strains of
rats were loaded on a Sephacryl S-200 column and eluted as described previously.[5]

Kinin released by various kininogenases   Citrated rat plasma (0.1 ml) was
incubated at 37°C for 15 min after acidified with N-HCl (pH 2.0), and
neutralized with N-NaOH and the volume of the mixture was adjusted to 1 ml
with 0.02 M tris buffer, pH 8.0, containing 0.1M NaCl, 0.5 mg o-phenanthroline and 1 mg EDTA-2Na.   Then the mixture was incubated respectively
with the following enzymes: 25 µl partially purified rat plasma kallikrein
(A_{280}=0.82),[5] 100 µl partially purified rat urinary kallikrein (A_{280}=11.0),[5]
25 µl snake venom kininogenase (SVK, A_{280}=1.87)[5] or 2 mg trypsin (bovine,
Type XI, Sigma).   After incubation for 1 hr the mixture was mixed with
2.33 ml EtOH heated at 70°C and stored at 70°C for 10 min.   The supernatant was evaporated and the residue was dissolved in 20 mM sodium
phosphate buffer, pH 7.0, containing 0.15 M NaCl and 0.1% gelatin.

Bioassay of kinins   The kinin released was assayed by using rat uterus
as described previously[3] with synthetic bradykinin (Peptide Institute,
Osaka) as a standard.   The kinin fraction collected from HPLC of the extract of the incubation mixture of B/N-Ka rat plasma with trypsin, was
also assayed on guinea pig ileum suspended in Tyrode's solution.   The contracting activity of the kinin extracted was compared with those of synthetic bradykinin, lysylbradykinin (Lys-bradykinin, Peptide Institute,
Osaka) and isoleucylseryl-bradykinin (Ile-Ser-bradykinin, a gift from
Dr. S. Sakakibara, Peptide Institute, Osaka).

Immunization and production of antisera   Rat HMW kininogen and its light
chain were prepared as reported previously.[6]   Rat LMW kininogen and
T-kininogen were purified as described previously.[7]   Each antiserum was
raised in rabbits (male 2-3 kg, Japanese white rabbit) for 7-11 weeks.[8]
Immunodiffusion was undertaken in 1.5% agarose gel in 0.05 M barbiturate
buffer, pH 8.2, at room temperature overnight.

RESULTS

The kinin release of plasmas of the three strains of rat, B/N-Ki, SD
and B/N Ka, were examined as shown in Figure 1. Plasmas of SD and B/N-Ki
rats released similar amount of kinin by rat plasma kallikrein, but B/N-
Ka rat plasma did not release significant amount. Plasmas of SD and B/N-
Ki rats released similar amount of kinin by urinary kallikrein and SVK
and it was larger than those by plasma kallikrein. B/N-Ka rat plasma
did not release significant amount of kinin by these enzymes, suggesting
also the deficiency of LMW kininogen. Trypsin released larger and variable
amount of kinin from plasmas of all the three strains of rat.

Then, the plasmas of the three strains of rat were examined by gel
filtration. Figure 2 shows the pattern of B/N-Ki rat plasma on a Sephacryl

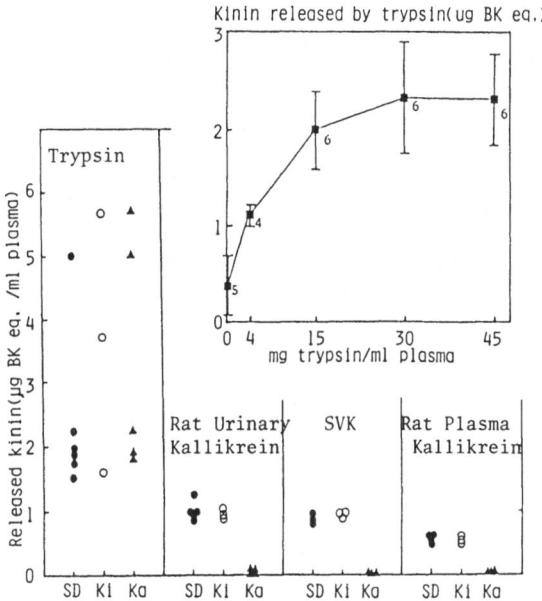

Figure 1. Kinin release of SD, B/N-Ki and B/N-Ka rat plasmas by
several kininogenases. The amount of kinin was assayed on rat
uterus and expressed as bradykinin equivalent in ml plasma.
Plasma was pretreated as acidification and conditions for incubation and sample preparation were described in the text.

S-200 column chromatography. The plasma of SD rat was eluted in a similar
pattern as B/N-Ki rat.[5] In the chromatogram of B/N-Ki, HMW kininogen was
eluted at the fractions of prekallikrein activity, and in these fractions
almost similar amount of kinin was released by plasma kallikrein, urinary
kallikrein, SVK and trypsin. The second peak of kininogen was found in
the lower molecular weight fraction where the clotting activity of
Factor XII was eluted. (Figure 2). From this fraction urinary kallikrein
and SVK released almost the same amount of kinin, but plasma kallikrein
did not release kinin from the fraction. Trypsin released larger amount
of kinin in these fractions, especially lower molecular weight fractions,
where urinary kallikrein or SVK did not release kinin, as shown in Figure
2.

In the chromatogram of B/N-Ka plasma there was no correcting activity
of HMW kininogen deficient plasma, and prekallikrein was eluted at the
fraction of Factor XII, as shown in Figure 3. In this figure there was no
significant kinin release by urinary kallikrein and SVK, but at the
corresponding fractions of kinin released by trypsin in B/N-Ki plasma,
there was large amount of the kinin activity by trypsin in B/N-Ka plasma.

These results suggest that there are three kininogens in normal rat
plasma and in B/N-Ka plasma there is a kininogen which released kinin only
by trypsin.

The kinin activity found in the above fractions of B/N-Ka plasma was
further examined as follows. The pooled fraction was incubated with
trypsin as described in the method section and the kinin was extracted as
shown in the inlet of Figure 4 and applied to HPLC. As shown in Figure 4,
retention time of the kinin was nearly the same as that of synthetic Ile-

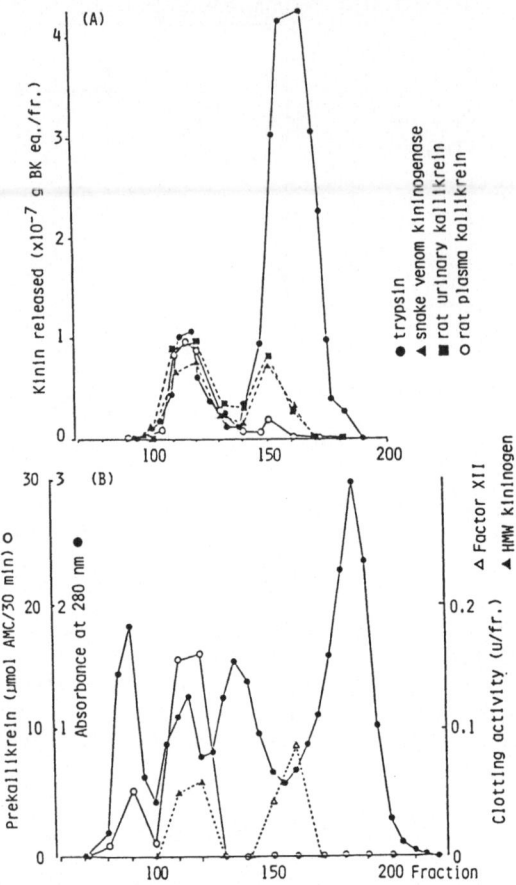

Figure 2. Gel filtration pattern of B/N-Ki plasma.
B/N-Ki plasma, 4 ml was allowed to a Sephacryl S-200 column
chromatography. Elution was performed with 0.02 M Tris-HCl
buffer, pH 8.0 containing 0.2 M NaCl, EDTA-2Na and polybrene,
and 1.2 ml fractions were collected. Details are seen in the
reference.[5]

Ser-bradykinin, so-called T-kinin, reported by Okamoto et al.[10] The
fractions from HPLC were assayed on rat uterus, and only this fraction
had a biological activity. The fraction was further examined on guinea
pig ileum for contracting activity, in comparison with synthetic bradykinin, Lys-bradykinin and Ile-Ser-bradykinin. The result indicates that
the kinin released could be Ile-Ser-bradykinin, as shown in Table I.

Table I. Contracting activities of the kinin released from B/N-Ka
plasma in comparison with synthetic kinins on rat uterus and guinea pig
ileum. (Bradykinin = 1)

	Rat uterus	Guinea pig ileum
Bradykinin	1.0	1.0
Lys-bradykinin	0.5	0.3
Ile-Ser-bradykinin	1.0	0.3
kinin fraction	1.0	0.3

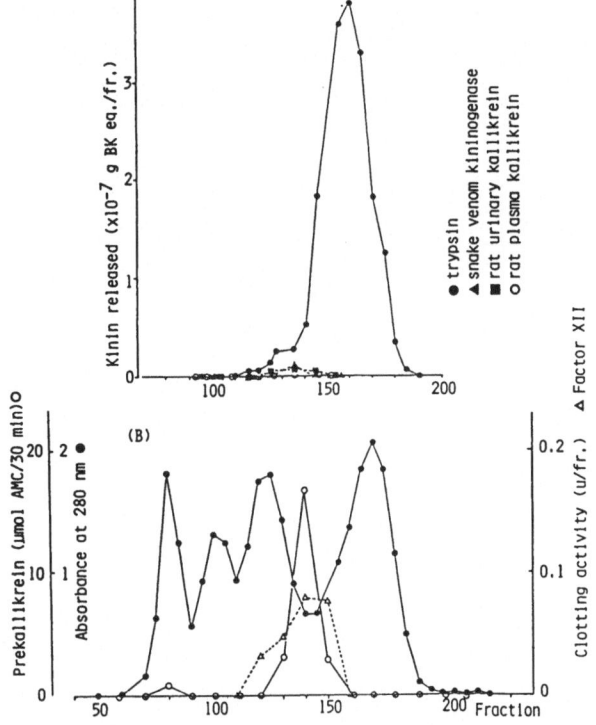

Figure 3. Gel filtration pattern of B/N-Ka rat plasma.
Conditions are the same as those for Figure 2.[5]

Antisera were raised in rabbits immunized with purified kininogens
from SD rat plasma.[6-7] Immunodiffusion was carried out as shown in Figure
5. With anti HMW kininogen-L-chain serum, which was monospecific to HMW
kininogen,[7] B/N-Ki and SD rat plasmas showed precipitation lines fused
each other, but B/N-Ka rat plasma showed no line (Figure 5(A). With anti
T-kininogen antiserum, all the three plasmas showed precipitation lines
fused each other (Figure 5 (B). Furthermore B/N-Ka plasma showed fused
line with that of purified rat T-kininogen (C). The result clearly indicates that B/N-Ka rat plasma is deficient in HMW kininogen antigen, but
contains T-kininogen antigen.

DISCUSSION

Functional deficiency of HMW kininogen in B/N-Ka rat plasma was
demonstrated as follows: (A) B/N-Ka plasma showed prolonged APTT and it
was not corrected by mixing with Fitzgerald plasma.[4] (B) Kinin-release
by kaolin activation of the plasma was as low as the limit of the bioassay.[3] (C) Kinin-release was also low when incubated with purified rat
plasma kallikrein. (D) There was no fraction containing correcting
activity of HMW kininogen deficient plasma among the fractions of
Sephacryl S-200 chromatography of B/N-Ka plasma, as shown in Figure 2.

In addition to HMW kininogen deficiency, functional deficiency of
LMW kininogen in B/N-Ka rat plasma was demonstrated as shown in Figure 1,
in that no kinin release by rat urinary kallikrein or SVK. In mammalian
plasma, such as human and bovine plasmas, as reviewed previously,[10] there
are two kininogens, one of which is HMW kininogen, a substrate for both

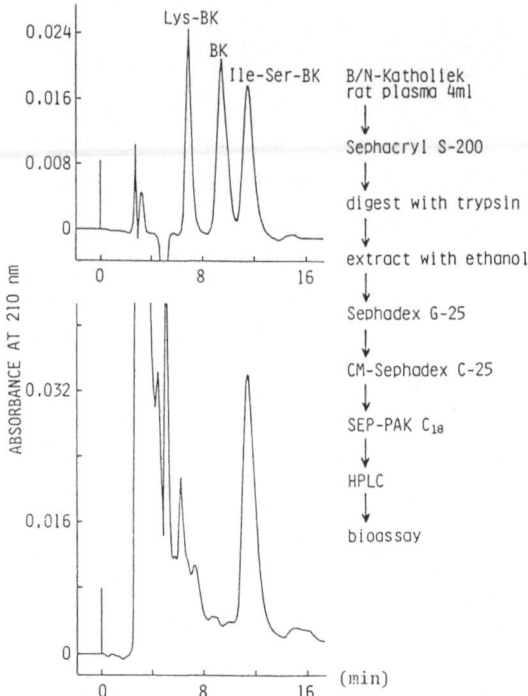

Figure 4.   HPLC pattern of the kinin released from B/N-Ka plasma by
trypsin. Kinin extraction procedure is illustrated on the
right side. ODS-Finepak Sil (46 x 250 mm) column with a guard
column (ERC-ODS, 6 x 30 mm) was eluted by a solvent, containing 20% CH_3CN, 0.01 M KH_2PO_4, 0.25 M Na_2SO_4, pH 2.7, at a
flow rate of 1 ml/min at 42°C and the eluate was monitored
at 210 nm (UVIDEC-100V).

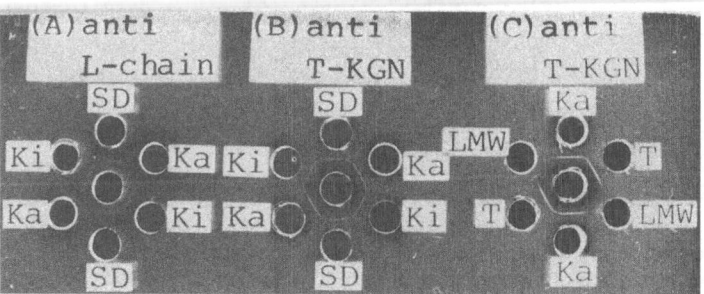

Figure 5.   Immunodiffusion of the plasmas of the three strains rats against
kininogen antisera.
Center wells contained 10 µl each antiserum to HMW kininogen
L-chain (A), and antiserum to T-kininogen (B) and (C). Surround-
ing wells contained 5 µl each plasma of SD rat (SD), B/N-Ka rat
(Ka), B/N-Ki rat (Ki), 2.4 µg LMW kininogen (LMW) and 2.2 µg
T-kininogen (T). Details are seen in the text.

plasma kallikrein and glandular kallikrein, and another is low molecular weight kininogen, a substrate for glandular kallikrein. In SD and B/N-Ki rats plasmas the amount of kinin released from LMW kininogen could be calculated by substraction of the amount of kinin released by plasma kallikrein from the kinin released by urinary kallikrein, since rat urinary kallikrein releases bradykinin from HWM kininogen and also LMW kininogen isolated from SD rat.[7]

The amount of kinin released by trypsin was larger than that released by urinary kallikrein or SVK in SD and B/N-Ki rat plasmas. The fact is uinque in rat plasma, and it is different feature from human and rabbit plasmas.[11] Even if large amount of trypsin was used, the amount of kinin released by trypsin was almost equal to that released by SVK in human or rabbit plasma. Bedi et al.[12] and Okamoto et al.[9] reported that rat plasma released Ile-Ser-bradykinin, T-kinin by acid protease or trypsin. In our gel-filtration study (Figure 2), there were fractions where the kinin activity was demonstrated only by trypsin in all the three strains of rat. Then it was proved that B/N-Ka rat plasma contained a precursor protein of T-kinin (Figure 4). In this report the assumption that rat plasma contains three kinds of kininogen was further confirmed, and furthermore, this was proved by the purification and the characterization of the three kininogens from SD rat plasma (H. Kato et al., in this book).

Antigenic survey for kininogens in rat plasma resulted in that B/N-Ka rat plasma contained only T-kininogen antigen and lacked HMW kininogen antigen. The result further supports that B/N-Ka-deficiency could be in HMW and LMW kininogens, but there is T-kininogen in the plasma.

ACKNOWLEDGEMENT

This work was partly supported by a Grant-in-Aid for Scientific Research (59480410) from the Ministry of Education, Science and Culture, Japan.

REFERENCES

1. E. Marks, B. Alving, and J. J. Pisano, The kallikrein-kinin system in the Brown Norway rat, Thrombosis Res. 31, 653-656, (1983).
2. J. Damas and A. Adam, Congenital deficiency in plasma kallikrein and kininogens in Brown Norway rat, Experientia, 36, 586-587, (1980).
3. S. Oh-Ishi, K. Satoh, I. Hayashi, K. Yamazaki, and T. Nakano, Differences in prekallikrein and high molecular weight kininogen levels in two strains of Brown Norway rat (Kitasato and Katholiek strain), Thrombosis Res. 28, 143-147, (1982).
4. S. Oh-Ishi, I. Hayashi, K. Satoh, and T. Nakano, Prolonged activated partial thromboplastin time and deficiency of high molecular weight kininogen in Brown Norway rat mutant (Katholiek strain), Thrombosis Res. 33, 371-377, (1984).
5. I. Hayashi, T. Ino, H. Kato, S. Iwanaga, T. Nakano, and S. Oh-Ishi, Demonstration of the third kininogen in high and low molecular weight kininogen-deficient Brown Norway rat, Thrombosis Res. 36, 509-516, (1984).
6. I. Hayashi, H. Kato, S. Iwanaga, and S. Oh-Ishi, Rat plasma HMW kininogen: A simple method for purification and its characterization, J. Biol. Chem. (in press).
7. K. Enjyoji, H. Kato, S. Iwanaga, I. Hayashi, and S. Oh-Ishi, Purification and characterization of two LMW kininogens from rat plasma, Seikagaku (in Japanese, Abstrc.), 56, 759, (1984).

8. I. Hayashi, T. Ino, H. Kato, S. Iwanaga, K. Yamazaki, K. Satoh, S. Oh-Ishi, and T. Nakano, Blood coagulation and plasma kinin system in HMW kininogen-deficient rat (B/N-Katholiek): Roles of rat HMW kininogen, Jap. J. Pharmacol. 36, Suppl., 75P, (1984) (Abstract).

9. H. Okamato and L. M. Greenbaum, Isolation and structure of T-kinin, Biophys. Biochem. Res. Commun., 112, 701-726, (1983).

10. E. Harbermann, Kininogens, in: Handbook of Experimental Pharmacology, eds. E. G. Erdos and A. F. Wilde, 25, pp. 250-228, Springer-Verlag, Berlin, (1970).

11. Y. Uchida and M. Katori, An improved method for determination of the total kininogen in rabbit and human plasma, Biochem. Pharmacol., 27, 1463-1470, (1978).

12. G. S. Bedi, J. Balwierczak, and N. Back, Purification and characterization of an acid protease and vasopeptide kinins from Murphy-strum lymphosarcoma, Adv. Exp. Med. Biol., 156B, 705-708, (1983).

AMINO ACID SEQUENCE OF THE LIGHT CHAIN OF HUMAN HIGH MOLECULAR MASS KININOGEN

Josef Kellermann, Friedrich Lottspeich, Agnes Henschen and
Werner Müller-Esterl

Max-Planck-Institut für Biochemie, D-8033 Martinsried and
Abteilung für Klinische Chemie und Biochemie der Universität
München, D-8000 München

SUMMARY

The light chain of human high molecular mass kininogen consists of 255
amino acid residues. The half-cystine residue which forms the single disulfide bridge to the heavy chain is located in position 225. The light
chain contains 9 O-glycosidically linked carbohydrate side chains. A comparison of the human high molecular mass kininogen light chain with the
bovine high molecular mass kininogen light chain reveals a pronounced
homology. However, in position 88 of the human sequence an insertion of
22 amino acid residues was found. This insertion and an amino acid exchange
in position 131 may explain the different behaviour of human and bovine high
molecular mass kininogen during plasma kallikrein digestion.

INTRODUCTION

Human high molecular mass kininogen is a single chain glycoprotein with
an apparent molecular mass of about 116 kDa as determined in SDS-gel electrophoresis. It is a plasmaprotein which plays an important role in the
contact phase activation of the intrinsic pathway of blood coagulation. By
the action of plasma kallikrein a vasoactive peptide kinin is liberated.
The remaining kinin-free molecule, which still exhibits clotting activity,
consists of two disulfide linked peptide chains, the heavy chain (M_r 62
kDa) and the light chain (M_r 58 kDa). It is in the light chain that the
clotting activity and the binding sites for plasma prekallikrein and/or
factor XI are located.

In the bovine high molecular mass kininogen an additional peptide,
the histidine-rich peptide, is liberated by the action of plasma-kallikrein
leading to the loss of clotting activity. In the case of bovine high
molecular mass kininogen the amino acid sequence of the light chain[1-4] and
the c-DNA sequence of the entire molecule[5] have been published.

RESULTS AND DISCUSSION

Human high molecular mass kininogen was isolated from human plasma and
cleaved with porcine pancreatic kallikrein, mercaptolysed and carboxymethy-

lated. The light chain was isolated from the cleavage mixture by ion exchange chromatography on CM-Sephadex C-50.[6] The light chain was pure by the criteria of amino acid analysis and SDS-gel electrophoresis. The amino acid analysis of the light chain of human high molecular mass kininogen is shown in Fig. 1. As in the bovine high molecular mass light chain a large amount of histidine, glycine and lysine was found. In the light chain only galactosamine could be detected. Therefore it was concluded that all the carbohydrate bound to the light chain was linked O-glycosidically.

The light chain was cleaved by a large number of reagents and enzymes, i.e. cyanogen bromide, hydroxylamine, trypsine, staphylococcal protease and thermolysine. The cleavage mixtures were fractionated by high-performance liquid chromatography using gel permeation and reversed phase columns, and the resulting fragments sequenced. In this way the complete amino acid sequence of the light chain of human high molecular mass kininogen could be established.[7] The complete sequence is shown in Fig. 2. The carbohydrate attachment sites were determined after deglycosilation of the peptides with anhydrous hydrogen fluoride. The half-cystine residue which forms the single disulfide bridge to the heavy chain was found in position 225.

Amino acid	a	b
Cys	0.4	1
Asp	27.9	28
Thr	16.2	19
Ser	17.3	21
Glu	31.6	31
Pro	14.0	20
Gly	29.5	29
Ala	7.4	7
Val	4.7	5
Met	3.6	4
Ile	9.7	10
Leu	11.9	12
Tyr	1.6	2
Phe	5.6	6
Lys	21.4	21
His	26.8	27
Arg	7.5	8
Trp	n.d.	4
Σ		255

Fig. 1. Amino acid analysis of human high molecular mass kininogen light chain. (a) uncorrected values, (b) values, found by amino acid sequence analysis.

A comparison between the human and the bovine high molecular mass kininogen is given in Fig. 3. It reveals a high degree of homology (62% identity). As in the bovine high molecular mass kininogen, the sequence at the
N-terminal half of the human light chain is rich in histidine, glycine and
lysine. Although this histidine-rich region, which is essential for clotting
activity, is released from the bovine molecule by the action of plasma kallikrein, no corresponding histidine-rich fragments are released from human
kininogen. A possible explanation for this may be the insertion of 22 amino
acid residues in position 88 of the human sequence. Furthermore, an amino
acid exchange where an arginine in the bovine light chain is replaced by a
lysine in the human light chain is found in position 131. At this position
plasma kallikrein cleaves the bovine high molecular mass kininogen light
chain, whereby the histidine-rich fragment is liberated and the clotting
activity is lost.

```
                                                    CHO
M K R P P G F S P F R K₁ S S R I G E I K E E T T V S P P H T(Q)M A P A Q

D E E R D S G K E Q G H T R R H D W G H E K Q R K H N L G H G H K H E R

D Q G H G H Q R G H G L G H G H E Q Q H G L G H G H K F K L D D D L E H

Q G G H VL D H G H K H K H G H G H G K H K N K G K K(N G K H N G W)K T E

                  CHO                    CHO        CHO                      CHO
H L A S S S E D S T(T P)S A Q T Q E K(T)E G P(T)P I P S L A K P G V(T)V

                  CHO          CHO                                    CHO
T F S D F Q D S D L I A(T)M M P P I S P A P I Q S D D D W I P D I Q T D

                                                      CHO
P N G L S F N P I S D F P D T T S P K C P G R P W K S V S E I N P T T Q

              255
M K E S Y Y F D L T D G L S
```

Fig. 2. Amino acid sequence of human high molecular mass kininogen light
         chain.

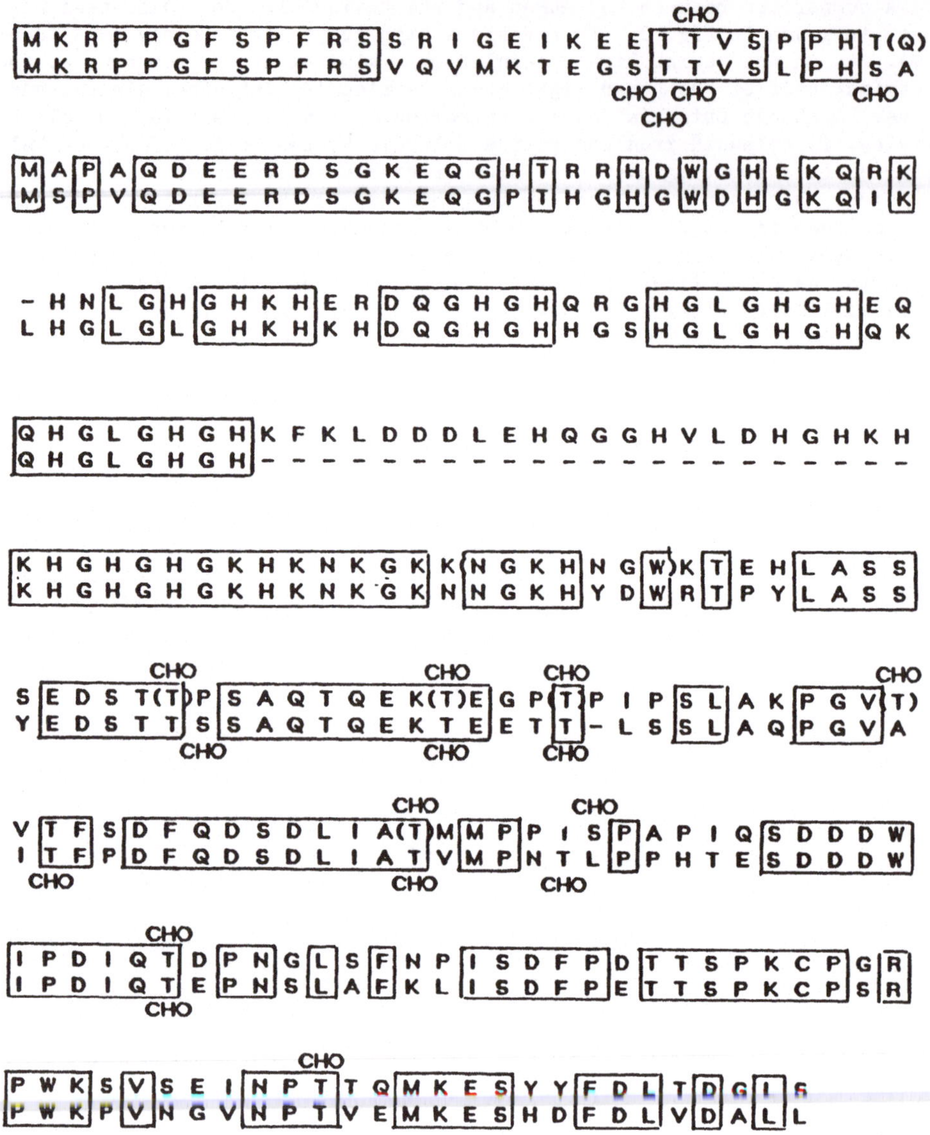

```
                                              CHO
M K R P P G F S P F R S S R I G E I K E E T T V S P P H T(Q)
M K R P P G F S P F R S V Q V M K T E G S T T V S L P H S A
                                    CHO CHO        CHO
                                        CHO

M A P A Q D E E R D S G K E Q G H T R R H D W G H E K Q R K
M S P V Q D E E R D S G K E Q G P T H G H G W D H G K Q I K

- H N L G H G H K H E R D Q G H G H Q R G H G L G H G H E Q
L H G L G L G H K H K H D Q G H G H H G S H G L G H G H Q K

Q H G L G H G H K F K L D D D L E H Q G G H V L D H G H K H
Q H G L G H G H - - - - - - - - - - - - - - - - - - - - -

K H G H G H G K H K N K G K K N G K H N G W K T E H L A S S
K H G H G H G K H K N K G K N N G K H Y D W R T P Y L A S S

        CHO                CHO        CHO                    CHO
S E D S T(T)P S A Q T Q E K(T)E G P T P I P S L A K P G V(T)
Y E D S T T S S A Q T Q E K T E E T T - L S S L A Q P G V A
      CHO                CHO        CHO

                        CHO              CHO
V T F S D F Q D S D L I A(T)M M P P I S P A P I Q S D D D W
I T F P D F Q D S D L I A T V M P N T L P P H T E S D D D W
CHO                        CHO        CHO

        CHO
I P D I Q T D P N G L S F N P I S D F P D T T S P K C P G R
I P D I Q T E P N S L A F K L I S D F P E T T S P K C P S R
        CHO

            CHO
P W K S V S E I N P T T Q M K E S Y Y F D L T D G I S
P W K P V N G V N P T V E M K E S H D F D L V D A L L
```

Fig. 3. Alignment of the amino acid sequence of the light chains of human high molecular mass kininogen (upper line) with the bovine high molecular mass kininogen.

REFERENCES

1. Y. N. Han, M. Komiya, S. Iwanaga, and T. Suzuki, J. Biochem., 77:55-68 (1975).
2. Y. N. Han, H. Kato, S. Iwanaga, and T. Suzuki, J. Biochem., 79:1201-1222 (1976).
3. Y. N. Han, H. Kato, S. Iwanaga, S. Oh-ishi, and M. Katori, J. Biochem., 83:213-221 (1978).
4. N. Hashimoto, Y. N. Han, H. Kato, and S. Iwanaga, S. Seikagaku (in Japanese), 49:896 (1977).

5. N. Kitamura, Y. Takagaki, S. Furuto, T. Tanaka, H. Nawa, and S. Naka-
    nishi, Nature, 305:545-548 (1983).
6. B. Dittmann, A. Steger, R. Wimmer, and H. Fritz, Hoppe-Seyler's Z.
    Physiol. Chem., 362:919-927 (1981).
7. J. Kellerman, F. Lottspeich, A. Henschen, and W.Müller-Esterl, Eur. J.
    Biochem., in preparation (1985).

AMINO ACID SEQUENCE OF THE LIGHT CHAIN OF HUMAN LOW MOLECULAR MASS

KININOGEN

Friedrich Lottspeich, Josef Kellermann, Agnes Henschen,
Günther Rauth and Werner Müller-Esterl

Max-Planck-Institut für Biochemie, D-8033 Martinsried and
Abteilung für Klinische Chemie und Biochemie der Universität
München, D-8000 München

SUMMARY

The light chain of human low molecular mass kininogen consists of 38
amino acid residues. The half-cystine residue which forms the disulfide
bridge to the heavy chain is located in the position 18. Alignment of the
low molecular mass kininogen light chain with corresponding sections of
other kininogens revealed that the N-terminal part of it is species specific and the C-terminal part is function specific. Furthermore, some internal homologies between various sections of the total molecule were
found. A statistically significant sequence homology between the low
molecular mass kininogen light chain and the C-terminal part of the ribonucleases was observed.

INTRODUCTION

Human low molecular mass kininogen is a single chain glycoprotein with
a molecular mass of about 68 kDa. Limited proteolysis of the low molecular mass kininogen with kallikreins liberates the kinin moiety from its in-
terior. The residual two-chain molecule is held together by a single disulfide bridge. The heavy chain (M_r 64 kDa) corresponds to the N-terminal
part of the original kininogen molecule and is, as it seems, identical to
the heavy chain of the high molecular mass kininogen, the light chain
(M_r 4 kDa) corresponds to the C-terminal part. So far, all the known
functions of low molecular mass kininogen can be explained as related to
the kinin liberation. In bovine low molecular mass kininogen the amino
acid sequence of the light chain[1] and the c-DNA sequence of the whole
molecule[2] are known.

RESULTS AND DISCUSSION

Low molecular mass kininogen from pooled human plasma[3] was cleaved
with porcine pancreatic kallikrein, mercaptolysed and carboxymethylated.
The light chain was isolated by high performance liquid chromatography on
a large pore size Vydac TP RP column using a 0.1% trifluoroacetic acid/
acetonitrile gradient. The light chain was obtained in high yield and was
pure by the criteria of amino acid analysis, gel electrophoresis and

N-terminal amino acid sequence analysis. In the amino acid analysis, given
in Fig. 1 neither glucosamine nor galactosamine could be detected, indicating that the light chain of human low molecular mass kininogen is devoid of
carbohydrate side chain. The complete amino acid sequence of the light
chain could be elucidated by teh combined results of a direct N-terminal sequence analysis and an analysis of the tryptic fragments.[4] To ascertain
the C-terminus a carboxypeptidase digest was performed. The complete
amino acid sequence is given in Fig. 2. In position 18 the half-cystine
residue which forms the disulfide bridge to the heavy chain was found.

The alignment of the light chain of human low molecular mass kininogen
with other kininogen light chain sequences is shown in Fig. 3. Compelte
identity between human high and low molecular light chains is observed up
to amino acid residue 11. Beyond that amino acid residue virtually no
homology can be detected. A similar result is obtained when comparing the
bovine high and low molecular mass kininogen light chain sequences. A complete identity up to amino acid residue 12 and no homology beyond that amino
acid residue can be found. When, however, the light chain sequences of
human and bovine low molecular mass kininogen are compared, no homology
can be detected in the N-terminal 10 amino acid residues, but in the C-
terminal part a strong homology is found.

This pattern of homology and the fact that the heavy chains of high
and low molecular mass kininogen are believed to be identical, suggests
that the C-terminal part of the light chain is responsible for the specific
function of high and low molecular mass kininogen, respectively. The first
11 or 12 amino acid residues of the light chain, however, are species specific.

Amino Acid	a	b
Cys	1.2	1
Asp		
Thr	2.1	2
Ser	5.8	6
Glu	7.2	7
Pro	2.9	3
Gly	2.9	3
Ala	2.9	3
Val	1.0	1
Met		
Ile	1.8	2
Leu	1.1	1
Tyr	1.1	1
Phe		
Lys	3.0	3
His	1.1	1
Arg	3.9	4
Trp	n.d.	
ξ		38

Fig. 1. Amino acid analysis of human low molecular mass kininogen light
chain. (a) Uncorrected values, (b) Assumed integers.

```
  1           5                10                15
Ser-Ser-Arg-Ile-Gly-Glu-Ile-Lys-Glu-Glu-Thr-Thr-Ser-His-Leu-Arg-Ser-Cys-

 20  21         25                30                25
Glu-Tyr-Lys-Gly-Arg-Pro-Pro-Lys-Ala-Gly-Ala-Glu-Pro-Ala-Ser-Glu-Arg-Glu-

Val-Ser
```

Fig. 2. Amino acid sequence of human low molecular mass kininogen light chain.

When comparing the low molecular mass kininogen light chain sequence with the other known kininogen sequences a statistically significant internal homology between position 77-103 and 390-435 additionally to the already described strong homology between position 103-224 and 225-346 was found.

A computer search of the light chain sequence of low molecular mass kininogen against the protein sequence data base of Dayhoff et al.[5] showed statistically significant relationship between the low molecular mass kininogen light chain and the C-terminal part of various ribonucleases and the N-terminal part of antithrombin III. The results are presented in Table 1.

In Fig. 4 a schematic representation of the low molecular mass kininogen and ribonuclease regions which are involved in the sequence alignment is shown. Statistically significant scores were obtained for the pairs AD and BC within the kininogen and the pairs AE and DE in the comparison with the ribonucleases. So far it is not known if this unexpected sequence homologies reflect any kind of functional relatedness or a similar tertiary structure or if these proteins are derived from a common evolutionary ancestor.

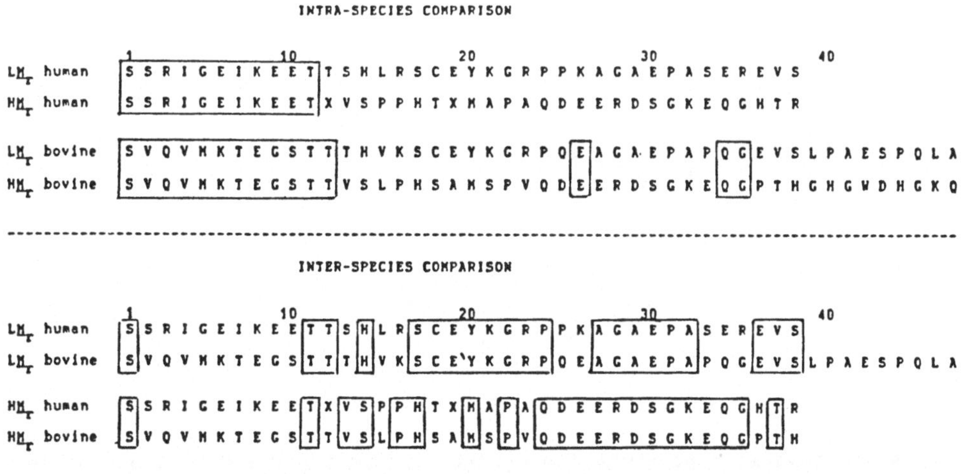

Fig. 3. Alignment of the amino acid sequence of the light chain of human low molecular mass kininogen with other kininogen sequences.

Table 1. Comparison Scores in Standard Deviation (SD) Units of Different
Ribonucleases (Carboxy-Terminal Part) and Human Antithrombin III
(Amino-Terminal Part) with Human (a) and (b) Low Molecular Weight
Kininogen Light Chain

	Score in SD units	
	(a)	(b)
Ribonuclease		
Ox, bison, water buffaloes, eland, topi, brindled gnu, sheep, and goat	5.6	4.3
Giraffe	4.5	2.2
Red deer, roe deer, fallow deer, reindeer, and moose	5.2	4.3
Pronghorn	7.3	3.6
Ox, seminal	5.6	4.3
Arabian and Bactrian camels	6.8	3.9
Pig	5.8	5.2
Hippopotamus	5.7	4.2
Pike whale	4.0	5.2
Horse	3.4	4.2
Chinchilla	4.7	5.5
Coypu	4.2	5.7
Guinea pig, A	5.8	4.6
Guinea pig, B	4.9	4.5
Muskrat	3.4	4.6
Golden hamster	4.0	3.9
Mouse	3.9	4.2
Rat	2.7	3.4
Two-toed sloth	2.6	1.5
Red kangaroo	4.4	3.1
Antithrombin-III (heparin cofactor) - Human	4.2	2.8

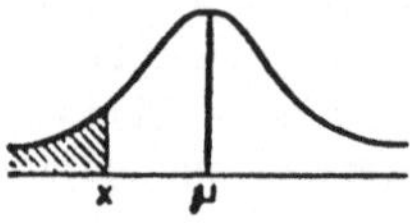

Normal distribution with mean μ and
standard deviation σ. The probability
of obtaining a score $>x$ is shown in
terms of z, the number of standard
deviation units from x to the mean,
$z=(x-\mu)/\sigma$.

z (SD units)	probability of a score $> x$
1.0	0.159
2.0	0.227×10^{-1}
3.0	0.135×10^{-2}
4.0	0.317×10^{-4}
5.0	0.287×10^{-6}
6.0	0.987×10^{-9}
7.0	0.128×10^{-11}

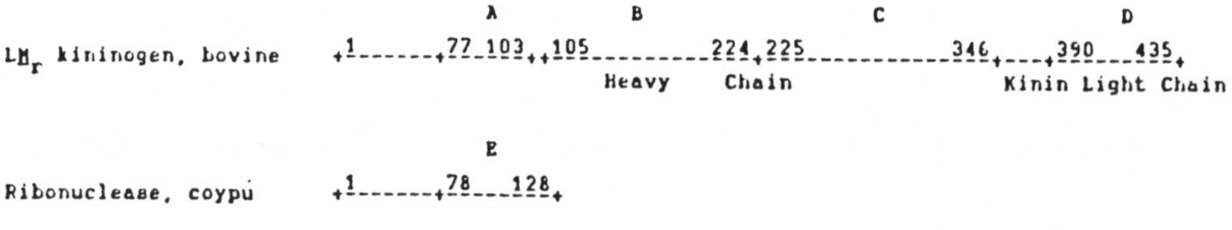

LM_r kininogen, bovine

```
                     A         B              C              D
 +1-------+77_103++105---------224,225--------346+---+390___435+
                     Heavy   Chain              Kinin Light Chain
```

Ribonuclease, coypu
```
                   E
 +1-------+78___128+
```

	B	C	D	E
A	-1.8	-0.9	3.9	5.1
B		15.1	-1.1	-1.3
C			-1.7	-1.2
D				5.6

Fig. 4. Schematic representation of the different parts of the bovine low
molecular mass kininogen and the C-terminal part of ribonuclease
from coypu.

REFERENCES

1. H. Kato, Y. N. Han, and S. Iwanaga, J. Biochem., (Tokyo), 82:377-385 (1977).
2. H. Nawa, N. Kitamura, T. Hirose, M. Asai, I. Inayama, and S. Nakanishi, Proc. Natl. Acad. Sci. USA, 80:90-94 (1983).
3. W. Müller-Esterl, M. Vohle-Timmermann, B. Boos, and B. Dittmann, Biochim. Biophys. Acta, 706:145-152 (1982).
4. F. Lottspeich, J. Kellermann, A. Henschen, G. Rauth, and W. Müller-Esterl, Eur. J. Biochem., 142:227-232 (1984).
5. M. O. Dayhoff, L. T. Hunt, W. C. Barker, B. C. Orcutt, L. S. Yeh, H. R. Chen, D. G. George, M. C. Blomquist, and G. C. Johnson, in: "Atlas of Protein Sequence and Structure, Vol. 5: Natl. Biomed. Res. Found., Georgetown Univ. Med. Center, Washington, DC (1982).

LIMITED PROTEOLYSIS OF HMW KININOGEN BY PLASMA KALLIKREIN IN MAN—

EVIDENCE FOR A PROCESSING MECHANISM DIFFERENT FROM THE BOVINE SYSTEM

Werner Müller-Esterl, Hans Hock, Günther Rauth,
Josef Kellermann*, Friedrich Lottspeich*, and Agnes Henschen*

Department of Clinical Chemistry and Clinical Bio-
chemistry, University of Munich, D-8000 Munich 2, FRG, and
*Max Planck Institute of Biochemistry, D-8033 Martinsried
Munich, FRG

SUMMARY

The limited proteolysis of human HMW kininogen by plasma kallikrein
has been studied. Kallikrein liberated bradykinin from HMW kininogen
(M_r 114 kDa) and generated a two-chain molecule with a heavy chain of
M_r 63 kDa and a light chain of M_r 58 kDa interconnected via a single
disulfide bridge. As proteolysis proceeded, a step-wise processing of
the initially formed light chain occurred giving rise to modified light
chains of M_r 45 and 41 kDa. Sequence analysis indicated that two polypeptides had been cleaved from the amino- and carboxy-terminal parts of
the 58 kDa light chain. Major part of the histidine-rich peptide which
is critical to surface binding of HMW kininogen was kept in the shortened
light chains. These findings are consistent with the observation that
trimming of the human HMW kininogen does not abolish its procoagulant
activity. By contrast, the bovine HMW kininogen is inactivated due to removal of the entire histidine-rich peptide. Hence, the proteolytic processing mechanisms for HMW kininogen are distinct in the human and the
bovine contact phase activation systems.

INTRODUCTION

High molecular weight (HMW) kininogen, a large precursor protein of
the kinins, circulates in plasma in complexed form with prokallikrein and/
or factor XI.[1] In the early events of contact phase activation, HMW
kininogen places the complexed proenzymes on subendothelial surfaces in
close vicinity to Hageman factor (F XII).[2] Binding of HMW kininogen to
the contact phase is mediated by the histine-rich peptide (HRP) present
in the light chain (L chain) of the molecule.[3] Subsequently, a reciprocal
activation of F XII and prokallikrein proceeds which triggers the intrinsic coagulation pathway via F XI.[4]

In the bovine system, activated plasma kallikrein cleaves HMW
kininogen under the release of bradykinin and fragment 1.2 including the
entire HRP.[5] Removal of the surface-binding portion results in a dissociation of the processed kininogen from the subendothelium thus

terminating contact phase activation.[3] Unlike the bovine molecule, the human HMW kininogen retains its procoagulant activity upon proteolytic processing by plasma kallikrein.[6-8] At present, the molecular basis of an envisaged alternative processing mechanism in man is not fully understood. This study was undertaken to elucidate the structural differences in the bovine and human kininogens responsible for the divergence of their cleavage patterns.

MATERIALS AND METHODS

HMW kininogen was purified from human plasma by ion-exchange chromatography on DEAE- and CM-Sephadex.[9] Plasma kallikrein was isolated from Cohn fraction IV-1 essentially following the procedure of Sampaio et al.[10] Analytical SDS electrophoresis[11] demonstrated that the purified proteins were largely homogeneous. For limited proteolysis of human HMW kininogen, 1.2 µg plasma kallikrein dissolved in 2 µl 0.1 M Tris, pH 8.0 was added to 120 µg HMW kininogen dissolved in 58 µl of the same buffer (molar ratio of enzyme to substrate 1:70). The samples were incubated at 37°C. After fixed time intervals (o, 15, 30, 60, 120, 180, 240, 300 min), aliquot samples of 10 µl were withdrawn, mixed with 10 µl sample buffer (2x) containing 10% (w/v) dithiothreitol,[11] and heated at 95°C for 5 min. Then, the samples were run on SDS gel electrophoresis in a linear 10 to 25% (w/v) polyacrylamide gradient gel.[11] Limited proteolysis of the isolated L chain (58 kDa) was performed under identical conditions except that the molar ratio of enzyme to substrate was 1:210.

To prepare the heavy (H) chain and the L chain, 10 mg HMW kininogen was incubated with 14 µg tissue kallikrein from porcine pancreas (molar ratio of enzyme to substrate 1:220) under identical conditions given above. The proteolysis was terminated after 15 min by the addition of 100 µl 1 M diisopropylfluorophosphate. Then, reductive cleavage of the disulfide bonds and carboxymethylation of the free thiol groups was done.[12] Separation of the H and the L chain (58 kDa) was accomplished by ion-exchange chromatography on SP-Sephadex.[6] To generate the modified L chain of 45 kDa, the same procedure was used except that plasma kallikrein was applied (molar ratio of enzyme to substrate 1:170). Proteolysis was allowed to proceed for 16 h. For the preparation of the modified L chain of 41 kDa, 10 mg of the isolated 45 kDa L chain was subjected to limited proteolysis by plasma kallikrein as described above. The reaction products were separated by gel filtration on AcA 44 (Rauth, G. and Müller-Esterl, W., in preparation). N-terminal amino acid sequence determinations of the L chain variants were performed by the Edman degradation method[13] in the presence of Polybrene.

RESULTS

Limited proteolysis of HMW kininogen by plasma kallikrein

Proteolytic processing of human HMW kininogen by plasma kallikrein progressively transformed the single-chain parent molecule into a two-chain molecule with the concomitant release of bradykinin. The time course of limited proteolysis was followed by SDS gel electrophoresis of the reaction components after reductive cleavage of their disulfide bonds (Figure 1). The virgin HMW kininogen of apparent M_r 114 kDa was converted into two major fragments representing the H chain of M_r 63 kDa and the L chain of M_r 58 kDa. As proteolysis proceeded, another fragment of M_r 45 kDa appeared (Figure 1).

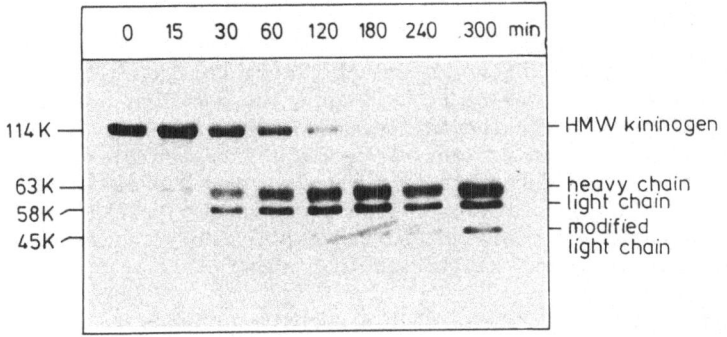

Figure 1. Time course of the limited proteolysis of human HMW kininogen
by plasma kallikrein followed by SDS electrophoresis in a
linear 10-25% polyacrylamide gradient gel in the presence of DTT.

Application of larger amounts of plasma kallikrein resulted in the
emergence of two closely spaced bands of M_r 45 and 41 kDa and the disappearance of the 58 kDa L chain, while the relative intensity of the H
chain of 63 kDa remained largely unaltered (not shown). This mode of chain
formation suggested that the initially formed L chain of 58 kDa was only a
transient product which was proteolytically trimmed to yield the modified
L chains of 45 and 41 kDa. The H chain was not prone to secundary proteolytic cleavage.

Isolation of the heavy and light chains

The two initially formed fragments of HMW kininogen, i.e., the H
chain of 63 kDa and the L chain of 58 kDa, were isolated by ion exchange
chromatography on SP-Sephadex following reductive cleavage of the disulfide
bonds. Analytical SDS electrophoresis of the purified proteins demonstrated that the two fragments were essentially homogeneous (Figure 2).
The isolated H and L chains were used for further fragmentation studies.

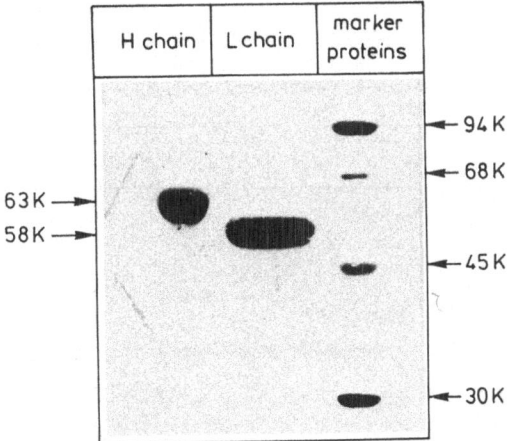

Figure 2. SDS electrophoresis of the isolated H and L chains from human
HMW kininogen in a 7.5% polyacrylamide gel. Marker proteins
are phosphorylase b (94 kDa), bovine serum albumin (68 kDa),
ovalbumin (45 kDa) and carbonic anhydrase (30 kDa).

Limited proteolysis of the isolated L chain

Incubation with catalytic amounts of plasma kallikrein resulted in a rapid converstion of the 58 kDa L chain into the modified L chain of 45 kDa (Figure 3). With prolonged incubation, the 45 kDa form was further processed to yield an L chain variant of 41 kDa. Thus, an identical pattern of L chain variants was generated from the isolated L chain (58 kDa) and from native HMW kininogen by proteolytic processing. Unlike the L chain, the purified H chain was resistant to further proteolytic breakdown by catalytic amounts of plasma kallikrein (not shown).

Amino-terminal sequence analysis of the L chain variants

From the proteolytic digests of HMW kininogen and its isolated fragments, the three L chain variants of 58 kDa, 45 kDa and 41 kDa were isolated (see Methods). N-terminal amino acid analysis revealed that Ser-Ser-Arg-Ile- was the only sequence present at the amino terminus of the 58 kDa L chain, while Gly-His-Gly-Leu- was present at the amino terminus of the 45 kDa L chain. Comparison of these sequences with the complete primary structure of the human HMW kininogen L chain (Kellermann et al., this volume) indicated that a glycopolypeptide of 68 amino acids containing a single carbohydrate attachment site had been removed from the amino terminus of the 58 kDa L chain to yield the shortened L chain of 45 kDa. This fragment was designated F 1.

The sequence analysis of the isolated 41 kDa L chain revealed the same amino terminus present in the 45 kDa form, i.e., Gly-His-Gly-Leu-. From this we concluded that a peptide of M_r close to 4 kDa must have been removed from the carboxy terminus of the 45 kDa L chain. Preliminary results from the N-terminal amino acid sequence analysis of the proteolytic digest of the 45 kDa L chain identify this fragment as a glycopolypeptide of 24 amino acids containing a single carbohydrate attachment site. This fragment derived from the C-terminal end of the 45 kDa L chain was designated F 2. Figure 4 summarizes the various H and L chains of human HMW kininogen including the predicted fragments F 1 and F 2.

DISCUSSION

The assignment of the cleavage sites for plasma kallikrein in the L chain of human HMW kininogen is given in Figure 5. The initial cleavages at position -9 (Lys-Arg) and -1 (Arg-Ser) release bradykinin and form a

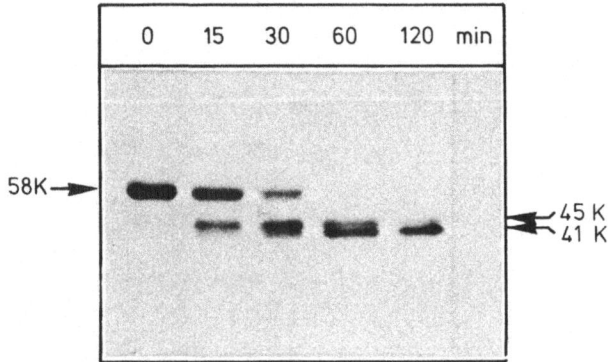

Figure 3. Time course of the limited proteolysis of the isolated 58 kDa L chain from human HMW kininogen by plasma kallikrein followed by SDS electrophoresis in a linear 10 to 20% polyacrylamide gradient gel.

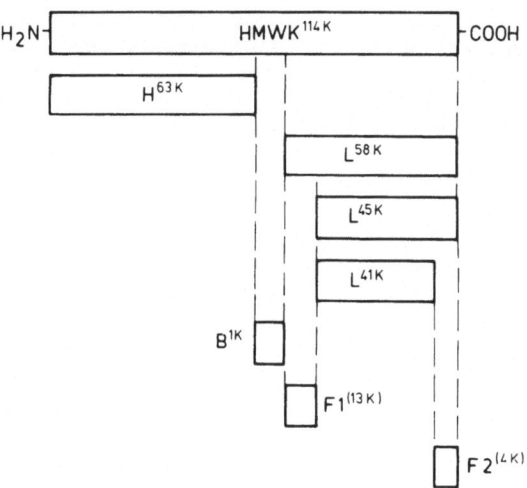

Figure 4. Schematic representation of the fragments formed from human HMW kininogen (HMWK) by proteolytic processing with plasma kallikrein. H, heavy chain; B, bradykinin; L, light chain variant; F, fragment.

two-chain kininogen molecule with a H chain of 63 kDa covalently linked to the L chain of 58 kDa by a single disulfide bridge. In a secondary cleavage (Arg-Gly), the glycopolypeptide F 1 corresponding to fragment 1 in the bovine molecule[3] is removed from the amino-terminus of the newly generated L chain. Major part of the histidine-rich peptide (corresponding to the bovine fragment 2)[3] is still present in the human 45 kDa L chain. Finally, a cleavage at position 231 (Lys-Ser) removed the C-terminal glycopolypeptide F 2 from the L chain of human HMW kininogen thus again keeping the histidine-rich portion. Hence, the step-wise proteolytic trimming of the human HMW kininogen by plasma kallikrein removes only peripheral segments of its L chain. In this way, major part of the HRP critical to contact phase binding is preserved in the processed molecule (Figure 5).

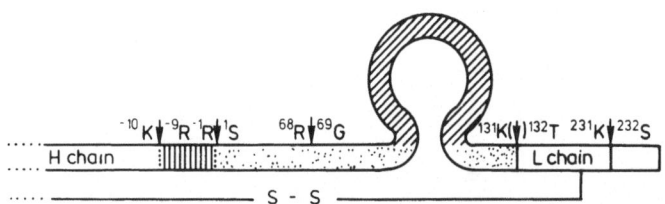

Figure 5. Assignment of the cleavage sites for plasma kallikrein in the human HMW kininogen molecule. ▦ bradykinin, ▨ extension loop, ▨ histidine-rich peptide. Numbers indicate the relative positions in the L chain.

Preservation of the surface-binding region easily explains why limited proteolysis of the human HMW kininogen L chain does not abolish its intrinsic procoagulant activity. By contrast, the bovine HMW kininogen molecule looses fragment 1.2 including the entire histidine-rich portion due to a single cut at position 110 (Arg-Thr). This renders the bovine molecule completely inactive. Figure 6 summarizes our current knowledge on the proteolytic processing mechanisms HMW kininogens undergo during contact phase activation in man and ox.

A simple explanation for the observed differences in the cleavage patterns of human and bovine HMW kininogen is provided by the comparison of the primary structures of their L chain portions. Amino acid sequence analysis indicates that the cleavage site in bovine HMW kininogen (Arg-Thr)[14] is semi-conserved in the human kininogen (Lys-Thr) and therefore does not per se preclude the cleavage by plasma kallikrein. The human HMW kininogen, however, has an extra portion of 22 amino acids not present in the bovine kininogen. This extension precedes the relevant peptide bond (Lys-Thr) in the human molecule, cf. Figure 5 (Kellermann, et al., this volume). Thus, it is conceivable that the extra loop provides a sterical hindrance so as to block the processing proteinase to cut at this particular position.

The results presented in this study do not allow any conclusions as to the physiological relevance of the in vitro experiments. Preliminary results from Western blotting and immunoprinting of plasma samples using specific antibodies against human kininogens suggest that a similar, if not identical fragmentation pattern of HMW kininogen occurs in human plasma.[15]

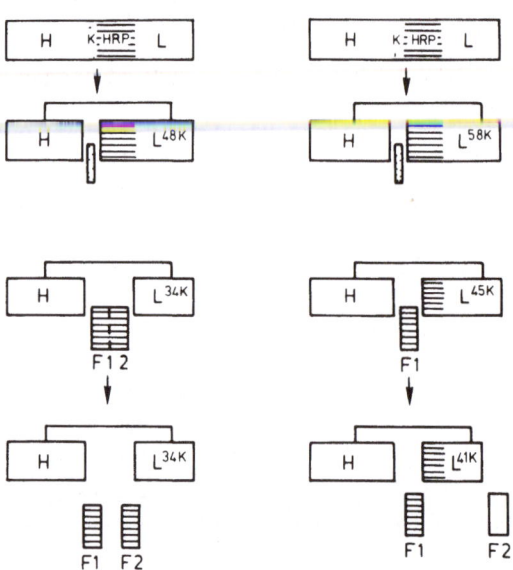

Figure 6.   Comparison of the proteolytic processing of HMW kininogen by plasma kallikrein in ox (left) and man (right). For abbreviations, see Figure 4.

REFERENCES

1. R. C. Wiggins, B. N. Bouma, C. G. Cochrane, and J. H. Griffin, Role of HMW kininogen in surface-binding and activation of coagulation factor XI and prekallikrein, Proc. Natl. Acad. Sci. USA, 74:4636-4640, (1977).

2. J. H. Griffin and C. G. Cochrane, Mechanisms for the involvement of HMW kininogen in surface-dependent reactions of Hageman factor, Proc. Natl. Acad. Sci. USA, 73:2554-2558, (1976).

3. T. Sugo, N. Ikari, H. Kato, S. Iwanaga, and S. Fujii, Functional sites of bovine HMW kininogen as a cofactor in kaolin-mediated activation of factor XII (Hageman factor), Biochemistry, 19:3215-3220, (1980).

4. R. L. Heimark, K. Kurachi, K. Fujikawa, and E. W. Davie, Surface activation of blood coagulation, fibrinolysis and kinin formation, Nature, 286:456-460, (1980).

5. Y. N. Han, M. Komiya, S. Iwanaga, and T. Suzuki, Studies on the primary structure of bovine HMW kininogen. Amino acid sequence of a fragment ("histine-rich peptide") released by plasma kallikrein, J. Biochem., 77:55-68, (1975).

6. D. M. Kerbiriou and J. H. Griffin, Human HMW kininogen. Studies of the structure-function relationships and of proteolysis of the molecule occurring during contact phase activation, J. Biol. Chem., 254:12020-12027, (1979).

7. S. Schiffman, C. Mannhalter, and K. Tyner, Human HMW kininogen. Effects of cleavage by kallikrein on protein structure and procoagulant activity, J. Biol. Chem., 255:6433-6438, (1980).

8. K. Mori and S. Nagasawa, Studies on human HMW kininogen. II. Structural change of HMW kininogen by the action of human plasma kallikrein, J. Biochem., 89:1465-1473, (1981).

9. B. Dittmann, A. Steger, R. Wimmer, and H. Fritz, A convenient large-scale preparation of HMW kininogen from human plasma, Hoppe-Seyler's Z. Physiol. Chem., 362:919-927, (1981).

10. C. Sampaio, S. C. Wong, and E. Shaw, Human plasma kallikrein. Purification and preliminary characterization, Arch. Biochem. Biophys., 165:133-139, (1974).

11. U. K. Laemmli, Cleavage of structural proteins during the assembly of the head of bacteriophage T4, Nature, 227:680-685, (1970).

12. A. Henschen and P. Edman, Large scale preparation of S-carboxymethyled chains of human fibrin and fibrinogen and the occurrence of σ-chain variants, Biochim. Biophys. Acta, 263:351-367, (1972).

13. P. Edman and G. Begg, A protein sequenator, Eur. J. Biochem., 1:80-91, (1967).

14. H. Kato, S. Nagasawa, and S. Iwanaga, HMW and LMW kininogens, Methods Enzymol., 80:172-198, (1981).

15. W. Müller-Esterl and M. Wimmer, Adv. Inflamm. Res., (1985, in press).

INTERACTION OF HUMAN LOW MOLECULAR WEIGHT KININOGEN WITH HUMAN MAST CELL

TRYPTASE

Lawrence B. Schwartz, Manfred Maier and Jocelyn Spragg

Medical College of Virginia, Richmond, VA 23298; Institute
of Medical Physiology, University of Vienna Medical Faculty
Vienna, Austria A-1090; Department of Medicine, Harvard
Medical School and Department of Rheumatology and Immunology
Brigham and Women's Hospital, Boston, MA 02115

Supported in part by grants AI-20487, HL-22939, AI-10356,
AM-05577 and RR-05669 from the National Institutes of Health

SUMMARY

The capacity of purified tryptase, the major neutral tryptic protease
of human lung mast cells, to serve as a kininogenase was examined with
purified human low molecular weight kininogen (LMWK) as the substrate.
Incubating of 25 mug of tryptase with LMWK for 2 to 30 minutes, with or
without heparin, yielded no net time-dependent kinin release as determined
on the estrous rat uterus. The 0.4 mug of kinin seen represented less than
10% of that released from excess LMWK by 5 mug of human urinary kallikrein
in 5 min. Incubation at pH 5.5 with or without heparin did not significantly alter this result. LMWK did not appear by SDS-PAGE to be cleaved by
tryptase either in the presence or absence of heparin. In contrast to its
action on HMWK, tryptase did not extensively cleave LMWK, or destroy its
reactivity with kallikrein.

INTRODUCTION

The possible role of kinins and the plasma kinin-forming system in
immunologic reactions has been addressed in many in vivo and in vitro
studies (reviewed in 1). While it has been shown that antigen-antibody
complexes themselves do not activate the plasma kinin-forming system in
vitro[2], there are studies to suggest that basophil and mast cell constituents, released in IgE-dependent reactions, interact with components of
this system (reviewed in 3). Reports that, in human systemic anaphylaxis
to hymenoptera venom, high molecular weight kininogen (HMWK) procoagulant
activity was diminished at times when Factor XII and plasma prekallikrein
were normal or less markedly diminished[4,5], suggest consumption of HMWK.
Whether kinin activity is generated in association with the reduction in
HMWK procoagulant activity has not been determined. Reports that kininogenase activity is released from immunologically challenged mixed human
leukocytes[6,7], human lung[8] and pulmonary mast cells[9,10] suggest HMWK may
be utilized to generate kinin during IgE-dependent reactions.

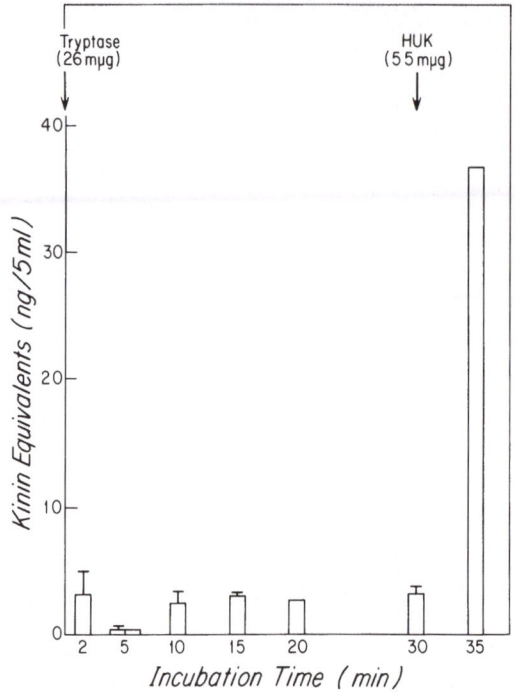

Fig. 1. Release of kinin from purified human
LMWK by purified human pulmonary mast
cell tryptase at physiologic pH. Human urinary kallikrein (HUK) was added after 30 minutes of incubation.

Tryptase, which is secreted in IgE-dependent reactions, is the major
neutral protease and protein component of human lung mast cells[11] and
accounts for over 90% of the TAMe esterase activity in dispersed human lung
cells containing at least 5% mast cells. It is an enzyme of MW = 144,000
with two alpha subunits of MW = 37,000 and two beta subunits of MW =
35,000[11]. Each subunit has one active site[11] and the alpha and beta sub-
units·share common antigenic determinants[12]. Purified tryptase, when incubated with purified, single-chain, functionally active HMWK[13], has been
shown to destroy HMWK without release of kinin and with loss of both its
procoagulant activity and its capacity to serve as a source of kinin in the
presence of kallikrein[14]. By electrophoresis of tryptase-treated HMWK in
polyacrylamide gels containing sodium dodecyl sulfate, it appeared that
tryptase extensively cleaved the procoagulant chain of HMWK[14] as recently
shown also for human neutrophil elastase[15] and human factor XI[16].

The other major human plasma kininogenase substrate, low molecular
weight kininogen (LMWK), is normally present at a concentration of 2 uM.
It has recently been purified as a single-chain, functionally active protein of MW = 66,000[17]. Because HMWK did not provide a substrate for kinin
release by tryptase, the study described herein was undertaken to examine
the capacity of purified tryptase to release kinin from purified human LMWK.

METHODS

p-Tosyl-L-arginine methyl ester (TAMe) and porcine heparin (Sigma,
St. Louis, MO); trypsin (Worthington, Freehold, NJ); and bradykinin (Bachem,
Torrance, CA) were purchased as indicated.

Tryptase was purified to apparent homogeneity from human pulmonary mast cells[11] and stored at -70°C. Immediately prior to assessment of its kininogenase activity, the capacity of tryptase to cleave TAMe was confirmed by a direct spectrophotometric assay[11,18] which had been calibrated with a standard trypsin preparation. The two tryptase preparations used had specific activities towards TAMe of 76.7 and 87.8 units/mg, representing 88% and 97%, respectively, of the activity of the freshly purified enzyme preparations. Purified human urinary kallikrein was prepared as described[19,20], quantified by radioimmunoassay[21] and stored at -70°C.

Human LMWK was also purified to apparent homogeneity from freshly frozen pooled human plasma[17] and aliquots were stored at -70°C. The kininogen was shown to be the intact single chain form of the substrate by SDS-PAGE under reducing conditions[17] and by resistance of the kinin moiety to inactivation by carboxypeptidase B[22]. Incubation with human urinary kallikrein for 30 minutes at pH 8.6 released approximately 0.6 pmoles of kinin from a pmole of substrate.

Porcine heparin was purified as described[23] and stored at -70°C as a 1.1 mg/ml solution.

Assays

The enzymatic release of biologically active kinin from purified LMWK was measured in the estrous rat uterus assay[24] standardized with bradykinin whose concentration had been determined by amino acid analysis.

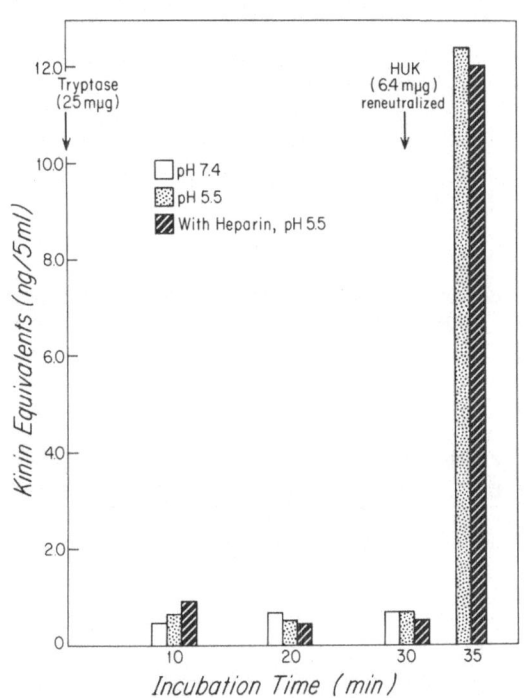

Fig. 2. Effect of acid pH and heparin on the release of kinin from purified low molecular weight kininogen by trytase. Human urinary kallikrein (HUK) was added after 30 minutes of incubation.

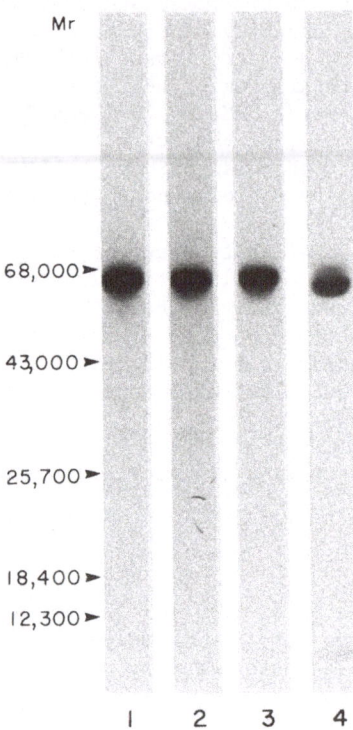

Fig. 3. SDS-PAGE of LMWK. Samples were denatured and reduced after incubation
for 30 minutes with substrate and
buffer (lane 1), substrate and tryptase (lane 2), substrate plus tryptase and heparin (lane 3), or substrate plus human urinary kallikrein
(lane 4).

Experiments conducted only at pH 7.4 were carried out in 0.04 M Tris-Cl
buffer containing 0.15 M NaCl and 0.02 M CaCl$_2$[23]. When experiments were
conducted in parallel at pH 5.5 and 7.4, 0.04 M sodium phosphate buffers
containing 0.10 M NaCl were used and adjusted to the same ionic strength
with additional NaCl. All incubations were carried out at 37°C.

SDS-PAGE was performed in a 5.17% acrylamide gradient slab gel as before[14]. Fourteen ug of LMWK were incubated at pH 7.4 and 37°C with 0.35
ug of tryptase for 0, 5, 30 and 240 minutes in the presence or absence of
2.0 ug of purified heparin. Samples were denatured and reduced before
electrophoresis.

RESULTS

In the initial experiments, 26 mug of tryptase (76.7 u/mg) were incubated in a final volume of 50 ul with 1.4 ug of purified LMWK at pH 7.4
for times ranging from 2 to 30 minutes. No more than 0.4 mug of kinin was
detected by bioassay at any time point and no net time-dependent kinin
production was observed (Fig. 1). When bradykinin was incubated with tryptase or LMWK for 30 minutes full biological activity was recovered, indicating that large amounts of kinin were not being generated and then degraded or adsorbed. Further, when 5.5 mug of human urinary kallikrein was

108

added to the LMWK-tryptase mixture after the 30-minute incubation period and incubation continued for 5 minutes more, 3.6 mug of kinin were generated (Fig. 1). This represents more than 9 times the amount of kinin detected in the LMWK-tryptase mixture and over 95% of the kinin generated when these concentrations of untreated LMWK and kallikrein were incubated together for 5 minutes. The addition of 400 mug of heparin to the incubation mixtures containing tryptase resulted in less than a 2-fold increase in the amount of kinin recovered.

Inexperiments to examine the possibility that kinin release by tryptase was optimal at pH 5.5[10], 25 mug of enzyme (87.8 units/mg) were incubated with 3 ug of kininogen at pH 7.4 or pH 5.5 for 10, 20, or 30 minutes in a 50 ul volume (Fig. 2). At pH 7.4, less than 0.7 mug of kinin were recovered at any time point and again no evidence for net kinin generation was obtained. When the incubations were carried out at pH 5.5, a small increment in kinin release was seen only at the 10-minute time point; the addition of heparin (400 mug) to the pH 5.5 incubation mixtures did not appreciably alter this result. In contrast, when 6.4 mug of urinary kallikrein was added to the incubation mixtures which had been reneutralized after 30 minutes incubation with tryptase, between 12.0 and 12.3 mug of kinin were recovered 5 minutes later (Fig. 2). This represents 17 times the amount of kinin detected with tryptase and LMWK alone and greater than 95% of the kinin generated when these preparations of kallikrein and kininogen were incubated together for 5 minutes in the absence of tryptase. Because no time-dependent generation of kinin by tryptase was observed, quantitative measurements of the Km and Vmax were not made.

The interaction of tryptase with LMWK was also examined directly by SDS-PAGE (Fig. 3). After reduction and alkylation, 14 ug of LMWK gave an apparent molecular weight of 66,000 with buffer (lane 1). The same molecular weight was seen after incubation for 30 minutes at 37°C with 350 mug of tryptase (lane 2). The addition of 2 ug of heparin to the LMWK-tryptase incubation mixture had no effect on the electrophoretic mobility of LMWK (lane 3). Extending the incubation time to 4 hours either with or without heparin yielded no detectable substrate cleavage. In contrast, incubation of 14 ug of LMWK with 32 mug of human urinary kallikrein for 30 minutes at 37°C led to almost complete disappearance of the MW = 66,000 band and to the appearance of one band at an apparent MW = 64,000 and another at an apparent MW less than 12,000 (lane 4).

DISCUSSION

The capacity of purified tryptase from human lung mast cells to cleave purified human plasma LMWK and to release kinin was directly determined by bioassay. When tryptase (14 nM catalytic subunit) and LMWK (0.4 or 0.9 uM) were incubated from 2 to 30 minutes at 37°C, at pH 7.4 and pH 5.5, with and without heparin (8 ug/ml), no net time-dependent generation of kinin activity was detected. In addition, essentially all of the kinin activity releasable by 2.3 or 2.7 nM human kallikrein from LMWK not previously exposed to tryptase was also released from tryptase-treated LMWK. Thus, in contrast to the degradation of HMWK by tryptase[14], the 30-minute incubations of LMWK with tryptase did not inactivate the capacity of LMWK to serve as a substrate for human urinary kallikrein (Figs. 1 and 2), suggesting that tryptase has little capacity to cleave the latter substrate in any way. This was directly demonstrated by SDS-PAGE (Fig. 3), in which no appreciable cleavage of LMWK was observed with tryptase under conditions where cleavage by urinary kallikrein was almost complete.

It is apparent from this work and the earlier study[14] that cleavage of either LMWK or HMWK by tryptase does not occur in vitro at physiologic pH. These results do not support a recent report that purified tryptase has kininogenase activity towards human kininogens at pH 5.5, but not at pH 7.4[10]. Because tryptase has a Ph optimum for esterase activity of 8.0 and for peptidase activity of 7.4[25], it is in fact unlikely that it would express proteolytic activity against kininogens at pH 5.5 and not at pH 7.4. The kinin release observed _in situ_ in challenged allergic nasal mucosa[26] may therefore be due to the IgE-dependent release of an as yet uncharacterized kininogenase, or to the release of other enzymes or cofactors[27] that can activate the plasma kinin-forming system, perhaps at an earlier step than kininogen cleavage.

ACKNOWLEDGEMENTS

The authors acknowledge the excellent technical assistance of T.R. Bradford, K.A. Kusiak, J. P. Whelan and R.S. Wolff.

REFERENCES

1. Spragg, J., Talamo, R.C. and Austen, K.F.: Immunochemistry of brady-kinin and immunologic activation of the kinin system. In: Brady-kinin, Kallidin and Kallikrein ed, by E.G. Erdos. Springer pp. 531-549 (1970).
2. Cochrane, C.G., Wuepper, K.D., Aiken, B.S., Revak, S.D. and Spiegel-berg, H.L.: The interaction of Hageman factor and immune complexes. J. Clin. Invest. 51: 2736 (1972).
3. Newball, H.H., Meier, H.L., Kaplan, A.P., Revak, S.D., Cochrane, C.G. and Lichtenstein, L.M.: Activation of Hageman factor by proteases released during antigen challenge of human lung. Trans. Assoc. Am. Phys. 94: 126 (1981).
4. Smith, P.L., Kagey-Sobotka, A., Bleecker, E.R., Traystman, R., Kaplan, A.P., Gralnick, H., Valentine, M.D., Permutt, S. and Lichtenstein, L.M.: Physiologic manifestations of human anaphylaxis. J. Clin. Invest. 66: 1072-1080 (1980).
5. Ratnoff, O.D. and Nossel, H.L.: Wasp sting anaphylaxis. Blood 61: 132-139 (1983).
6. Newball, H.H., Talamo, R.C. and Lichtenstein, L.M.: Release of leuko-cyte kallikrein mediated by IgE. Nature 254: 635-636 (1975).
7. Newball, H.H., Berninger, R.W., Talamo, R.C. and Lichtenstein, L.M.: Anaphylactic release of a basophil kallikrein-like activity. I. Purification and characterization. J. Clin. Invest. 64: 457-465 (1979).
8. Newball, H.H., Meier, H.L., Kaplan, A.P., Revak, S.D., Cochrane, C.G. and Lichtenstein, L.M.: Anaphylactic release of human lung kinin-generating activities (LK-A'S). Fed. Proc. 39: 906A (1980).
9. Proud, D., Schulman, E.S., MacGlashan, D.W., Pierce, J.V. and Newball, H.H.: Anaphylactic release of a kininogenase from purified human lung mast cells. Clin. Res. 30: 165A (1982).
10. Proud, D. and Lichtenstein, L.M.: Human lung mast cell kininogenase: Apparent identity to tryptase. Fed. Proc. 43: 1807A (1984).
11. Schwartz, L.B., Lewis, R.A. and Austen, K.F.: Tryptase from human pulmonary mast cells. Purification and characterization. J. Biol. Chem. 256: 11939-11943 (1981).
12. Schwartz, L.B.: Monoclonal antibodies against human mast cell tryptase demonstrates shared antigenic sites on subunits of tryptase and selective localization of the enzyme to mast cells. J. Immunol. (In press).
13. Maier, M., Austen, K.F. and Spragg, J.: Characterization of the pro-coagulant chain derived from human high molecular weight kininogen (Fitzgerald factor) by human tissue kallikrein. Blood 62: 457-463 (1983).

14. Maier, M., Spragg, J. and Schwartz, L.B.: Inactivation of human high molecular weight kininogen by human mast cell tryptase. J. Immunol. 130: 2352-2356 (1983).

15. Kortmann, H., Bönner, G., Müller-Esterl, W., Jochum, M. and Fritz, H.: Limited and unspecific proteolysis of kininogens in acute necrotizing pancreatitis (ANP). Abstracts of the Kinin '84 Savannah International Congress, Oct. 21-25 (1984).

16. Colman, R.W.: Regulation of the plasma kallikrein-kininogen system. Abstracts of the Kinin '84 Savannah International Congress, Oct. 21-25 (1984).

17. Maier, M., Austen, K.F. and Spragg, J.: Purification of single chain human low molecular weight kininogen and demonstration of its cleavage by human urinary kallikrein. Anal. Biochem. 134: 336-346 (1983).

18. Walsh, K.A.: Trypsinogens and trypsins of various species. Methods in Enzymology XIX: 41-63 (1970).

19. ole-MoiYoi, O., Spragg, J. and Austen, K.F.: Structural studies of human urinary kallikrein (urokallikrein). Proc. Natl. Acad. Sci. USA 76: 3121-3125 (1979).

20. ole-MoiYoi, O., Pinkus, G.S., Seldin, D.C., Spragg, J. and Austen, K.F.: Structure, functional characteristics and immunohistochemical localization of human glandular kallikreins from kidney and pancreas. In: Plasma and Cellular Modulatory Proteins ed. by D.H. Bing and R.A. Rosenbaum. Boston Center for Blood Research pp. 183-201 (1981).

21. Silver, M.R., ole-MoiYoi, O., Austen, K.F. and Spragg, J.: An active site radioimmunoassay for urokallikrein and demonstration of a latent form of the enzyme. J. Immunol. 124: 1551-1555 (1980).

22. Spragg, J. and Austen, K.F.: The preparation of human kininogen. III. Enzymatic digestion and modification. Biochem. Pharmacol. 23: 781-791 (1974).

23. Schwartz, L.B., Kawahara, M.S., Hugli, T.E., Vik, D., Fearon, D.T. and Austen, K.F.: Generation of C3a anaphylatoxin from human C3 by human mast cell tryptase. J. Immunol. 130: 1891-1895 (1983).

24. Orange, R.P. and Austen, K.F. The biological assay of slow reacting substances--SRS-A, bradykinin, prostaglandins. In: Methods in Immunology and Immunochemistry, Vol. V ed. by C.A. Williams and M.W. Chase. Academic Press pp. 145-149 (1976).

25. Schwartz, L.B. and Austen, K.F.: Structure and function of the chemical mediators of mast cells. Prog. Allergy 34: 271-321 (1984).

26. Proud, D-, Togias, A., Naclerio, R.M., Crush, S.A., Norman, P.S. and Lichtenstein, L.M.: Kinins are generated in vivo following nasal airway challenge of allergic individuals with allergen. J. Clin. Invest. 72: 1678-1685 (1983).

27. Hojima, R.L.: In vitro activation of the contact (Hageman Factor) system of plasma by heparin and chondroitin sulfate E. Blood 63: 1453-1459 (1984).

INDEPENDENT CONSUMPTION OF HIGH AND LOW MOLECULAR WEIGHT KININOGENS

IN VIVO

Yasuhiro Uchida and Makoto Katori

Department of Pharmacology, Kitasato University School of
Medicine, Sagamihara, Kanagawa 228, Japan

SUMMARY

The levels of high molecular weight (HMW) kininogen and pre-kallikrein in rat plasma were markedly reduced after single injection of bromelian (10 mg/kg, i.v.) and gradually recovered over a 72 hour period. The level of low molecular weight (LMW) kininogen, however, was not changed during this period.

Rat pleurisy was induced by intrapleural injection of λ-carrageenin. The levels of HMW kininogen and prekallikrein, but not of LMW kininogen, in the exudate were markedly decreased, when compared with those in plasma of the same animals.

After pretreatment with disulfiram, oral administration of ethanol (2 g/kg) or intravenous injection of acetaldehyde (10 mg/kg) to rats caused significant decrease in the plasma level of LMW kininogen with no significant effect on the plasma HMW kininogen and prekallikrein levels.

These results suggest that HMW and LMW kininogens may be consumed separately in vivo and play different roles.

INTRODUCTION

The presence of both HMW and LMW kininogens in plasma has been reported.[1] More recently, the discovery of a hereditary deficiency of kininogens in plasma accelerated the study of the roles and HMW kininogen was demonstrated to be a cofactor in the activation of coagulating factor XII (Hageman factor) with prekallikrein.[2-5] The role of LMW kininogen in vivo, however, has not been discussed previously.

The present paper reports that HMW and LMW kininogens in plasma were independently consumed in different conditions.

MATERIALS AND METHODS

Stem bromelain (10 mg/kg), a thiol protease from pineapple stems, was injected into rat tail vein under light ether anesthesia.

Rat pleurisy was induced by one-tenth ml of 2% λ-carrageenin into the right pleural cavity of male SD-strain rats (specific pathogen free, 8-10 weeks old). Exudate accumulation and cell migration were observed during the 24 hour period.

Disulfiram (150 mg/kg; Nakarai Chemical Col, Osaka), an aldehyde dehydrogenase inhibitor, was given orally to Wistar-strain rats (8-10 weeks old) and 24 hours later rats were administered by ethanol (2 g/kg, p.o.) or acetaldehyde (10 mg/kg, i.v.).

Blood was collected under light ether anesthesia from the carotid artery of rats into plastic tubes containing 1/10 volume of 3.8% sodium citrate. Plasma was obtained by centrifugation at 1000 g at 20°C for 15 minutes and stored at -70°C until use.

Prekallikrein determination

Plasma prekallikrein was activated with kaolin and acetone and plasma kallikrein was assayed using Z-Phe-Arg-MCA (Peptide Institute Inc., Osaka) as substrate according to the method of Oh-ishi and Katori.[6] One arbitrary unit was 1×10^{-7} M AMC released during 10 minutes at 37°C. The difference in the amidolytic activities in the presence of between soy bean trypsin inhibitor (SBTI) and lima bean trypsin inhibitor (LBTI) (Worthington Biochemical Co., Freehold, New Jersey) was considered as the plasma kallikrein activity.

Determination of HMW and LMW kininogens

HMW kininogen level in plasma and the exudate of the pleurisy was measured by the amount of kinin released after the activation of factor XII with glass powder (Ballotini #14; Jencons., England) in the presence of o-phenanthroline (O-PT; Wako Pure Chemical, Tokyo), as described by Uchida and Katori.[7] LMW kininogen level was determined after depletion of HMW kininogen by glass powder in the absence of O-PT and acid denaturation of the HMW kininogen-depleted plasma by measuring the amounts of kinin release following trypsin treatment (1 mg/ml plasma).

This assay method was recently criticized because of insufficient release of kinin from kininogens by trypsin.[8] However, increase in the amount of trypsin up to 10 mg/ml plasma generated the same amount of kinin (2.3 ± 0.1 ug BK equivalent/ml original plasma) from the acid-treated rat plasma as that released by 1 mg/ml of trypsin (2.1 ± 0.1 ug BK equivalent/ ml plasma), when assayed on rat uterus. Thus, the original method was used in this experiment.

RESULTS AND DISCUSSION

Decrease in HMW kininogen and prekallikrein

Single intravenous injections of stem bromelain (10 mg/kg) to rats caused transient fall of systemic blood pressure for 15 minutes and the levels of HMW kininogen and prekallikrein were reduced to one thirtieth and one twelfth, respectively, whereas the LMW kininogen level was not significantly reduced (Table 1). This was attributed to the activation of factor XII in plasma by bromelain.[9] The reduced levels of HMW kininogen and prekallikrein in plasma did not recover until 72 hours after bromelian injection.[9]

Table 1. Plasma levels of prekallikrein and HMW and LMW kininogens after i.v. injection of bromelain or saline into rats

	kininogen (ng BK q./mg protein)*		prekallikrein** (cpm)
	HMW	LMW	
saline	12.0 ± 1.2	9.7 ± 1.4	5395 ± 540
bromelain	0.4 ± 0.0	7.3 ± 1.4	439 ± 174

* expressed as ng BK released/mg protein.

**expressed as counts of ^{3}H-MeOH released from ^{3}H-TAME after activation.

Each value indicates mean ± SE from four to seven rats.

In the carrageenin-induced rat pleurisy, the evels of HMW kininogen and prekallikrein in the exudate at 3 hours after carrageenin were markedly decreased when expressed in terms of nanograms and arbitrary units per milligram protein, respectively, as shown in Table 2, whereas the levels of HMW kininogen and prekallikrein in plasma of the pleurisy rats were not different from those of the normal healthy rats. This may indicate that the plasma prekallikrein was activated and bradykinin was released in the pleural cavity.[10] Prekallikrein in plasma was proved to be activated by carrageenin probably through the activation of factor XII in vitro.[10] Thus, the reduction can be interpreted as the consumption. The low levels of HMW kininogen and prekallikrein in the pleural exudate were observed during the entire course of pleurisy. Conversely, LMW kininogen in the exudate remained at the same level as that in plasma throughout the course of the pleurisy.

From these two findings, HMW kininogen was preferentially consumed, when prekallikrein or factor XII was activated in the body.

Table 2. Levels of prekallikrein and HMW and LMW kininogens in the pleural exudate and plasma in rat carrageenin-induced pleurisy and control rats

	plasma (control rats)	plasma (pleurisy rats)	exudate (pleurisy rats)
HMW kininogen	13.1 ± 1.3	10.9 ± 0.9	0.005*
LMW kininogen	13.5 ± 1.3	11.5 ± 1.0	8.1 ± 0.7
prekallikrein	43.5 ± 5.5	43.3 ± 2.9	9.0 ± 0.5**

* Kininogen levels wrre expressed as ng bradykinin released/mg protein.
**Prekallikrein level was expressed as an arbitrary unit of amidase activity of generated plasma kallikrein in terms of mg protein.

The values are means ± SE from five animals.

Decrease in LMW kininogen

When Wistar-strain rats, pretreated by disulfiram (150 mg/kg p.o.), were given by oral administration of ethanol (2 g/kg), the plasma level of LMW kininogen was significantly reduced, comparing with that in control rats, whereas those of HMW kininogen and prekallikrein were not different from those in the control rats (Figure 1). When pretreatment with disulfiram was omitted, the reduction of HMW kininogen was not observed. This indicates that acetaldehyde caused the reduction. In fact, intravenous injection of acetaldehyde (10 mg/kg) to the disulfiram-treated rats caused further decrease of LMW kininogen. The HMW kininogen and prekallikrein levels were not significantly reduced (Figure 1). These results well agreed with those in other paper.[11]

In in vitro system, in which hog pancreas kallikrein was incubated with human plasma and the residual levels of both kininogens were assayed, increasing doses of the tissue kallikrein consumed preferentially LMW kininogen. The HMW kininogen was consumed only when most of LMW kininogen was consumed (Figure 2).

These observations suggest that a tissue kallikrein may be released by acetaldehyde formed following ethanol ingestion under the inhibition of acetaldehyde dehydrogenase by disulfiram in rats. This may explain flushing after ingestion of alcohol in man as well.

These results mentioned above clearly indicate that HMW and LMW kininogens may be consumed separately in vivo and thus play different roles.

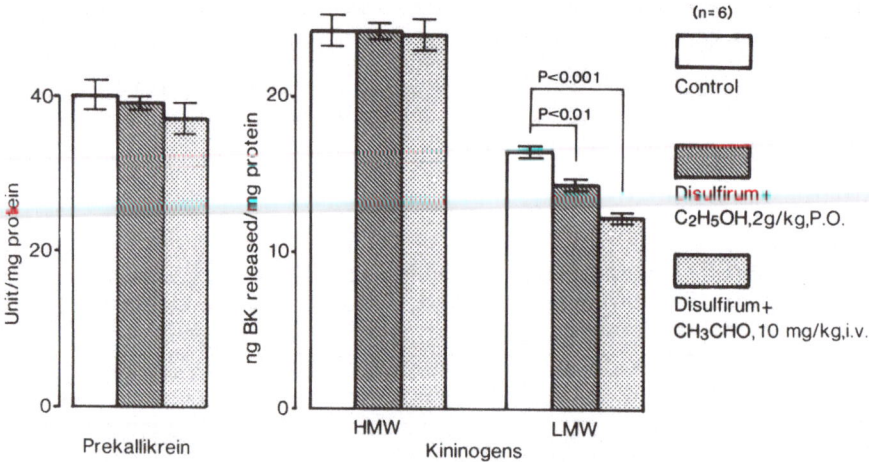

Figure 1. Significant reduction of LMW kininogen in plasma after administration of ethanol (2 g/kg, p.o.) or acetaldehyde (10 mg/kg, i.v.)

Rats were pretreated with disulfiram (150 mg/kg, p.o.) 24 hours before the experiments.

The ordinate at the left panel shows an arbitrary unit of AMC released/mg protein. That at the right panel indicates kininogen levels in plasma, expressing an ng bradykinin/mg protein. Each column indicated mean ± SE from six animals. Only the LMW kininogen level was consumed significantly.

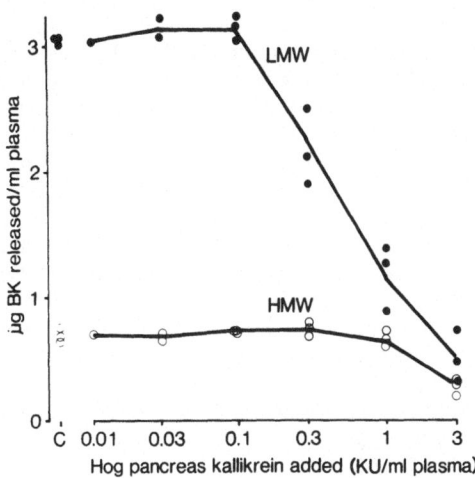

Figure 2. Preferential consumption of LMW kininogen in human plasma
after addition of hog pancreas kallikrein in vitro.

The ordinate shows ug BK released/ml original plasma. Bradykinin released was assayed by enzyme immunoassay. The abscissa
indicates kallikrein unit/ml human plasma added.

ACKNOWLEDGEMENT

The authors wish to thank Mr. N. Sunahara, Dainippon Pharmaceutical
Co. for the generous gift of the bradykinin enzyme immunoassay kits.

REFERENCES

1. E. Haberman, Kininogens, in: Handbook of Experimental Pharmacology,
    XXV, ed. by E. G. Erdoes, Springer-Verlag, Berlin, pp. 250-288,
    (1970).
2. K. D. Wuepper, Prekallikrein deficiency in man, J. Exp. Med., 138:
    1345-1355, (1973).
3. H. Saito, O. D. Ratnoff, R. Waldmann, and J. P. Abraham, Fitzgerald
    trait: Deficiency of a hitherto unrecognized agent, Fitzgerald
    factor, participating in surface-mediated reactions of clotting,
    fibrinolysis, generation of kinins, and the property of diluted
    plasma enhancing vascular permeability (PF/DIL), J. Clin. Invest.,
    55:1082-1089, (1975).
4. R. W. Colan, A. Bagdasarian, R. C. Talamo, C. F. Scott, A. M. Seavey,
    J. A. Guimaraes, J. V. Pierce, and A. P. Kaplan, Williams trait:
    Human kininogen deficiency with diminished levels of plasminogen
    proactivator and prekallikrein associated with abnormalities of
    the Hageman factor-dependent pathways, J. Clin. Invest., 56:1650-
    1662, (1975).

5. S. Oh-ishi, A. Ueno, Y. Uchida, M. Katori, H. Hayashi, H. Koya, K. Kitajima, and I. Kimura, Abnormalities in the contact activation through factor XII in Fujiwara trait: A deficiency in both high and low molecular weight kininogens with low level of prekallikrein, Tohoku J. Exp. Med., 133:67-80, (1981).

6. S. Oh-ishi and M. Katori, Fluorometric assay for plasma prekallikrein using peptidylmethylcoumarinylamide as a substrate, Thrombosis Res., 14:551-559, (1979).

7. Y. Uchida and M. Katori, Differential assay method for high molecular weight and low molecular weight kininogens, Thrombosis Res., 15:127-134, (1979).

8. H. Okamoto and L. M. Greenbaum, Kininogen substrates for trypsin and cathepsin D in human, rabbit and rat plasmas, Life Sci., 32:2007-2013, (1983).

9. S. Oh-ishi, Y. Uchida, A. Ueno, and M. Katori, Bromelain, a thiol-protease from pineapple stem, depletes high molecular weight kininogen by activation of Hageman factor (factor XII), Thrombosis Res., 14:665-672, (1979).

10. Y. Uchida, K. Tanaka, Y. Harada, A. Ueno, and M. Katori, Activation of plasma kallikrein-kinin system and its significant role in pleural fluid accumulation of rat carrageenin-induced pleurisy, Inflammation, 7:121-131, (1983).

11. K. Hatake, Behavior of the kallikrein-kinin system on alcohol ingestion, Jpn. J. Alcohol & Drug Dependence, 19:32-62, (1984) (in Japanese).

URINARY KININOGEN: A POSSIBLE REGULATOR OF KININ FORMATION IN NORMAL INDIVIDUALS AND SUBJECTS WITH ESSENTIAL HYPERTENSION, END-STAGE RENAL AND LIVER DISEASE

Marc S. Weinberg, W. M. Trebbin, and Richard J. Solomon

Department of Medicine, Roger Williams General Hospital and Providence Veterans Administration Medical Center, Brown University Division of Biology and Medicine, Providence Rhode Island 02908

SUMMARY

Most previous studies have not significantly correlated urinary kallikrein to urinary kinins. We investigated whether urinary kininogen might influence kinin formation within the urine. On an ad-lib diet the 24 hour excretion of total and intact kininogen, kinins and kallikrein was determined in 24 control subjects, 20 untreated essential hypertensives, 12 with end-stage renal disease and 8 subjects with liver disease. Kallikrein and kinins were measured by a direct radioimmunoassay. Total kininogen was determined from the sum of preformed kinins and kinins generated after trypsin (intact kininogen). Cross reactivity between purified human low molecular weight kininogen and bradykinin antiserum was 3%. Total and intact kininogen were significantly correlated with kinins in controls, essential hypertension and liver disease. In essential hypertension, end-stage renal and liver diseases kinins were significantly decreased. This was associated with a reduction in kininogen but not kallikrein in essential hypertension and liver disease, and a reduction in kallikrein but not kininogen in end-stage renal disease. Thus, renal kinin generation in various states may be affected by either or both kininogen and kallikrein.

INTRODUCTION

The kallikrein-kininogen-kinin system has been postulated to play an important role in the regulation of blood pressure and modulation of salt and water transport.[1] However, the parameters reflecting the activity of the renal kallikrein-kininogen-kinin system have not been completely defined. With rare exceptions, urinary kallikrein activity has not been correlated to simultaneously measured urinary kinins, and therefore may not reflect the activity or concentration of the kidney.[1,2] Other factors such as urinary pH, cation concentrations, kallikrein inhibitors and osmolality have been postulated to play a role in the regulation of the activity of the kallikrein-kininogen-kinin system.[3]

Several studies have reported the presence of kininogen in human urine.[4-8] However, there is very little data investigating the physiological importance of urokininogen, which has not usually been considered to play an important role in the regulation of kinin formation. We raised the hypothesis that urinary kininogen may be important in regulating kinin generation within the urine. This situation will be satisfied if kininogen is present in urine in a concentration which obeys a first order rate for kinin formation. In order to evaluate this hypothesis, we measured various components of the renal kallikrein-kininogen-kinin system in normal subjects and pathological states such as essential hypertension, end-stage renal and liver diseases, were urinary levels of kallikrein or kininogen are altered.

METHODS

Subjects were evaluated at the Roger Williams General Hospital and Providence Veterans Administration Medical Center after giving informed consent. We evaluated four groups of subjects; normal controls, and patients with essential hypertension, and end-stage renal and liver diseases. Normals, essential hypertensives, and subjects with liver disease were on no medications for three weeks. Those with end-stage renal disease were taken off medications for a minimum of one day. Patients were encouraged to void frequently throughout the day. Twenty-four hour urines were collected untreated and in HCl-pepstatin in order to preserve urinary kinins and kininogen.[9,10] Total kallikrein was analyzed in untreated urine, while total and intact kininogen and endogenous kinins were measured in treated urines.

Total (active and inactive) urinary kallikrein was determined by a radioimmunoassay using rabbit anti-human urinary kallikrein serum kindly supplied by Dr. Narendra B. Oza (Boston, MA), as previously reported.[11] Urinary kinins were analyzed by a radioimmunoassay using rabbit anti-bradykinin serum generously supplied by Dr. Colin Johnston (Melbourne, Australia).[12] Total kininogen was determined from the sum of preformed kinins and kinins generated after trypsininzation of intact kininogen. Total and intact kininogen were reported in ugkinins/day. The cross reactivity between purified human low molecular weight kininogen (generously supplied by Drs. John Pisano and Jack Pierce, Bethesda, Maryland), and bradykinin antiserum was 3%.

Because the group with liver disease was small compared to the other groups, two separate analyses were performed. Controls, hypertensives and subjects with end-stage renal disease were in the first analysis, while controls and volunteers with liver disease were in the second group. Statistical analysis was performed using multiple and univariate analysis of variance or covariance followed by specialized multiple comparison tests.[13] Since differences in subject age and urinary sodium rather than group conditions might be responsible for observed differences in group means, covariance analysis was performed for kallikrein. Age and urinary sodium had no effect on or correlation to total and intact kininogen or endogenous kinins; thus no covariates were used for these analyses. Partial correlations with age and urinary sodium as covariates were performed[14] between endogenous urinary kinins and other variables in normal volunteers. Significance was reported when $p < .05$. All data is the mean±SEM.

RESULTS

The components of the kallikrein-kininogen-kinin system are shown in Table 1 for normals, and subjects with untreated hypertension, end-stage renal and liver diseases. As can be seen there were significant alterations in kallikrein, kinins, and total and intact kininogen between normals and subjects with essential hypertension, end-stage renal and liver disease.

In normal subjects, the twenty-four hour urinary excretion of total and intact kininogen were 34.0+6.3 and 12.2+2.2 ug kinins, respectively. Assuming 1 mg low molecular weight kininogen generates 11.2 ug kinins,[15] the concentrations of total and intact urinary kininogen were approximately 3 and 1 ug kininogen/ml, respectively.

Using partial correlations with urinary sodium and age as covariates, urinary kinins were significantly correlated to both total and intact kininogen in normals and untreated essential hypertensives. In liver disease, the correlations were significant only when urinary sodium and age were not used as covariates.

In Figure 1 alterations in urinary kallikrein, endogenous kinins, and total and intact kininogen are shown for normal controls and subjects with untreated hypertension and end-stage renal disease. Figure 2 contains alterations in components of the kallikrein-kininogen-kinin system in controls and individuals with liver disease.

As can be seen kinins were significantly decreased in hypertensives, end-stage renal and liver diseases. Reduced kinins were associated with a significant decrease in total kininogen but not kallikrein in hypertensives and liver disease. While intact kininogen was significantly decreased in hypertensives, it was arithmetically, but non-significantly decreased in liver disease. Reduced kinins were associated with a decrease in kallikrein but not kininogen in end-stage renal disease.

Table 1. Components of the Kallikrein-Kininogen-Kinin System in Controls, Essential Hypertension (EH), End-Stage Renal Disease (ESRD), and Liver Disease (LIVER). N represents the number of individuals in each group, while * = P .05. Intact and total kininogen is reported in ug kinins/day

Group (N)	Kallikrein (ug/day)	Kinins (ug/day)	Intact Kg (ug/day)	Total Kg (ug/day)
CONTROLS (24)	130.0+12.5	21.8+4.7	12.2+2.2	34.0+6.3
EH (20)	173.6+34.1	8.0+1.9*	3.3+0.8*	11.3+2.4*
ESRD (12)	2.5+ 0.8*	0.9+0.4*	81.5+60.3	82.3+60.2
LIVER (7)	80.0+41.5	6.8+3.8*	7.2+ 2.6	14.0+ 4.6*

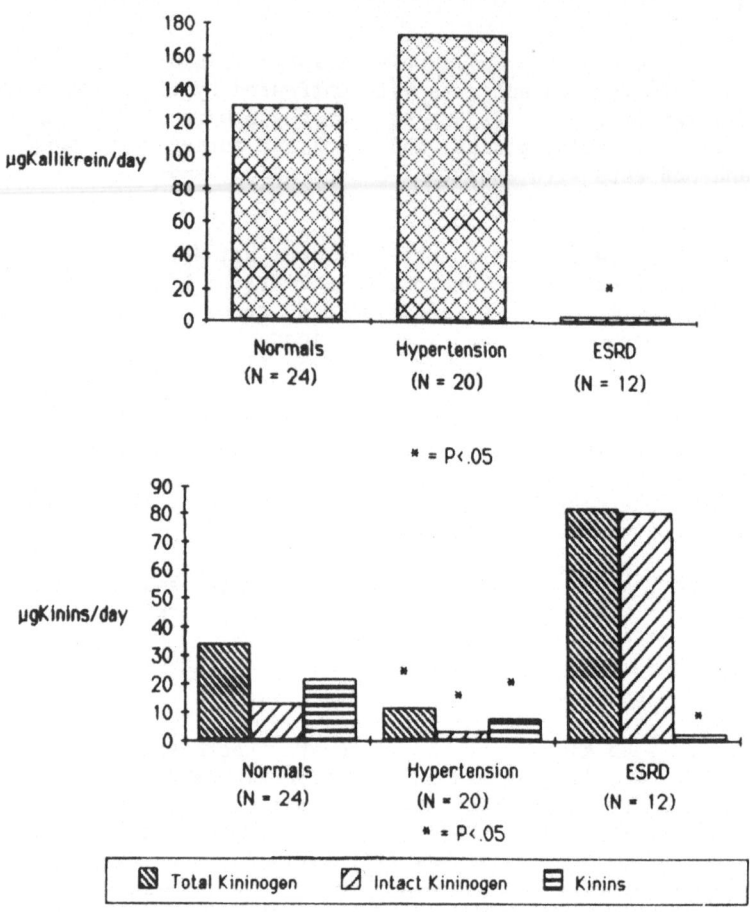

Figure 1. Urinary excretion of kallikrein, kinins, and total and intact kininogen in normals, untreated essential hypertensives, and subjects with end-stage renal disease.

DISCUSSION

This is the first study reporting the urinary excretion of total kininogen, intact kininogen, kinins and total kallikrein in normals and subjects with various human diseases. There were three findings of physiological importance in this study. First, urinary levels of intact kininogen were calculated to be approximately 1 ugkininogen/ml urine. The Km for the reaction between human urinary kallikrein and human low molecular weight kininogen has been reported to be 9.0 - 12.5 uMolar[16,17] or 0.63 - 1.0 mg/ml. Therefore, in this study intact urinary kininogen was approximately one thousand times less its Km, supporting the possibility of first order kinetics in the reaction between kallikrein and kininogen.

Secondly, there was a highly significant correlation between preformed kinins and urinary total and intact kininogen in normals, untreated essential hypertensives, and liver disease. This relationship supports the possibility that intact kininogen might influence the formation of kinins within the urine. Thus, kininogen, along with pH, cations, osmolality, kininases, kallikrein, and kallikrein inhibitors may be important in the generation of kinin formation within the tubule.

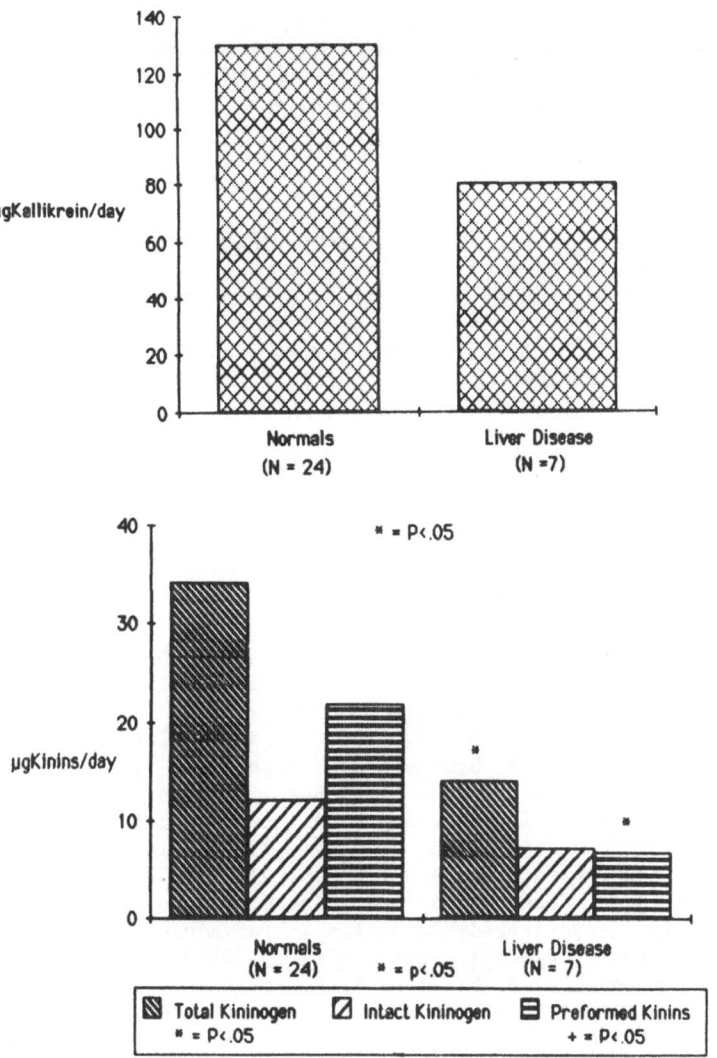

Figure 2. Urinary excretion of kallikrein, kinins, and total and intact kininogen in normals and subjects with liver disease.

Thirdly, decreased urinary kinins were found in hypertension, end-stage renal and liver diseases. However, in these diseases a different pathogenesis accounts for the deficiency in kinins. On one hand, in end-stage renal disease reduced kinins were associated with sufficient substrate (kininogen) but a lack of enzyme (kallikrein). On the other hand, in hypertension and liver disease the deficiency in urinary kinins was associated with normal kallikrein excretion but reduced total and intact kininogen. Although intact kininogen was decreased in liver disease, the lack of statistical significance may be due to the small group size. Thus, these data suggest that kallikrein alone may not be sufficient for the generation of kinins within the urinary space.

Therefore, renal kinin formation in various pathological conditions may be affected by either kininogen and/or kallikrein. Because of the potential importance of kininogen and possibility of first order kinetics in the reaction between human urinary kallikrein and low molecular weight kininogen, an evaluation of alterations in the excretion of urinary kininogen along with kinins is warranted.

REFERENCES

1. N. G. Levinsky, The renal kallikrein-kinin system, Circ. Res., 44: 441-451, (1979).
2. O. A. Carretero and A. G. Scicli, The renal kallikrein-kinin system, Am. J. Physiol., 238:F247-255, (1980).
3. W. Lieberthal, N. B. Oza, D. B. Bernard, and N. G. Levinsky, The effect of cations on the activity of human urinary kallikrein, J. Biol. Chem., 257:10827-10830, (1982).
4. J. J. Pisano, J. Corthorn, K. Yates, and J. V. Pierce: The kallikrein-kinin system in the kidney, Controv. Nephrol., 12:116-125, (1978).
5. J. L. Hulthen, J. F. Dymling, and B. Hokfeit, Kinins in relation to kallikrein activity, kininogen, electrolytes, aldosterone and catecholamines in urine from normal individuals, Acta. Physiol. Scand., 110:307-314, (1980).
6. D. Proud, M. Perkins, J. V. Pierce, K. N. Yates, P. F. Highet, P. L. Herring, M. Mangkornkanok/Mark, R. Bahu, F. Carone, and J. J. Pisano, Characterization and localization of human renal kininogen, J. Biol. Chem., 256:10634-10639, (1981).
7. M. S. Weinberg, C. A. St. Martin, P. Azar, M. Taylor, W. M. Trebbin, and R. J. Solomon, Urokininogen: A possible regulator of the kallikrein-kinin system, Clin. Res., 32:459A, (1984).
8. W. Muller-Esterl, I. Juso, and H. Fritz, Quantitation and differentiation of human kininogens by enzyme-linked immunosorbent assays (ELISA), Fresenius Z. Anal. Chem., 317:733-734, (1984).
9. V. Hial, H. R. Keiser, and J. J. Pisano, Origin and content of methionyl-lysyl-bradykinin, lysyl-bradykinin and bradykinin in human urine, Biochem. Pharmacol., 25:2499-2503, (1976).
10. M. S. Weinberg, N. B. Oza, and N. G. Levinsky, Components of the kallikrein-kinin system in rat urine, Biochem. Pharmacol., 33:1779-1782, (1984).
11. N. B. Oza, W. Lieberthal, D. B. Bernard, and N. G. Levinsky, Antibody that recognizes total human urinary kallikrein, Radioimmunological determination of inactive kallikrein, J. Immunol., 126: 2361-2364, (1983).
12. W. Lieberthal, L. Arbeit, N. B. Oza, D. B. Bernard, and N. G. Levinsky, Reduced ratio of active-to-total urinary kallikrein in essential hypertension, Hypertension, 5:603-609, (1983).
13. B. E. Huitema, The analysis of covariance and alternatives, John Wiley & Sons, New York, NY, pp. 238-240.
14. F. N. Kerlinger and E. J. Pedhazer, Multiple regression in behavioral research, Holt, Rinehart & Winston, Inc., New York, NY, pp. 83.
15. W. Muller-Esterl, M. Vohle-Timmermann, B. Boos, and B. Dittman, Purification and properties of human low molecular weight kininogen, Biochim. Biophys. Acta., 706:145-152, (1982).

16. M. Maier, K. F. Austen, and J. Spragg, Kinetic analysis of the interaction of human issue kallikrein with single chain human high and low molecular weight kininogens, Proc. Natl. Acad. Sci., 80:3928-3932, (1983).

17. J. V. Pierce and J. A. Guimaraes, Further characterization of highly purified human plasma kininogens, in: The Chemistry and Biology of the kallikrein-Kinin System in Health and Disease by J. J. Pisano and K. F. Austen, eds., U. S. Government Printing Office, Washington, D. C., pp. 121-128, (1977).

MONOCLONAL ANTIBODIES TO RAT PLASMA KININOGEN

Gurrinder S. Bedi and Nathan Back

Department of Biochemical Pharmacology
State University of New York at Buffalo
Buffalo, New York 14260

SUMMARY

Spleen cells from Balb/c mice immunized with purified rat plasma kininogen were fused to P-3 mouse myeloma cells. Positive clones were identified by enzyme linked immunosorbent assay (ELISA), cloned successively two times with limiting dilution and expanded as ascites tumors. Five hybridomas were developed that produced monoclonal antibodies against plasma kininogen. Two of the secreted antibodies were of the $IgG_1(k)$ isotype and the remaining three were of the $IgG_1(\lambda)$, $IgG_{2A}(k)$ and $IgM(k)$ isotypes respectively. The specificity of the monoclonal antibodies was confirmed by the immunoprecipitation of kininogen with the antibodies coupled to Sepharose-4B followed by SDS-polyacrylamide gel electrophoresis. These monoclonal antibodies recognize at least two distinct epitopes on rat plasma kininogen.

INTRODUCTION

Kininogens are plasma proteins that contain the peptide sequence of the vasoactive kinin polypeptides bradykinin, lysyl-bradykinin and methionyl-lysyl-bradykinin. Two molecular species of kininogen, low molecular weight (LMW) and high molecular weight (HMW), have been reported in the plasma of various mammalian species.[1] Kininogens from rat plasma and from a transplanted rodent solid tumor have been isolated, purified and characterized by this laboratory.[2-4] These kininogens are substrates for kinin-forming proteases from rodent transformed and malignant cells.[5-9] At the Kinin '81 meeting in Munich we reported on a new vasopeptide with a novel sequence formed by the action of a Murphy-Sturm lymphosarcoma tumor acid protease on rat plasma kininogen.[10] The Ile-ser-bradykinin-leu sequence of this vasopeptide suggested the presence of a kininogen in rat plasma that may lack the conventional lys-arg bond present in LMW kininogen of other species.[11] Subsequently Okamoto and Greenbaum[12] isolated and characterized an undecapeptide, termed "T-kinin", after treatment of rat plasma with trypsin also having the novel sequence ile-ser around the bradykinin. In the present study we have prepared monoclonal antibodies against purified rat plasma kininogen containing this novel vasopeptide. These antibodies will complement chemical and physical methods used to study structural and functional features of rat plasma kininogens.

MATERIAL AND METHODS

Rat plasma kininogen was purified as described earlier.[2] Dulbecco's modified Eagles' Medium, horse serum, antibiotics and fungizone were obtained from Gibco (Grand Island, N.Y.). Polyethylene glycol (4000), and 2,6,10,14-tetramethylpentadecane (Pristane) were purchased from Aldrich Chemical Co. (Milwaukee, WI). Thymidine, hypoxanthine, aminopterine, Hepes, Tris and o-phenylene diamine were supplied by Sigma Chemical Co. (St. Louis, MO). Peroxidase conjugated antimouse immunoglobulins (IgA, IgG and IgM) were purchased from Cappel Laboratories (Conchranville, PA). Selective growth medium (HAT) contained hypoxanthine (100 μM), aminopterine (0.4 μM) and thymidine (48 μM) in Dulbecco's modified medium with 10% (vol/vol) horse serum.

Immunization of Mice and Cell Fusion

Male Balb/c mice were immunized by subcutaneous injection of 50 μg of rat plasma kininogen emulsified with an equal volume of Freund's complete adjuvant. One week later the injection was repeated but with incomplete adjuvant substituted for complete. Two weeks after the second injection the mice were bled from the tail vein and assayed for antibody titer. Three days prior to fusion, the mice received an intraperitoneal injection of 50 μg of kininogen in saline solution. The spleen from the donor mouse was removed under sterile conditions and rinsed twice with Dulbecco's modified Eagle medium (DMEM). The spleen cells were released by forcing the tissue through a coarse wire gauze screen and then twice through a fine mesh screen. The cells were collected by centrifugation at 500-600 xg for 10 min, resuspended in 10 ml of ice cold 0.83% ammonium chloride and incubated on ice for 5 min. The cells were mixed with 10 ml ice cold DMEM, collected by centrifugation at 600 xg for 10 min, the pellet washed twice with 10 ml of DMEM, resuspended in 10 ml of DMEM and then counted.

Cell fusion was performed using a slightly modified procedure of Kennett et al.[13] as described earlier for the production of monoclonal antibodies to rat plasma kallikrein.[14] Mouse P3-X63-AG8-653 myeloma cells (2×10^7), washed and resuspended in serum free-DMEM, were pelleted with immune spleen cells (1×10^8). The pellet was resuspended in 100 μl ice cold Hepes buffered DMEM (HDMEM) and mixed gently with 500 μl of 60% polyethylene-glycol (final PEG concentration 50%). After 1.5 min the cells were mixed gently with 10 ml DMEM and centrifuged for 10 min at 1000 xg.

The packed cells were diluted with 20 ml DMEM containing 10% horse serum (DMEMHS), poured into a 100 mm petri dish and incubated at 37°C. After 30 min the cells were diluted with additional 28 ml DMEMHS and mixed with 48 μl of 1000 x HAT (13.6 mg hypoxanthine, 1.16 mg thymidine, and 0.18 mg aminopterin/ml). One ml was distributed to each well of two 24-well Costar tissue culture plates. Cells were grown at 37°C in a humidified 5% CO_2 atmosphere and after seven days additional 1 ml HAT medium was added to each well and thereafter one-half ml was added. The medium in each well was replaced carefully with fresh HAT medium twice a week. During the following two weeks, the HAT medium gradually was replaced by HT medium, and finally replaced by HAT-free medium.

Hybrid cells surviving HAT nutritional selection were tested for antibody production, and positive wells were cloned by limiting dilution in P-3 myeloma cells-conditioned medium. Cells from selected wells from the second cloning were expanded in tissue cultures and grown as ascites tumors by injection of 5×10^6 cells into the peritoneal cavity of male Balb/c mice primed with 2,6,10,14-tetramethylpentadecane.

Enzyme-Linked Immunosorbant Assay (ELISA)

For ELISA[15] coaster microtiter vinyl plates were coated with 10 µg/ml kininogen in 0.1 M sodium bicarbonate buffer, pH 9.6 at 37°C for 2-3 h. Non-specific binding to microtiter plate surface was blocked by soaking the wells in 0.5% bovine serum albumin in phosphate buffered saline (PBS). After four washings with PBS containing 0.2% Tween-20, the plates were incubated for 1-2 h at 37°C with culture supernatants or ascites fluid diluted in PBS. Unbound antibodies were washed 4 times with wash buffer (0.02 M Tris-HCl, pH 8.0, containing 0.2% Tween-20). The specificity-bound antibodies then were reacted for 1 h with 100 µl of 1:500 dilution of goat antimouse immunoglobulin peroxidase conjugate (Cappel Labs). Excess conjugate was removed, washed four times with wash buffer, soaked 3-5 min, and washed four more times prior to the addition of substrate. One hundred µl of 0.2% o-phenylenediamine, 0.015% H_2O_2 in 65mM phosphate-17 mM citrate buffer, pH 4.5, then was added and plates incubated at 37°C. After 30 min the reaction was stopped by the addition of 50 µl of 4 M H_2SO_4 and read at 495 nm after dilution with water.

Radioiodination of Kininogen and Measurement of Affinity

Iodination was carried out by chloramine-T procedure[16] using 5 µg of rat plasma kininogen in 20 µl of 0.1 M sodium phosphate, pH 7.2 with 0.5 mCi [^{125}I]Na. The labeled product was purified by gel filtration on a 0.9x10 cm column of Sephadex G-75. The specific activity of [^{125}I] kininogen was 35-40 µCi/µg.

For radioimmunoassays all reagents and subsequent dilutions were made in 0.05 M sodium phosphate buffer, pH 7.5, containing 0.1% bovine serum albumin. Radioimmunoassay mixture contained 0.1 ml radiolabeled kininogen, 0.1 ml of buffer or a dilution of unlabeled kininogen and 0.2 ml of serial dilutions of antibody-containing fluid. After incubation for 16 h at 4°C, 0.1 ml of sheep antimouse IgG and 0.5 ml of 15% polyethylene glycol in phosphate buffer was added. After 2 h at 4°C the tubes were centrifuged at 3000 g for 30 min. The pellet was counted in a Packard γ-counter Model 5210. For the measurement of affinity the dilution of antibodies required to give 50% maximal binding determined was used in similar incubations with various concentrations of unlabeled kininogen. The results were calculated according to Scatchard[17] in order to determine binding affinity.

RESULTS

Hybrid cell growth was present in all 48 culture wells generated from this single fusion experiment. Supernatants from 4 wells were strongly positive by the ELISA test and a supernatant from another well was slightly positive. Hybrid cells from these five wells were subcloned by limiting dilution at a cell density of one cell per well in 96-well microtiter dishes. After 3 weeks in culture, clones generated by limiting dilutions were rescreened by ELISA. Selected positive subclones were expanded and those with the highest antibody activity from each cell line were employed for ascites production in Balb/c mice primed with pristane to obtain large amount of antibodies. Culture medium from actively growing cultures of clones C4G7, D6H7, B5H10 and B2E2 showed half-maximum ELISA values at supernatant dilutions of 50 to 100 fold. More than a thousand-fold increase in titer of antibodies was observed in the ascites fluid from these clones with 50% ELISA values at approximately 10^{-5}-fold dilutions. However, ascites fluid from clone B3F4 showed a low titer with half-maximum ELISA value at 600-fold dilution. Antibody titration curves for the five clones are shown in Figure 1.

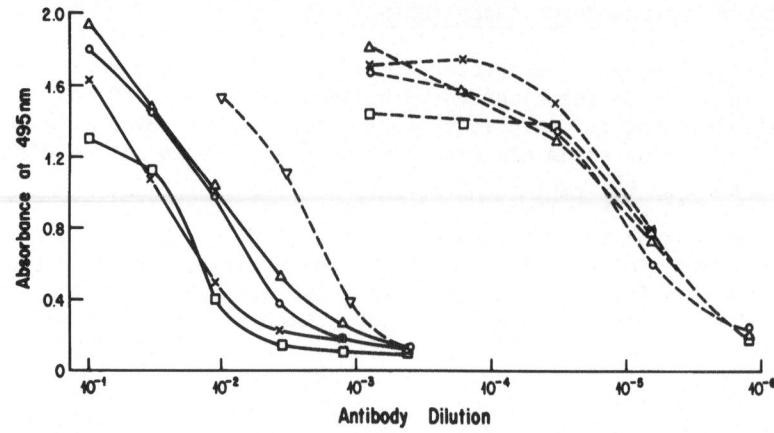

Fig. 1. Antibody titer of monoclonal antibodies to rat plasma kininogen.
ELISA was performed in microtiter plates coated with rat plasma
kininogen using suitable dilutions of culture medium (solid
lines) or ascites fluid (broken lines) from the following clones:
C4G7 (o), D6H7 (Δ), B5H10 (□), B2E2 (x) and B3F4 (∇).

Immunoglobulin Class and Subclass of Antibodies

The immunoglobulin type and subclass of antibodies in the supernatant
of culture media of cloned hybrid cells were determined by Ouchterlony
immunodiffusion with precipitating antisera. Two of the antibodies are of
the IgG_1 k isotype and one each of the IgG_1 λ, IgG_{2a}k and IgMk isotype,
respectively.

Affinity of Antibodies

The binding of [^{125}I] kininogen to monoclonal antibodies was investigated in the presence of various concentrations of unlabeled rat plasma
kininogen (Fig. 2). The binding data thus obtained were subjected to
Scatchard analysis. As shown in Fig. 2 (inset), linear relationships were
observed for all five antibodies, thus confirming their monoclonal nature.
The mean dissociation constant (K_d) values calculated from these plots
ranged between 0.58×10^{-9} M to 5.4×10^{-9} M. Table 1 summarizes the
characteristics of these monoclonal antibodies.

Determination of Distinct Epitopes on Kininogen

Two methods were used to determine the number of spatially distinct
epitopes recognized by the monoclonal antibodies. The first method was
based on an ELISA double antibody binding system developed by Friguet et
al.[18] It is presumed that when two monoclonal antibodies recongnizing
spatially distinct epitopes are used at saturating concentration the ELISA
value obtained should be equal to the sum of individual values. For each
pair of antibodies, the addivity index can be expressed as "percent
addivity" calculated by the following relation described by Friguet et
al.[18]

$$A.I. = \frac{A_{1+2} - \frac{A_1 + A_2}{2}}{A_1 + A_2 - \frac{A_1 + A_2}{2}} \times 100$$

where A_1, A_2 and A_{1+2} are the ELISA absorptions with the first antibody alone, the second antibody alone, and the 2 antibodies together respectively. Antibody pairs which recognize same antigenic site will have 0% A.I., and those with distinct binding sites 100% A.I. The results obtained are summarized in Table 2.

The second method was based on the direct competition between the two antibodies for [125I] kininogen. Excess protecting antibody was preincubated overnight at 4°C with [125I] kininogen and then the mixture added to microtiter wells coated with second monoclonal antibody. Presumption was made that if the protecting antibody recognizes the same antigenic determinant as recognized by coating antibody, no binding of labeled-antigen will be observed on microtiter plates. The results of this assay are summarized in Table 3.

No radioactive antigen binding was observed for antibody pairs KNG-C4G7-D6H7 and B5H10-B2E2 when either of the antibody pairs was used as coating antibody or as protective antibody. No distinct results could be obtained with antibody B3F4. An unrelated antibody, KAL-B3C9 against rat plasma kallikrein, when used as protective antibody, did not inhibit binding with any of the specific antibody used as coating antibodies. Based on these two experiments antibodies can be grouped into at least two general groups according to the site recognized.

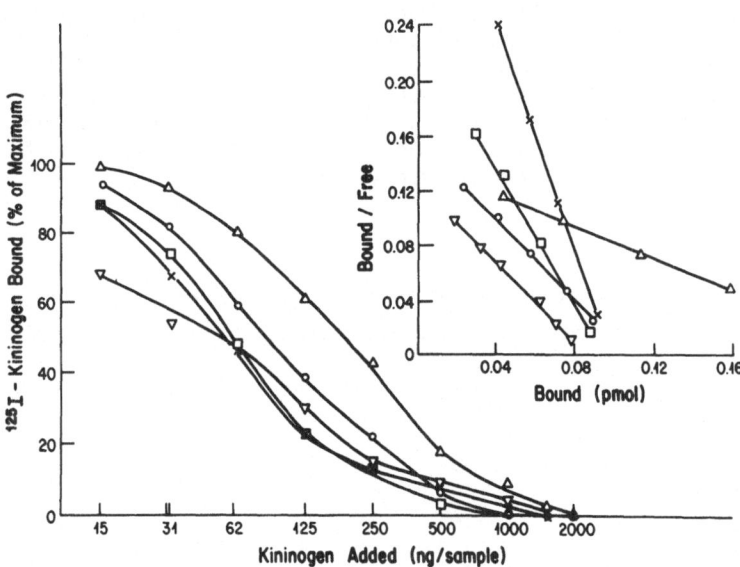

Fig. 2. Displacement of ^{125}I-labeled kininogen by unlabeled rat plasma kininogen. Monoclonal antibodies used were C4G7 (o), D6H7 (Δ) B5H10 (□), B2E2 (x), and B3F4 (∇). Scatchard plots of binding of rat plasma kininogen to monoclonal antibodies are shown in inset.

Table 1. Characteristics of the Monoclonal Antibodies

Monoclonal Antibody	Antibody Type		Titer[a]		Inhibition Constant (NG)[b]	K_d (nM)[c]
	Heavy Chain	Light Chain	Culture Medium	Ascites Fluid		
KNG–C4G7	IgG_1	λ	100	8.0×10^4	85	1.72
KNG–D6H7	IgG_1	k	90	9.0×10^4	180	5.44
KNG–B5H10	IgG_1	k	65	1.5×10^5	60	0.78
KNG–B2E2	IgG_{2a}	k	50	1.5×10^5	55	0.58
KNG–B3F4	IgM	k	10	5.0×10^2	80	1.80

[a]Amount of dilution required to obtain half maximal ELISA value.
[b]Amount of unlabeled kininogen required to give 50% inhibition of ^{125}I-labeled kininogen binding as determined from displacement curves of radio-immunoassays.
[c]K_d is the apparent equilibrium dissociation constant (avidity) of antibody-kininogen complex determined from Scatchard analyses of radioimmunoassay data.

Specificity of the Antibodies

The specificity of the monoclonal antibodies was determined by immuno-affinity purification of rat plasma kininogen. A crude kininogen prepara-tion was incubated overnight with monoclonal antibodies coupled to CNBr-activated Sepharose-4B. The bound material was eluted with 0.1 M glycine-HCl buffer, pH 2.5. Analysis of the eluate on SDS-polyacrylamide gel electrophoresis showed a single protein band with electrophoretic mobility similar to that of kininogen purified by conventional procedure (Figure 3). The eluted material was identified as kininogen by bioassay, on the iso-lated perfused rat uterus muscle preparation.[2]

Table 2. Percent Addivity Index of Monoclonal Antibodies

Ascites Fluides	C4G7	D6H7	B5H10	B2E2	B3F4
C4G7	–	13	50	50	42
D6H7	13	–	52	47	13
B5H10	50	52	–	17	0
B2E2	50	47	17	–	15
B3F4	42	17	0	15	–

Table 3. Determination of Distinct Epitopes on Rat Plasma LMW-Kininogen by Competitive Binding of Monoclonal Antibodies

Coating Antibody	Competing Antibody					Control[b]
	C4G7	D6H7	B5H10	B2E2	B3C9[a]	
	Binding of [^{125}I] kininogen (% of Control)					
KNG–C4G7	0	13	97	102	113	100
KNG–D6H7	0	0	68	72	90	100
KNG–B5H10	89	91	0	0	100	100
KNG–B2E2	100	99	12	0	93	100

[a]Unrelated monoclonal antibody against rat plasma kallikrein.
[b]No competing antibody used.

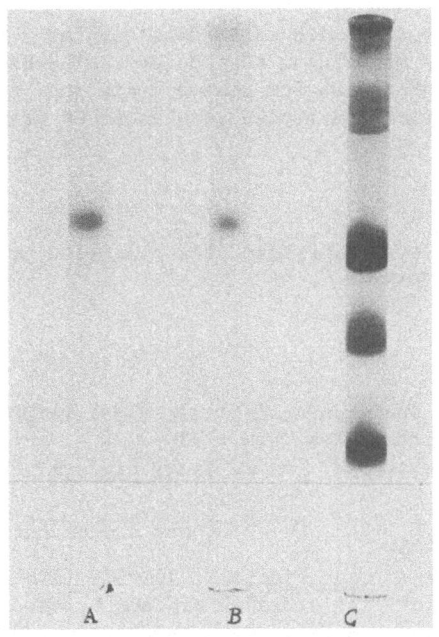

Fig. 3. SDS-polyacrylamide gel electrophoresis of rat plasma kininogen purified by immunoaffinity chromatography (A), and by conventional multistep purification procedure (B). Molecular weight markers shown in (C) are: Transferrin (90,000), bovine serum albumin (68,000), ovalbumin (45,000) and chymotrypsinogen A (25,000).

DISCUSSION

Generation of site-specific monoclonal antibodies is an important step towards understanding the structure-function relationship of closely related proteins. The presence of different species of kininogen in rat plasma raises interesting questions about the interrelationship of these plasma proteins. Monoclonal antibodies which recognize unique determinants on various forms of kininogens will be useful for immunological, biochemical and localization studies of these related proteins and for studies involving interaction of plasma kininogens with other components of the blood coagulation "cascade" system. We have used the hybridoma technique to produce five monoclonal antibodies against rat plasma kininogen. The specificity of the antibodies was confirmed by direct immunoprecipitation of the kininogen by these antibodies.

For monoclonal antibodies to be useful as site-specific probes it is essential that these antibodies should be directed against distinct epitopes. By two separate experimental approaches adopted it was concluded that these antibodies recognized at least two distinct epitopes. Although monoclonal antibodies C4G7 and D6H7 blocked the binding of one another to kininogen, suggesting that these were directed against the same or overlapping antigenic sites, they originated from different clones because both have distinct globulin-light chain. Similarly, although antibody pair B5H10 and B2E2 recognized overlapping antigenic sites, both have distinct immunoglobulin subclass. Because of low binding of monoclonal antibody B3F4 we could not define distinctly the epitope specificity for B3F4.

None of the five monoclonal antibodies interacted with human HMW and LMW-kininogen, but all except one interacted identically with Murphy-Sturm lymphosarcoma tumor kininogen (unpublished data).

Our preliminary studies with antibodies coupled to Sepharose-4B clearly show that these monoclonal antibodies can be used to develop an affinity purification procedure for plasma kininogen, thereby eliminating lengthy multistep purification procedures described previously.[2]

ACKNOWLEDGEMENT

Supported in part by U.S. Public Health Service Grant No. CA 38270, National Cancer Institute.

REFERENCES

1. H. Z. Movat, in: "Bradykinin, Kallidin and Kallikrein," E. G. Erdos, ed., Springer-Verlag, New York (1979).
2. G. S. Bedi, J. Balwierczak, and N. Back, Biochem. Pharmac., 32:2061-2069 (1983).
3. J. Balwierczak, G. S. Bedi, and N. Back, Adv. Expt. Med. and Biol., 156B:727-740 (1983).
4. H. C. Li and N. Back, Prep. Biochem., 561-579 (1980).
5. N. Back and R. Steger, in: "Bradykinin and Related Peptides," F. Sicuteri, M. Rocha e Silva, and N. Back, eds., Plenum Press, New York (1970).
6. N. Back and R. Steger, in: "Vasopeptides: Chemistry, Pharmacology and Pathophysiology, N. Back and F. Sicuteri, eds., Plenum Press, New York (1972).
7. P. P. LeBlanc and N. Back, J. Natl. Cancer Inst., 54:1107-1114 (1975).
8. H. C. Li, W. F. McLimans, and N. Back, Biochem. Pharmac., 26:1187-1195 (1975).

9. G. S. Bedi, J. Balwierczak, and N. Back, <u>Biochem. Pharmac.</u>, 32:2071-2077 (1983).

10. G. S. Bedi, J. Balwierczak, and N. Back, <u>Adv. Expt. Med. and Biol.</u>, 156B:705-726 (1983).

11. G. S. Bedi, J. Balwierczak, and N. Back, <u>Biochem. Biophys. Res. Commun.</u>, 112:621-628 (1983).

12. H. Okamoto and L. M. Greenbaum, <u>Biochem. Biophys. Res. Commun.</u>, 112:701-708 (1983).

13. R. H. Kennett, T. J. McKearn, and K. B. Bechtol, <u>in</u>: "Monoclonal Antibodies and Hybridomas: A New Dimension in Biological Analysis," Plenum Press, New York (1980).

14. G. S. Bedi and N. Back, <u>Hybridoma</u>, 3:287-292 (1984).

15. E. Engvall, <u>in</u>: "Methods in Enzymology, H. V. Vanakis and J. J. Langone, eds., Vol. 70A, Academic Press, New York (1980).

16. W. M. Hunter and F. C. Greenwood, <u>Nature</u>, 194:495-496 (1962).

17. G. Scatchard, <u>Ann. N. Y. Acad. Sci.</u>, 51:660-672 (1949).

18. B. Firguet, L. Djavadi-Ohaniance, J. Pages, A. Bussard, and M. Goldberg, <u>J. Immunol. Meth.</u>, 60:351-358 (1983).

HYDROLYSIS OF RAT HIGH MOLECULAR WEIGHT KININOGEN BY PURIFIED RAT URINARY

KALLIKREIN: IDENTIFICATION OF BRADYKININ AS THE KININ FORMED

J. P. Girolami*, F. Alhenc-Gelas**, M. L. Dos Reis**,
J. L. Bascands*, J. M. Suc**, P. Corvol**, and J. Menard**

*Inserm U 133, Route de Narbonne, 31062 Toulouse, France
**Inserm U 36, 17 rue du Fer à Moulin, 75005 Paris, France

SUMMARY

We have previously reported that, although human urinary kallikrein,
like glandular kallikreins for other species, releases lysyl-bradykinin
from homologous and heterologous substrates, rat urinary kallikrein released a kinin which migrated like bradykinin in CM-cellulose chromatography and polyacrylamide gel electrophoresis (BBA677,471,1981). In the
study we definitively established the nature of the kinin produced by rat
urinary kallikrein by using purified enzyme and substrate, HPLC, radioimmunoassay and N-terminal analysis. Rat urinary kallikrein was purified to
apparent homogeneity by a procedure which included affinity chromatography
on aprotinin agarose. The kinin produced by rat urinary kallikrein acting
on either pure rat high molecular weight kininogen or rat plasma or semi-
purified bovine and dog plasma was identified as bradykinin. This observation provides the evidence of species differences in the specificity of
glandular kallikreins acting on kininogens.

INTRODUCTION

Kallikreins are serine proteases which release the vasodilator kinins,
bradykinin (BK) (Arg-Pro-Gly-Phe-Ser-Pro-Phe-Arg) and Lys-bradykinin (LBK)
from the precursors called kininogens. Kallikreins are found in plasma and
several organs such as salivary gland, pancreas, kidney and brain. The
tissular (or glandular) kallikreins differ from plasma kallikreins. They
do not react with antibodies against each other indicating large differences
in the structure of their molecules. Moreover the enzymatic properties of
both classes of kallikrein are different. Although both plasma and glandular kallikreins are able to release kinins in blood or tissues, they differ
by substrate specificity, sensitivity to proteases inhibitors and the nature
of the kinin which they release. It is generally admitted that plasma
kallikrein hydrolyses a Lysyl-Arginine bond in high molecular weight (HMW)
kininogen and releases bradykinin (BK), whereas glandular kallikreins act
on Low molecular weight (LMW) kininogen and release a Lysyl bradykinin
(LBK). Lysyl bradykinin was in fact identified as the kinin produced by
horse and human urinary kallikrein acting on homologous substrate.[1,2]
Human and rabbit urinary kallikreins also release LBK from bovine kininogen.[3,4] However such a distinction between the nature of the products

formed by glandular and plasma kallikreins may not be true in the rat. We indeed reported that rat urine acting on bovine or rat semipurified kininogen released a kinin which migrated like BK and not LBK on polyacrylamid gel electrophoresis and on CM-cellulose chromatography.[3] Recently it was also reported that high concentration of trypsin release from rat plasma a new kinin called T-kinin which has the structure of an Ile-Ser-bradykinin. We decided to further precise the nature of the kinin released by rat urinary kallikrein from rat kininogen by using: completely purified enzyme and substrate, purification on high performance liquid chromatography, radioimmunoassay of kinins and N-terminal aminoacid analysis. In this paper we report that rat urinary kallikrein hydrolyses homologous HMW kininogen and releases a kinin which is identical to bradykinin.

MATERIALS AND METHODS

Bradykinin triacetate, Lysyl bradykinin and Met-Lys-bradykinin were from Bachem, DEAE Sephacel and Sephadex G100 were purchased from Pharmacia, Aprotinin-Agarose was provided by Dr. E. Sache, Choay Chimie S2266 and S2244 were from Kabi Vitrum, dansyl chloride and dansyl aminoacids were from Sigma, Micropolyamide sheets F1700 were supplied by Schleicher and Schull.

Collection of Urine

Six liters of urine were collected from female Sprague Dawley rats and centrifuged for 10 min at 1000 x g. The proteins were precipitated with ammonium sulfate at 80% saturation, then dialyzed against water and lyophilized.

Purification of Urinary Kallikrein

The kallikrein was purified by a three step procedure which included ion exchange chromatography, aprotinin affinity chromatography and gel filtration[5] (Table 1).

Kallikrein Activity Assay

Kallikrein in the column effluents was monitored by its amidolytic activity using the synthetic substrate S2266 (Val-Leu-Arg-pNa).[6] The results are expressed in nanomoles of S2266 hydrolyzed per minute of incubation per ml. The kininogenase activity was also determined and measured as previously described.[3]

Proteins Measurement

Proteins in the column effluents were monitored by their absorbance at 280 nm. Proteins concentration was determined by the method of Lowry et al.[7]

Polyacrylamide Gel Electrophoresis

Vertical gel electrophoresis was performed as previously described.[8] Acrylamide concentration in the gels was 2%.

Isoelectric Focusing

Isoelectric focusing was carried out in an LKB Multiphor apparatus. Gels contained 5% acrylamide, 2% bis acrylamide and 1% ampholine pH 3 to 6. The cathode wick buffer eas ethylenediamine (4 ml/l) and the anode wick buffer was 0.02% sulfuric acid.

Purification of Rat HNW Kininogen

Rat HMW kininogen was purified to apparent homogeneity from rat plasma as described elsewhere.[9] The purified kininogen has a kinin content of 10-12 µg BK per mg of protein, as determined after trypsin hydrolysis.

Generation of Kinin by Rat Urinary Kallikrein (RUK) From Rat HMW Kininogen and Various Kininogen Preparations

HMWK was hydrolyzed by RUK in the following conditions: 12 µg of protein corresponding to 12 ng of bradykinin equivalents were incubated with 1 µg of purified urinary kallikrein for 30 min at 37ºC. The reaction was then stopped with cold 95% ethanol (4/1,V/v). Following centrifugation at 2000 x g for 10 min the supernatant was evaporated and the residue was resuspended in 0,1M phosphate buffer pH 7. Rat plasma, dog and bovine semi purified substrate were prepared as previously described.[3] 15 mg containing 2000 µg of bradykinin generating capacity were also incubated with RUK in the same conditions than described for HMWK.

High Performance Liquids Chromatography Separation

The kinin produced was analysed on HPLC. HPLC was performed on a water HPLC apparatus (model 600) using a C 18 ubondapack column. The elution was made with 18% acetonitrile in 0.04 M triethylammonium formate pH 3,15 at a flow rate of 0,7 ml/min and 0,3 ml fractions were collected. The kinins were detected with a bradykinin radioimmunoassay.[3] Bradykinin Lysyl bradykinin and Met-Lys-bradykinin (MLBK) were run to calibrate the system. The antibodies raised against BK recognized longer analogs such as LBK and MLBK but none of the BK fragments.

N-Terminal Group Analysis by Dansylation

The kinins purified on HPLC were dansylated according to the method of Gray and Hartley[10] and hydrolysed. The hydrolysate was dissolved in acetone acetic acid (3/2, v/v) and spotted on micropolyamide sheet (5x5 cm). A two dimensional ascending chromatography was performed in the following solvent systems. Solvent I: water formic acid (50/1 v/v) solvent II: Benzene: acetic acid (9/1 v/v). One picomole of each dansylated aminoacid can be detected on the sheet by UV light absorption.

RESULTS AND DISCUSSION

Purification of RUK

The results of the purifications are shown in Table 1. DEAE Sephacel chromatography allowed a 13 fold purification. Recovery of kallikrein was 91%, as determined by kininogenase activity. A small amount of amidolytic activity was not retained on the column (Fig. 1a), no kininogenase activity was detectable on these fractions. This non kallikrein amidolytic activity might be identical to esterase A. The fractions corresponding to kallikrein were pooled. The kallikrein isolated from DEAE Sephacel was devoid of uro-kinase activity. After affinity chromatography, a contaminant with a MW of 68000 was present together with kallikrein on SDS gel electrophoresis. This contaminating protein was eliminated by gel filtration on Sephadex G100 (Fig. 1c).

Table 1.   Purification of Rat Urinary Kallikrein

	Protein (mg)	Specific Amidolytic Activity μmoles/min/mg	Specific Kininogenase Activity (μg/min/mg)	Recovery*	Purification*
Crude Enzyme	3114	0.101	1.73	100	1
DEAE Sephacel Chromatography	220	0.895	22.5	91	13
Iniprol Agarose Affinity	2.62	10.8	352.	25	307
Sephadex G100 Chromatography	0.68	39.86	910	10.2	526

*Calculated on the basis of kininogenase activity.

Fig. 1.   a: DEAE Sephacel chromatography of urinary proteins column 5x30 cm sample applied : 2.5 g proteins in 40 ml of 0.1M phosphate buffer pH 5; fraction volume 10 ml, flow rate 80 ml/h. (---) absorbance at 280 nm; (......) conductivity; (———) amidolytic activity.

   b: Affinity chromatography of kallikrein purified on DEAE Sephacel (----) Absorbance at 280 nm   (......) pH (———) amidolytic activity.   Elution : step 1 : 0.1 M sodium phosphate, buffer pH 7.8,   step 2 : 0.1 M sodium phosphate buffer pH 6, step 3 : 0.1 M acetate buffer pH 3.5.

   c: Sephadex G100 filtration of kallikrein purified by DEAE Sephacel and affinity chromatography fraction volume : 3 ml flow rate : 19 ml/h buffer 0.01 M sodium phosphate buffer pH 7, 1 M in NaCl.

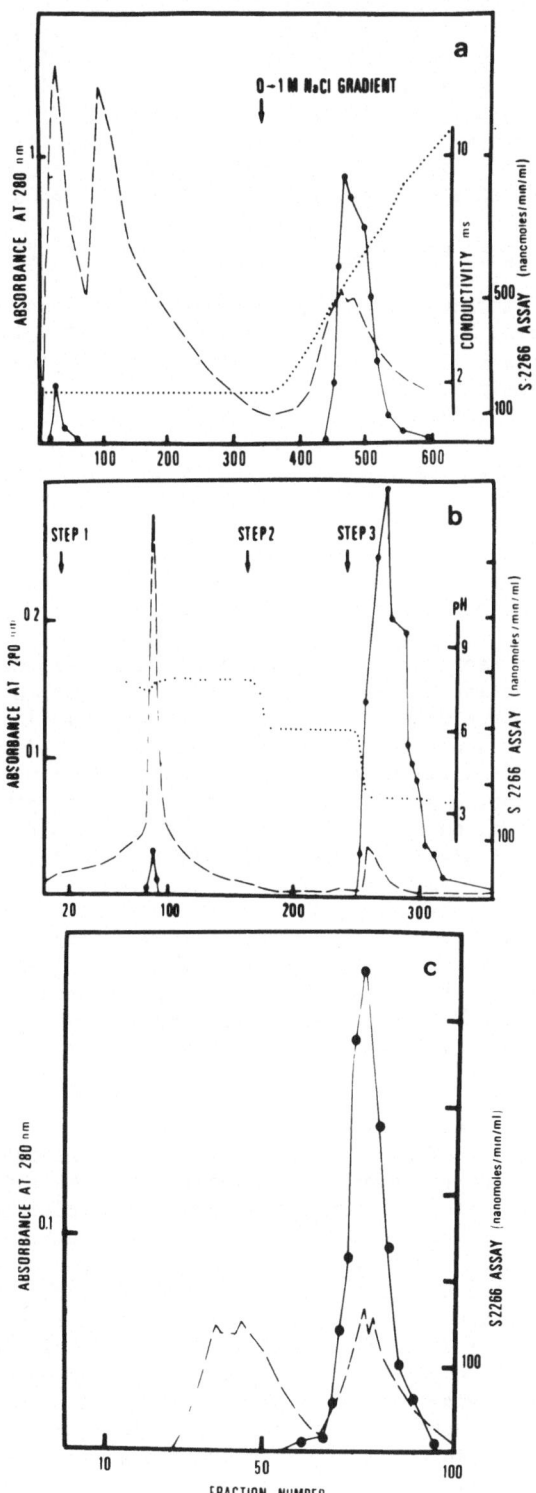

Characterization of Purified Urinary Kallikrein

The purified kallikrein displayed two bands on SDS disc gel electrophoresis with molecular weight of 28 and 29000 respectively (Fig. 2). On isoelectric focusing two main components of PI 3.90 and 4.08 (Fig. 2) were separated. The specific activities of purified kallikrein were 910 µg kinin/min/mg of proteins when citrate dog plasma is used as substrate, 420 µg kinin/min/mg of protein on bovine plasma and 909 µg kinin/min/mg of protein on rat HMW kininogen. The specific activity estimated by the amidolytic assay was 39,86 µmoles of S2266 hydrolyzed/min/mg of protein.

Hydrolysis of Kininogens and Identification of Generated Kinins

Hydrolysis of rat HMWK by pure urinary kallikrein was substrate and enzyme dependent (Fig. 3). HMW kininogen was not completely exhausted by RUK, the kinins released event after a prolonged incubation time up to 1 hour were approximately 50% of the amount of kinins liberated by trypsin. When the product of kallikrein with rat HMWK was analyzed on reversed phase HPLC and radioimmunoassay, immunoreactivity was only detected as a single peak with a retention time identical to that of bradykinin (Fig. 4). When LBK was incubated together with rat urinary kallikrein and kininogen, it was recovered in a separate peak with a recovery around 95% confirming that no aminopeptidase activity was present in the preparations. The N-terminal amino acid analysis of the kinin purified on HPLC showed that the N-terminal amino acid had the same R_f than arginin in Table 2.

In spite of the fact that the separation of standard dansyl arginine and dansyl lysine was incomplete in the systems used, the addition of standard arginine to the unknown sample gave a single well limited spot whereas two confluent spots were observed when dansyl lysine was added to the sample instead of dansyl arginine. When pure rat urinary kallikrein was incubated with rat, dog or bovine plasma. The kinin generated had the same retention time on HPLC (16 min) than BK and its N-terminal residue had the same R_f than bradykinin. The N-terminal amino-acid was clearly different from the other amino-acid tested including isoleucine and serine.

The kinin produced by rat urinary kallikrein acting on homologous substrate was identified as bradykinin by the following arguments 1) it is recognized by the antibody against BK, 2) it has the same retention time than BK on HPLC, 3) the N-terminal amino acid is arginine. A new kinin, Ileu-Ser-BK or T kinin was recently discovered in the rat.[11] The kinin produced by RUK on HMW kininogen is however bradykinin and not T kinin or Ser Bradykinin. It is in fact considered that T kinin is produced by trypsin from plasma protein substrate called T kininogen. The fact that rat UK releases BK from HMW kininogen or rat plasma, whereas glandular kallikrein from at least three other species release LBK from homologous or heterologous substrate (1-2-4) shows, that species specificity occurs in the reaction between glandular kallikreins and kininogens. The rat appears to be an exception among other species since it does not release LBK. Differences in the structure of kininogens between the rat and other species, specially in the pre-BK sequence of the molecule can explain that the nonapeptide BK is produced in one case and the decapeptide LBK in the other. However rat UK releasesalso BK from bovine and dog substrate. The primary structure of bovine high and low molecular weight kininogen has been established and it appears that both kininogens have a Met Lys bradykinin sequence in their molecule.[12] It therefore appears that rat urinary kallikrein cleaves as Lys-Arg bond in bovine kininogen whereas human urinary kallikrein cleaves a Met-Lys bond in the same molecule.[3] Our study demonstrated that BK is the kinin produced by urinary kallikrein in the rat and that species differences occur in the specificity of glandular kallikrein.

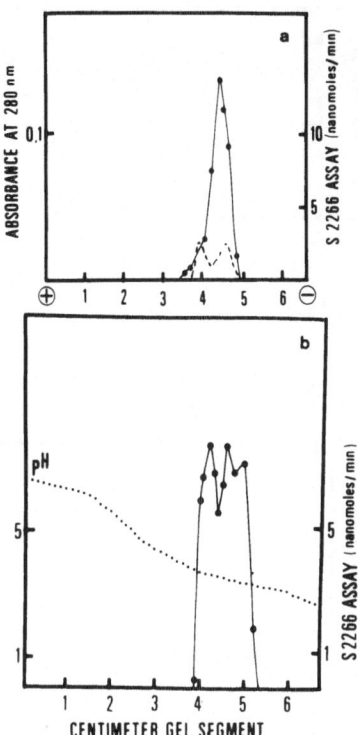

Fig. 2. SDS page electrophoresis (a) and isoelectrofocusing (b) of purified rat urinary kallikrein.

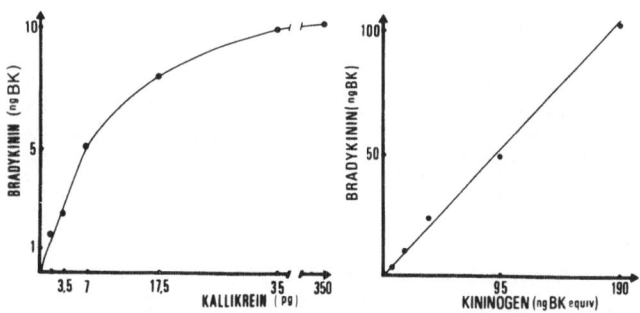

Fig. 3. Hydrolysis of rat HMW kininogen by rat urinary kallikrein.
   (a) Incubation of 20 µg of HMW kininogen with various amount of
        kallikrein for 30 min at 37°C in 0.5 ml of phosphate buffer
        pH 8.5, 3 mM EDTA and 3 mM o-phenanthroline.
   (b) Incubation of various amounts of kininogen with 1 µg of
        kallikrein.

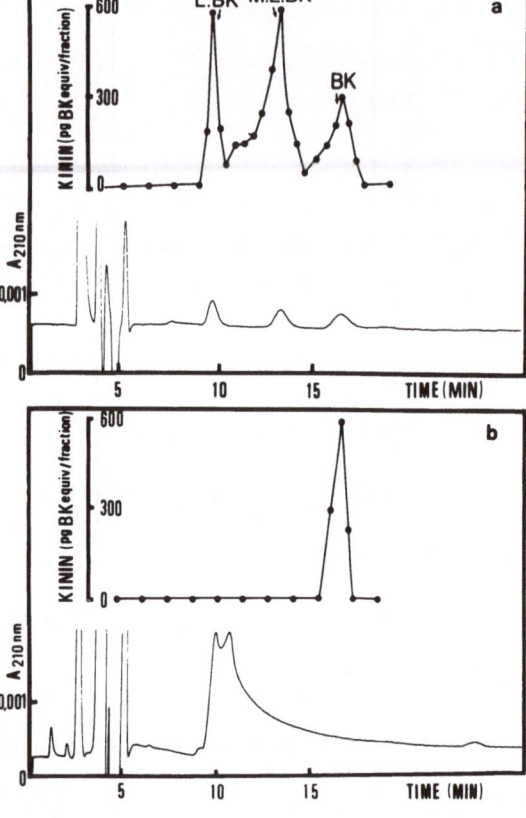

Fig. 4. Reverse phase HPLC of standard kinins (a) and of the kinin produced by rat urinary kallikrein on rat HMW kininogen (b).

Table 2. N-Terminal Analysis

Chromatography of Different Dansyl Amino Acids

Dansyl Aminoacid	RF1	RF2
Arginine	0.9	0.01
Lysine	0.9	0.15
Methionine	0.25	0.22
Isoleucine	0.3	0.66
Proline	0.39	0.77
Serine	0.70	0.20

Amino Terminal Analysis of Peptides Liberated By
Rat Urinary Kallikrein From Various Kininogen Preparations

Kininogen Source	RF1	RF2
Pure HMWG	0.88	0.0
Bovine plasma	0.87	0.0
Dog plasma	0.88	0.0
Rat plasma	0.87	0.0

ACKNOWLEDGMENTS

This study was supported in part by the Fondation pour la Recherche
Médicale. The authors wish to thank C. Mora and C. Sabardu for technical
assistance in preparing the manuscript.

REFERENCES

1. J. V. Pierce and M. E. Webster, Human plasma kallidins: Isolation and
   chemical studies, Biochem. Biophys. Res. Commun., 5:353-357 (1961).
2. E. S. Prado, M. E. Webster, and J. L. Prado, Kallidin (Lysyl-bradykinin),
   the kinin formed from horse plasma by horse urinary kallikrein,
   Biochem. Pharmacol., 20:2009-2015 (1971).
3. F. Alehnc-Gelas, J. Marchetti, J. Allegrini, P. Corvol, and J. Menard,
   Measurement of urinary kallikrein activity species differences in
   kinin production, Biochem. Biophys. Acta, 677:477-488 (1981).
4. J. Marchetti, Personal communication.
5. Nib. Oza, V. M. Amin, R. K. McGregor, A. G. Scicli, and O. A. Carretero,
   Isolation of rat urinary kallikrein and properties of its antibodies, Biochem. Pharmacol., 25:1607-1612 (1976).
6. E. Amunsen, J. Putter, P. Friberger, M. Knos, M. Lars Braten, and G.
   Claeson, Methods for the determination of glandular kallikrein by
   means of a chromogenic tripeptide substrate, in: "Kinins-II," S.
   Fujii, H. Moriya, and T. Suzuki, eds., Plenum Press (1979).
7. O. M. Lowry, N. J. Rosebrough, A. L. Faar, and R. J. Randall, Protein
   measurement with the folin phenol reagent, J. Biol. Chem., 193:265-
   275 (1951).
8. V. K. Laemmli, Cleavage of structural proteins during the assembly of
   the head of bacteriphage T4, Nature, 227:680-685 (1970).
9. M. L. Dos Reiss, F. Alhenc-Gelas, J. Allegrini, D. Kerbiriou, P. Corvol,
   and J. Menard, High molecular weight kininogen (HMW Kg) in the rat.
   Complete purification antibodies. Demonstration of lack of immunoreactive kininogen in a strain of Brown-Norway rats, Biochim.
   Biophys. Acta (Submitted).
10. W. R. Gray and B. S. Hartley, Determination of N-terminal amino acid
    by the dansyl method, Biochem. J., 89:379-393 (1963).
11. H. Okamoto and L. M. Greenbaum, Isolation and structure of T-Kinin,
    Biochem. Biophys. Res. Comm., 112:701-708 (1983).
12. H. Nawa, N. Kitamura, T. Mirose, M. Asai, S. Inayama, and S. Nakanishi,
    Primary structures of bovine liver low molecular weight kininogen
    precursors and their two mRNAs, Proc. Natl. Acad. Sci. USA, 80:90-
    94 (1983).

REDUCED OR UNCHANGED COFACTOR FUNCTION OF HUMAN HIGH MOLECULAR WEIGHT

KININOGEN INDUCED BY HUMAN PLASMA KALLIKREIN

Harald Thidemann Johansen and Kjell Briseid

Department of Pharmacology, Institute of Pharmacy, University
University of Oslo, Blindern, Oslo 3, Norway

SUMMARY

Plasma kallikrein activated spontaneously during the purification of
prekallikrein (I) and acetone-activated plasma kallikrein (II) were at pH
7.4 both capable of reducing the capacity of purified human high molecular
weight kininogen (HMrK) to function as cofactor in the contact phase activation of factor XII in a crude plasma preparation. At pH 6.8 only I had
such an effect. SDS polyacrylamide gel electrophoresis with reduction indicated that both I and II contained kallikrein as a cleaved three-chain
molecule. I contained in addition a Mr 49,000 fraction reflecting possibly
uncleaved heavy chain. The registration of reduced cofactor function of
HMrK induced by plasma kallikrein is discussed in view of the assay procedure
used.

INTRODUCTION

Several reports in the literature state that the capacity of human
high molecular weight kininogen (HMrK) to function as a cofactor in the
contact phase activation of factor XII remains unchanged after treatment
with plasma kallikrein.[1-4] The cofactor-active light chain part of the
HMrK molecule was found to be very slowly digested by plasma kallikrein.[5]
The interactions, however, between HMrK and plasma kallikrein are not yet
fully elucidated: Chan et al.[6] reported on an extensive loss of the cofactor
activity of HMrK that went parallel with the kallikrein-induced release of
bradykinin, whereas Scott et al.[7] described HMrK as a pro-cofactor needing
activation by plasma kallikrein to gain functional activity. In a recent
paper Johansen and Briseid[8] reported on the reduction at different rats of
the cofactor activity of HMrK induced by different preparations of human
plasma kallikrein. In the present work we have studied in parallel the
effects on HMrK of plasma kallikrein activated spontaneously during the isolation of prekallikrein,[8] and plasma kallikrein purified after acetone activation, and stated to contain a cleaved heavy chain.[9]

METHODS

Plasminogen-free rat citrated plasma with benzamidine was prepared and
acetone-treated as described previously.[10]

147

High molecular weight kininogen (HMrK) was isolated from fresh human citrated plasma.[5] The preparations used had specific activities of 10-13 (µg bradykinin/A 280).

Spontaneous plasma kallikrein   Plasma prekallikrein was partially purified.[11] Kallikrein activated spontaneously during the purification procedure was isolated as described previously.[8]

Acetone-activated plasma kallikrein was prepared according to Nagase and Barrett.[9]

Substrate for assay of factor XIIa (prekallikrein activator, PKA). Human prekallikrein was partially purified,[11] and kallikrein eventually generated during the purification procedure was removed.[8]

Assay of esterase activity was carried out with benzoyl arginine ethylester (BAEe) as substrate.[10] One esterase unit corresponds to 1 µmol ester split per min. at 25°.

Assay of amidolytic activity was carried out with the tripeptide substrate H-D-Pro-Phe-Arg-pNA 2 HCl (S-2302). The substrate was dissolved 2 mM in distilled water. The enzyme preparations were diluted in tris buffer 50 mM, pH 7.9, so that a mixture of 400 µl diluted test and 200 µl substrate solution produced a rise in O.D. at 405 nm in the range 0.1-0.4 in 2 min. One amidase unit corresponds to 1 µmol p-nitroanilide split per min. at 25°.

Assay of HMrK functionally active as cofactor for the activation of factor XII   At 25° 80 µl of prekallikrein (6.0 BAEe esterase units per ml) were incubated with 20 µl of activator preparation (acetone-treated plasminogen-free rat plasma freshly diluted 1+5 v/v with 5 mM phosphate, 150 mM NaCl buffer of pH 7.4, and incubated 1+1 v/v with a suspension of kaolin 20 mg/ml in 150 mM NaCl for 2 min. at 25°). Aliquots were withdrawn after 20 sec., and after 3 min. and 20 sec., and the rate of activation of S-2302 amidase was determined. The amount of activated factor XII was calculated as PKA units per ml plasma, one PKA-U being the amount of activator that activates one S-2302 unit of prekallikrein per min. at 25°. When HMrK was introduced in connection with the dilution of the plasma preparation, the increased level of activated factor XII reflected the cofactor capacity of the added HMrK.

Assay of plasminogen activator (PGA) was carriedout by the fibrin plate method.[12,10]

Polyacrylamide gel electrophoresis of proteins was carried out as described previously.[8]

Isoelectric focusing of proteins was run in a 5% polyacrylamide gel containing Pharmalyte® 3-10, for 3000 volthours.

Chemicals used are referred to in previous papers.[8,10,13]

RESULTS

Plasma Kallikrein

All plasma kallikrein preparations tested produced two bands in SDS polyacrylamide gel electrophoresis without reduction, one main band corresponding to a Mr of about 83,000 and a weaker band of Mr about 80,000. Run in SDS polyacrylamide gels with reduction both kallikrein activated spontaneously during prekallikrein purification,[8] and kallikrein purified from acetone-activated plasma[9] yielded bands correspondign to molecular weights of 22,000, 31,000, 34,000 and 36,000, indicating the presence of kallikreins I and II as three-chain enzymes.[9] The spontaneous kallikrein yielded in addition a protein band with a Mr close to 49,000, possibly reflecting the presence also of uncleaved heavy chain.

Isoelectric focusing of the kallikrein preparations showed microheterogeneity in the pH-range 8.05-8.60. Four peaks were regularly present corresponding to pH 8.11, 8.25, 8.33 (the strongest one) and 8.38.

Freshly prepared preparations of spontaneously activated plasma kallikrein showed different degrees of plasminogen activator activity when related to the esterase (BAEe) or amidase (S-2302) activities present. The PGA activities regularly declined during storage at -70°, whereas the esterase and amidase activities were more stable.[8] The PGA activities obtained with the acetone-activated plasma kallikrein[9] were always low, usually not exceeding 200 CTA mU/BAEe esterase unit, whereas the same ratio for kallikrein activated spontaneously and tested freshly made, was about 600.[8]

The two kinds of preparations compared in the present work (Fig.'s 2 and 3) showed about the same PGA activities after storage of several months at -70°C; CTA mU/BEe esterase unit being assayed to 193 and 211 for acetone activated kallikrein and spontaneous kallikrein respectively.

Effect of Different Plasma Kallikrein Preparations on the Cofactor Activity of High Molecular Weight Kininogen

In the undiluted crude plasma preparation used as a source of factor XII HMrK is protected from destruction by acetone-activated proteases by the presence of benzamidine 7.5 mM. During the kaolin treatment of the diluted plasma a partial destruction of the HMrK cofactor activity takes place, reducing the extent of activation of factor SII correspondingly.[13] Purified HMrK added prior to the kaolin activation procedure will stoichiometrically increase the yield fo factor XII a (Fig. 1).

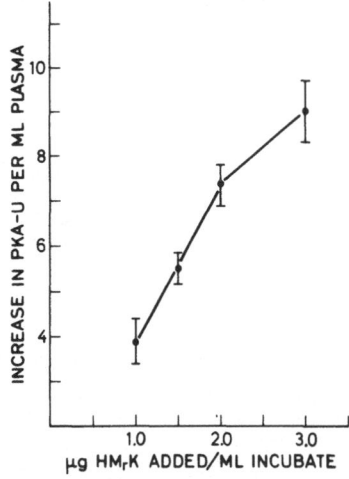

Fig. 1.   Assay of HMrK as a cofactor for the activation of factor XII in a plasma preparation. Increase in prekallikrein activator (PKA) activity caused by the addition of different amounts of HMrK to diluted plasma. HMrK amounts stated refer to ml kaolin incubate. Kallikrein assayed as S-2302 amidase.

Fig.'s 2 and 3 demonstrate the cofactor effects remaining in HMrK after treatment with the two different kinds of kallikrein preparation for different periods of time. Parallel control incubates of HMrK with buffer solution showed no change in HMrK cofactor activity during the experimental periods.

When HMrK was incubated with plasma kallikrein at pH 7.4 both acetone-activated and spontaneously activated kallikrein were able to reduce the cofactor activity obtainable with HMrK, and at about the same rate (Fig. 2). When the incubations were carried out at pH 6.8, however, only the spontaneously activated kallikrein was capable of reducing the cofactor activity of HMrK to some extent (Fig. 3, I), whereas the acetone-activated kallikrein rather caused an increase in the HMrK cofactor activity (Fig. 3, II).

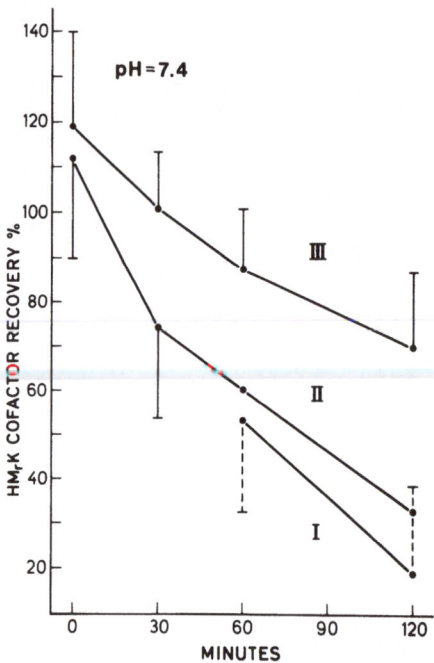

Fig. 2. Plasma kallikrein induced loss of cofactor activity of HMrK as a function of time, pH 7.4. Incubates of HMrK and plasma kallikrein were tested for HMrK cofactor activity remaining after 30, 60 or 120 minutes. I: Acetone-activated plasma kallikrein. HMrK 4.8 µg/ml incubated with kallikrein 0.10 BAEe esterase U/ml corresponding to 0.34 S-2302 amidase U/ml. II: Spontaneously activated plasma kallikrein. HMrK 7.2 µg/ml incubated with kallikrein as in I. III: Acetone-activated plasma kallikrein. HMrK 7.2 µg/ml incubated with kallikrein as in I.

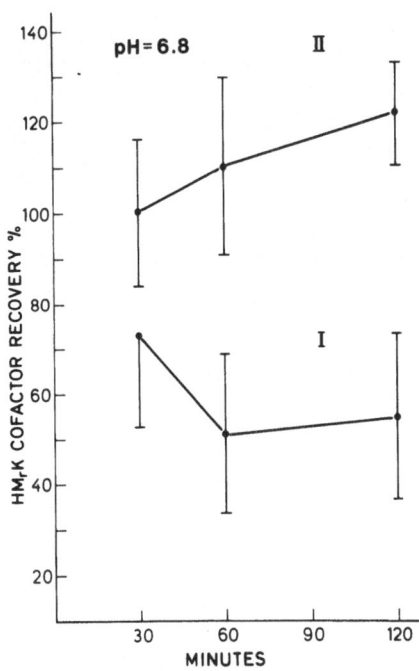

Fig. 3.   Plasma kallikrein induced loss of cofactor activity of HMrK as
a function of time, pH 6.8.   Apart from the lower pH used for
the incubates, the experiments designed as those presented in
Fig. 2.   The concentration of HMrK was the same for both kallikrein
preparations tested.   I: Spontaneously activated plasma kallikrein.
II: Acetone-activated plasma kallikrein.

DISCUSSION

In the present work plasma kallikrein prepared by two different methods
were both found capable of altering purified HMrK in such a way that the
reaction product had a significantly reduced capacity to function as a
cofactor in the contact phase activation of factor XII.   The kallikrein
preparations tested had PGA activities of the same order of size at the
time they were tested in the cofactor assay.   A crude acetone-activated
plasma preparation was used as the source of factor XII.   The results
provide evidence that the kallikrein preparations invstigated were either
themselves capable of causing a destruction of the cofactor activity in
HMrK, or the induced cleavage of HMrK would render the HMrK molecule more
susceptible to destruction by proteases present in the plasma preparation.
Further, the possibility of an inhibiting effect by clealvled HMrK in the
crude assay system used, instead of a destruction of its cofactor effect,
can not be excluded.   In the present work we used rat plasma instead of
human plasma because the precision of the cofactor assays was thereby improved, but otherwise the two kinds of plasma seemed to function similarly
in our assay procedure.   The fact that both acetone-activated plasma kallikrein[9] and kallikrein activated spontaneously during the purification of
prekallirein[8] were capable of reducing the cofactor effect of HMrK at pH
7.4, whereas only the spontaneously activated enzyme was effective at pH
6.8, indicates the presence of functional differences between the two preparations.

In SDS polyacrylamide gel electrophoresis without reduction both preparations showed the same protein pattern: one main band and one weaker band
corresponding to Mr values of 83,000 and 80,000 respectively.   As shown

by Nagase and Barrett[9] we found that the acetone-activated kallikrein in
SDS polyacrylamide gels with reduction yielded protein bands that indicated
the presence of the two forms of kallikrein as three-chain molecules.
In the spontaneously activated plasma kallikrein we could in addition regis-
ter a protein band corresponding to a Mr close to 49,000. This band might
reflect the presence also of some uncleaved kallikrein heavy chain.

The plasma kallikrein induced reduction of the cofactor activity of
HMrK observed in the present work might seem surprising, considering the
clear evidence in the literature that the light chain part of the HMrK
molecule retains full cofactor capacity.[1-5] As discussed above treatment
of HMrK with plasma kallikrein might not necessarily in a direct manner
destroy its cofactor activity, but rather induce alterations in the HMrK
molecule that renders it more susceptible to destruction in the plasma
system used. Further work is required to settle this problem.

REFERENCES

1. R. E. Thompson, R. Mandle, Jr., and A. P. Kaplan, Characterization
    of human high molecular weight kininogen. Procoagulant activity
    associated with the light chainof kinin-free high molecular weight
    kininogen, J. Exp. Med., 147:488-499 (1978).
2. D. M. Kerbiriou and J. H. Griffin, Human high molecular weight kinino-
    gen. Studies of structure-function relationships and of proteolysis
    of the molecule occurring during contact activation of plasma, J.
    Biol. Chem., 254:12020-12027 (1979).
3. S. Schiffman, C. Mannhalter, and K. D. Tyner, Human high molecular
    weight kininogen. Effects of cleavage by kallikrein on protein
    structure and procoagulant activity, J. Biol. Chem., 255:6433-6438
    (1980).
4. M. Silverberg, J. E. Nicoll, and A. p. Kaplan, The mechanism by which
    the light chain of cleaved HMW-kininogen augments the activation
    of prekallikrein, factor XI and Hageman factor, Thromb. Res.,
    20:173-189 (1980).
5. R. E. Tghompson, R. Mandle, Jr., and A. P. Kaplan, Studies of binding
    of prekallikrein and factor XI to high molecular weight kininogen
    and its light chain, Proc. Natl. Acad. Sci. U.S.A., 76:4862-4866
    (1979).
6. J. Y. C. Chan, H. Z. Movat, and C. E. Burrowes, High molecular weight
    kininogen: its inability to correct the clotting of kininogen-defi-
    cient plasma after cleavage of bradykinin by plasma kallikrein,
    plasmin or trypsin, Thromb. Res., 14:817-824 (1979).
7. C. F. Scott, L. D. Silver, M. Schapira, and R. W. Colman, Cleavage
    of human high molecular weight kininogen markedly enhances its
    coagulant activity, J. Clin. Invest., 73:954-962 (1984).
8. H. T. Johansen and K. Briseid, Reduced cofactor function of human high
    molecular weight kininogen induced by human plasma kallikrein,
    Acta Pharmacol. et Toxicol., 55:25-32 (1984).
9. H. Nagase and A. J. Barrett, Human plasma kallikrein. A rapid purifi-
    cation method with high yield, Biochem. J., 193:187-192 (1981).
10. H. T. Johansen and K. Briseid, Separation of plasma kallikrein and
    a kallikrein-like plasminogen activator generated by acetone in
    rat plasma, Acta Pharmacol. et Toxicol., 52:371-380 (1983).
11. K. Laake and A. M. Venneröd, Determination of factor XII in human
    plasma with arginine proesterase (prekallikrein). I. Preparation
    and properties of the substrate, Thromb. Res., 2:393-407 (1973).
12. F. Haverkate and P. Brakman, in: "Progress in Chemical Fibrinolysis
    and Thrombolysis, J. F. Davidson, M. M. Samama, and P. C. Desnoyers,
    eds.

13. K. Briseid and H. T. Johansen, Activation of factor XII in human plasma: Protection by benzamidine of the cofactor function of high molecular weight kininogen, <u>Acta Pharmacol. et Toxicol.</u>, 53:344-352 (1983).

STUDIES ON THE ANTIGENIC DETERMINANTS OF HUMAN LOW MOLECULAR WEIGHT

KININOGEN

Tytti Kärkkäinen, Ann-Christine Syvänen and Ulla Hamberg[*]

Department of Biochemistry, University of Helsinki
Unioninkatu 35, SF-00170 Helsinki 17, Finland
*Deceased

INTRODUCTION

The antigenic reactivity of proteins is located in restricted parts
of the molecule forming the antigenic determinants that react with the
binding sites of the antibody molecule.[1] Low molecular weight (LM_r) and
high molecular weight (HM_r) kininogens are immunologically related molecules with common antigenic determinants in the heavy chain of both
proteins.[2-4] We have further characterized the nature of these determinants
using a kinin-free LM_r kininogen isolated from Cohns plasma fraction IV
(H_C antigen).[5,6] As shown recently[7] the determinant structure of kininogen reside in the polypeptide backbone of the molecule and is not influenced by the partial removal of carbohydrates. This antigen has a
heterogeneous light chain which can be isolated after reduction and
carboxymethylation. An antiserum produced against the native H_C antigen
recognizes all native forms of kininogen in human plasma.

This investigation concerns isolation of antibodies against the conformational and sequential determinants of the native H_C kininogen by
immunoadsorption. Antigenic response was also studied after reduction and
separation of the polypeptide chain without carboxymethylation. High
performance liquid chromatography (HPLC) was also used to separate tryptic
and S. ureus V8 protease released peptides of the antigen. These peptides
were analyzed by radioimmunoassay using antiserum against the native
antigen and against the reduced and carboxymethylated antigen.

MATERIALS AND METHODS

Preparation of H_C antigen and antisera

The kinin-free low molecular weight kininogen (H_C antigen) was isolated
from Cohns fraction IV according to the method used in 5,6,8 containing
both conformational and sequential determinants of the heavy chain.
Antisers against the H_C kininogen and the reduced and carboxymethylated
kininogen were produced in rabbits as before.[5,6]

Separation of the heavy chain from the reduced H$_C$ kininogen

Reduction and separation of the heavy chain of a kinin-free LM$_r$ kininogen was performed as described by Bouvet et al.[9] About 1 mg of immunoreactive kininogen was dissolved in 150 µl of 0.55M Tris-HCl buffer pH 8.2 and 150 µl of 4M 2-merkaptoaethanol (Fluka) was added. After 1h at room temperature the sample was applied to a Sephadex G-100 column (0.5 x 27 cm) equilibrated with 1N acetic acid and previously calibrated with an equal amount of reduced and ^{14}C-carboxymethylated kininogen heavy chain prepared as described by Syvänen et al.[5] Pooling of the heavy chain was performed from the 0.3 ml fractions following the elution curve obtained with ^{14}C-labelled heavy chain. Acetic acid was removed by gel filtration in a PD-10 prepacked column (Pharmacia). The protein pool was lyophilized. The absence of the light chain was checked by SDS-gel electrophoresis in a 12-22.5% gradient polyacrylamide slab gel.

Enzymatic cleavage of H$_C$ antigen

H$_C$ antigen (1 mg) was cleaved by 10 µg of trypsin (TRTPCK, Worthington) in 0.5 ml of 0.1M Tris-HCL buffer pH 8.0 and by 30 µg of S. aureus V8 protease (Miles) in 0.5 ml of 0.05 M ammonium acetate overnight at 37°C.

Separation of cleavage peptides by HPLC

HPLC was performed on a Milton ROY apparatus on a Hibar RP-18 column using a linear gradient 0-70% CH$_3$CN in 10mM sodium phosphate pH 4.3 as described before.[5] Peptide containing fractions were collected and lyophilized. Lyophilized fractions were dissolved in 500 µl of 0.05 M phosphate buffer pH 7.5 and 5 µl and 50 µl samples were tested by kininogen RIA (see below).

Radioimmunoassay (RIA)

Kininogen was radioidinated (Na[125]I, IMS 30, Amersham) according to Greenwood et al.[10] using Chloramine-T. Free Na[125]I was removed by gel filtration on Sephadex G-25 using 0.05 sodium phosphate buffer pH 7.5 and a column washed with 1 ml of 1% bovine albumin (Sigma, RIA grade). RIA was performed as described earlier[5] except that the antigen-antibody complex was precipitated with 20% polyethylene glycol (PEG 4000, Fluka) containing 1.5 mg/ml bovine γ-globulins (Sigma G-5009) at +4°C according to (11). Radioactivity was measured with an RIAGAMMA 1271 Counter (LKB Wallac). In the RIA assays antiserum against the unreduced kininogen was diluted 1:20000 whereas antiserum against the reduced and carboxymethylated kininogen was diluted 1:2000.

SDS-polyacrylamide gel electrophoresis (SDS-PAGE)

SDS-PAGE was performed according to Laemmli[12] in a 12-22.5% slab gel with 80 V voltage overnight. HMW and LMW molecular weight markers were obtained from Pharmacia.

RESULTS AND DISCUSSION

Isolation of antibodies against conformation and sequence dependent determinants

Figure 1 illustrates the separation of antibodies produced against different antigenic determinants in LM$_r$ kininogen. An immunoadsorbent column containing immobilized reduced and carboxymethylated (RCM) heavy

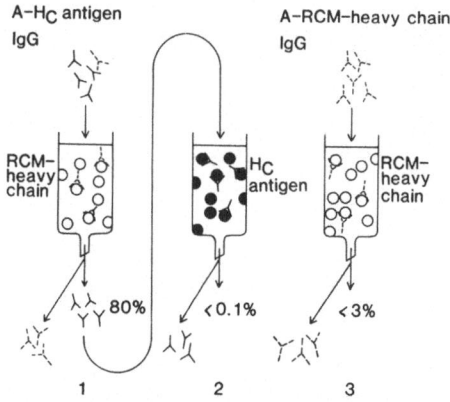

Figure 1. Schematic representation of separation of kininogen antibodies against conformational (—) and sequential (---) determinants.

chain retained 20% antibodies which would correspond to the antibodies against the sequence dependent determinants. All antibody activity was adsorbed to the column prepared from immobilized H_C kininogen.

Reduced heavy chain of H_C antigen

The molecular masses by SDS-gel electrophoresis obtained for the reduced and carbozymethylated (lane 1) and the reduced (lane 2) H_C antigen are similar as shown by Figure 2. It also shows the absence of the light chain in the heavy chain preparations after separation on Sephadex G-100.

The reduced and carboxymethylated heavy chain loses the antigenic response against the conformation dependent determinants of the native heavy chain. Present findings show that when submitted to only reduction the heavy chain still contains some dominating conformation dependent determinants manifested by parallel inhibition curves in RIA (Figure 3) when compared with the unreduced H_C antigen using antiserum against the intact H_C antigen. This is an indication that the light chain does not influence the dominating determinants of H_C antigen.

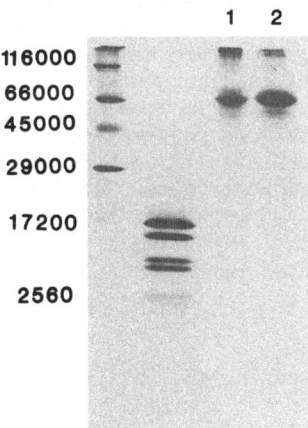

Figure 2. SDS-gradient polyacrylamide gel electrophoresis (12-22.5% slab gel) of the heavy chain of 25 µg of (1) reduced and carboxy-methylated and (2) reduced H_C kininogen showing the absence of the light chain removed after gel filtration. Molecular weight markers of the left.

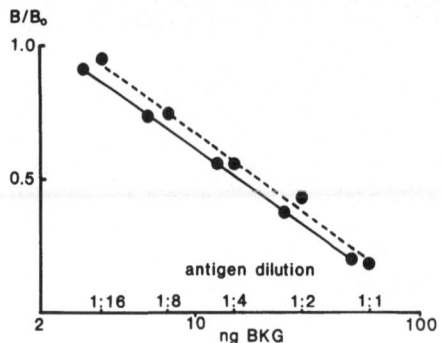

Figure 3. Radioimmunoassay inhibition curves of ($\bullet$ —— $\bullet$) H_C kininogen
and ($\bullet$ -- $\bullet$) the reduced and isolated H_C kininogen heavy chain
using antiserum against H_C kininogen containing the conformation
dependent determinants. B/B_0 is the ratio of ^{125}I labelled
H_C antigen bound in the presence and absence of inhibitor.

Enzymatic cleavage products of H_C kininogen separated by HPLC

When H_C kininogen is digested with trypsin or S. aureus V8 protease,
cleaved peptides can be separated by HPLC as illustrated in Figure 4.
Tryptic peptides were collected in 53 fractions and each lyophilized and
redissolved fraction was measured by RIA. When antiserum against the
unreduced H_C kininogen was used, no immunoreactive peptide fraction was
observed. The same applies for the 56 fractions collected from the
separation of peptides produced by S. aureus V8 protease (Figure 4b).
However, when anti-RCM kininogen serum was used in RIA immunoreactive
fractions were observed between fractions 42-49 (peak fraction 46) in
S. aureus V8 protease peptides and in fractions 45-52 (peak fraction 50)
of the tryptic peptides. These immunoreactive peptides probably represent
antigenic sites of kininogen, but need further studies.

The present findings demonstrate that antigenic determinants of both
conformational and sequential type are present in the LM_r kininogen
molecule. The conformational determinants depend of the intact disulfide
bonds and dominate the antigenic structure (Figure 1). The affinity constant of H_C kininogen antibodies is three orders of magnitude larger for
the native molecule than for the reduced and carboxymethylated heavy
chain.[5] The role of a single disulfide bond linking the heavy and the
light chains for the antigenic structure of the native kininogen is unknown, but present results suggest that reduction alone reduces antigenic
response of the heavy chain. Antiserum prepared against the reduced and
carboxymethylated heavy chain reacted identically with the native plasma
kininogen and the reduced antigen suggesting the presence of an antigenic
site of sequential type.

The determinants dominating the antigenic structure reside primarily
in the heavy chain of kininogen yielding a higher association constant of
the antiserum when the antigen is not submitted to chemical modifications.
This suggests that the kinin-free LM_r kininogen isolated from Cohns
fraction IV is a suitable antigen for preparation of LM_r antiserum. It
also further stresses the fact as shown before[6] that the heavy chain is
unusually resistant to proteolysis by activated plasma kallikrein.

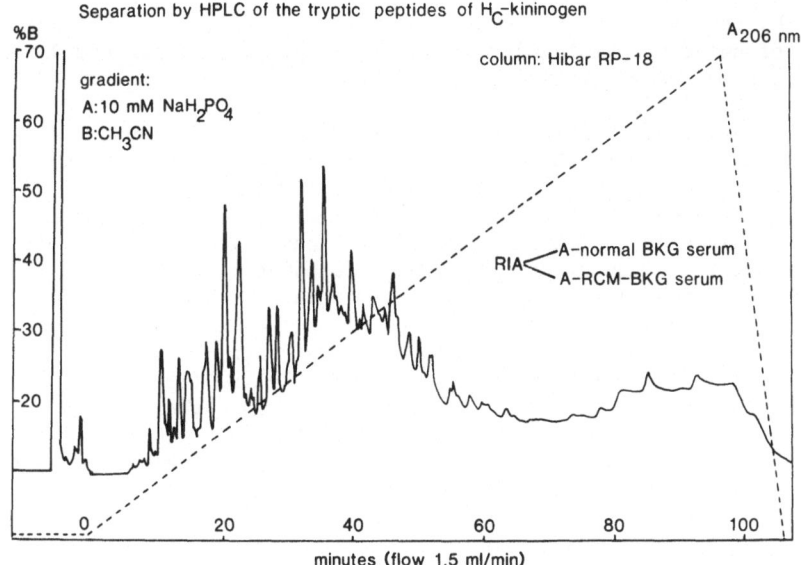

Separation by HPLC of the tryptic peptides of H_C-kininogen

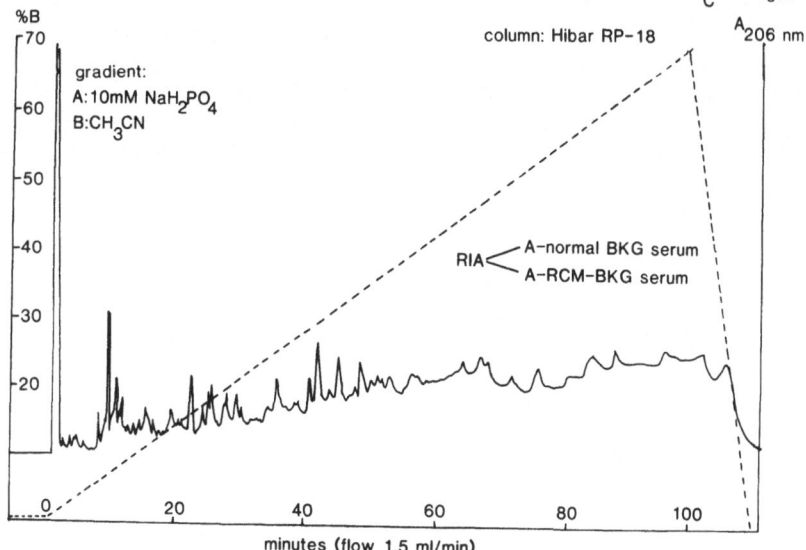

Separation by HPLC of the peptides from cleavage with S.aureus V8 protease of H_C-kininogen

Figure 4. Separation by high performance liquid chromatography of peptides from H_C antigen (1 mg) obtained after digestion with a) trypsin and b) <u>S. aureus</u> V8 protease in a gradient (---) of CH_3CN in sodium phosphate buffer pH 4.3. The adsorbance (——) was measured at 206 nm.

REFERENCES

1. M. Z. Atassi, Precise determination of the entire antigenic structure of lysozyme: Molecular features of protein antigenic structures and potential of surface-stimulation synthesis - a powerful new concept for protein binding sites, <u>Immunochemistry</u>, 15:909-926, (1975).
2. H. Z. Habal, B. J. Underdown, and H. Z. Movat, Further characterization of human plasma kininogen, <u>Biochem. Pharmac.</u>, 24:1241-1243, (1975).

3. D. M. Kerbiriou, B. N. Bouma, and J. H. Griffin, Immunochemical studies of human high molecular weight kininogen and of its complexes with plasma prekallikrein and kallikrein, J. Biol. Chem., 255:3952-3958, (1980).

4. A.-C. Syvänen, U. Turpeinen, S. Siimesmaa, and U. Hamberg, A radio-immunoassay for the detection of molecular forms of human plasma kininogen, FEBS Lett., 129:241-245, (1981).

5. A.-C. Syvänen, T. Kärkkäinen, and U. Hamberg, Conformation and sequence dependent antigenic determinants in human low molecular weight kininogen, Mol. Immunol., 20:669-678, (1983).

6. T. Kärkkäinen, A.-C., Syvänen, U. Turpeinen, and U. Hamberg, Isolation and immunologic properties of a heterogeneous antigen with the characteristics of the heavy chain of human low molecular weight kininogen, Mol. Immunol., 19:179-189, (1982).

7. U. Turpeinen, Studies on the antigenicity and carbohydrates of human low molecular weight kininogen, Mol. Immunol., 20:1411-1418, (1983).

8. T. Kärkkäinen, Immunopurification of human plasma kininogens, Mol. Immunol., in press.

9. J.-P. Bouvet, J. Pillot, and P. Liacopoulos, Human myeloma light chains with increased molecular weight: high frequency among λ chains, Mol. Immunol., 20:397-407, (1983).

10. F. C. Greenwood, W. M. Hunter, and J. S. Glover, The preparation of ^{131}I-labelled human growth hormone of high specific radioactivity, Biochem. J., 89:114-123, (1963).

11. B. Desbuquois and G. D. Aurbach, Use of polyethylene glycol to separate free and antibody-bound peptide hormones in radioimmuno-assays, J. Clin. Endocrinol., 33:732-738, (1971).

12. U. K. Laemmli, Cleavage of structural proteins during the assembly of the head of bacteriophage T4, Nature, 227:680-685, (1970).

KININOGEN BY THE SRI METHOD IN HUMAN SERUM DURING AN ACUTE PHASE INFLAMMA-

TORY REACTION

Ulla Hamberg*+, Tytti Kärkkäinen* and Thomas Tallberg**

*Department of Biochemistry, University of Helsinki,
Unioninkatu 35, SF-00170 Helsinki 17, Finland and **Laboratory
of Immunology, Helsinki University Central Hospital
Mannerheimintie 172, SF-00280 Helsinki 28, Finland
+Deceased

INTRODUCTION

The concentration of several serum proteins changes during the acute
phase in inflammatory states.[1] Kininogen belongs to this group of acute
phase reactants as shown in our earlier studies and also with plasma from
patients with rheumatoid arthritis.[2] In early studies plasma kininogen
was measured exclusively by estimation of the bradykinin equivalent by bioassay on the isolated rat uterus or guinea pig ileum.[3] More recently a
bradykinin enzyme immunoassay,[4] radioimmunoassay[5] and rocket immunoelectrophoresis[6] were reported for the determination of HM_r kininogen in plasma.
A method designated to determination of the total plasma and serum kininogen by single radial immunodiffusion (SRI) was recently presented by us in
detail.[7] The SRI method was compared with and correlated to kininogen determined by the bradykinin equivalent and gives the corresponding normal
values in human plasma and serum. This presentation deals with its application in a study of kininogen investigated in a serum material collected
from patients during periods of treatment with immunotherapy in renal cell
carcinoma.[8-12] An inflammatory reaction provoked during the treatment was
shown by the increase of a_1-acid glycoprotein and some other acute phase
reactants.

THE SRI METHOD

As antigen for immunization the SRI method utilizes the conformation
dependent determinants of the heavy chain common to both plasma kininogens.
This unusual kinin-free LM_r-kininogen antigen (the H_C antigen) isolated
from Cohns plasma fraction IV contains the intact disulfide bond between
the protease resistant heavy chain and a heterogeneous light chain (for
details see 13). The SRI method has the advantage of measuring total plasma
or serum kininogen independently of the presence or absence of kinin segment
in the molecule, but provides an antiserum with higher association constant
(3.8×10^9 M^{-1}) compared with the antiserum produced with the reduced and
carboxymethylated protein (1.1×10^6 M^{-1}). It has higher avidity for the
native kininogen shown by the 400 times larger amount of reduced and carboxymethylated kininogen needed to produce 50% inhibition in radioimmunoassay.

The carefully controlled monospecific anti-kininogen serum was applied using the same concentration in the agar plate determined by the titer. When the titer is greater than 1.0 mg/ml, 2.5% (v/v) of antiserum is sufficient, but titers lower than 0.8 mg/ml necessitate 5% (v/v) concentration of antiserum in the plate. The bradykinin equivalent 4.30 ± 0.52 mg/ml (± 2 SD) corresponds to the SRI value 0.260 ± 0.052 mg/ml (± 2 SD) in normal plasma. In serum the corresponding SRI value was 0.313 ± 0.044 mg/ml (± 2 SD) for pooled serum. In each SRI determination a standard of normal human plasma was used avoiding possible errors derived from applying purified kininogen preparations.[7]

THE BRADYKININ EQUIVALENT

The determination of the bradykinin equivalent in plasma samples has been described in detail before.[7,14] Bradykinin was released with trypsin (Worthington TRL/TPCK), extracted into boiling ethanol, collected from the supernatant after centrifugation and subsequently dried under reduced pressure. After redissolving into the original plasma volume with ice cold saline bradykinin was assayed on the isolated guinea pig ileum. The amount of bradykinin per ml plasma, designated the bradykinin equivalent, was a direct measure of the kininogen content.

PATIENT SERUM SAMPLES

Serum samples were obtained from patients with renal cell carcinoma receiving active specific immunotherapy with polymerised autologous tumor tissue and supportive measures (for details see 8-12). The samples were kept frozen at -20°C until assayed. The SRI kininogen was determined over a period of averagely 20 months during treatment. The bradykinin equivalent was determined in patient serum with increased SRI kininogen. Due to lack of material the assay could not always be performed with those samples showing the highest SRI kininogen values, but in all cases kininogen was higher than normal.

RESULTS AND DISCUSSION

The average increase of kininogen is illustrated in Fig. 1 over 1-26 months of treatment in four patient sera. In general the highest kininogen increase was found after beginning the treatment as seen in Fig. 2. Alpha-1-acid glycoprotein followed the similar pattern. The parallel increase of this typical acute phase protein indicates that an inflammatory reaction was provoked (Fig. 1) sustained by the increase of some other typical acute phase reactants also measured in parallel such as haptoglobin, C3c and a_1-antitrypsin, while albumin remained within the normal range in all cases. The inflammatory response therefore is verified with one exception (HL Fig. 1) for unknown reasons.

The bradykinin equivalent was in all cases lower than the calculated corresponding to the high SRI kininogen (Table 1). This indicates that the kallikrein-kinin system has been activated releasing bradykinin. Contrary to these findings Sharma et al.[2] found high bradykinin equivalents in patients with rheumatoid arthritis and were able to show that the kininogen, determined in their cases by the rat uterus method, was normalized with anti-inflammatory drugs verifying the inflammatory response. In neither case kallikrein was measured in the patient materials. By the SRI method kininogen does not escape detection regardless of proteolytic degradation of the molecule by limited proteolysis in serum. As shown in our earlier studies[7,13] the heavy chain of HM_r and LM_r kininogens is remarkably resistant

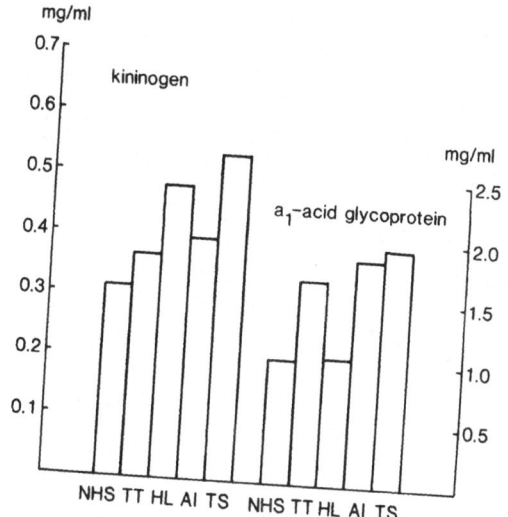

Fig. 1. Kininogen and α_1-acid glycoprotein by single radial immunodiffusion (mg/ml) in acute phase inflammatory patient sera. Number of samples: Kininogen : TT n=11, HL n=5, AI n=7, TS n=4. α_1-acid glycoprotein: TT n=11, HL n=5, AI n=7, TS n=2.

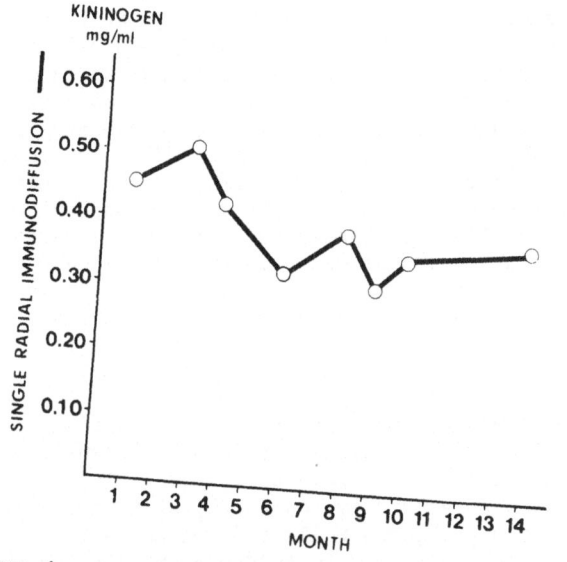

Fig. 2. Kininogen in acute phase patient serum (A.I.) during treatment of active specific immunotherapy over 1-14 months. Kininogen was measured by single radial immunodiffusion (mg/ml).

Table 1. SRI Kininogen and the Bradykinin Equivalent in Patient Serum Samples

| Patient | Month of Treatment | SRI Proteins mg/ml | | | Bradykinin Equivalent (ug/ml) | |
| | | Albumin | α_1-acid glycopr. | Kininogen | Calculated | Found |
		35-55	0.55-1.40	0.269-0.357		
A.I.	1	34.2	3.20	0.456	7.46	3.14
T.S.	5	35.2	1.76	0.410	6.71	4.00
	6	32.0	-	0.640	10.47	-
	7	-	-	0.441	7.21	1.96
T.T.	8	44.3	1.54	0.435	7.12	5.38
	18	-	2.41	0.366	5.99	2.37
H.L.	18	40.5	1.09	0.552	9.03	4.39

to proteolysis while the light chain suffers some cleavage at the N-terminal end apparently by activated plasma kallikrein after first releasing the bradykinin segment. The SRI method is therefore independent of that first step removing the active peptide from kininogens following the activation of kallikrein. Possible errors caused by an escape of bradykinin necessary for the estimation of kininogen by the bradykinin equivalent are avoided. The events occurring during the acute phase reaction would be more accurately described by SRI than by bioassay alone. As shown by Suzuki et al.[15] when prekallikrein was not yet activated in pregnancy the high kininogen measured by the bradykinin equivalent corresponded to our results of increased SRI kininogen (for details see Kärkkäinen et al. this volume). So far there is no evidence of any hidden determinants or confromational change for the antigen (H_c) applied to prepare the antiserum. We have shown recently that purified LM_r kininogen measured by the SRI method is antigenically unchanged after releasing the bradykinin segment by incubation with pancreas kallikrein.[7] Using four times concentrated normal human serum (NHS) antigenic identity could be shown between NHS and all four patient sera when tested against anti-H_C-kininogen serum[13] (Fig. 3).

It is tempting to assume that the molecule accounting for the increase in patient serum is the HM_r kininogen. It is well known[3] that HM_r releases bradykinin more easily after kallikrein activation. The lowest bradykinin equivalents (Table 1) were generally found only after prolonged treatment apparently followed by a prolonged kallikrein effect also affecting LM_r kininogen.[7] There is some preliminary evidence obtained by isoelectric focusing of patient sera with high SRI kininogen (Fig. 2, 3 months). The part of HM_r kininogen (pI 4.7-4.8) slightly increased compared with NHS. In our recent work and as shown by Maki et al.[16] HM_r kininogen also increases during pregnancy. The resistance to proteolysis of the heavy chain common to HM_r and LM_r kininogen may give a more accurate account of the events in inflammatory states. The use of the antiserum against the native kininogen heavy chain in SRI and RIA[7] appears to be the method of choice to study kininogen levels even in pathological states when activation of plasma kallikrein is highly probable.

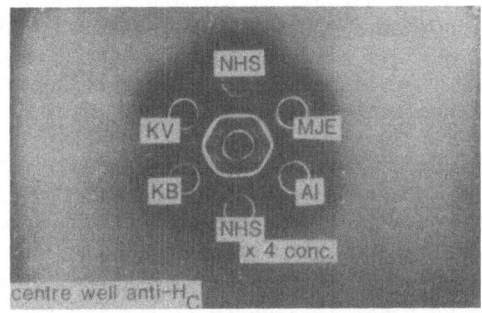

Fig. 3. Double immunodiffusion analysis showing identity between four
different patient sera and normal human serum against anti-H_C-
kininogen serum.

ACKNOWLEDGEMENTS

This investigation was supported by grants from the Societas Scienti-
arum Fenniae, Signe and Ane Gyllenberg's Foundation and Magnus Ehrnrooths
Foundation.

REFERENCES

1. A. Koj, Acute-phase reactants, in: "Structure and Function of Plasma
     Proteins," A. C. Allison, ed., Plenum Publishing Corporation (1974).
2. J. N. Sharma, J. J. Zeitlin, P. M. Brooks, W. W. Buchman, and W. C.
     Dick, The action of aspirin on plasma kininogen and other plasma
     proteins in rheumatoid patients: Relationship to disease activity,
     Clin. Exp. Pharmacol. Physiol., 1:347–354 (1980).
3. C. G. Cochrane and J. H. Griffin, The biochemistry and pathophysiology
     of the contact system in plasma, Adv. Immuno., 33:241–306 (1982).
4. A. Ueno, S. Oh-Ishi, T. Kitagawa, and M. Katori, Enzyme immunoassay of
     bradykinin, Adv. Pxp. Med. Biol., 120A:195–202 (1979).
5. D. Proud, J. V. Pierce, and J. J. Pisano, Radioimmunoassay of human
     high molecular weight kininogen in normal and deficient plasma,
     J. Lab. Clin. Med., 95:563–574 (1980).
6. B. N. Bouma, D. M. Kerbiriou, R. A. A. Vlooswijk, and J. H. Griffin,
     Immunological studies of prekallikrein, kallikrein and high molecular
     weight kininogen in normal and deficient plasmas and in normal plasma
     after cold dependent activation, J. Lab. Clin. Med., 96:693–709
     (1980).
7. U. Hamberg and T. Kärkkäinen, Determination of human plasma kininogen
     by a single radial immunodiffusion method and the bradykinin equiva-
     lent, Clin. Chim. Acta, 142:211–220 (1984).
8. Th. Tallberg, Cancer immunotherapy by means of polymerized autologous
     tumour tissue with special reference to some patients with pulmonary
     tumour, Scand. J. Respir. Dis. Suppl., 89 (1974).
9. H. Tykkä, Active specific immunotherapy with supportive measures in the
     treatment of advanced palliatively nephrectomized renal adenocarci-
     noma. A controlled clinical study, Academic dissertation, Scand. J.
     Urol. & Neephrol. Suppl., 63 (1981).
10. H. Tykkä, K. Oravisto, M. Turunen, and Th. Tallberg, Disappearance of
     lung metastases during immunotherapy in five patients juffering from
     renal carcinoma, Scand. J. Respir. Dis., 123, Suppl. 89 (1974).
11. H. Tykkä, K. Oravisto, T. Lehtonen, S. Sarna, and Th. Tallberg, Active
     specific immunotherapy of advanced renal-cell carcinoma, Eur. Urol.,
     4:250 (1978).

12. J. A. Neidhart, S. G. Murphy, L. A. Hennick, and H. A. Wise, Active specific immunotherapy of stage IV renal cell carcinoma with aggregated tumour antigen adjuvant, Cancer, 46:1128-1134 (1980).
13. A.-C. Syvänen, T. Kärkkäinen, and U. Hamberg, Conformation and sequence dependent determinants of human low molecular weight kininogen, Molec. Immunol., 20:669-678 (1983).
14. U. Hamberg, Kininogen in human plasma after fibrinolytic activation, Scand. J. Clin. Lab. Invest. Suppl., 107:37-47 (1969).
15. S. Suzuki, T. Murakoshi, and W. Sakamoto, Studies on the various causal factors related to hypercoagulability in the field of obstetrics with special reference to the onset of DIC as viewed from the changing of kinin-kallikrein system and fibrinopeptide A, Adv. Exp. Med. Biol., 156A:1055-1065 (1983).
16. M. Maki, K. Soga, and K. Gotoh, The kinin-forming enzyme system in pregnancy and obstetrical DIC, in: "Disseminated Intravascular Coagulation," T. Abe and M. Yamaka, eds., Karger, Bibliotheca Haematologica, 49:239-246 (1983).

KININOGEN AS A PREGNANCY-ASSOCIATED PLASMA PROTEIN

Tytti Kärkkäinen and Ulla Hamberg[*]

Department of Biochemistry, University of Helsinki
Unioninkatu 35, SF-00170 Helsinki 17, Finland
*Deceased

INTRODUCTION

Pregnancy induces marked changes in plasma protein concentrations. Some proteins are secreted by the placenta into the maternal circulation and are thus called pregnancy-specific plasma proteins. Pregnancy-specific beta-1-glycoprotein (SP1) was the first protein of this group.[1] Other plasma proteins also undergo changes during normal pregnancy and in response to contraceptive doses of estrogens.[2,3] In early studies several authors reported determination of kininogen during pregnancy, delivery and puerperium[4-6] indicating increased kininogen during pregnancy, decreasing values during labor and increasing kininogen content in puerperium. In all these studies kininogen was determined by the estimation of the bradykinin equivalent by bioassay on the rat uterus or guinea pig ileum. Suzuki[7] found in a preliminary report a 100% increase of plasma kininogen compared with non-pregnancy levels showing that bradykinin was not released from kininogen during the pregnancy periods. In particular interest has more recently been focused on the HM_r (high molecular weight) kininogen due to its function as a cofactor in the activation of F XII and the onset of coagulation. Maki et al.[8] reported increase of HM_r kininogen during pregnancy and decrease with the start of labor which suggested that the vasoactive bradykinin was relesed during labor through the activation of plasma kallikrein and brought back to normal level after delivery. Similar findings were recently reported by Suzuki et al.[9] applying the bradykinin equivalent to determine kininogen while Maki et al.[8] were first to utilize immunological determination with HM_r specific antiserum in pregnancy.

This investigation concerns the study of kininogens in plasma samples taken during pregnancy applying a single radial immunodiffusion (SRI) method recently developed in our laboratory[10] and radioimmunoassay.[11,12] The distribution of LM_r and HM_r kininogens was estimated by isoelectric focusing and SRI.

MATERIALS AND METHODS

Plasma Samples

Pooled normal blood bank plasma CPD (citrate, phosphate, dextrose) plasma was obtained from the Finnish Red Cross Blood Transfusion Service

(FRC). Single donor blood from normal and pregnant women was taken from healthy volunteers using 10 ml plastic tubes containing 1 ml of ACD anti-coagulant (citric acid, trisodium citrate, dextrose). All plasma samples were centrifuged 20 min at 1000 g +4°C.

Preparation of Antigens and Antisera

Immunologically pure kinin-free LM_r kininogen (H_C antigen) from Cohns fraction IV was prepared as described earlier.[11,13,14] Antiserum (titre 1,1 mg/ml) was developed in a rabbit against this antigen containing the conformation dependent determinants of the kininogen heavy chain[11] using 200 µg antigen injections every fortnight in Freunds complete adjuvant.

Immunologically pure kininogen ws isolated from normal pooled blood bank plasma (FRC) using QAE-Sephadex A-50[11] and SP-Sephadex C-50 chromatography[15] for the isolation of HM_r light chain after reduction and alkylation. Antiserum against the HM_r light chain was developed in a rabbit as above. The cross-reactivity with the heavy chain was less than 0.1%.

Single Radial Immunodiffusion (SRI)

The quantitative determination of total plasma kininogen was performed as described in detail recently.[10] Pregnancy-specific SP1, ceruloplasmin, α_1-acid glycoprotein, fibrinogen, α_1-antitrypsin and transferrin were measured using commercial M-Partigen or NOR-Partigen plates (Behringwerke, FRG) using Standard Human-Serum (ORDT 06/07), Protein-Plasma-Standard (OTFI 06/07) or β_1-SP1-Glycoprotein Standard (OTFL 02/03) (Behringwerke) as standards.

Radioimmunoassay (RIA)

Kininogen was radioiodinated with carrier-free Na ^{125}IMS 30, Amersham) using Chloramine-T.[11] Free ^{125}I was removed bygel filtration on Sephadex G-25 (Pharmacia). Total plasma kininogen ws measured using the same antiserum as for SRI diluted 1:20 000 with RIA-buffer (0.05 M sodium phosphate pH 7.5 containing 1% bovine albumin). Immunologically pure H_C kininogen prepared as described before was used as standard.

HM_r kininogen in plasma was measured using antiserum (diluted L;1400) against the reduced and alkylated light chain of HM_r kininogen as described above. The RIA assay for HM_r and total plasma kininogen ws performed as in (11,12).

Isoelectric Focusing

Isoelectric focusing of 2 ml of pregnancy plasma was performed in an LKB 8101 column (110 ml) using 1% Ampholine (LKB Products) in a linear sucrose gradient at +4°C as described earlier.[13] Kininogen was measured by SRI in 1 ml fractions.

Protein Determination

The protein content of plasma samples was measured by the method of Lowry et al.[16] using human albumin (Kabi) as standard.

RESULTS AND DISCUSSION

Pregnancy-Associated SP1 and Kininogen

Some proteins also known as acute phase reactants and the pregnancy-specific SP1 were measured in pregnancy plasma by SRI in comparison with total plasma kininogen and the corresponding pooled CPD plasma values (Table I). The appearance of SP1 was observed after 11 weeks of pregnancy (MK) with the highest value 0.24 mg/ml after 40 weeks (KK). Similarly the highest increase (150%) occurred with kininogen after 37 weeks. The increase of SP1 during pregnancy is almost linear while kininogen reaches a plateau between 19-32 weeks. Both proteins attain the maximum value in the last month of pregnancy (Table I, MK, AK). Kininogen decreased during puerperium as also shown with SP1 and remained somewhat increased (0.35 mg/ml, Table I) compared with the normal value 0.26 mg/ml and was almost unchanged in another case 3 days after delivery (SH, not shown).

As seen in Table I in no case alpha-1-acid glycoprotein was increased above normal. This clearly distinguishes the reaction of kininogen in pregnancy from that of kininogen as an acute-phase reactant in inflammation (see Hamberg and Kärkkäinen, this volume).

The protein content measured during the first trimester was 83 mg/ml (Range 79-87 mg/ml, 4 samples) and during the last trimesters 77 mg/ml (range 57-112 mg/ml, 23 samples).

Single RIA determinations of HM_r kininogen in normal plasma yielded the average value 96 mg/ml (16 samples). This compares favorably with 90 mg/ml obtained by Proud et al.[18] In pregnancy plasma samples HM_r content was 119-135 mg/ml between 32-39 weeks. This is in agreement with the results of Maki et al.[8] Lack of methodological details and different methods used so far leave the comparison of HM_r kininogen in pregnancy uncertain.

Antigenic identity between the pregnancy plasma and normal plasma was shown by parallel inhibition curves in RIA using the anti-H_C-kininogen serum responding to the conformational determinants in the heavy chain of all normal plasma kininogens.[10] The same applies to the specific RIA determination of HM_r kininogen using the antiserum prepared against the light chain of HM_r kininogen. These results demonstrate that both LM_r and HM_r kininogen in pregnancy plasma are antigenically identical with the kininogens in normal plasma.

pI Distribution of Heterogeneous LM_r and HM_r Kininogen

The focusing profile of pregnancy plasma is given in Fig. 1 and shows that 89% of kininogen focused between pI 4.2-4.6. No kininogen is found at pI 4.7 with 2 ml of normal plasma as shown before.[13] The pI 4.2-4.6 are therefore derived from LM_r kininogen. In the pregnancy plasma sample with increased total plasma kininogen 11% was found in the pI 4.7-4.8 fractions, the pI range of HM_r kininogen.[19] This result may indicate that HM_r kininogen has increased during pregnancy which would be in keeping with the results of Suzuki,[7] Maki et al.[8] and Suzuki et al.[9] As suggested by Maki et al.[8] an increase of prekallikrein and HM_r would contribute together with oxytocin to the physiological mechanism of labor.

ACKNOWLEDGEMENTS

This investigation was supported by grants from the Signe and Ane Gyllenberg Foundation and the Magnus Ehrnrooth Foundation, Helsinki, Finland.

Table I. Kininogen (mg/ml) in Plasma During Various Periods of Pregnancy Determined by SRI in Comparison with SPl, Alpha-1-Antitrypsin, Ceruloplasmin, Fibrinogen, Transferrin and Alpha-1-Glycoprotein

Normal Ranges[X]	Mg/Ml	0[XX]	2.0-4.0	0.15-0.60	2.00-4.50	2.0-4.0	0.5-1.40	0.21-0.31
Sample	Weeks	SPl	Alpha-1-Anti-Trypsin	Cerulo-Plasmin	Fibrinogen	Trans-Ferrin	Alpha-1-Acid Glyco-Protein	Kininogen
MK I	11	0.02	2.53	0.43	3.28	1.95	0.41	0.32
II	15	0.04	2.87	0.45	3.40	2.20	0.41	0.41
III	19	0.05	3.23	0.49	3.52	2.40	0.37	0.49
IV	23	0.08	3.50	0.57	4.06	2.65	0.41	0.53
V	27	0.12	3.50	0.49	3.92	2.65	0.37	0.54
VI	32	0.16	3.50	0.49	4.18	2.85	0.37	0.54
VII	37	0.23	3.88	0.53	4.60	3.10	0.41	0.65
AK I	37	0.23	4.00	–	7.12	–	0.48	0.57
II	39	0.20	4.80	–	7.98	–	0.40	0.58
Puerperium 3 Days		0.07	4.60	–	4.49	–	0.84	0.35
Normal CPD-Plasma		0	2.28	0.26	4.16	1.83	0.60	0.26

X Putnam (17)

XX Rohn (1)

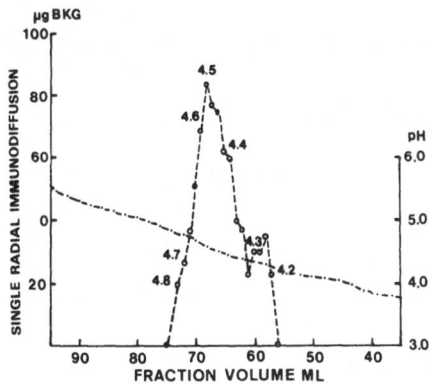

Fig. 1. Isoelectric focusing in the pH gradient 3.5-5 (---) (70h, +4°C) of 2 ml single donor pregnancy plasma. Total plasma kininogen (BKG) was measured by SRI (o-o) in 1 ml fractions. Kininogen content was 0.52 mg/ml (SH).

REFERENCES

1. H. Bohn, Nachweis und characterisierung von schwanger-schaftsproteinen in der menschlichen placenta, sowie ihre quantitative immunologische bestimmung im serum schwangerer frauen, Arch. Gynäk., 210:440-457 (1971).
2. C.-B. Laurell, S. Kullander, and J. Thorell, Rate of plasma protein normalization after partutrition and withdrawal of oral contraceptives, Scand. J. Clin. Lab. Invest., 26:345-348 (1970).
3. P. O. Ganrot, Variation of the concentrations of some plasma proteins in normal adults, in pregnant women and in newborns, Scand. J. Clin. Lab. Invest., 29(Suppl.):83-88 (1972).
4. C. R. Diniz and I. F. Carvalho, A micromethod for determination of brady-kininogen under several conditions, Ann. NY Acad. Sci., 104:77-89 (1963).
5. P. Periti and F. Gasparri, Bradykininogen in the blood of women during pregnancy, labor and puerperium, in: "Hypotensive Peptides," E. G. Erdös, N. Back, and F. Sicuteri, eds., Springer Verlag, New York (1966).
6. B. Wiegershausen, I. Paegelow, E. Neumayer, and H. Walter, Kininogengehalt in plasma und fruchtwsser, Acta Biol. Med. German., 19:61-71 (1967).
7. S. Suzuki, The evaluation of the role of the kallikrein-kinin systems with coagulation factors during pregnancy, delivery and puerperium, Abstr. VII Int. Cong. Thromb. Haem., 1052 (1979).
8. M. Maki, K. Soga, and K. Gotoh, The kinin-forming enzyme system in pregnancy and abstetrical DIC, in: "Disseminated Intravascular Coagulation," T. Abe and M. Yamanaka, eds., Karger, Bibliotheca Haematogica, 49:239-246 (1983).
9. S. Suzuki, T. Murakoshi, and W. Sakamoto, Studies on the various causal factors related to hypercoagulability in the field of obstetrics - With special reference to the onset of DIC as viewed from the changing of kinin-kallikrein system and fibrinopeptide A, Adv. Exp. Med. Biol. 156B:1055-1065 (1983).

10. U. Hamberg and T. Kärkkäinen, Determination of human plasma kininogen by a single radial immunodiffusion method and the bradykinin equivalent, Clin. Chim. Acta, 142:211-220 (1984).

11. A.-C. Syvänen, T. Kärkkäinen, and U. Hamberg, Conformation and sequence dependent determinants in human low molecular weight kininogen, Mol. Immunol., 20:669-678 (1983).

12. A.-C. Syvänen, U. Turepinen, S. Siimesmaa, and U. Hamberg, A radioimmunoassay for the detection of molecular forms of human plasma kininogen, FEBS Lett., 129:241-245 (1981).

13. T. Kärkkäinen, A.-C. Syvänen, U. Turpeinen, and U. Hamberg, Isolation and immunologic properties of a heterogeneous antigen with the characteristics of the heavy chain of human plasma kininogen, Mol. Immunol. 19:179-189 (1982).

14. T. Kärkkäinen, Immunopurification of human plasma kininogens, Mol. Immunol., In Press (1985).

15. D. M. Kerbiriou and J. Griffin, Human high molecular weight kininogen. Studies of structure-function relationships and of proteilysis of the molecule occurring during contact activation of plasma, J. Biol. Chem., 254:12020-12027 (1979).

16. D. H. Lowry, N. J. Rosebrough, A. L. Farr, and R. J. Randall, Protein measurement with the folin phenol reagent, J. Biol. Chem., 193:265-275 (1951).

17. F. W. Putnam, alpha, beta, gamma, omega - the roster of the plasma proteins, in: "Plasma Proteins," F. W. Putnam, ed., Vol I, Academic Press, New York (1975).

18. D. Proud, J. V. Pierce, and J. J. Pisano, Radioimmunoassay of human high molecular weight kininogen in normal and deficient plasma, J. Lab. Clin. Med., 95:563-574 (1980).

19. T. Nakayasu and S. Nagasawa, Studies on human kininogen. I. Isolation, characterization and cleavage by plasma kallikrein of high molecular weight (HMW) kininogen, J. Biochem., 85:249-258 (1979).

HEMODYNAMICS OF THE ISOLATED PERFUSED RAT KIDNEY IN THE ABSENCE AND PRESENCE

OF KALLIKREIN SUBSTRATE

Manfred Mair, Zydi Zhegu and Bernd R. Binder

Laboratory for Clinical-Experimental Physiology at the
Department of Medical Physiology, University of Vienna
Austria

SUMMARY

Rat kidneys were isolated and perfused for 120 minutes at 80mm Hg with Krebs-Henseleit buffer containing 7gm% bovine albumin fraction V. Analysis of the bovine albumin revealed the presence of a contaminating kallikrein substrate which exhibited a MW of 55.000 upon gelfiltration on Sephadex G-200, similar to the reported MW of bovine low molecular weight kininogen. The mean values for renal perfusate flow rate (RPF) and glomerular filtration rate (GFR) in kidneys perfused with this bovine albumin depleted of the kallikrein substrate were significantly lower when compared to standard perfusions. In two other groups of isolated kidneys perfused with kallikrein substrate depleted bovine albumin, purified bovine low molecular weight kininogen (bLMWK, 8.5µg protein in 50µl per minute) or synthetic bradykinin (Bk, 1 ng in 10µl per minute) were infused after the first 30 minute clearance period into the renal artery. The induced hemodynamic changes were similar in that RPF and GFR significantly increased. These studies show that depletion of bovine albumin from kallikrein substrate results in a concomitant decrease of RPF and GFR, while overall renal function is unaffected. Infusion of both bLMWK or BK to kallikrein substrate depleted bovine albumin has similar effects resulting in a simultaneous increase in RPF and GFR. This suggests that endogenous kallikrein from the perfused kidney releases kinin from infused bLMWK and indicates that kinin primarily affects the afferent arterioles.

INTRODUCTION

A variety of factors and their interactions are believed to affect glomerular afferent and efferent capillaries and hence glomerular hemodynamics. One of these factors is the renal kallikrein kinin system but its function within the kidney is not clearly understood.[1]

Kinin induced vasodilatation has been studied by several investigators and has been implicated in functional vasodilatation of various glands, the intestine, the kidney and the placenta.Rev. [2,3] In most of these experiments, exogenous kinins were given on the assumption that they can reproduce the effects evoked by the activation of the endogenous kallikrein-kinin system. In the kidney, however, this has been criticized, since the site of kinin induced vasodilatation and kallikrein induced kinin generation appear to be different.[2] Other investigators studied the renal kallikrein kinin system by administration of inhibitors of the converting enzyme[4] or of kallikrein[5], another approach which does not allow definite conclusions.

We are interested in the renal kallikrein-kinin system and its relation to renal hemodynamics, since experiments on hemorrhagic hypotension suggested to us that this vasodilatory system might contribute to functional vasodilatation during autoregulation of renal blood flow and GFR.[5,6] We now would like to present experiments which extend our observation and support a rather specific action of the renal kallikrein-kinin system on renal hemodynamics.

MATERIALS AND METHODS

Kidneys were obtained from male Sprague-Dawley rats weighing 280-340g anesthetized by an intraperitoneal injection of sodium thiopental (Pentothal[R], 5-6mg/100g body weight). The animals were fasted overnight prior to surgery but had free access to water. The procedure and apparatus for perfusing isolated kidneys was that described in detail by Bowman and Maack[7] with few modifications. The perfusate consisted of Krebs-Henseleit bicarbonate buffer containing 7g% bovine albumin (Armour Pharmaceutical Company, Fraction V). After dialysis for 18-24 hours against the same buffer, glucose, creatinine and L-amino acids were added[8] and, after equilibration with 5% CO_2 in O_2, the pH was adjusted to 7.4 - 7.5. The perfusate was then filtered through a 0.45μm pore size membrane filter (Metrizel[R], Gelman). Seventy five ml each were used for the preperfusion fluid and the recirculating perfusion fluid.[8] During the experiments the perfusate was saturated with a mixture of 95% O_2 - 5% CO_2 and kept at 37-38°C.

After initiation of perfusion 50-100μl (appr. 16μCi) of ^{3}H-labelled polyethylene glycol (^{3}H-PEG, molecular weight 4.000, specific activity 1.6mCi/g, New England Nuclear Corp.) was added to the perfusate and a 20 min time period was allowed for pressure and flow equilibration and to obtain steady urine flow. Eight clearance periods of 15 min each were then started and midpoint samples of perfusate were obtained. A perfusion pressure of 80 ± 2mm Hg was maintained by adjusting the speed of the perfusion pump.

PERFUSION EXPERIMENTS

Standard perfusions: ten kidneys were perfused using bovine albumin fraction V in a concentration of 7g% in the perfusion medium.

Perfusions with incubated perfusate: For these experiments the bovine albumin was incubated for 6 hours with insolubilized rat urinary kallikrein, purified according to the method of [9] at 37°C in order to deplete the active kallikrein substrate. Complete depletion was checked and the albumin was used for perfusion as described above.

Perfusions with incubated perfusate and infusion of purified bovine low molecular weight kininogen: In this group of ten kidneys perfused with kallikrein substrate depleted albumin purified bovine low molecular weight kininogen[10] was continuously infused into the renal artery after the second clearance period at a rate of 8.5µg protein in 50µl per minute.

Perfusions with incubated perfusate and infusion of bradykinin: In this group of 10 kidneys perfused with kallikreinl substrate depleted albuminl synthetic bradykinin (1 ng in 10µl per minute) was infused instead of kininogen under otherwise identical conditions as described above.

DETERMINATIONS

The perfusate flow rate was directly read off from an inline flow meter. The clearance of ^{3}H-PEG was taken as a measurement of GFR. The radioactivity was determined in a Beckman Gamma 9000 scintillation counter. Concentration of Na^+ in perfusate and urine samples was determined by flame photometry. Urine samples were collected in preweighed vials and the volume was determined gravimetrically.[7] Kininogen (kallikrein substrate) concentration was determined in the guinea pig ileum – or estrous rat uterus – bioassay after incubation of 100-500µl of sample with an excess of purified rat urinary kallikrein (10µl, 100ng) for 5 minutes unless otherwise indicated. The concentration is given as ng BK generated per ml of sample.

RESULTS

The hemodynamic and renal functional parameters obtained with the standard perfusion technique in 10 kidneys are shown in Fig. 1.

Careful analysis of the fresh perfusion medium revealed the presence of a kallikrein substrate which released kinin upon incubation with purified rat urinary kallikrein. Gelfiltration experiments showed that this kallikrein substrate had a molecular weight of 55.000 similar to the reported molecular weight of bovine low molecular weight kininogen.[10] The mean concentration of the substrate in the bovine albumin fraction V was found to be 60ng/ml. Various batches of albumin were therefore treated with insolubilized rat urinary kallikrein (100-500µl, 1-5µg).

In a series of perfusion experiments we then used the perfusion medium depleted of the kallikrein substrate. Fig. 2 and Table 1 show the hemodynamic and functional parameters of these perfusion experiments in comparison to the standard perfusions. These studies show that depletion of the perfusion medium from Kallikrein substrate results in a concomitant decrease of perfusate flow rate and GFR while overall renal function is unaffected.

Experiments were then conducted to see whether or not we could reconstitute this depleted perfusion medium with the kallikrein substrate. Infusion of bovine low molecular weight kininogen at a constant rate of 8.5µg protein in 50µl per minute after the second clearance period was followed by an increase in kallikrein substrate concentration in the perfusate (not shown). It also induced significant changes in hemodynamics and function of the IPRK which are shown in Fig. 3 and 4 in comparison to the group of perfusions with depleted perfusate alone. These studies show that infusion of purified bLMWK increases both perfusate flow rate and GFR.

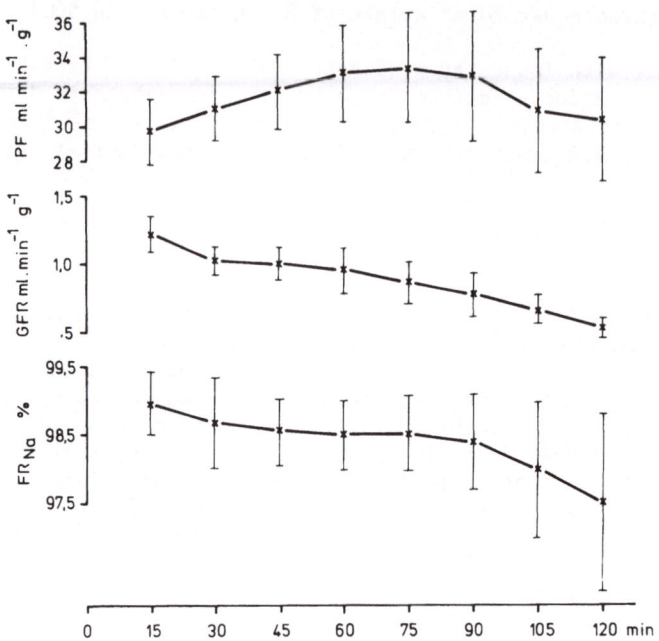

Figure 1. Perfusate flow (PF), glomerular filtration rate (GFR) and fractional sodium reabsorption (FR_{Na}) of 10 isolated perfused kidneys under standard conditions, mean values and standard deviations.

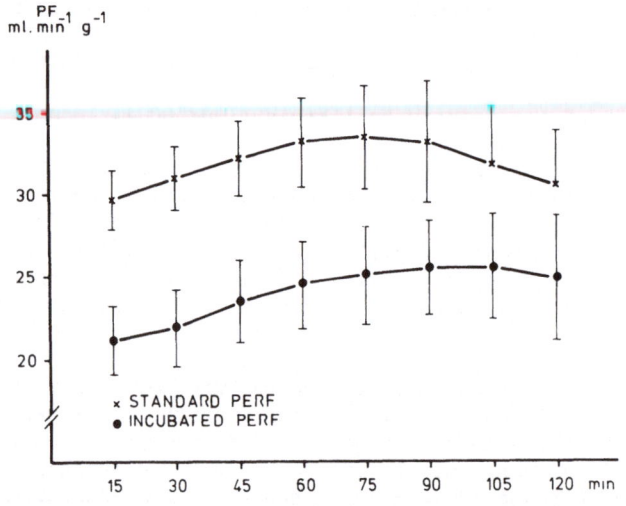

Figure 2. Perfusate flow rate of 10 isolated perfused kidneys employing standard perfusate (X) or kallikrein substrate depleted perfusate (•).

Table 1

Perfusions with incubated perfusate

Min.	15	30	45	60	75	90	105	120
GFR $ml.min^{-1}.g^{-1}$	0.94[d] ±0.12	0.89[c] ±0.13	0.81[d] ±0.11	0.8[b] ±0.11	0.8 ±0.13	0.72 ±0.13	0.65 ±0.16	0.58 ±0.22
FF %	4.16 ±0.68	4.08[b] ±0.61	3.5 ±0.64	3.34 ±0.66	3.24[a] ±0.64	2.87[a] ±0.61	2.55[a] ±0.49	2.33[a] ±0.82
V $\mu l.min^{-1}$	35 ±18.5	50.2 ±21.1	50.8 ±21.2	48.9 ±16.9	49.5 ±18.1	45.5 ±13.6	37.2 ±10.2	31 ±10.8
FR_{Na} %	98.76 ±0.74	98.41 ±0.95	98.34 ±0.91	98.37 ±1.11	98.1 ±1.03	97.97 ±0.92	97.85 ±1.18	97.75 ±1.42
U_{Na} x V $mmol.min^{-1}$	1.7 ±1.19	2.15 ±1.25	2.16 ±1.15	2.24 ±1.35	2.43 ±1.28	2.32 ±1.0	1.99 ±0.88	1.7 ±0.8

Renal functional parameters of kidneys perfused with kallikrein substrate depleted perfusate. Significant differences to standard perfusions are a = $p < 0.05$, b = $p < 0.01$, c = $p < 0.005$, d = $p < 0.001$. Mean and S.D.

177

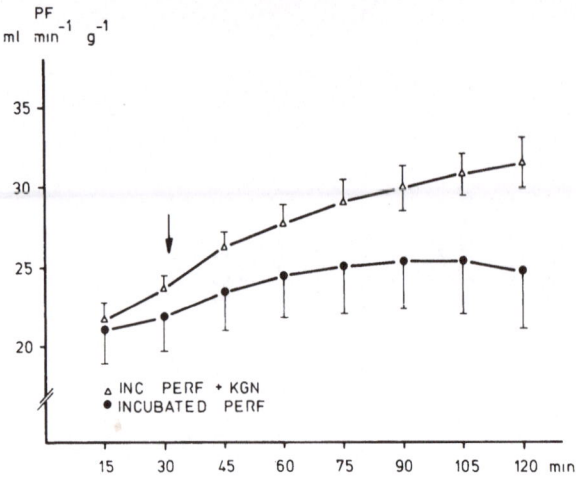

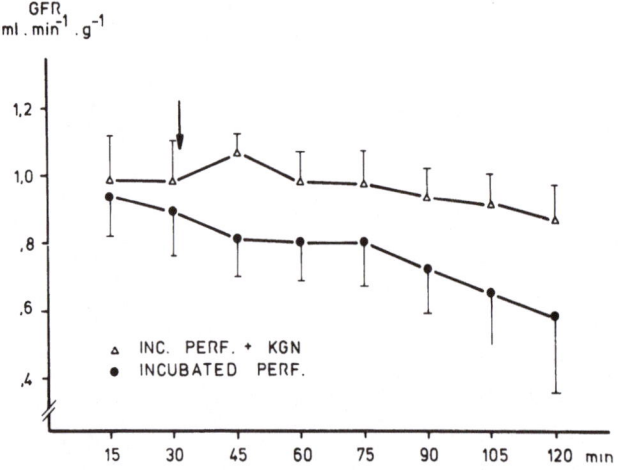

Figure 3 (top) and Figure 4 (bottom). Perfusate flow rate and
glomerular filtration rate of kidneys perfused with
kallikrein substrate depleted perfusate in the presence (△)
or absence (●) of purified bovine low molecular weight
kininogen.

Almost identical results were obtained when synthetic bradykinin was
infused into the renal artery of another group of 10 perfused kidneys
(not shown).

DISCUSSION

Although the values for renal functional parameters obtained with the
standard perfusion technique meet the standards required in renal physiology they decline during the course of the perfusion. The decline in GFR
and sodium reabsorption has been attributed mainly to changes in intrarenal
physical factors.[11] However, it is also possible that accumulation of a
vasoconstricting or consumption of a vasodilating agent causes the decline
in RPF and GFR.

Our studies in fact show that the bovine albumin fraction V used as oncotic agent for perfusion of isolated rat kidneys contains a kallikrein substrate. This substrate has physiochemical and functional properties similar to bovine low molecular weight kininogen. Isolated kidneys were therefore perfused with this bovine albumin fraction V depleted of the kallikrein substrate. These kidneys exhibit a reduced perfusate flow rate and glomerular filtration rate together with an increased resistance, when compared to experiments with substrate containing perfusion medium. In contrast, addition of synthetic bradykinin or purified bovine low molecular weight kininogen to the substrate depleted albumin restores the original values for perfusate flow rate and glomerular filtration rate and decreases resistance.

The similarity of the hemodynamic changes induced by perfusion with either kininogen or bradykinin suggests that the isolated perfused rat kidney secretes kallikrein and releases kinin from the added kininogen. From the resulting pattern of RPF and GRF a specific site of action for the released kinin can be postulated. This is explained in Figure 5, which depicts a simplified glomerulus. Although the regulation of the renal circulation is mediated by neural, humoral or intrarenal physical factors, it is ultimately dependent on resistance changes resulting from the construction or relaxation of vascular smooth muscle. The hydraulic pressure within glomerular capillaries depends upon afferent and efferent arteriolar resistances, increasing with selective efferent constriction or afferent dilatation (Figure 5).

Our conclusion is therefore consistent with the interpretation that the simultaneous decrease of flow and glomerular filtration rate seen after depletion of the perfusate of kallikrein substrate and the simultaneous increase of these parameters after reconstitution with bradykinin or low molecular weight kininogen suggests that the released endogenous kinin primarily affects the afferent arteriole.

SELECTIVE ALTERATION OF AFFERENT RESISTANCE (R_A)

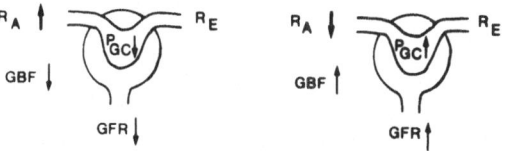

SELECTIVE ALTERATION OF EFFERENT RESISTANCE (R_E)

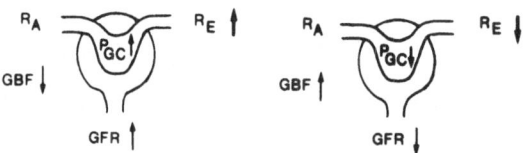

Figure 5. The effect of resistance-changes on glomerular blood flow (GBF) and glomerular filtration rate (GFR).

ACKNOWLEDGEMENTS

The authors acknowledge the excellent technical assistance of Ingrid Jerabek, Gunther Reissert, Eva Holtzl and Dr. H. Rana and thank H. Hitschmann for typing the manuscript.

REFERENCES

1. J. Schnermann and J. P. Briggs, Participation of renal cortical prostaglandins in the regulation of glomerular filtration rate, Kidney Int., 19:802-815, (1981).
2. O. A. Carretero and A. G. Scicli, Possible role of kinins in circulatory homeostasis. State of the art review, Hypertension Suppl. I Vol., 3:I-4-I-12, (1981).
3. M. Seino, O. A. Carretero, R. Albertini, and A. G. Scicli, Kinins in regulation of uteroplacental blood flow in the pregnant rabbit, Am. J. Physiol., 242:H142-H147, (1982).
4. C. I. Johnston, B. Clappison, B. P. McGrath, P. G. Matthews, J. A. Millar, and W. P. Anderson, Kallikrein, kinins and blood pressure - effects of angiotensin-converting enzymes inhibition, Prog. Biochem. Pharmacol., 17:123-133, (1980).
5. M. Maier, M. Starlinger, Z. Zhegu, H. Rana, and B. R. Binder, The effect of the protease inhibitor aprotinin on renal hemodynamics in the pig, Hypertension, January (1985).
6. M. Maier, M. Starlinger, M. Wagner, D. Meyer, and B. R. Binder, The effect of hemorrhagic hypotension on urinary kallikrein excretion, renin activity, and renal cortical blood flow in the pig, Circ. Res., 48:386-392, (1982).
7. R.H. Bowman and T. Maack, Effect of albumin concentration and ADH on H_2O and electrolyte transport in perfused rat kidney, Am. J. Physiol., 226:426-430, (1974).
8. G. DeMello and T. Maack, Nephron function of the isolated perfused rat kidney, Am. J. Physiol., 231:1699-1707, (1976).
9. M. Maier, E. Polivka, and B. R. Binder, Application of hydrophobic interaction chromatography for purification of pig urinary kallikrein. Characterization of the enzyme and its antibody, Hoppe-Seyler's Z. Physiol. Chem., 362:883-896, (1981).
10. M. Yano, H. Kato, S. Nagasawa, and T. Suzuki, An improved method for the purification of kininogen-II from bovine plasma, J. Biochem., 62:386-388, (1967).
11. T. Maack, Physiological evaluation of the isolated perfused rat kidney, Am. J. Physiol., 238:F71-F78, (1980).

ACTIVE KALLIKREIN, PREPROKALLIKREIN, AND KALLIKREIN-INHIBITOR COMPLEX

Julie Chao, Lee Chao, Cheryl M. Woodley, William Gerald and
Harry S. Margolius

Departments of Pharmacology, Biochemistry and Medicine
Medical University of South Carolina, Charleston, SC

SUMMARY

Active kallikreins isolated from various exocrine and endocrine tissues
were identified by a monoclonal antibody in Western blot analyses to be
~ 38,000 dalton proteins. Kallikreins isolated from rat pancreas, kidney,
submandibular gland, brain, spleen and urine were indistinguishable with
respect to molecular weight and immunological characteristics. Preprokallikreins were synthesized in a cell-free translation system directed by mRNAs
and immunoprecipitated by affinity-purified kallikrein antibody. Analysis
of the precipitates by SDS-polyacrylamide gel electrophoresis revealed
a ~ 37,000 dalton polypeptide in kidney, brain and submandibular gland
translation products. This 37,000 dalton kallikrein precursor was hybrid-
arrested by a kallikrein cDNA encoding tissue kallikrein which was isolated
from a rat submandibular gland cDNA library. The immunoprecipitates of
products directed by pancreaticv mRNA showed a major protein with Mr of
~ 30,000. An endogenous ~ 92,000 dalton component in rat urine and kidney
was also identified by a monoclonal antibody to tissue kallikrein and represents a kallikrein-inhibitor complex. These results indicate that tissue
kallikreins can be initially synthesized as 37,000 or 30,000 dalton prepro-
peptides and then converted into a 38,000 dalton active form by proteolytic
processing and glycosylation. The active kallikrein is capable of binding
to an inhibitor to form a 92,000 dalton complex.

INTRODUCTION

Tissue kallikreins have been identified in and isolated from the
kidney, salivary glands, pancreas, gastrointestinal mucosa, colon, sweat
glands and urine.[1,2] Recently, tissue kallikrein or kallikrein-like serine
proteases have been found at several new sites such as brain,[3] spleen,[4]
vasculature,[5] and erythrocyte membranes.[6] Tissue kallikreins from any
of these organs within a species appear to be nearly identical to the enzyme
at any of the other sites. They are acidic glycoproteins with PI's near
4.0.[1,2] The mature active kallikrein at any site is probably formed from
the preproenzyme following proteolytic cleavage and glycosylation. Despite
the similarity in size, charge, immunological characteristics and physicochemical properties of tissue kallikreins at various exocrine and endocrine
tissues, the primary translation products of tissue kallikrein and their
regulation at various sites are not well understood. Using specific

monoclonal and polyclonal antibodies to rat tissue kallikrein, we have isolated and identified active tissue kallikrein, the preproenzyme, as well as an endogenous tissue kallikrein-inhibitor complex.

METHODS

Enzyme Purification and Antibody Isolation

Tissue kallikreins were purified as described previously from rat urine,[7] brain,[3] and spleen.[4] Kallikreins from kidney were affinity-purified as described previously by a kallikrein monoclonal antibody-affinity column.[3,4] Polyclonal anti-rat urinary kallikrein antisera were generated in a sheep or rabbits[7] and monoclonal mouse anti-kallikrein antibodies were developed and characterized.[8] Monoclonal antibodies from ascitic fluid or polyclonal antibodies from sheep antiserum were affinity purified on a kallikrein-affinity column as described.[3] Submandibular gland, pancreas or kidney tissue extracts were prepared according to published procedures.[4] Protein concentration was determined by the method of Lowry et al.[9] using bovine serum albuin as standard.

Poly(A$^+$) mRNA Isolation and Cell-Free Translation

RNA from submandibular gland, pancreas and kidney was prepared according to the guanidium thiocyanate extraction procedure of Chirgwin et al.[10] Brain RNA ws isolated as described previously.[3] Polyadenylated RNA was isolated by two cycles of chromatography on an oligo (dT)-cellulose column. Cell-free translations directed by mRNAs from rat brain, submandibular gland, pancreas and kidney were carried out using [^{35}S] methionine as the radiolabel in a rabbit reticulocyte lysate as described.[3] The translation products were then immunoprecipitated with affinity purified polyclonal antibodies and analyzed on SDS-polyacrylamide gels followed by fluorography.[3]

Western Blot Analysis

Purified rat tissue kallikreins from urine, brain, spleen, kidney or tissue extracts from submandibular gland and pancreas were electrophoresed on a gradient (7.5-17.5%) polyacrylamide gel containing 0.1% SDS and transferred to nitrocellulose as previously described.[3] The free binding sites on the nitrocellulose were blocked with 3% BSA in 10 mM Tris-HCl, 0.9% NaCl, pH 7.5 for 45 min at 40°C. Affinity purified monoclonal antibodies were iodinated with the lactoperoxidase method.[11] Kallikreins were directly bound by ^{125}I-monoclonal antibodies (1 x 10^6 cpm/ml) in blot buffer (20 mM Tris, pH 7.5, 100 mM NaCl, 1% BSA, 0.2% Nonidet P-40) for 2 hr at 4°C. The nitrocellulose was washed with blot buffer 4 times at 4°C, dried, and autoradiographed.

Hybrid-Arrested Translation

Hybrid-arrested translation of rat submandibular gland mRNA by a tissue kallikrein cDNA probe was carried out as described.[12] Six µg of total RNA was mixed with 0.5 µg of single stranded M13 phage carrying rat tissue kallikrein cDNA[13] in a total volume of 3 µl. The solution was heated to 100°C for 1 min and quick-frozen in a dry-ice ethanol bath. To the tube was added formamide to 80%; 1,4-piperazine diethanesulfonic acid, pH 6.4, to 10 mM, and NaCl to 0.4 M in a final volume of 25 µl. The mixture was incubated at 48°C for 2 h and hybridization terminated by adding 0.2 ml of ice cold water containing 25 µg of yeast tRNA. The sample was divided into two equal portions and one was heated to 100°C for 1.5 min, then quick chilled in a dry-ice ethanol bath. The nucleic acid was precipitated, dried and resuspended in 5 µl water for translation assay.

RESULTS

Monoclonal Antibody Identification of Tissue Kallikreins

Tissue kallikreins were purified from rat urine, brain, spleen and
kidney. The purified kallikreins were analyzed by Western blotting using
a specific monoclonal antibody (V_4D_{11}) to rat urinary kallikrein. Figure
1 shows the direct binding of ^{125}I-monoclonal antibody to purified kallikreins from urine (lane 1), brain (lane 2), spleen (lane 3), kidney (lane
4). The specificity of the monoclonal antibody was clearly demonstrated
in the binding of a single tissue kallikrein in pancreatic (lane 5) and
submandibular gland extract (lane 6). The electrophoretic mobilities of
these tissue kallikreins are similar with their molecular weights estimated
to be 38,000. We have found previously that tissue kallikreins of various
origins are indistinguishable with respect to size, charge, immunological
characteristics, pH optimum and substrate specificity or susceptibility
to various inhibitors.[3,4,7]

Identification of Preprokallikrein in a Cell-Free Translation System

In the rabbit reticulocyte system, polyadenylated mRNAs from pancreas,
kidney, brain and submandibular gland were used to direct cell-free protein
synthesis. These primary biosynthetic products were immunoprecipitated
from the total translation products by affinity-purified sheep anti-kallikrein antibodies. The ^{35}S-methionine labeled proteins were visualized
by fluorography as shown in Figure 2. Control total translation products
(lane 1) or immunoprecipitates with the sheep antibodies in the absence

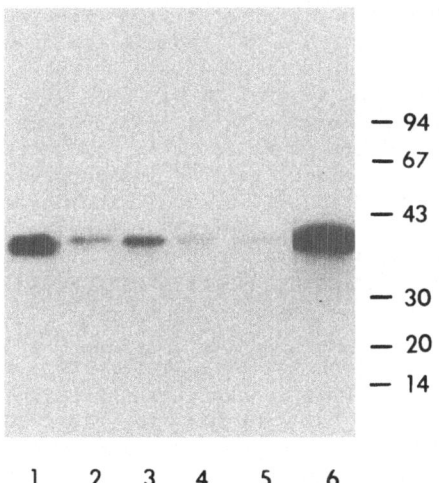

1   2   3   4   5   6

Fig. 1. Western blot analysis of rat tissue kallikreins. Purified kallikreins obtained from urine (lane 1), brain (lane 2), spleen (lane
3) and kidney (lane 4) (~ 5 µg each) as well as pancreatic (lane
5) (500 µg) or submandibular gland extracts (lane 6) (50 µg) were
analyzed by Western blotting using ^{125}I-monoclonal anti-kallikrein
antibody (V_4D_{11}) as described. The antibody binding was visualized
by autoradiography.

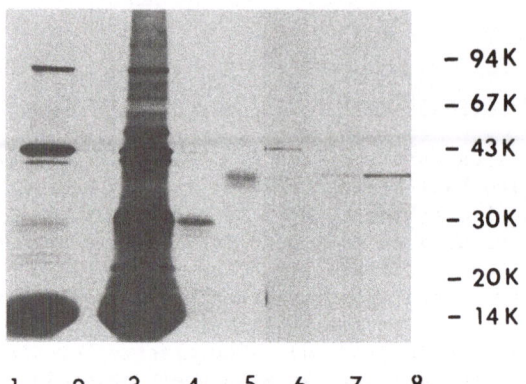

Fig. 2. Identification of kallikrein immunoreactive translation products.
Purified (polyA$^+$) mRNAs were translated in vitro and analyzed as
described. Lane 1, control, reaction containing no mRNA; lane
2, control immunoprecipitate with affinity-purified sheep anti-
rat urinary kallikrein; lane 3, polypeptides from pancreatic mRNA-
directed translation; lane 4, immunoprecipitates of pancreatic
mRNA-directed translation products; lane 5, ^{125}I-rat urinary kallikrein A & B; lane 6, immunoprecipitates of kidney; lane 7, immunoprecipitates of brain; and lane 8, immunoprecipitates of submandibular gland mRNA-directed translation products. Molecular weight
markers in kilodaltons are indicated.

of added mRNA (lane 2) show a non-specific protein band with Mr of ~ 46,000
as was also seen in the immunoprecipitates from translation products (lanes
4 & 6). Pancreatic mRNA-directed total translation products and the products
immunoprecipitated by the sheep antibodies are shown in lanes 3 and 4.
A predominant protein bnad and several minor bands with Mr's of ~ 28-30,000
as well as a larger polypeptide with Mr of ~ 43,000 was precipitated from
pancreatic translation products (lane 4). The immunoprecipitable translation
products of kidney (lane 6), brain (lane 7) and submandibular gland (lane
8) are similar in size with Mr's of ~ 37,000. They have similar electrophoretic mobility to purified ^{125}I-labeled rat urinary kallikrein (lane 5,
upper band is kallikrein A, and lower band is kallikrein B), while the biosynthetic products from pancreas are species with Mr's of ~ 30,000 and
43,000.

The 37,000 dalton immunoprecipitable protein is also hybrid-arrested
in a translation assay by a specific rat tissue kallikrein cDNA. Figure
3 shows that hybridization of rat submandibular gland RNA with a kallikrein
cDNA prevents the synthesis of a polypeptide with Mr of 37,000 (lane 2)
while the control heat-melted sample has no specific effect on kallikrein
translation (lane 1). The results demonstrate clearly that this 37,000
dalton biosynthetic polypeptide represents preprokallikrein. The conclusion
is based on the fact that this 37,000 dalton protein was not only recognized
by kallikrein antibody but also was hybrid-arrested by a tissue kallikrein
cDNA. Thes eprimary synthetic products represent kallikrein precursors
since no processing enzymes are present in the rabbit reticulocyte translation system.

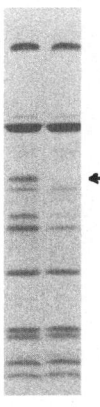

1 2

Fig. 3. Hybrid-arrested translation of rat submandibular kallikrein mRNA.
Single-stranded DNA carrying rat tissue kallikrein cDNA was hybridized with total RNA from rat submandibular gland. The sample
was divided into two equal portions. The control was heated at
100°C to melt the hybrid while the other was not heated before
translation. Both samples were translated in a rabbit reticulocyte
lysate cell-free system and analyzed on a SDS-polyacrylamide gel.
Lane 1, control polypeptides synthesized in the presence of rat
submandibular gland RNA hybridized with kallikrein cDNA, but heated
to 100°C before translation. Lane 2, same as lane 1 except the
sample was translated without heating. The arrow indicates the
position of the kallikrein translation product with Mr of ~ 37,000.

Identification of Endogenous Kallikrein-Inhibitor Complexes

An endogenous kallikrein-inhibitor complex with Mr of ~ 92,000 was
identified in urine and kidney by Western blot analyses using a specific
monolconal antibody to rat tissue kallikrein (Figure 4). The ^{125}I-labeled
monoclonal antibody binds directly to a   38,000 dalton protein in the pancreatic extract (lane 1), purified urinary kallikrein (lane 2), submandibular
gland extract (lane 3), rat urine (lane 4) and kidney extract (lane 5).
In addition, a higher molecular weight entity with Mr of 92,000 in urine
and kidney was also recognized by this monoclonal antibody. Because the
results of the cell-free translation assays (Figure 2) show that tissue
preprokallikreins vary only from 30,000 to 43,000 daltons, this 92,000 dalton
protein recognized by the specific monoclonal antibody to tissue kallikrein
is not a kallikrein precursor and likely represents a kallikrein-inhibitor
complex.

DISCUSSION

The present report shows that rat tissue kallikreins from brain, spleen,
kidney, pancreas, submandibular gland and urine are generally indistinguishable with respect to size, charge and immunological characteristics.
However, tissue kallikrein belongs to a large family of arginyl-esteropep-
tidases including the γ-subunit of nerve growth factor, an epidermal growth
factor-binding protein, β-nerve growth factor endopeptidase, tonin and
arginyl esterase A.[13-18] These kallikrein-related proteins are expressed
in submandibular gland and have enzymatic similarities and immunological
cross-reactivity. By using a monoclonal antibody to rat urinary kallikrein
which has no evident cross-reactivities with any related kallikrein-like

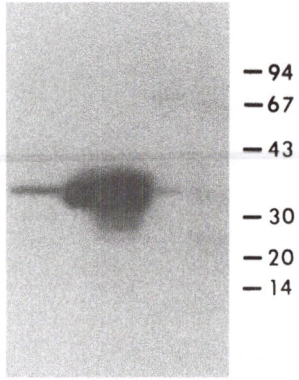

| | | | | |
|1|2|3|4|5|

Fig. 4. Western blot analysis of kallikrein-inhibitor complex in urine
and kidney. Rat urine (1 ml) and rat kidney homogenate (5 ml,
~ 12 mg/ml) were immunoprecipitated with 0.1 ml of sheep anti-
kallikrein antiserum. The immunoprecipitates were separated in
a linear SDS-polyacrylamide gel. The experimental conditions are
similar to that described in the legend to Figure 1. Lane 1, rat
pancreatic extract; lane 2, purified rat urinary kallikrein; lane
3, rat submandibular gland extract; lane 4, immunoprecipitated
rat urine; lane 5, immunoprecipitated rat kidney extract. Note
the endogenous kallikrein-inhibitor complex with Mr of ~ 92,000.

proteases, we have specifically identified kallikrein from various sites
in Western blot analyses as a ~ 38,000 dalton protein.

The kallikrein precursors were immunoprecipitated and identified from
a cell-free translation system. The preprokallikrein translation product
of kidney, brain and submandibular gland appears to be similar in size with
Mr of ~ 37,000. This 37,000 dalton polypeptide can also be hybrid-arrested
by a kallikrein cDNA. These results indicate clearly that this protein
represents preprokallikrein of kidney, brain and submandibular gland. The
kallikrein translation product of pancreas revealed two proteins with Mr's
of ~ 30,000 and a minor protein with a Mr of ~ 43,000. The 30,000 dalton
pancreatic kallikrein precursor may be the same as the 29,227 dalton rat
pancreatic preprokallikrein deduced from a pancreatic kallikrein cDNA sequence.[18] Whether this 30,000 dalton pancreatic preprokallikrein is the
precursor of the active 38,000 dalton pancreatic kallikrein remains to be
determined.

The results from cell-free translation studies indicated kallikrein
precursors ranging from Mr of 30,000 to 43,000. Therefore, the ~ 92,000
dalton protein identified in urine and kidney extract by a specific kalli-
krein-monoclonal antibody may represent a SDS-stable kallikrein-inhibitor
complex. This inhibitor may play an important regulatory role in tissue
kallikrein activity and metabolism. The localization and characterization
of this kallikrein inhibitor will be a subject of much interest. In summary,
the results indicate tht tissue kallikrein is initially synthesized as a
37,000 dalton preprokallikrein in kidney, brain and submandibular gland
and a 30,000 or 43,000 dalton polypeptide in pancreas and then converted
into a 38,000 dalton active form by proteolytic processing and glycosylation. The active kallikrein is capable of binding to a kallikrein inhibitor
to form a 92,000 dalton complex in vivo.

REFERENCES

1. F. Fiedler, Enzymology of glandular kallikreins, in: "Handbook of Experimental Pharmacology," Vol. 25, Supplement, Springer-Verlag, New York (1979).

2. J. J. Pisano, Chemistry and biology of the kallikrein-kinin system, in: "Proteases and Biological Control, Vol. 2, Cold Spring Harbor Conferences on Cell Proliferation," E. Reich, D. B. Rifkin,, and E. Shaw, Cold Spring Harbor (1975).

3. J. Chao, C. Woodley, L. Chao, and H. S. Margolius, Identification of tissue kallikrein in brain and in the cell-free translation product encoded by brain mRNA, J. Biol. Chem., 58:15173-15178 (1983).

4. J. Chao, L. Chao, and H. S. Margolius, Isolation of tissue kallikrein in rat spleen by monoclonal antibody-affinity chromatography, Biochem. Biophys. Acta, (In Press, 1984).

5. H. Nolly and M. C. Lama, Vascular kallikrein: A kallikrein-like enzyme present in vascular tissue of the rat, Clin. Sci., 63:249S-251S (1982).

6. J. Chao, L. Chao, and H. S. Margolius, Identification of a kallikrein-like latent serine proteinase in human erythrocyte plasma membranes, Biochem. Biophys. Res. Commu., 121:722-729 (1984).

7. J. Chao and H. S. Margolius, Isozymes of rat urinary kallikrein, Biochem. Pharmacol., 28:2071-2079 (1979).

8. C. M. Woodley, J. Chao, H. S. Margolius, and L. Chao, Specific identification, stimulation or inhibition of rat tissue kallikrein with monoclonal antibodies, Kinin '84, Abstract, p. 150 (1984).

9. O. H. Lowry, N. J. Rosebrough, A. L. Farr, and R. J. Randall, Protein measurement with the folin phenol reagent, J. Biol. Chem., 193:265-275 (1951).

10. J. M. Chirgwin, A. E. Przybyla, R. J. McDonald, and W. J. Rutter, Isolation of biologically active ribonucleic acid from sources enriched in ribonuclease, Biochemistry, 18:5294-5299 (1979).

11. K. Shimamoto, J. Chao, and H. S. Margolius, The radioimmunoassay of human urinary kallikrein and comparisons with kallikrein activity measurements, J. Clin. Endocrinol. Metab., 51:840-848 (1980).

12. W. L. Gerald, J. Chao, and L. Chao, Sex dimorphism and hormonal regulation of rat tissue kallikrein mRNA (Manuscript Submitted, 1984).

13. W. L. Gerald, J. Chao, and L. Chao, isolation and analysis of a cDNA clone Encoding Rat Submaxillary Gland Kallikrein, DNA, 3:86 (1984).

14. A. J. Mason, B. A. Evans, D. R. Cox, J. Shine, and R. I. Richards, Structure of mouse kallikrein gene family suggests a role in specific processing of biologically active peptides, Nature, 303:300-307 (1983).

15. M. A. Bothwell, H. Wyndham, and E. M. Shooter, The relationship between glandular kallikrein and growth factor processing proteases of mouse submaxillary gland, J. Biol. Chem., 254:7287-7294 (1979).

16. J. Chao, Purification and characterization of rat urinary esterase A, a plasminogen activator, J. Biol. Chem., 258:4434-4439 (1983).

17. R. P. McPartland, R. Rapp, M. K. Joseph, and D. L. Sustarsic, Isolation and partial characterization of rat urinary esterase A_2, Biochem. Biophys. Acta, 742:100-108 (1983).

18. G. H. Swift, J.-C. Dagorn, P. L. Ashley, S. W. Cummings, and R. J. MacDonald, Rat pancreatic kallirkein mRNA: Nucleotide sequence and amino acid sequence of the enclosed preproenzyme, Proc. Natl. Acad. Sci. USA, 79:7263-7267 (1982).

CHARACTERIZATION OF RAT KALLIKREIN-LIKE MULTIGENE FAMILY AND ITS EXPRESSION

IN THE SUBMANDIBULAR GLAND

Lee Chao, William Gerald and Julie Chao

Departments of Biochemistry and Pharmacology
Medical University of South Carolina
Charleston, SC

SUMMARY

A cDNA clone encoding rat tissue kallikrein was isolated from a sub-mandibular cDNA library. The kallikrein cDNA clone was used as a probe to analyze the complexity of the kallikrein-like gene family and its expres-sion. The results indicate that rat kallikrein-like genes identified with this probe belong to a very large and highly homologous multigene family. A number of these genes, perhaps as many as a dozen or so, are expressed in the submandibular gland.

INTRODUCTION

Tissue kallikrein belongs to a multigene family which encodes a group of structurally related serine proteases including the gamma subunit of nerve growth factor, the epidermal growth factor binding protein, gamma renin, tonin and esterase A. Many of these proteins are expressed in the submaxillalry gland of the mouse[1] and the submandibular gland of the rat (see Woodley et al., this volume). Earlier studies have established the role of NGF γ subunit and EGF, respectively.[2,3] The function of the remaining kallikrein-like proteins is not clear at this time. REcent studies have indicated that these kallikrein-related proteases may be excellent candidates for processing peptide hormones.[4]

To investigate the complexity of the expressed kallikrein genes we have constructed a cDNA library from rat submandibular gland poly A+ RNA. A kallikrein cDNA was identified and used to probe additional kallikrein-like cDNA clones from this library. We have also used the kallikrein cDNA as a probe to screen a lambda Charon 4A library constructed with genomic DNA from a rat submandibular gland. The results show that the rat kallikrein-like genes form a large and highly homologous family. It also appears that most of the kallikrein-like genes are expressed in the submandibular gland. Gene structure and sequence comparisons suggest that at least one of the kallikrein-like genes, a pseudogene, may have evolved recently from an active kallikrein-like gene.

MATERIALS AND METHODS

RNA Isolation and cDNA Synthesis

Total RNA was isolated from rat submandibular gland by the guanidinium thiocyanate procedure.[5] Polyadenylated RNA (poly A+) was purified by two cycles of chromatography on an oligo dT-cellulose column. The first strand cDNA synthesis was carried out with AMV reverse transcriptase using oligo dT primers and the second strand was synthesized with the same enzyme without primers. The staggered ends were made blunt with Klenow fragment of DNA polymerase I and subsequently phosphorylated with T4 polynucleotide kinase. The double-stranded cDNA was inserted into the Sma I site of pUC8 and transformed into E. coli JM83.[6] White colonies containing inserts were picked for further testing. The cDNA library was screened with an immuno-logical screening procedure as described by Helfman et al.[7] using affinity-purified anti-kallikrein antibodies followed by I-labeled protein A.

Rat Genomic Library Construction and Screening

Rat submandibular gland DNA and Charon 4A phage DNA were purified as described by Maniatis et al.[8] The purified rat DNA partially digested with EcoR 1 and sized in 0.45% agarose gel. DNA fragments ranging from 16 to 20 Kb were recovered and inserted into the EcoR 1 site of Charon 4A.[9] The rat genomic library was amplified once and screened with the appropriate cDNA probes using the in situ hybridization procedure described by Benton and Davis.[10]

DNA and RNA Hybridization Analyses

The procedures for DNA hybridization were according to those described by Maniatis et al.[8] RNA filter hybridization was carried out by the method of Thomas.[11]

DNA Sequence Analysis

The dideoxy method of Sanger[12] was used for DNA sequencing with M13 vectors of Messing[13] and commercially available primers.

RESULTS

A cDNA library was constructed from purified rat submandibular gland poly A RNA using AMV reverse transcriptase. The cDNA inserts were placed under the control of lac Z promoter and a ribosome binding site in the ex-presion plasmid pUC8.[13] The library was screened with affinity-purified anti-kallikrein antibody to identify those clones that synthesize kalli-krein. Several clones were identified as positives by this procedure. One of these clones, RSK1105, was analyzed in detail and sequenced. This clone was identified as a kallikrein cDNA clone because the amino acid sequence predicted by this clone is identical to that of the rat submandibular kalli-krein and the nucleotide sequence agrees with an earlier report of rat pan-creatic kallikrein cDNA.[14]

Immunological screening procedures can only identify about one-sixth of the potential kallikrein or kallikrein-like cDNA clones within a library. About half of the clones cannot be expressed correctly due to a 50% chance that an insert is introduced into the vector in the wrong orientation. For those inserts with correct orientations, about two-thirds may be ligated into the vector in the wrong reading frame. Thus proteins produced from these inserts are useless for immunoscreening. To identify all kallikrein and kallikrein-like clones within our cDNA library, we have used RSK1105 as a probe to screen the cDNA library by Southern hybridization. The results in Figure 1 show that additional clones in the library were identified and that these clones vary in signal intensity when probed with the kallikrein cDNA insert, RSK1105. After extensive rescreening we have narrowed the kallikrein-like clones from the submandibular library to 19. DNA from these clones were purified and the inserts were excised from the vector by double digestion with EcoR 1 and BamH 1. The linearized vector and insert DNA were separated in a 1.5% agarose gel and analyzed by Southern hybridization. The cDNA clones have various insert sizes as indicated in Figure 2A. In addition, several clones, such as RSK799, RSK3363, and RSK3441, have internal EcoR 1 or BamH 1 cleavage sites. The results of Southern hybridization are shown in Figure 2B. Note the varying degree of hybridization of the cDNA clones to the RSK1105 probe with clones RSK3390 and RSK3305 being the strongest. RSK799, RSK1600 and RSK1908 generated moderate signals while the remainder of the clones gave very weak signals. These clones are being sequenced at this time. Our preliminary results indicate that the kallikrein-like cDNA clones from therat submandibular gland may represent a group of related genes with sequence homologies ranging from 30 to 80%.

The results presented in Table 1 suggest that a group of closely related genes are present in the rat genome as a gene family and that many or all of these gene family members are expressed in the rat submandibular DNA. The length of the genomic DNA inserts range from 16 to 20 kb. The genomic clones were amplified once and plated on agar plates. RSK1105 DNA was nick-translated in the presence of ^{32}P-dCTP and used as a probe. A total of 4.5 million phage plaques were screened which represent about 2.5 genome equivalents of rat DNA.[8] Instead of 2 to 3 kallikrein genes we have identified 34 kallikrein or kallikrein-like genomic clones. We have analyzed these genomic clones in detail by restriction mapping. Our preliminary results indicated that at least 18 different kallikrein-like genomic clones can be recognized. We have tentatively divided these genomic clones into six classes as shown in Table 1. These results are in agreement with the observation made in the mouse where kallikrein-like multigene family has been identified earlier. Several representative genomic clones are being analyzed by restriction mapping and sequencing to study the organization and the evolution of the rat kallikrein-like gene family.

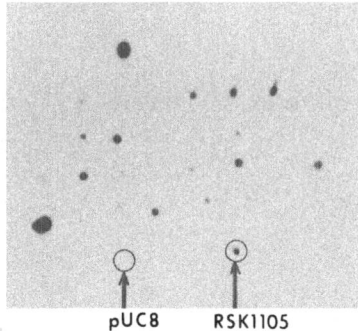

pUC8   RSK1105

Fig. 1. In situ hybridization of kallikrein-like cDNA clones from rat submandibular gland. The kallikrein cDNA clones were replicated onto nitrocellulose filters and screened with RSKG1105 as a probe. Shown above is the autoradiogram of the filter following in situ hybridization. The signals generated by RSK1105 and the vector pUC8 are indicated.

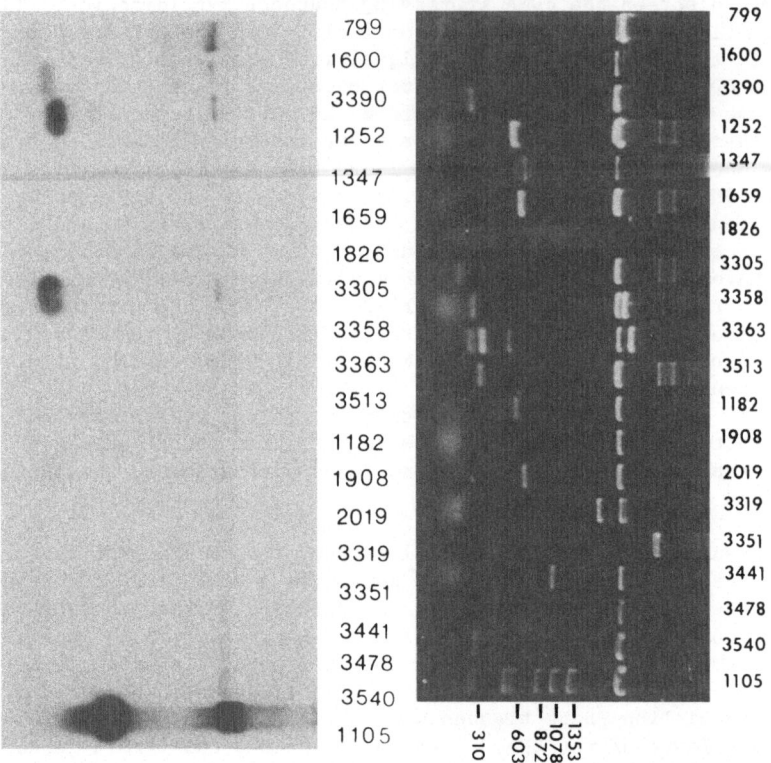

Fig. 2. Analysis of submandibular kallikrein cDNA clones. Nineteen positive kallikrein cDNA clones were purified and cleaved with EcoR 1
and BamH 1. The vector and insert DNA were separated in a 0.9%
agarose gel for Southern hybridization using RSK1105 as a probe.
2A, agarose gel separation of kallikrein-like DNA. The clone
numbers are indicated above and the molecular weight hybridization
pattern of the cDNA clones. 2B, Southern blot analysis of the cDNA
clones with RSK1105 insert as the probe.

Table 1.   Classification of Kallikrein-Like Genomic Clones

Type	Number	Characteristic Fragment
Class I Clones	5	12,000 bp
Class II Clones	9	9,000 bp
Class III Clones	5	8,500 bp
Class IV Clones	4	6,000 bp
Class V Clones	1	5,000 bp
Class VI Clones	10	undefined

Characteristic fragment indicates the common EcoR I fragment that is hy-
bridizable tothe kallikrein cDNA probe.

DISCUSSION

Several interesting facts have emerged from this study. First, the rat kallikrein gene, like that of the mouse, belongs to a closely related multi-gene family. Furthermore, most of the members of this multigene family are expressed in the submandibular gland. This is not surprising since several kallikrein-like proteins, such as the gamma subunit of the nerve growth factor, the epidermal growth factor binding protein, gamma renin and tonin, are known to be synthesized in the submandibular gland. Further analysis of the submandibular cDNA clones may eventually lead to the identification of the individual genes as well as their protein products in this glandular tissue.

It is of special interest to note that strong sequence homology has been maintained among the kallikrein gene family members. Extensive sequence homology within a gene family are thought to occur by concerted evolution. In this senario mutations of the gene family member are corrected by gene conversion where a portion of an allele may be replaced in a non-reciprocal exchange within the gene family. However, it is not known if there is any selective advantage by maintaining such a high degree of sequence homology within a given gene family. Alternatively, the homogeneity of the kallikrein genes may indicate a recent origin of the gene family. It is possible, for example, that the kallikrein gene family is derived from a single primordial kallikrein gene by repeated gene duplications that generate the six major kallikrein archtypes as the first significant event in kallikrein gene evo-lution. Further modification by base substitutions and rearrangement within each archtype eventually gave rise to the modern day kallikrein gene family. In a sense the kallikrein gene family may be regarded as a young gene family in evolution. In support of this notion, we have recently sequenced a kalli-krein pseudogene and compared its sequence divergence against the coding region of the kallikrein cDNA. We noted a total of 35 substitutions in 384 bp compared. Eighteen substitutions are replacement type with 10 of these occurring at the first condon, 7 at the second codon and 1 at the third codon. The other 17 substitutions are silent. Based on the assumption ad-vanced by Efstratiadis et al.[15] regarding the rate of multigene evolution, the kallikrein pseudogene may have diverged from the active gene approximate-ly 6 million years ago. This is clearly an overestimate since the rate of mutation in pseudogenes is known to be much higher.[16] We may therefore ten-tatively conclude that at least one member of the gene family has diverged very recently as compared to the mammalian divergence time of 85 million years ago. Further studies are needed to give a definitive picture of the kallikrein gene family organization and evolution.

ACKNOWLEDGEMENT

This work was supported in part by grants HL 29397 and HL 33552 from the National Institutes of Health.

REFERENCES

1. A. J. Mason, B. A. Evans, D. R. Cox, J. Shine, and R. I. Richards, Structure of mouse kallikrein gene family suggests a role in specific processing of biologically active peptides, Nature, 303:300-307 (1983).
2. E. A. Berger and E. M. Shooter, Evidence for pro-B-nerve growth factor, a biosynthetic precursor to B-nerve growth factor, Proc. Natl. Acad. Sci. USA, 76:6294-6298 (1979).

3. P. Frey, R. Forand, T. Magiag, and E. M. Shooter, The biosynthetic precursor of epidermal growth factor and the mechanism of its processing, Proc. Natl. Acad. Sci. USA, 76:6294-6298 (1979).

4. J. Shine, A. J. Mason, B. A. Evans, and R. I. Richards, The kallikrein multigene, Quant. Biol., 48:419-426 (1983).

5. J. M. Chirgwin, A. E. Przybyla, R. J. McDonald, and W. J. Rutter, Isolation of biologically active ribonucleic acid from sources enriched in ribonuclease, Biochemistry, 18:5294-5299 (1979).

6. J. Vieira and J. Messing, The pUC plasmids, an M13 mp7-derived system for insertion mutagenesis and sequencing with synthetic universal primers, Gene, 19:259-268 (1982).

7. D. Helfman, J. Feramisco, J. Fiddes, G. Thomas, and S. Hughes, Identification of clones that encode chicken tropomysin by direct immunological screening of cDNA expression library, Proc. Natl. Acad. Sci. USA, 80:31-35(1983).

8. T. Maniatis and E. Fritsch, in: "Molecular Cloning, A Laboratory Manual," Cold Spring Harbor Laboratory, pp. 270-294, 382-389, 455-467 (1982).

9. F. R. Blattner, B. G. Williams, A. E. Blechl, K. D. Thompson, H. E. Faber, L. A. Furlong, D. J. Grunwald, D. O. Kiefer, D. D. Moore, J. W. Schumm, E. L. Sheldon, and O. Smithies, Charon phages: Safer derivatives of bacteriophage lambda for DNA cloning, Science, 196:161-169 (1977).

10. W. D. Benton and R. Davis, Screening gt recombinant clones by hybridization to single plaques in situ, Science, 196:180-182 (1977).

11. P. Thomas, Hybridization of denatured RNA transferred or dotted to nitrocellulose paper, in: "Methods in Enzymology, Vol. 100," R. Wu, L. Grossman, and K. Moldave, eds., Academic Press, pp. 255-266 (1983).

12. F. Sanger, S. Nicklen, and A. Coulson, DNA sequencing with chain terminating inhibitors, Proc. Natl. Acad. Sci. USA, 74:5463-5467 (1977).

13. J. Messing, New M13 vectors for cloning, in: "Methods in Enzymology, Vol. 101," R. Wu, L. Grossman, and K. Moldave, eds., Academic Press, pp. 325-331 (1983).

14. G. Swift, J. Dagorn, P. Ashley, S. Cummings, and R. J. McDonald, Rat pancreatic kallikrein mRNA: Nucleotide sequence and amino acid sequence of the encoded preproenzyme, Proc. Ntl. aCad. Sci. USA, 79: 7263-7267 (1982)

15. A. Efstratiadis, J. W. Posakony, C. O'Connell, R. A. Sprtiz, J. K. DeRiel, B. G. Forget, S. M. Weisman, J. L. Slightom, A. E. Blechl, F. E. Baralle, C. C. Shoulders, and N. J. Proudfoot, The structure and evolution of the human B-globin gene family, Cell, 21:653-668 (1980).

16. W. H. Li, T. Gojobori, and M. Nei, Pseudogenes as a paradigm of neutral evolution, Nature, 292:237-239(1981).

PROCESSING OF APOLIPOPROTEIN B-100 OF HUMAN PLASMA LOW DENSITY LIPOPROTEINS

BY TISSUE AND PLASMA KALLIKREINS

Alan D. Cardin*, Richard L. Jackson**, Virginia H Donaldson+,
Julie Chao++, and Harry S. Margolius++

From *the Division of Lipoprotein Research, Department of
Pharmacology and Cell Biophysics, University of Cincinnati
College of Medicine, Cincinnati, Ohio 45267-0575; **The Merrell
Dow Research Institute, Merrell Dow Pharmaceuticals, Inc.
Cincinnati, Ohio 45215; +the Children's Hospital Research
Foundation, Cincinnati, Ohio 45267; and ++the Departments of
Pharmacology and Medicine, Medical Unviersity of South
Carolina, Charleston, South Carolina 29425

SUMMARY

Human plasma low density lipoporteins (LDL) are the major carriers of
cholesterol and cholesteryl esters in the circulation. Their increased
levels correlate positively with increased risk of coronary artery disease.
LDL contain a single major apolipoprotein of apparent molecualr weight (Mr) =
550,000, designated apolipoprotein B-100 (apoB-100), and ins ome LDL preparations, minor components termed apoB-74 (410,000) and apoB-26 (145,000). The
structural relationship of the apoB-74 and -26 proteins to the apoB-100 has
remained obscure and their roles in cholesterol metabolism are unknown. In
the present study, we show that the addition of kaolin to plasma anticoagulated with EDTA induces the proteolytic cleavage of apoB-100. As a result,
two apoB peptides are produced with Mr indistinguishable from plasma apoB-74
and -26. The specific cleavage of apoB-100 was mimicked in vitro by purified
human plasma and tissue kallikreins. In contrast, thrombin, factor Xa,
plasmin, trypsin, and chymotrypsin did not produce these peptides when incubated with LDL. The findings of the study suggest that apoB-74 and -26
are proteolytic fragments of apoB-100 and that the endogenous protease has
a kallikrein-like specificity for DLD-apoB-100. The role of plasma and
tissue kallikreins in cholesterol metabolism remains to be determined.

INTRODUCTION

Apolipoprotein B (apoB)[1] is a major constituent of the triglyceride-
rich chylomicrons and very low density lipoproteins (VLDL) and of the

---

[1]The abbreviations used are: ApoB, apolipoprotein B; VLDL, very low density
lipoproteins; LDL, low density lipoproteins; SDS, sodium dodecyl sulfate;
EDTA, disodium salt of ethylenediaminetetraacetic acid; PPACK, D-phenyl-
alanyl-L-Prolyl-L-arginine chloromethylketone.

cholesteryl ester-rich low density lipoproteins (LDL). ApoB plays a central role in the transport of cholesterol (free and esterified), triacylglycerols and phospholipids in the circulation.[1] The chylomicrons of intestinal lymph contain a single species of apoB termed apoB-48 plus various other apoprotein constituents.[2] ApoB-48 has an apparent molecular weight (Mr) of 265,000 as determined by electrophoresis in SDS.[2] The VLDL and LDL are of hepatic origin and cotnain a high moelcular weight species of apoB termed apoB-100 (Mr $\simeq$ 550,000). Unlike VLDL, however, LDL has two additional apoB peptides termed apoB-74 (410,000) and apoB-26 (145,000). Although evidence suggests that apoB-48 and apoB-100 are under separate genetic regulation,[3] the origin of apoB-74 and -26 in LDL and their roles in lipid metabolism have remained obscure. The present study focuses on the structural relation of the apoB-100, -74, and -26 apoproteins. The present findings show that human plasma and tissue kallikreins cleave apoB-100 into two peptides which appear identical to plasma apoB-74 and -26. The potential role of kallikreins in the metabolism of the cholesteryl ester-rich low density lipoproteins is discussed.

METHODS

Materials

Highly purified human thrombin (50 units/mg of protein) was a generous gift from Dr. J. W. Fenton (Division of Laboratories and Research, New York State Department of Health, Albany, NY). Human urinary (tissue) kallikrein was purified to homogeneity as described previously.[4,5] Its activity was 74 α-N-tosyl-L-arginine methylesterase units/mg of protein. Human plasma kallikrein, purified by the method of Nagase and Barrett[6] and Donaldson et al.,[7] had an activity of 58 units/mg of protein as determined in the clotting assay described previously.[8] All buffer solutions were prepared with deionized distilled water. Kaolin was obtained from Fisher Scientific Company and PPACK from Calbiochem.

Blood Collection, Plasma Isolation, and Lipoprotein Purification

Blood (25 ml) was collected by venipuncture from normal fasting donors into plastic syringes fitted with an 18-gauge needle. The blood contained a final EDTA concentration of 0.5% (w/v). To obtain plasma, blood was transferred to nitrocellulose tubes and spun at 6000 x g to remove cells. To prevent degradation of apoB by exogenous enzymes introduced during lipoprotein isolation, the plasma was adjusted with PPACK, aprotinin, NaN$_3$, and phenylmethylsulfonyl fluoride to final concentrations of 1 μM, 100 kallikrein-inhibitory units/ml, 0.01% and 0.5 mM, respectively. LDL (d = 1.02-1.05 g/ml) were isolated from plasma by sequential ultracentrifugal flotation in salt solutions of KBr as described previously.[9]

Digestion of ApoB-100 with Thrombin and Kallikreins

Enzmic digests were performed at an enzyme:apoB-100 protein ratio of 1:100 (w/v) at 37°C with 100 g of LDL protein (apoB) in 0.1 ml of 10 mM Tris-HCl, 0.15 M NaCl, pH 7.4, 0.01% NaN$_3$. In some experiments, bovine serum albumin was included in the incubation at a final concentration of 25 mg/ml. Thrombin digests were terminated by adjusting the samples to 1 μM in PPACK. Kallikrein digests were terminated by mixing the samples with 0.235 ml of an electrophoresis sample buffer consisting of 10 mM Tris-HCl, 1.4% SDS, 1 mM EDTA, 8.6 M urea, 1.4% 2-mercaptoethanol, 29% sucrose, and 0.04% bromphenol blue. The samples were then heated at 60°C for 15 min and subjected to gel electrophoresis. ApoB peptides were separated on 3-6% pore-gradient polyacrylamide gels as previously described.[10]

Immunoblot Analysis

After polyacylamide gel electrophoresis, the gel was soaked for 10 min in 25 mM Tris-HCl, 192 mM glycine, pH 8.3 containing 20% (v/v) methanol (transfer buffer). Proteins were electrophoretically transferred from the gel to nitrocellulose paper (0.45 μm, Bio-Rad Corporation) for 3 h at 200 mA in transfer buffer.[11] The nitrocellulose was soaked overnight in 10 mM Tris-HCl, 0.15 M NaCl, pH 7.4, containing 3% BSA (Buffer A) to quench the remaining protein binding sites.[12] The nitrocellulose was then incubated for 3 h with a goat antiserum containing a polyclonal antibody to apoB-100 diluted 1:500 in Buffer A. The nitrocellulose was washed three times for 5 min per wash in Buffer A containing 0.05% Tween-20. The nitrocellulose was incubated for 1 h with a rabbit anti-goat peroxidase-conjugated IgG (Miles-Yeda Limited) diluted 1:1000 in Buffer A, and then washed as described above. ApoB peptides were visualized by the reaction of peroxidase with the HRP color reagent (Bio-Rad Laboratories) containing 4-chloro-1-napthol.

Other Methods

Goat antiserum containing a polyclonal antibody to apoB-100 was prepared as previously described.[9] Protein was determined by the method of Lowry et al.[13] with bovine serum albumin as standard and by amino acid analysis. Gel densitometry was performed on a Zeineh soft laser scanning desnitometer (Biomed Instruments, Inc., Chicago, IL). Quantitative densitometric scans were conducted in the linear range of the optical response with respect to peptide mass. Apparent molecular weights of peptides were determined by extrapolation from a standard plot of the logarithm of the molecular weights versus the electrophoretic mobility of standard proteins. The protein standards were thyroglobulin (670,000 and 330,000 molecular weight forms), ferritin half-unit (220,000), bovine serum albumin dimer (134,000), phosphorylase b (94,000), and bovine serum albumin monomer (67,000).

RESULTS

Fig. 1 is an immunoblot analysis of two LDL preparations obtained from different normal donors. The LDL of Donor 1 (lane a) contains a single polypeptide termed apolipoprotein B-100 (apoB-100) while the LDL of Donor 2 (lane b) contains two additional peptides termed apoB-74 and apoB-26. These proteins were detected with a polyclonal antiserum to apoB-100 (see Methods). The results show that the apoB-74 and -26 polypeptides are apoB-100 related antigens. The apparent molecular weights of the apoB-100, -74, and -26 proteins are 550,000 ± 6,000, 410,000 ± 5,000, and 145,000 ± 3,000, respectively (mean and S.D. of twelve different preparations). The apoB-74 and -26 proteins were isolated by preparative gel electrophoresis. Amino acid mass analysis shows that these polypeptides are present in a 1.0:1.0 (mole/mol) ration in LDL (Fig. 1, lane b). The stoichiometries of these peptides in LDL, their antigenic relatedness to apoB-100, and the sum of their apparent molecular weights (555,000 ± 8,000) indicate that apoB-74 and -26 are fragments of apoB-100 (550,000 ± 6,000).

In the next series of experiments, apoB-100 in LDL was digested with various enzymes to determine if proteolysis might explain how apoB-74 and -26 arise in plasma LDL. The degradation products were analyzed by gradient-gel electrophoresis and their mobilities were compared to apoB-74 and -26. Incubation of LDL containing only apoB-100 (Fig. 1, lane a) with either plasmin, trypsin, or chymotrypsin under conditions of limiting enzyme, time, and temperature resulted in multiple fragments not resembling plasma apoB-74 and -26 (not shown). However, thrombin generated a single cleavage of apoB-

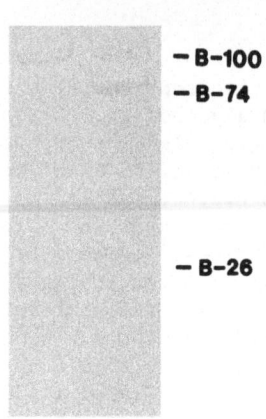

Fig. 1. Immunoblot analysis of the apoB polypeptides of human plasma LDL. Lane a shows the apoB-100 polypeptide present in the LDL of Donor 1; lane b, the apoB-100, -74, and -26 peptides present in the LDL of Donor 2.

100 to yield two major peptides. Fig. 2, lane a of the gradient-gel shows apoB-100, -74, and -26 of plasma LDL. ApoB-74 and -26 constitute approximately15% of the total apoB mass in this LDL preparation. Lane b shows the two apoB peptides T_1 and T_2 which result from thrombin cleavage. Like apoB-74 and -26, T_1 and T_2 comprise 15% of the total apoB mass on the gel. It is known that the electrophoretic mobility of apoB increases with increasing protein mass applied to the gel.[2,9] Since, however, the T_1, T_2, apoB-74, and -26 peptides are present in equivalent amounts, the mobilities of the thrombin-derived apoB peptides (lane b) can be compared to those of the plasma peptides (lane a). Such a comparison indicates that the mobilities of T_1 and T_2 are similar but not identical to apoB-74 and -26. The

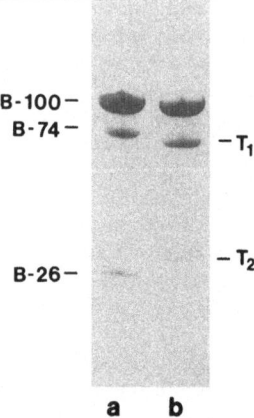

Fig. 2. Polyacrylamide gel electrophoresis of thrombin-treated LDL. Lane a shows apoB-100, -74, and -26 of plasma LDL; lane b, (from top to bottom) apoB-100 and its thrombin degradation products, T_1 and T_2.

T_1 and T_2 peptides have apparent molecular weights of 385,000 and 170,000 respectively. In other experiments not shown, factor Xa generated two apoB peptides with mobilities like those of T_1 and T_2.

In contrast to thrombin and factor Xa, purified human plasma and tissue kallikreins degraded apoB-100 to yield two peptides, K_1 and K_2, with mobilities like those of apoB-74 and -26 (Fig. 3). Lane a shows the gradient-gel pattern of plasma LDL containing apoB-100, -74, and -26; lanes b and c show the K_1 and K_2 peptides obtained by degradation of apoB-100 with tissue and plasma kallikreins, respectively.

To compare the mobilities of the thrombin and kallikrein peptides of apoB-100 more closely with apoB-74 and -26, mixing experiemnts were performed (Fig. 4). The mixing of thrombin-treated LDL with either kallikrein-treated LDL (lane a) or plasma LDL (lane b) shows that the T_1 and T_2 peptides do not comigrate during electrophoresis with K_1, K_2, apoB-74 or -26. However, the mixing of kallikrein-treated LDL with plasma LDL (lane c) shows that the K_1 and K_2 peptides comigrate with authentic plasma apoB-74 and -26.

In view of the results with purified kallikreins, it was of interest to determine if contact activation of plasma in the presence of EDTA would generate peptides in plasma LDL with apoB-74 and -26 mobilities. Subjects were chosen who were previously identified as having only apoB-100 in their LDL. Their plasmas, anticoagulated with EDTA (see Methods), were aliquoted into plastic tubes containing increasing amounts of kaolin and incubated at room temperature. The lipoproteins of d < 1.063 g/ml of each plasma sample was isolated by ultracentrifugation and then analyzed by gradient-gel electrophoresis. As shown in Fig. 5, the amount of peptides with apoB-74 (and apoB-26, data not shown) mobilities increased with increasing kaolin up to 30 μg kaolin/ml plasma. LDL isolated from plasma in the absence of kaolin had only apoB-100. These results show that surface activation of plasma enzymes by kaolin can generate two peptides in LDL with electrophoretic mobilities indistinguishable from apoB-74 and -26.

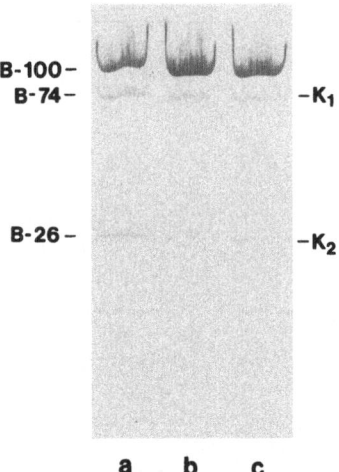

a   b   c

Fig. 3.   Gradient-gel electrophoresis of kallikrein-treated LDL B-100. Lane a shows apoB-100, -74, and -26 of plasma LDL; lanes b and c show the K_1 and K_2 peptides of LDL which result from the cleavage of apoB-100 by tissue and plasma kallikreins, respectively.

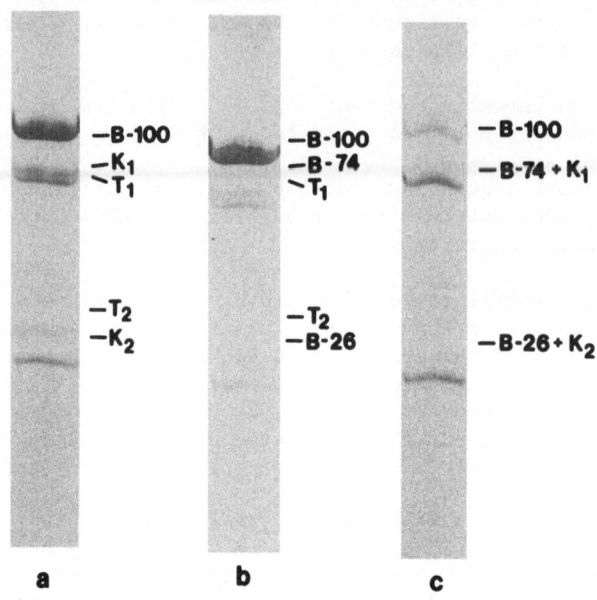

Fig. 4. Mixing experiments comparing the mobilities of the apoB peptides of the thrombin- and kallikrein-treated LDL samples with apoB-74 and -26 peptides of plasma. Lane a, kallikrein-treated LDL (apoB-100, K_1 and K_2) plus thrombin-treated LDL (apoB-100, T_1, and T_2); lane b, thrombin-treated LDL plus plasma LDL (apoB-100, -74, and -26); lane c, kallikrein-treated LDL plus plasma LDL B-100, -74, and -26.

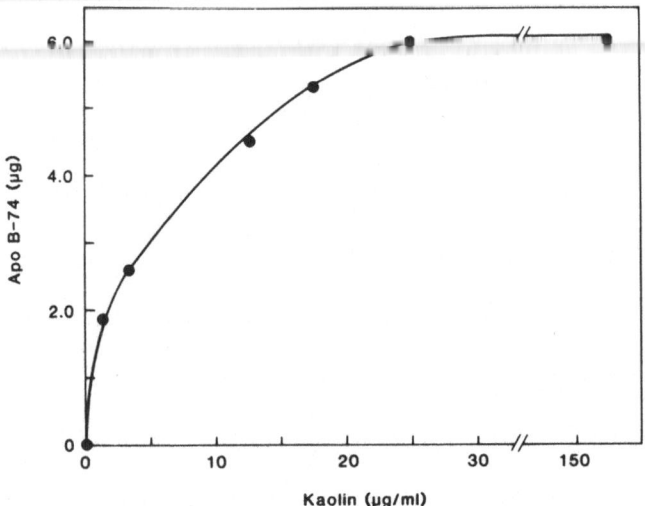

Fig. 5. The addition of kaolin to plasma generates apoB peptides in LDL with electrophoretic mobilities indistinguishable from plasma apoB-74 and -26.

DISCUSSION

We previously reported that the presence of the apoB-74 and -26 peptides in LDL can be diminished by the mixing of serine protease inhibiters with blood at the moment of blood collection.[10] In the present study, we show that peptides with apoB-74 and -26 mobilities can be generated in LDL by the addition of kaolin to plasma anticoagulated with EDTA. This finding suggests that the endogenous protease is surface activated via a factor XIIa dependent-like reaction independent of a Ca^{2+} requirement. In reconstitution experiments conducted under physiological conditions of pH, temperature, ionic strength, LDL, albumin and enzyme concentrations, both purified human plasma and tissue kallikreins cleaved apoB-100 into two peptides (K_1 and K_2) that comigrated with apoB-74 and -26 during gel electrophoresis. More recent studies have confirmed that the K_1 and K_2 peptides have amino acid compositions, NH_2-terminal sequences and reactivities to anti-apoB monoclonal antibodies that are indistinguishable from those of authentic plasma apoB-74 and -26. Although the identity of the endogeneous protease is unknown, it is clear that its specificity is identical to the in vitro specificity of kallikrein(s) for apoB-100 of LDL.

Kaolin activates factor XII (factor XIIa) and factor XIIa converts plasma prekallikrein to kallikrein. Experiments are currently in progress to determine if kallikrein can act in plasma to process apoB-100 via this pathway. Moreover, an immunoreactive tissue kallikrein in serum has been reported.[14] It is not known, however, if this tissue kallikrein interacts with plasma lipoproteins. In a recent study, Paskhina et al.[15] reported tha t plasma kallikrein, prekallikrein, and kinins were preferentially absorbed to LDL and not VLDL. This observation might explain the reported absence of apoB-74 and -26 in VLDL[2] and, further, raises the question of whether there is a circulatory pool of lipoprotein-associated kallikreins that act preferentially on apoB-100 and not kininogen.

Atherosclerosis, a disease of the vessel wall,[16] is exacerbated by high LDL levels.[1,16] Interestingly, purified tissue kallikrein processes the apoB-100 polypeptide chain. The effect of this processing on LDL metabolism is currently not known. Moreover, it is not known how the apoB-100 processing activity of tissue kallikrein relates to the kininogenase and esterase activities of the enzyme in its purified and membrane-bound forms. How this activity might bear on the regulation of LDL metabolism is of interest as Nolly and Lama have reported the existence of a kallikrein-like activity in rat vascular tissue.[17]

ACKNOWLEDGEMENTS

We gratefully acknowledge the assistance of Robin Wright in preparing the manuscript for publication and Gwen Kraft in preparing the figures. This work was supported in part by grant nos. HL-31387, HL-30999, HL-17705, HL-29566, HL-15690, HL-29397; by the Children's Hospital Research Foundation (V.H.D.) and the American Heart Association (A.D.C.). J.C. and A.D.C. are Research Career Development and New Investigator Awardees, respectively, of the National Heart, Lung, and Blood Institute.

REFERENCES

1. J. L. Goldstein and M. S. Brown, The low-density lipoprotein pathway and its relation to atherosclerosis, Ann. Rev. Biochem., 46:897-930 (1977).

2. J. P. Kane, D. A. Hardman, and H. E. Paulus, Heterogeneity of apolipoprotein B: Isolation of a new species from human chylomicrons, Proc. Natl. Acad. Sci. USA, 77:2465-2469 (1980).

3. M. J. Malloy, J. P. Kane, D. A. Hardman, R. L. Hamilton, and K. B. Dalal, Normotriglyceridemic abetalipoproteinemia: Absence of the B-100 apolipoprotein, J. Clin. Invest., 67:1441-1450 (1981).

4. K. Shimamoto, J. Chao, and H. S. Margolius, The radioimmunoassay of human urinary kallikrein and comparisons with kallikrein activity measurements, J. Clin. Endocrinol. Metab., 51:840-848 (1980).

5. J. Chao, S. Tanaka, and H. S. Margolius, Inhibitory effects of sodium and other monovalent cations on purified versus membrane-bound kallikrein, J. Biol. Chem., 258:6461-6465 (1983).

6. H. Nagase and A. J. Barrett, Human plasma kallikrein: A rapid purification method with high yield, Biochem. J., 193:187-192 (1981).

7. V. H. Donaldson, R. A. Harrison, F. A. Rosen, D. H. Bing, G. Kindness, J. Canar, C. J. Wagner, and S. Awad, Variability in purified dysfunctional C_1-inhibitor protein frompatients with hereditary angioneurotic edema, J. Clin. Invest., 75:1-9 (1985).

8. H. Saito, O. D. Ratnoff, and V. H. Donaldson, Defective activation of clotting, fibrinolytic, and permeability-enhancing systems in human Fletcher trait plasma, Circ. Res.,34:641-651 (1974).

9. A. D. Cardin, K. R. Witt, C. L. Barnhart, and R. L. Jackson, Sulfhydryl chemistry and solubility properties of humanplasma apolipoprotein B, Biochemistry, 21:4503-4511 (1982).

10. A. D. Cardin, K. R. Witt, J. Chao, H. S. Margolius, V. H. Donaldson, and R. L. Jackson, Degradation of apolipoprotein B-100 of human plasma low density lipoproteins by tissue and plasma kallikreins, J. Biol. Chem., 259:8522-8528 (1984).

11. H. Towbin, T. Staehelin, and J. Gordon, Electrophoretic transfer of proteins from polyacrylamide gels to nitrocellulose sheets: Procedure and some applciations, Proc. Natl. Acad. Sci. USA, 76:4350-4354 (1979).

12. J. M. Gershoni and G. E. Palade, Protein blotting: Principles and applciations, Anal. Biochem., 131:1-15 (1983).

13. O. H. Lowry, N. J. Rosebrough, A. L. Farr, and R. J. Randall, Protein measurement with the folin phenol reagent, J. Biol. Chem., 193:265-275 (1951).

14. K. Shimamoto, R. K. Mayfield, H. S. Margolius, J. Chao, W. Stroud, and A. P. Kaplan, Immunoreactive tissue kallikrein in human serum, J. Lab. Clin. Med., 103:731-738 (1984).

15. T. S. Paskhina, L. R. Polyantseva, A. V. Krinskaya, T. P. Egorova, V. Ph. Nartikova, I. M. Karmansky, and R. I. Yakubovskaya, Components of KKKK system in plasma and edematous fluids of patients with nephrotic syndrome (NS): Compensatory and pathogenetic role of kinins in nephrotic syndrome, Adv. Exp. Med. Biol., 156B:1119-1125 (1983).

16. R. Ross, The arterial wall and atherosclerosis, Ann. Rev. Med., 30:1-15 (1979).

17. H. Nolly and M. C. Lama, Vascular kallikrein: A kallikrein-like enzyme present in vascular tissue of the rat, Clin. Sci. (Lond.), 63:249s-251s (1982).

TRANSPORTING EPITHELIA AS TARGETS FOR KININ EFFECTS

A.W. Cuthbert and L.J. MacVinish

Department of Pharmacology
University of Cambridge
Hills Road
Cambridge, CB2 2QD

Running title: Kinins and epithelial function

One approach which can be used to discover the function(s) of the
kallikrein-kinin system is to make the assumption that tissue kallikrein
can generate lysyl bradykinin (LBK, kallidin) in tissues, where it then
acts as local hormone. If this be true then it follows that novel effects
of kinin may be discovered in tissues where kallikrein is especially localized. Consideration of these effects may then allow some conclusions to be
drawn about the roles of the kallikrein-kinin system in either physiological
or pathological states.

Many epithelia are shown to be rich sources of tissue kallikrein (for
example in kidney, pancreas, salivary glands, alimentary tract, liver) and
much evidence has accrued about the localization of the enzyme in epithelia
at the histochemical level. On the other hand rather little is known about
the ways in which epithelial functions are modified by kinins.

Circumstantial evidence for the involvement of the K-K system in electrolyte homeostasis came from studies of urinary kallikrein excretion in
both normal and pathological states[1,2]. One effort to obtain more definitive evidence of a link between ion transporting processes and the presence
of the K-K system in an epithelium was made by Margolius and his colleagues,
using the toad urinary bladder. It was found that kallikrein inhibitors
reduced transepithelial sodium transport in the bladder[3], a tissue rich in
kallikrein-like enzymes. In 1981 Margolius spent an extended period in my
laboratory, specifically to look for possible effects of kinins on sodium
transport in a mammalian epithelium. It was already known that the mammalian
intestine contained kallikrein[4], thus fitting at least one of the criteria
given above.

Chloride secretion not sodium absorption

We found, rather quickly, that application of LBK to the basolateral
face of isolated rat colon epithelium, voltage clamped at zero potential,
caused a large inward current to flow. The direction of the current indicated that the tissue had responded by increasing the absorption of cations,
or by secreting anions or by a mixture of these two. The essential features
of the response to kinin are illustrated in Fig. 1. The response is rapid,

but occurred only when the peptide was added to the basolateral side of the tissue. Responses were sensitive to loop diuretics, such as frusemide and piretanide, giving the first clue that active transport of chloride was involved. Inhibitors of fatty acid cyclo-oxygenase, such as indomethacin, attenuated responses to LBK, while not affecting responses to prostaglandins of the E series.

We have gone on to do detailed studies of the kinin effects on rat colon[5-9] and have concluded that eicosanoid formation is necessary for the totality of the response but is not mandatory, while calcium ions have an essential but, as yet, incompletely defined role in the stimulation of chloride secretion. Our results, together with those of Manning et al.[10], plus the early preliminary studies of Hardcastle et al.[11] establish kinins as extremely potent stimulants of chloride secretion in the mammalian gut.

It is not our aim to describe these detailed studies here, rather it is our intention to show, briefly, how transepithelial ion transport can be measured, and how we have used standard methods to ask similar questions about other, less amenable, kallikrein containing epithelia.

Short-circuit currents and radiotracer fluxes

Many epithelia when bathed on both sides by identical salt solutions exhibit a transepithelial potential. Clearly these potentials cannot arise from chemical gradients since the bathing solutions on either side of the tissue are identical. The chambers in which the tissues are held are usually constructed in ways such that no hydrostatic gradients exist across the epithelium. Thus, in the absence of chemical or hydrostatic gradients, if ion movements across the tissue are entirely passive no transepithelial potential will be generated. The presence of a potential is indicative of active ion transport.

Under open circuit conditions the isolated rat colon epithelium has a transepithelial potential of a few millivolts, with the basolateral side positive with respect to the apical side. Thus an anion passing outwards across the epithelium moves up an electrical gradient. Addition of kinin to the tissue causes an increase in the transepithelial potential, commonly up to 10-12 millivolts. In the in vitro experimental situation it is not logical to study the effects of kinins on ion transport in a situation where the potential is allowed to vary in this way, as the changing potential will either increase or decrease the electrical gradient against which the ions are moving. This was appreciated long ago by Ussing and Zerahn[12] who used an external electrical circuit to keep the transepithelial potential at zero. The current flowing in the external circuit is called the short circuit current (SCC). Thus the current which flows in the absence of electrical, chemical and hydrostatic gradients is due to electrogenic (rheogenic) ion transport. Furthermore, the area under the current x time record is indicative of the charge carried across the tissue by active transport. It is an easy matter to convert current x time to chemical equivalents using the Faraday relationship. The equivalence between SCC and active transport of ions across an epithelium can be investigated using simultaneous measurements of SCC and ion fluxes using radioactive tracers.

Not withstanding the points made above some epithelia show electroneutral ion transport, which is active (i.e. energy requiring) but does not generate a SCC, for example electroneutral NaCl absorption. This type of transport can, however, be detected by measurements of ion flux. Fig. 2 illustrates a simple version of the processes of electrogenic chloride secretion and electroneutral NaCl absorption.

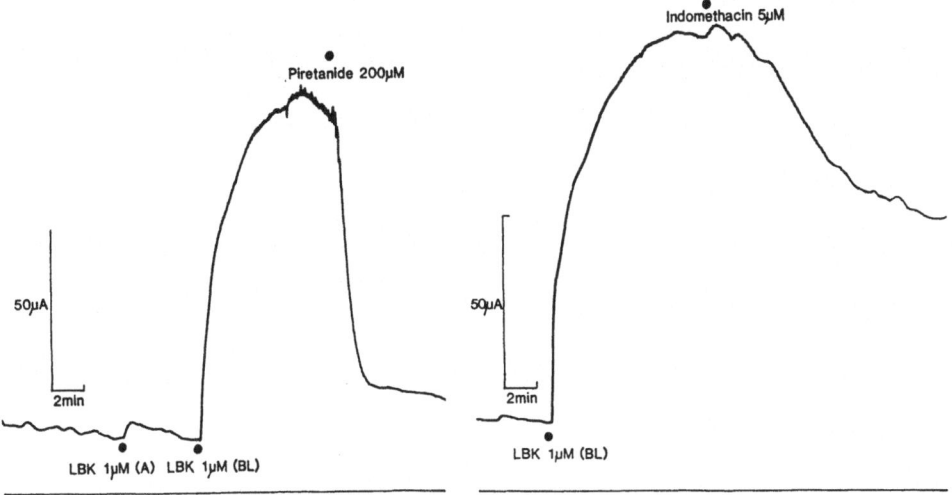

Fig. 1. SCC records from two preparations of colonic epithelia taken from
the same animal, each 0.6 cm^2. Horizontal line indicates zero
SCC. Lysylbradykinin (LBK) was added to either the solution bathing
the apical (A) or basolateral (BL) surface. Piretanide was added
to the basolateral bathing fluid only and indomethacin was added to
both sides of the tissue.

In our experiments with kallidin on the rat colon the increase on
chloride movement into the apical solution was 4.09 uEq cm^{-2} h^{-1}, a value
corresponding to 137% of the integrated SCC, that is more than sufficient
to explain the SCC responses. However, when Na fluxes were also taken into
account it was found that kallidin caused a small but significant reduction
in electroneutral NaCl absorption.[6] Making allowance for this the chloride
flux exceeds SCC by around 125%. It is not unusual for agents which cause
electrogenic chloride secretion to inhibit electroneutral NaCl absorption
at the same time.[14] Reference to the models given in Fig. 2 implies that
agents increasing tissue cAMP content will increase both electrogenic
chloride secretion and reduce electroneutral NaCl absorption. it is clear
from our studies and those of others that chloride is the major current
carrier involved in the SCC response to kinin, the excess movement of
chloride in the basolateral to apical direction may be balanced by exchange
for HCO$_3$'.

Increased Intracellular Calcium

A number of secretagogues increase electrogenic chloride secretion in
mammalian epithelia, and some appear to do this by increasing intracellular
calcium. Indeed, as with cAMP, increased Ca$_i$ both increases electrogenic
chloride secretion as well as reduces electroneutral NaCl absorption.[14]
Recently we have developed a way of increasing the calcium permeability of
the basolateral face of face colon epithelium using the photodynamic action
of erythrosine B[15]. Consequently calcium ions flood into the cells causing
an irreversible stimulation of electrogenic chloride secretion.

Fig. 3 illustrates an example of the photodynamic effect of erythrosine
B on rat colon, together with a summary of sets of flux studies with both
^{22}Na and ^{36}Cl. Electrogenic chloride secretion is stimulated while electroneutral NaCl absorption is virtually abolished. It is noticeable that
the change in electrogenic chloride movement caused by calcium entry is
almost exactly balanced by the SCC responses, making a strong case that

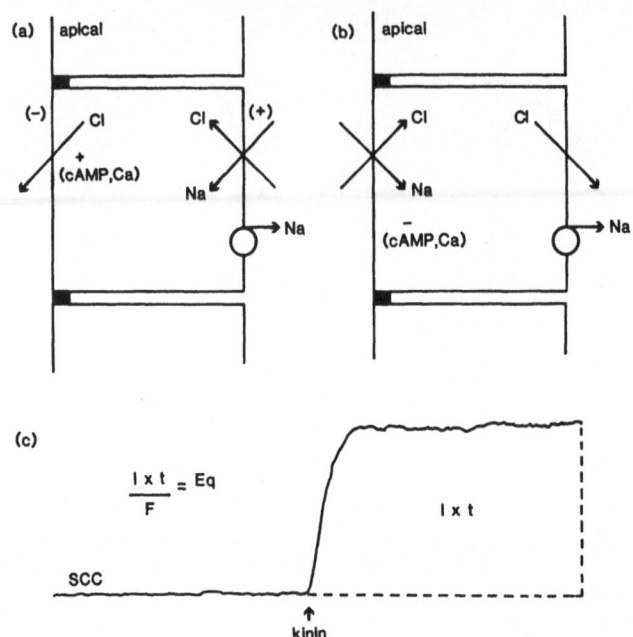

Fig. 2. Simple models for electrogenic chloride secretion (a) and electroneutral NaCl absorption (b) taken from 13. In (a) chloride enters
through the basolateral face of the cell using a contransport
mechanism, driven by energy stored in the sodium gradient. This
process is sensitive to frusemide. Na ions are returned through
the basolateral face by the sodium pump, while chloride exits
through the apical face through cAMP or Ca_i sensitive channels.
The transepithelial transfer of anions leads to a transepithelial
potential, apical side negative. Under short circuit conditions
chloride ions can continue to flow unassociated with cations, the
chemical asymmetry so developed being dealt with by electrode
processes in the external circuit. Under open circuit conditions
the transepithelial potential provides an electrical gradient for
the flow of cations. (b) In electroneutral transport Na and Cl
enter through the apical surface using a contransport mechanism
which is inhibited by cAMP or Ca_i. Chloride ions leave the cell
passively through the basolateral face, while Na ions are pumped
out by the sodium pump. No transepithelial potential or SCC is
developed. (c) Schematic of a SCC response to kinin in the colon.
The enclosed area equals the total extra charge transfer caused by
kinin. This can be calculated from I x t/F, where F is the Faraday.
Simultaneous measurements of net fluxes of various ions allows
the ion(s) carrying SCC to be identified.

chloride actually carries the increased SCC following irradiation. The
real point of showing this data is to emphasize that electroneutral transport does not generate a SCC and the possibility has to be faced that some
epithelia may respond to kinins without a change in SCC. It is important,
as other epithelia are investigated for sensitivity to kinins, that both
ion fluxes, as well as SCCs, are measured.

Kinins and the Kidney

In his paper in Kinins III[16] Pisano states that intraarterial injections into the kidney of kinins and inhibitors of kallikrein or kininases
have led some to believe that kinins are natriuretic and diuretic, and

206

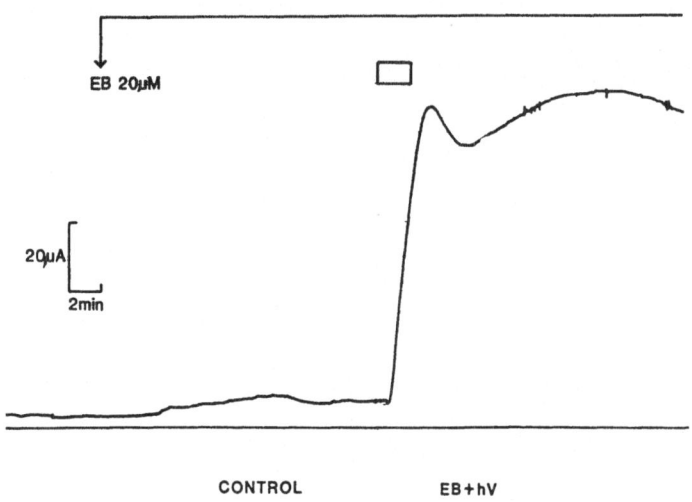

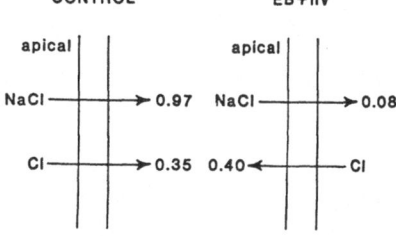

Fig. 3. SCC in a single preparation of colonic epithelium (0.6 cm^2).
Tissue was exposed to erythrosine B (EB), 20 uM, on the basolateral
side as indicated. There was no response until the tissue was
illuminated with white light (indicated by open box). The increase
in SCC remained after illumination had ceased. On the right is
shown the mean results of 24 flux experiments with either ^{36}Cl or
^{22}Na. Illumination in the presence of EB virtually abolished
electroneutral NaCl absorption while chloride absorption unassociated with sodium was changed to secretion. Thus the change in
chloride movement unassociated with Na is 0.75, while integration
of the areas under the SCC response curves gave a value of 0.82.
All figures refer to uEq 0.6 cm^{-2} (20 min)$^{-1}$. The results support
the view that SCC responses are due to chloride secretion. Additionally the responses are sensitive to loop diuretics, such as
frusemide.

others to believe they are antinatriuretic and antidiuretic. This parlous
state of affiars results, in part, from the difficulty of examining any
agent on such a complex organ as the kidney. On the other hand it seems
fairly clear that kinins are generated in the distal part of the nephron,
although the precise localization of the kallikrein responsible and the
source of the kininogen remains obscure.[17-21] We have tried to ask the
question does kinin affect electrogenic ion transport in the collecting
duct and from which face does the kinin act? To do this we employed a
technique which has been pioneered by Handler and his colleagues.[22,23]

Briefly, we prepared suspensions of pig renal papillary collecting
tubule (RPCT) cells[24] and formed primary cultures of these on previous
substrates coated with collagen. After the monolayers of epithelial cells
had become confluent they were mounted in special chambers for SCC recording. Our preliminary results can be summarized as follows, and Fig. 4
illustrates some typical results.

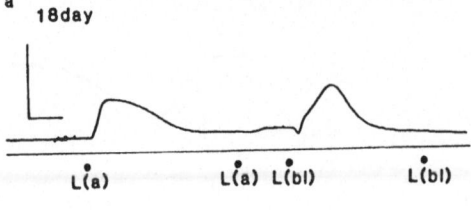

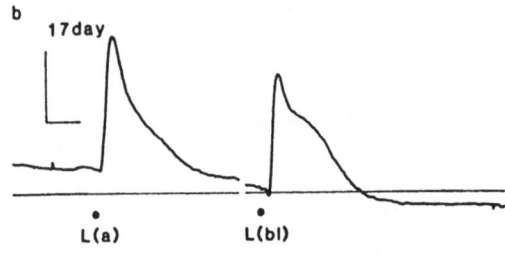

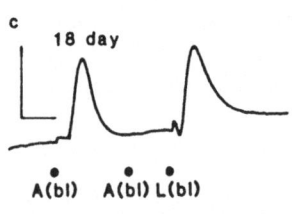

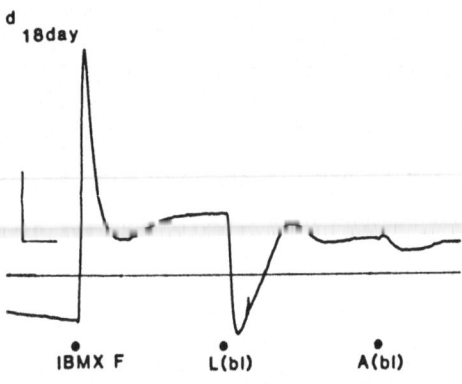

Fig. 4. Characteristics of the responses to lysylbradykinin in RPCT monolayers. Examples of records from four separate monolayers, each
of 0.2 cm^2, are shown. In each the horizontal line indicates
zero SCC, calibrations are 1 uA and 2 min. L refers to lysylbradykinin (1 uM) and A to arginine vasopressin (0.5 uM). The side to
which these agents were added is indicated as apical (a) or basolateral (bl). The features illustrated are as follows: (a) Shows
that responses to L show no sidedness, i.e., responses are obtained
with both basolateral and apical application of kinin. Although
the responses are transient a further response cannot be obtained
without washing away the kinin, presumably because of receptor
desensitization. (b) The form of the responses to kinin can vary
considerably. In this example there is evidence for a peak plus
plateau type response on SCC, perhaps indicating more than one

mechanism of action. (c) Arginine vasopressin produces similar responses to kinin, again with apparent receptor desensitization. Results in this trace suggest that there are different receptors for A and L, as a response to L could be obtained after the responses to A were desensitized. (d) Here the SCC was increased by a combination of IBMX (100 uM) and forskolin (10 uM). During the plateau, when presumably tissue cAMP levels were increased, the effects of L were reversed and those due to A were either abolished or marginally reversed. This suggests that L may affect SCC by more than one mechanism, one of which may involve cAMP.

(a) Monolayers had the morphology of collecting tubule cells. Cells were joined by tight junctions and showed apical microvilli on the free face (away from the collagen).
(b) Monolayers had small (-0.1 mV) transepithelial potentials and small resting SCCs (2.0 uA cm^{-2}).
(c) Responses, in the form of transient, inward currents were obtained in responses to kinin applied to either the apical or basolateral face of the tissue. Desensitization to the effects of kinin on one face did not preclude the effects of kinin applied to the opposite face.
(d) Unlike kinins, ADH was active only when applied to the basolateral surface. Desensitization to the effects of kinin did not prevent responses to ADH.
(e) The SCCs were sensitive to frusemide and were abolished by removing chloride from the bathing fluid.
(f) The effects of kinins were virtually abolished by indomethacin.
(g) Agents which increased tissue cAMP also caused an increase in SCC. In this situation the responses to kinin were reversed (i.e., transient fall in SCC).

Our tentative conclusions are that receptors for kinins occur on both faces of primary cultures of RPCT cells, and these are distinct from receptors to ADH. Kinins can stimulate electrogenic ion transport in collecting tubule cells, likely of chloride but possibly involving other ions too. The effect may be dependent on eicosanoid synthesis. The generation of kinin in the tubule lumen nd on the antelumenal face may be important for modulation of ion transporting activity in the collecting duct.

ACKNOWLEDGEMENT

L. J. McV. was supported by grant number HL17705 from the National Institutes of Health.

REFERENCES

1. R. G. Geller, H. S. Margolius, J. J. Pisano, and H. R. Keiser, Effects of mineralocorticoids, altered sodium intake and adrenalectomy on urinary kallikrein in rats, Circulation Res., 31:857-861 (1972).
2. H. S. Margolius, D. Horwitz, J. J. Pisano, and H. R. Keiser, Urinary kallikrein excretion in hypertensive man. Relationships to sodium uptake and sodium-retaining steroids, Circulation Res., 35: 820-825 (1974).
3. G. G. Orce, G. A. Castillo, and H. S. Margolius, Inhibition of short circuit current in toad urinary bladder by inhibitors of glandular kallikrein, Am. J. Physiol., 239:F459-F465 (1980).

4. A. Zimmerman, R. Geiger, and H. Kortmann, Similarity between a kinino-genase (kallikrein) from human large intestine and human urinary kallikrein, Hoppe-Seyler's Z. Physiol. Chem., 360:1767-1773 (1979).

5. A. W. Cuthbert, and H. S. Margolius, Kinin effects on electrolyte transport in rat colon, J. Physiol., 319:45P (1981).

6. A. W. Cuthbert and H. S. Margolius, Kinins stimulate net chloride se-cretion by rat colon, Brit. J. Pharmacol., 75:587-598 (1982).

7. A. W. Cuthbert, P. V. Halushka, H. S. Margolius, and J. A. Spayne, Role of calcium ions in kinin-induced chloride secretion, Brit. J. Phar-macol., 82:587-595 (1984).

8. A. W. Cuthbert, P. V. Halushka, H. S. Margolius, and J. A. Spayne, Mediators of the secretory response to kinins, Brit. J. Pharmacol., 82:597-607 (1984).

9. A. W. Cuthbert, P. V. Halushka, D. Kessel, H. S. Margolius, and W. C. Wise, Kinin effects on chloride secretion do not require eicosanoid synthesis, Brit. J. Pharmacol., 83:549-554 (1984).

10. D. Manning, S. H. Snyder, J. F. Kachur, R. J. Miller, and M. Field, Bradykinin receptor-mediated chloride secretion in intestinal func-tion, Nature, 299:256-259 (1982).

11. J. Hardcastle, P. T. Hardcastle, R. J. Flower, and P. A. Sandford, The effect of bradykinin on the electrical activity of rat jejunum, Experientia, 34:617-618 (1978).

12. H. H. Ussing and K. Zerahn, Active-transport of sodium as the source of electric current in the short-circuited isolated frog skin, Acta Physiol. Scand., 23:110-127 (1951).

13. R. A. Frizzell, M. Field, and S. G. Schultz, Sodium-coupled chloride transport by epithelial tissue, Am. J. Physiol., 236:F1-F8 (1979).

14. M. Donowitz, Ca^{2+} in the control of active intestinal Na and Cl trans-port: Involvement in neurohumoral action, Am. J. Physiol., 245:G165-G177 (1983).

15. A. W. Cuthbert, Calcium dependent chloride secretion in rat colon epi-thelium, J. Physiol., In press (1984).

16. J. J. Pisano, Observations on the kallikrein-kinin system in the kidney, in: "Kinins III. Adv. Exp. Med. & Biol.," 156B:929-938 (1983).

17. T. B. Orstavik, K. Nustad, P. Brandtzaeg, and J. V. Pierce, Cellular origin of urinary kallikreins, J. Histochem. Cytochem., 24:1037-1039 (1976).

18. D. Proud, M. Perkins, J. V. Pierce, K. N. Yates, P. F. Highet, P. L. Herring, M. M. Mark, R. Bahn, F. Carone, and J. J. Pisano, Character-ization and localization of human renal kininogen, J. Biol. Chem., 256:10634-10639 (1981).

19. D. Proud, M. A. Kepper, and J. J. Pisano, Distribution of immunoreactive kallikrein along the rat nephron, Am. J. Physiol., 244:F510-F515 (1983).

20. K. Tomita and J. J. Pisano, Binding of ^3H bradykinin in isolated nephron segments of the rabbit, Am. J. Physiol., 246:F732-F737 (1984).

21. K. Tomita, H. Endou, and F. Sakai, Localization of kallikrein-like activity along a single nephron in rabbits, Pflugers. Arch., 389:91-95 (1981).

22. J. S. Handler, F. M. Perkins, and J. P. Johnson, Studies of renal cell function using cell culture techniques, Am. J. Physiol., 238:F1-F9 (1980).

23. F. M. Perkins and J. S. Handler, Transport properties of toad kidney epithelia in culture, Am. J. Physiol., 241:C154-C159 (1981).

24. F. C. Grenier, T. E. Rollins, and W. L. Smith, Kinin-induced prosta-glandin synthesis by renal papillary collecting tubule cells in culture, Am. J. Physiol., 241:F94-F104 (1981).

PURIFICATION AND PARTIAL CHARACTERIZATION OF CAT COLON AND SUBMANDIBULAR

GLAND KALLIKREINS

Hiroyuki Fujimori*, Peter R. Levison*, and Melville Schachter

*Alberta Heritage Foundation for Medical Research Fellows
Department of Physiology, University of Alberta, Edmonton
Alberta, Canada   T6G 2H7

SUMMARY

Kallikreins from cat colon and submandibular gland have been purified
by acetone fractionation of tissue extracts, DEAE-Sephacel ion-exchange
chromatography, ρ-aminobenzamidine Sepharose 4B affinity chromatography
and gel filtration on Sephadex G-75. They were of similar M.W.,
approximately 40,000, and each comprised five forms by isoelectricfocusing
(pI 4.1-4.8). Both enzymes were potent kininogenases and exhibited
similar specificities with synthetic ester and amide substrates. They
were susceptible to a range of protease inhibitors. Surprisingly, neither
was sensitive to aprotinin yet both were partially inhibited by soya-bean
trypsin inhibitor. They were indistinguishable in our immunological tests.

An acidic esterase (pI 2.2-3.5) of M.W. 120,000 was isolated from cat
stomach by the same procedure. While it exhibited weak immunologic similarity to cat submandibular gland kallikrein, it had negligible kininogenase
activity and different substrate and inhibitor specificities to the two
kallikreins. It is concluded that similar tissue kallikreins are present
in the colon and submandibular gland of the cat but are distinct from this
cat stomach esterase.

INTRODUCTION

Tissue kallikreins (EC 3.4.21.35) are a group of serine proteases
that release the biologically active peptides, kinins, from their precursor, kininogen. Tissue kallikreins (kinino-genases) have been purified and extensively characterized from a number of mammals including man,
pig and rat, and exhibit a high degree of homology from different tissues
of different mammals.[3,11]

Abbreviations used are: CCK, cat colon kallikrein; CSE, cat stomach
esterase; CSK, cat submandibular gland kallikrein; ELISA, enzyme-linked
immunosorbent assay, τ-AMCHA, trans-4-(amino-methyl)-cyclohexane
carboxylic acid.

Of the kallikreins in the cat, purification and characterization have been reported only for the submandibular gland enzyme.[6] Using immuno-cytochemical techniques, this enzyme has been localized in the cat sub-mandibular gland.[7,14] Kallikrein-like immunoreactivity has been demon-strated in the mucosa of cat colon[13] and cat stomach[2] using antiserum against purified cat submandibular gland kallikrein. However, neither of these enzymes has been characterized. In the present study, we report the purification and partial characterization of kallikrein from the mucosa of cat colon (CCK) and comparie it with cat submandibular gland kallikrein (CSK). We were unable to isolate kallikrein from cat stomach.

MATERIALS AND METHODS

Materials

Materials used included DEAE-Sephacel, Sephadex G-50, Sephadex G-100, ГН-Sepharose 4B, Sephacryl S-200 SF (Pharmacia); diisopropylfluorophosphate, 5,5'-dithiobis-(2-nitrobenzoic acid), bradykinin triacetate, trypsin inhibitors (soya-bean) type I-S, (lima-bean) type II-L, (chicken egg-white) type IV-0, chymostatin, leupeptin, pepstatin, τ-AMCHA, ρ-aminobenzamidine dihydrochloride, Tos-Lys-CH_2Cl, Bz-Arg-OEt, Tos-Arg-OMe, 1-ethyl-3-(3-dimethylaminopropyl) carbodiimide, pharmalyte pH 2.5-5.0 (Sigma); Cbz-Lys-SBzl (Cambridge Research Biochemicals Ltd.); D-Val-Leu-Arg-ρNa, S2266 (Helena Laboratories); aprotinin (Bayer AG). Partially purified dog kininogen was prepared from heated dog plasma modified from the method of Moriwaki and Schachter.[10] Prior to lyophilisation, the preparation was acidified to pH 2.0 for 20 min at room temperature and then neutralized, centrifuged and the supernatant dialysed against distilled H_2O. Antiserum to purified CSK was raised in New Zealand rabbits.[12] ρ-Aminobenzamidine was coupled to CH-Sepharose 4B using 1-ethyl-3-(3-dimethylamino-propyl) carbodiimide according to the manufacturer's instructions.

Methods

Preparation of tissue extracts   Cats of either sex (3-6 kg) were anaesthetised by intraperitoneal injection of 35 mg sodium pentobarbital/kg. The colon and stomach contents were washed out with H_2O and the mucosa dissected out. The submandibular glands were washed with 0.9% (w/v) NaCl. Tissues were cut into small pieces and frozen with liquid N_2. Samples were homogenised with at least 5 vol. distilled H_2O at room temperature in a glass homogeniser and allowed to stand for 15 h at room temperature (2 h for stomach). The suspensions were centrifuged for 60 min at 4°C and 70,000 g, and the supernatant solutions were used for further puri-fication.

Assay techniques   Kallikrein was routinely assayed spectro-photometrically using 0.1 mM-Cbz-Lys-SBzl as substrate. Enzymic hydrolysis was monitored at 412 nm in 0.1 M-Tris/HCl, pH 8.0, at 37°C, with the use of 5,5'-dithiobis-(2-nitrobenzoic aiid) as chromogen for the benzylmercaptan. One unit of activity hydrolysed 1 μmol of substrate/min under the conditions described. D-Val-Leu-Arg-ρNa hydrolysis was measured using 0.1 mM-sub-strate at 405 nm under similar conditions. Hydrolysis of 1 mM-Bz-Arg-OEt and 1 mM-Tos-Arg-OMe was measured in 0.1 M-Tris/HCl buffer, pH 8.0, at 25°C at 253 nm and 247 nm respectively, as described by Fukuoka et al.[6] The kinetic constant K_m was determined for the hydrolysis of Cbz-Lys-SBzl and D-Val-Leu-Arg-ρNa in 0.1 M-Tris/HCl buffer, pH 8.0, at 37°C.

Kinin-releasing activity was measured in 0.1 M-Tris/HCl buffer, pH 8.0, at 37°C using 10 mg crude dog kininogen as substrate in a final

volume of 0.5-1.0 ml. The liberated kinin was estimated by contraction of
an isolated guinea-pig ileum segment suspended in a 10 ml bath of oxygenated
Krebs-Henseleit solution containing 6 mM-glucose, 1 μM-atropine sulphate
and 1 μM-pyrilamine maleate maintained at $37^{o}C$ with 1 g of tension. Contractions were recorded via an isometric force transducer. Synthetic bradykinin was used as the standard and kinin-forming activity was expressed in
terms of μg of bradykinin equivalent.

Protein was determined by absorption measurement at 280 nm. One
A_{280} unit is that amount of protein showing an absorbance of 1.0 when contained in 1.0 ml of solution. Isoelectricfocusing was performed with a
110 ml column (LKB) using pH 2.5-5.0 ampholine. Apparent M.W. was
determined by gel filtration on columns of either Sephadex G-100 or
Sephacryl S-200 SF. The effects of various protease inhibitors on
enzyme activity were determined by incubating equal volumes of inhibitor
solution with enzyme for 5 min at $25^{o}C$ and assaying an aliquot using
Cbz-Lys-SBzl as described previously. Double diffusion analysis was
carried out in 1% (w/v) agarose in 0.9% (w/v) NaCl for 20 h at $4^{o}C$. The
distance between wells was 3 mm (4.5 mm diameter) and 20 μl each of
antigen and CSK-antiserum were applied, separately. The precipitin lines
were observed directly. ELISA was performed using Dynatech Immulon 2
microtiter plates using antigen (0.2 ml) containing 10^{-2}-10^{-6} A_{280} units
of protein and either 0.1% (v/v) CSK-antiserum or 0.1% (v/v) normal
rabbit serum.

PROCEDURE FOR PURIFICATION OF CAT TISSUE KALLIKREINS

All procedures were conducted at $4^{o}C$ unless otherwise state.

Acetone fractionation

Tissue extracts (see Materials and Methods) were slowly adjusted to
35% (v/v) saturation with cold acetone and stirred gently for 40 min. The
precipitate was removed by centrifugation and the supernatant brought to
80% (v/v) saturation with cold acetone. After stirring gently for 40 min,
the precipitated material was collected by centrifugation, dissolved in
50 mM-Tris/HCl buffer, pH 8.0, and dialysed against 100 vol. of the same
buffer for 16 h.

DEAE-Sephacel ion-exchange chromatography

The solution was passed through a DEAE-Sephacel column (2/6 cm x 17 cm)
equilibrated with 50 mM-Tris/HCl buffer, pH 8.0. The column was washed
with at least 4 bed vol. of the same suffer and adsorbed material eluted
with a linear gradient of 0-0.4 M-NaCl in the same buffer (500 ml). Active
fractions were pooled, concentrated by dialysis against solid sucrose and
the concentrated solution dialysed against 100 vol. of 50 mM-Tris/HCl
buffer, pH 8.0, for 16 h. The elution profile for CCK is shown in Figure 1.

ρ-Aminobenzamidine-Sepharose 48 affinity chromatography

The enzyme solution was passed through a ρ-aminobenzamidine-Sepharose
4B column (2.6 cm x 10 cm) equilibrated with 50 mM-Tris/HCl buffer, pH 8.0,
at a flow rate of 25 ml/hr. The column was washed with at least 4 bed vol.
of the same buffer and adsorbed material eluted with a linear gradient of
0-2.0 m-NaCl in the same buffer (400 ml) at a flow rate of 25 ml/h and
fraction size of 5 ml. Active fractions were pooled, concentrated by
dialysis against solid sucrose and the concentrated solution dialysed
against 100 vol. of 5 mM-ammonium formate buffer, pH 8.0, for 16 h.

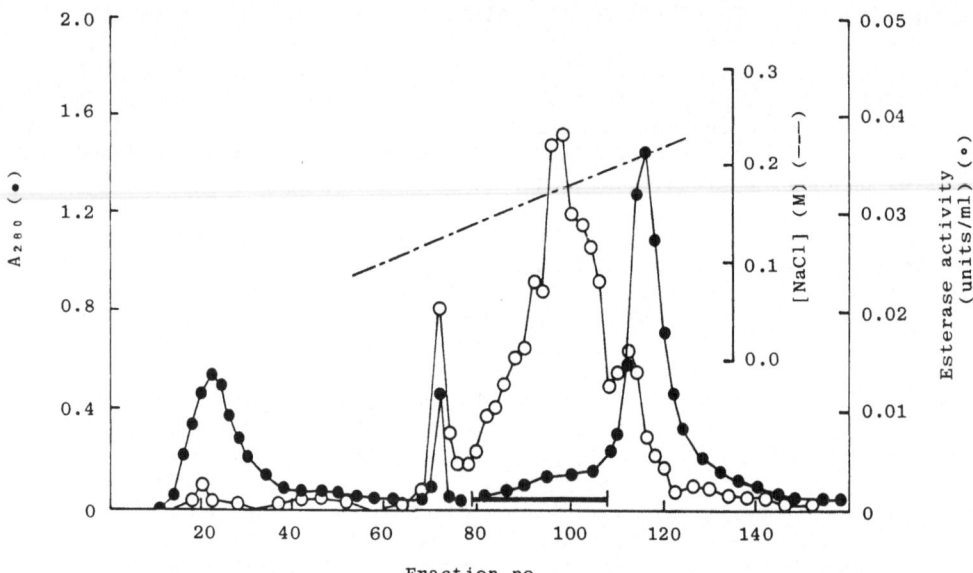

Figure 1. Chromatography of cat colon extract on DEAE-Sephacel.
For conditions, see the text. Fractions were pooled as indicated by the horizontal bar. Fraction volume 5 ml (10 ml for
fractions nos. 1-60).

Sephadex G-75 gel chromatography

The non-diffusable material was applied to a Sephadex G-75 column
(2.6 cm x 85 cm) equilibrated with 5 mM-ammonium formate buffer, pH 8.0.
Active fractions were pooled, concentrated by dialysis against solid
sucrose and the concentrated enzyme solution dialysed against 100 vol. of
5 mM-ammonium formate buffer, pH 8.0, for 16 h. The enzyme preparation
was stored at -20°C until further use.

RESULTS AND DISCUSSION

We have developed a scheme for the isolation of cat tissue kallikreins.
By following this scheme, CSK was purified with apparent M.W. 41,200 and comprised five forms (pI 4.15-4.76) by preparative isoelectricfocusing.
These, and our other findings, are in close agreement with those reported
by Fukuoka et al.[6] for CSK. Unlike many tissue kallikreins, CSK was not
significantly inhibited by aprotinin. This precluded the use of aprotinin-
Sepharose, a matrix commonly employed for the isolation of kallikreins[4]
as an affinity absorbent. Instead, the matrix ρ-aminobenzamidine-
Sepharose 4B was used and found to be satisfactory.

The apparent M.W. of 38,300 for CCK (Table 1) was similar to that of
CSK (41,200). These are typical values for most tissue kallikreins thus
far characterised[3] but where significantly lower than M.W. 120,000 obtained
for CSE. Isoelectricfocusing of CCK resolved 5 forms (pI 4.08-4.61) which
is similar to the pattern observed for CSK but distinct from the more
acidic CSE. In our bioassay system, CCK released 87 µg-bradykinin
equivalents/min/A_{280}, which although 4-fold less than CSK (350 µg-
bradykinin equivalents/min/A_{280}) was nevertheless a very potent

kininogenase. On the other hand, CSE was a doubtful or very weak kininogenease, releasing 0.42 µg-bradykinin equivalents/min/A_{280} which is at least 8,000-fold less than CSK. Studies on stomach kallikreins of rat[16] and man,[17] and a cathepsin D-like enzyme from rat stomach[8,9] have been reported. All these preparations were kininogenases but their kinin-releasing ability was not quantitatively defined for comparison.

Of some interest is the fact that whereas high esterolytic activity was present in crude extracts of stomach mucosa, submandibular gland and colon mucosa, the former had little or no kininogenase activity. We were somewhat surprised by this observation in view of the apparent immunocyto-chemical localisation of this enzyme in the mucous cells of the gastric mucosa as well as in those of the intestine and colon.[13]

Comparing the ratios of rates of hydrolysis of Cbz-Lys-SBzl/Bz-Arg-OEt, D-Val-Leu-Arg-pNa/Bz-Arg-OEt and Bz-Arg-OEt/Tos-Arg-OMe for CCK and DSK (Table 2), we observed similar values for CCK and CSK but strikingly different ratios for CSE. The ratios for Bz-Arg-OEt/Tos-Arg-OMe of 1.78 for CCK and 2.26 for CSK were similar to the ratio of 1.25-2.78 reported previously for CSK.[6] On the other hand, the ratios obtained for Cbz-Lys-SBzl/Bz-Arg-OEt and Bz-Arg-OEt/Tos-Arg-OMe for CSE of 2.34 and 0.24 respectively were similar to those of 1.90 and 0.66 respectively obtained for the hydrolysis of these substrates by cat pancreatic trypsin.[5]

In terms of K_m (Table 2), D-Val-Leu-Arg-pNa was a better substrate than Cbz-Lys-SBzl for CCK, CSK and CSE. The K_m values of 14.3 µM, 33.3 µM and 19.2 µM obtained for hydrolysis of D-Val-Leu-Arg-pNa by CCK, CSK and CSE respectively were similar to those obtained for porcine pancreatic kallikrein (22 µM) and lower than the K_m value obtained for cat pancreatic trypsin (125 µM).[5]

Whilst CSE was inhibited by all protease inhibitors tested with the exception of chymostatin and t-AMCHA (Table 3), CCK and CSK were more specific in their inhibition profiles and were unaffected by the trypsin inhibitors from lima-bean and egg-white, pepstatin and Tos-Lys-CH_2Cl. Aprotinin is generally regarded as a tissue kallikrein inhibitor although it does exhibit some species variation.[4] Aprotinin did not inhibit CSK, as

Table 1. Characterisation of cat colon kallikrein (CCK), cat submandibular gland kallikrein (CSK) and cat stomach esterase (CSE)

	CCK	CSK	CSE
Molecular weight	38,300	41,200	120,000
pI (25°C)	4.08	4.15	2.23
	4.22	4.30	3.30
	4.34	4.45	
	4.46	4.60	
	4.61	4.76	
pH optimum	9.15	9.0-9.15	7.96
Kinin-releasing activity (µg-BK-min/A_{280})	86.9	350	0.042
ELISA (CSK-antiserum)	+	+	+

Table 2. Substrate specificity of cat colon kallikrein (CCK), cat submandibular gland kallikrein (CSK) and cat stomach esterase (CSE)

	CCK	CSK	CSE
Relative rates of hydrolysis:			
Cbz–Lys–SBzl/Bz–Arg–OEt	0.86	0.59	2.34
D–Val–Leu–Arg–ρNa/Bz–Arg–OEt	0.126	0.11	0.018
Bz–Arg–OEt/Tos–Arg–OMe	1.78	2.26	0.24
K_m (μM):			
Cbz–Lys–SBzl	76.0	110	64.5
D–Val–Leu–Arg– Na	14.3	33.3	19.2

Table 3. Effects of various protease inhibitors on the hydrolysis of 0.1
mM–Cbz–Lys–SBzl by cat colon kallikrein (CCK), cat submandibular
gland kallikrein (CSK) and cat stomach esterase (CSE) in 0.1
M–Tris/HCl buffer, pH 8.0, at 37°C. See the Materials and Methods
section for experimental details

	Inhibitor amount	% Inhibition		
		CCK*	CSK+	CSE‡
Aprotinin	100 KIU §	15	N.D.‖	65
Soya–bean trypsin inhibitor	2.5 mg	44	65	63
Lima–bean trypsin inhibitor	2.5 mg	N.D.	8	63
Egg–white trypsin inhibitor	2.5 mg	N.D.	N.D.	43
Leupeptin	0.5 mg	88	62	98
Chymostatin	0.5 mg	N.D.	12	19
Pepstatin	0.5 mg	N.D.	N.D.	23
Tos–Lys–CH$_2$Cl	1.0 mM	23	5	74
Diisopropylfluorophosphate	5.0 mM	N.D.	5	N.D.
τ–AMCHA	0.5 mg	N.D.	5	N.D.

* 5.7 munits/ml (Cbz–Lys–SBzl units

+ 6.0 munits/ml (Cbz–Lys–SBzl units)

‡ 11.0 munits/ml (Cbz–Lys–SBzl units)

§ Kallikrein inhibitor units (See Fritz and Wunderer, 1983, for definition)

‖ Non-detectable

was also observed by Kukuoka et al.[6] It had only weak activity towards CCK but partially inhibited CSE. Cat pancreatic trypsin, however, was completely inhibited by aprotinin.[5] In our experiments, CCK, CSK and CSE were all partially inhibited by soya-bean trypsin inhibitor. This observation may explain the early conclusion of Seki et al.[15] that kallikrein in the colon resembles plasma kallikrein.

Double immunodiffusion analysis (Figure 2a) of CCK and CSK using antibodies raised against purified CSK[12] demonstrated their immunological identity with single sharp precipitin lines. No precipitin line could be detected with CSE; however all three enzymes corss-reacted by ELISA (Fibure 2b) with CSK-antiserum, with CCK and CSK equally reactive but CSE at least 500-fold less reactive.

These studies provide a protocol for purification of the cat tissue kallikreins and present further characterisation data for these enzymes. The presence of kallikrein in the colon of the cat has been demonstrated by immunocytochemical techniques.[13] The present study confirms that this immunoreactive material is a typical cat tissue kallikrein resembling CSK. Studies on CSE from cat stomach suggest it to be a serine protease having similar purification properties to a cat tissue kallikrein. It is, however, not a typical cat tissue kallikrein and further characterisation is required before this enzyme can be classified.

ACKNOWLEDGEMENTS

We thank the Medical Research Council of Canada, the Alberta Heart Foundation and the Alberta Heritage Foundation for Medical Research for research grants. Grateful acknowledgement is made to Dr. E. Diener of the Department of Immunology for the loan of preparative isoelectric-focusing equipment. We also thank David Longridge and Saleem Qureshy for valuable assistance.

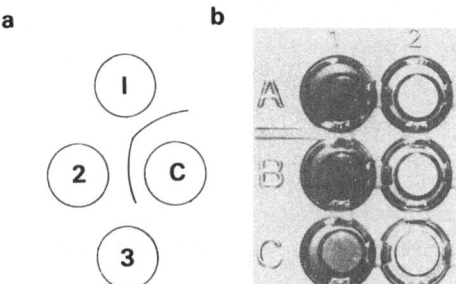

Figure 2. (a) Immunodiffusion, and (b) ELISA of cat colon (CCK) and sub-mandibular gland kallikrein (CSK) and cat stomach esterase (CSE)

For conditions see the text. (2) Well 1, 3.8×10^{-4} A_{280} units CSK; Well 2, 1.1×10^{-4} A_{280} units CCK; Well 3, 1.0×10^{-4} A_{280} units CSE; Well C, 20.0% (v/v) antiserum to CSK.
(b) Row A, 2×10^{-4} A_{280} units CSK; Row B, 7×10^{-5} A_{280} units CCK; Row C, 2×10^{-3} A_{280} units CSE; Column 1, 0.1% (v/v) antiserum to CSK; Column 2, 0.1% (v/v) normal rabbit serum.

REFERENCES

1. E. Amundsen, J. Putter, P. Friberger, M. Knos, M. Larsbraten, and G. Glaeson, Methods for the determination of glandublar kallikrein by means of a chromogenic tripeptide substrate, Adv. Exp. Med. Biol., 120A:83-95, (1979).
2. A. G. Billing, C. Moriwaki, M. W. Peret, and M. Schachter, Studies on the localization of some serine proteases (kallikrein, acrosin) in the digestive and reproductive tract, J. Physiol. 328:49P, (1982).
3. F. Fiedler, Enzymology of glandular kallikreins, in: Bradykinin, kallidin and kallikrein, ed. by E. G. Erdös, Handb. Exp. Pharmacol., 25 Suppl., Springer-Verlag, pp. 103-161, (1979).
4. H. Fritz, & G. Wunderer, Biochemistry and applications of aprotinin, the kallikrein inhibitor from bovine organs, Arzneim.-Forsch./Drug Res., 33:479-484, (1983).
5. H. Fujimori, P. R. Levison, & M. Schachter, Purification and partial characterisation of cat pancreatic and urinary kallikreins. Comparison with other cat tissue kallikreins and related pro-teases, Adv. Exp. Med. Biol., (in press, 1985).
6. Y. Fukuoka, Y. Hojima, S. Miyaura, & C. Moriwaki, Purification of cat submaxillary kallikrein, J. Biochem., 85:549-557, (1979).
7. Y. Hojima, B. Maranda, C. Moriwaki, & M. Schachter, Direct evidence for the location of kallikrein in the striated ducts of the cat's submandibular gland by the use of specific antibody, J. Physiol., 268:793-801, (1977).
8. M. Kobayashi, & K. Ohata, Property of kinin-forming enzyme in rat stomach, Jap. J. Pharmacol., 31:369-373, (1981).
9. M. Kobayashi, T. Shikimi, S. Miyata, & K. Ohata, Studies on kinin-forming enzyme in rat stomach, Jap. J. Pharmacol., 29:947-950, (1979).
10. C. Moriwaki, & M. Schachter, Kininogenase of the guinea-pig's coagulating gland and the release of bradykinin, J. Physiol., 219:341-353, (1971).
11. M. Schachter, Kallikreins (kininogenases) - A group of werine pro-teases with bioregulatory actions, Pharmacol. Rev., 31:1-17, (1980).
12. M. Schachter, M. W. Peret, C. Moriwaki, & J. A. A. Rodrigues, Locali-zation of kallikrein in usbmandibular gland of cat, guinea pig, dog and man by the immunoperoxidase method, J. Histochem. Cytochem., 28:1295-1300, (1980).
13. M. Schachter, M. W. Peret, A. G. Billing, & G. D. Wheeler, Immuno-localization of the protease kallikrein in the colon, J. Histochem. Cytochem., 31:1255-1260, (1983a).
14. M. Schachter, G. D. Wheeler, R. W. Matthews, M. W. Peret, & C. Moriwaki, Ultrastructural immunolocalization of kallikrein in apical granules of striated duct cells of cat submandibular gland, J. Histochem. Cytochem., 31:342-347, (1983b).
15. T. Seki, T. Nakajima, & E. G. Erdös, Colon kallikrein, its relation to the plasma enzyme, Biochem. Pharmacol., 21:1227-1235, (1972).
16. K. Uchida, M. Niinobe, M. Kato, & S. Fujii, Purification and pro-perties of rat stomach kallikrein, Biochim. Biophys. Acta, 614:501-510, (1980).
17. S. Uetsuji, M. Yamamura, M. Yamamoto, K. Uchida, H. Kushiro, J. Kodama, & S. Fujii, Human stomach kallikrein. Agents and Actions, 9:Suppl., pp. 137-142, (1982).

PURIFICATION AND PARTIAL CHARACTERIZATION OF CAT PANCREATIC AND URINARY

KALLIKREINS - COMPARISON WITH OTHER CAT TISSUE KALLIKREINS AND RELATED

PROTEASES

Hiroyuki Fujimori*, Peter R. Levison*, and Melville Schachter

*Alberta Heritage Foundation for Medical Research Fellows
Department of Physiology, University of Alberta, Edmonton
Alberta, Canada   T6G 2H7

SUMMARY

Kallikreins have been purified from cat pancreas and urine by methods similar to those described previously for cat colon and submandibular gland kallikreins.[6] The pancreatic kallikrein (M.W. 41,200, pI 4.75) was similar to the urinary kallikrein (M.W. 34,300 pI 4.35-4.70) in pH optimum, substrate specificity and inhibition profile. Both enzymes were potent kininogenases and immunologically similar. These enzymes closely resembled the kallikreins from cat colon and submandibular glands. A trypsin (M.W. 18,800) was isolated from cat pancreas and shown to be distinct from the group of kallikreins in all parameters tested. We attempted purification of cat renal kallikrein, but were unable to isolate any such enzyme. The major acidic esterase of cat kidney cortex (M.W. 59,000, pI 4.91) was purified and was distinct from both the cat tissue kallikreins and trypsin. The origin of cat urinary kallikrein remains unclear, but in the light of our findings, it may result from renal filtration of blood-borne tissue kallikreins rather than from intrarenal synthesis.

INTRODUCTION

Kallikreins (EC 3.4.21.35) are a group of related serine proteases which release biologically active peptides, kinins, from kininogens (see recent reviews by Fiedler[4] and Schachter[19]).

Abbreviations used are: CCK, cat colon kallikrein; CPK, cat pancreatic kallikrein; CPT, cat pancreatic trypsin; CRE, cat renal esterase; CSK, cat submandibular gland kallikrein; ELISA, enzyme-linked immunosorbent assay; t-AMCHA, trans-4-(amino-methyl)-cyclohexane carboxylic acid.

Few studies have been reported on kallikreins of the cat. The submandibular gland enzyme has been isolated and is the one best characterised at present.[6,7] In a previous study, we reported the purification of cat colon kallikrein (CCK) and cat submandibular gland kallikrein (CSK) and demonstrated their similar biological, chemical and immunological properties.[6] We reported the purification and partial characterisation of cat pancreatic (CPK) and urinary (CUK) kallikreins. A trypsin has also been isolated from cat pancreas (CPT) and compared with cat kallikreins.

Urinary kallikrein is generally regarded to originate from renal synthesis in the distal nephron.[2,11,15,19] In the cat kidney, however, we have failed to find any such enzyme. We do, however, report the purification and partial characterisation of the major acidic esterase from cat kidney cortex (CRE) using the procedure for the purification of cat tissue kallikrein.[6] It is, however, clearly a different enzyme. For example, it lacks kininogenase activity and fails to cross-react immunologically with other kallikreins.

MATERIALS AND METHODS

Materials

Materials used included DEAE-Sephacel, Sephadex G-50, Sephadex G-75, Sephadex G-100 (Pharmacia); diisopropylfluorophosphate, 5,5'-dithiobis-(2-nitrobenzoic acid), bradykinin triacetate, trypsin inhibitors (soyabean) type I-S, (lima-bean) type II-L, (chicken egg white) type IV-0, antipain, chymostatin, leupeptin, pepstatin, τ-AMCHA, EDTA, Tos-Lys-CH$_2$Cl, Bz-Arg-OEt, Tos-Arg, OMe, Bz-DL-Arg-ρNa, pharmalyte pH 2.5-5.0, Tween 20 and Triton X-100, aprotinin-agarose (Sigma); Cbz-Lys-SBzl (Cambridge Research Biochemicals Lts.); D-Val-Leu-Arg-ρNa, S2266 (Helena Laboratories); aprotinin (Bayer AG). ρ-Aminobenzamidine Sepharose 4B and partially purified dog kininogen were prepared as described previously.[6] Antiserum to purified CSK was raised in New Zealand rabbits.[20] CSK was purified as described previously.[6]

Methods

Preparation of tissue extracts   Cats of either sex (3-6 kg) were anaesthetised by intraperitoneal injection of 35 mg pentobarbital/kg. The bladder contents were aspirated with a sterile syringe. Urine was stored at -20°C until use. The pancreas and kidneys were removed and the pancreas, kidney cortex and medulla were cut into small pieces and frozen with liquid N$_2$. Pancreas samples were homogenised with at least 5 vol. of distilled H$_2$O at 4°C in a glass homogeniser and stood for 15 h at room temperature. The suspension was centrifuged for 60 min at 4°C and 70,000 g, and the supernatant used for purification.

Assay techniques   Kallikrein was routinely assayed spectrophotometrically using 0.1 mM-Cbz-Lys-SBzl as substrate. Enzymic hydrolysis was monitored at 412 nm in 0.1 M-Tris/HCl buffer, pH 8.0, at 37°C, with the use of 5,5'-dithiobis-(2-nitrobenzoic acid) as chromogen. One unit of activity hydrolysed 1 µmol of substrate/min under the conditions described. D-Val-Leu-Arg-ρNa hydrolysis was measured using 0.1 mM-substrate at 405 nm under similar conditions. Hydrolysis of 1.0 mM-Bz-Arg-OEt, 1.0 mM-Tos-Arg-OMe and 1.0 mM-Bz-DL-Arg-ρNa was measured in 0.1 M-Tris/HCl buffer, pH 8.0, at 25°C at 253 nm, 247 nm and 405 nm respectively, as described by Fukuoka et al.[7] The kinetic constant, K_m, was determined for the hydrolysis of

Cbz-Lys-SBzl and D-Val-Leu-Arg-ρNa in 0.1 M-Tris/Hcl buffer, pH 8.0, at 37°C. Kinin-releasing ability of enzyme samples was determined by bioassay on an isolated guinea-pig ileum preparation, using a dog kininogen substrate.[6] Protein was determined by absorption measurement at 280 nm. One A_{280} unit is that amount of protein showing an absorbance of 1.0 when contained in 1.0 ml of solution. Isoelectricfocusing was performed with a 110 ml column (LKB) using pH 2.5-5.0 ampholine. Apparent M.W. was determined by gel filtration on a column of Sephadex G-100. The effects of various protease inhibitors on enzyme activity were determined as described previously.[6] Double diffusion analysis and ELISA of enzyme preparations using CSK-antiserum and normal rabbit serum were carried out as described previously.[6]

Purification of Cat Pancreatic Kallikrein and Trypsin

Cat pancreatic tissue extract was chromatographed on DEAE-Sephacel as described previously.[6] The elution profile is shown in Figure 1. Four peaks of esterolytic activity were bound to the column, and the major peak (peak II), eluting between fraction nos. 113-128, further purified by ρ-aminobenzamidine-Sepharose 4B and Sephadex G-75 chromatography as described previously.[6]

Non-bound material from the DEAE-Sephacel step (Figure 1, fraction nos. 5-18) was pooled and concentrated by dialysis against solid sucrose and the concentrate dialysed against 100 vol. of 0.05 M-Tris/HCl buffer, pH 8.0, containing 1.0 mM-CaCl$_2$, for 16 h at 4°C. The enzyme solution was passed through an aprotinin-agarose column (1.6 cm x 25 cm) equilibrated with 0.05 M-Tris/HCl buffer, pH 8.0, containing 1.0 mM-CaCl$_2$, at a flow rate of 30 ml/h. The column was washed with at least 4 bed vol. of the same buffer and adsorbed material eluted with 1.0 mM-HCl, pH 3.0, containing 1.0 mM-CaCl$_2$ and 2.0 M-NaCl at a flow rate of 30 ml/h and fraction size of 5 ml. Active fractions were pooled and stored at -20°C.

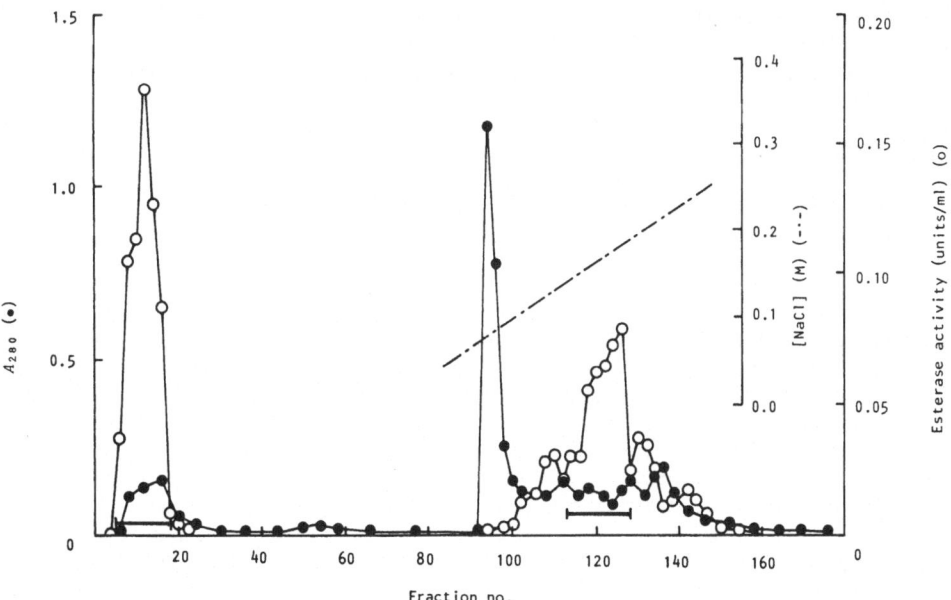

Figure 1. Chromatography of cat pancrease extract on DEAE-Sephacel.

For conditions see the text. Fractions were pooled as indicated by the horizontal bar. Fraction vol. 5 ml (10 ml for fraction nos. 1-70).

Purification of Cat Urinary Kallikrein

Cat urine was dialysed against 100 vol. of distilled H_2O for 16 h at 4°C. The non-diffusable material was fractionated with cold acetone (40-75%, v/v) and the precipitated material used for further purification. The active material was applied to a DEAE-Sephacel column (2.6 cm x 17 cm) previously equilibrated with 0.05 M-Tris/HCl buffer, pH 8.0, and washed with the same buffer until the A_{280} of the eluate was less than 0.002. The bound material was eluted initially stepwise with 0.05 M-Tris/HCl buffer, pH 8.0, containing 0.1 M-NaCl until the A_{280} of the eluate was less than 0.002, and then with a linear gradient of 0.1-0.5 M-NaCl in 0.05 M-Tris/HCl buffer, pH 8.0, as described previously.[6] A single peak of esterolytic activity was bound to the column. This was further purified by DEAE-Sephacel, ρ-aminobenzamidine-Sepharose 4B and Sephadex G-75 chromatography as described previously.[6]

Purification of Cat Renal Esterase

Kidney cortex was homogenised with 3 vol. of distilled H_2O and the homogenate frozen and thawed. Homogenisation was repeated and distilled water (2 vol.) added to the suspension. The mixture was stirred gently for 2 h at room temperature, then frozen and thawed. Triton X-100 was added to a final concentration of 0.5% (v/v) and the suspension stirred for 16 h at room temperature. The extract was centrifuged for 45 min at 4°C and 70,000 g and the precipitate discarded. The supernatant was fractionated with cold acetone (40-75%, v/v). This material was chromatographed on DEAE-Sephacel.[6] A single peak of esterolytic activity was bound to the column and this material chromatographed on ρ-amino-benzamidine-Sepharose 4B[6] but did not bind to this matrix. The step was repeated with the same result and the active material chromatographed on Sephadex G-75.[6] Active material was further purified by preparative isoelectricfocusing yielding three peaks of esterolytic activity, corresponding to pI values of 3.06, 4.91 and approximately 8.0. The major component of pI 4.91 was chromatographed on a column (3.0 cm x 65 cm) of Sephadex G-50 previously equilibrated with 5.0 mM-ammonium formate buffer, pH 8.0. Active fractions eluting in the void volume were pooled and stored at -20°C.

DISCUSSION

Using the procedure previously reported for the purification of tissue kallikreins from cat colon (CCK) and submandibular gland (CSK),[6] we have isolated kallikreins from cat pancreas and urine. A large fraction of esterolytic activity was not bound to the DEAE-Sephacel column during isolation of CPK (Figure 1) and this was used for further purification of CPT, since it is well established that bovine trypsin binds strongly to acidic ion-exchangers[21] it seems unlikely that CPT would bind to an anionic ion-exchange matrix. CPT bound strongly to aprotinin-agarose, unlike the cat tissue kallikreins, which were marginally affected by this inhibitor. It was found that DEAE-Sephacel chromatography of a crude CUK preparation was a very efficient purification step if performed twice. Initially, all adsorbed esterolytic activity was eluted stepwise with 0.1 M-NaCl in 0.05 M-Tris/HCl buffer, pH 8.0, and contaminating protein desorbed using NaCl gradient. Active material was rechromatographed on DEAE-Sephacel in the usual manner. Cat kidney cortex was subjected to homogenisation, freezing and thawing, and detergent treatment in order to disrupt cell membranes and release any membrane-bound material. It has been observed that kallikrein in rat kidney is membrane-bound[3] and therefore such treatment was deemed important. After acetone fractionation, the esterase content of the kidney extract increased significantly, an observation in keeping with the acetone activation observed during the purification of dog,[13] human,[12] and procine renal kallikreins.[14] The DEAE-Sephacel fraction was not inhibited by ρ-aminobenzamidine, unlike the cat tissue kallikreins, and preparative isoelectricfocusing of this material distinguished three peaks of esterolytic activity. The fraction of pI 4.91, which is in the range of pI values typical of cat tissue kallikreins, was used for further purification of CRE.

The apparent M.W. of 41.200 for CPK and 34,300 for CUK (Table 1) were similar to those of CSK (˜1,200) and CCK (38,300) reported previously.[6] These values differ from M.W. 18,800 and 59,000 for CPT and CRE respectively. In our bioassay, CUK released 328 μg-bradykinin equivalents/min/A_{280}, which was similar to that of CSK (350 μg-bradykinin equivalents/min/A_{280}), CPK was not as potent a kininogenase as CUK, releasing 92 μg-bradykinin equivalents/min/A_{280}, which was similar to 87 μg-bradykinin equivalents/min/A_{280} released by CCK.[6] CPT released only 1.2 μg-bradykinin equivalents/min/A_{280}, much less than that released by cat tissue kallikreins. The kininogenase activity of trypsin has been well documented[17] and it has been reported that crystalline bovine trypsin is at least 10-fold less potent at releasing kinin from a bovine kininogen preparation than a very crude preparation of human salivary kallikrein.[9] No kinin-releasing ability was detectable in our CRE preparation. A crude homogenate of cat kidney cortex did not contain detectable kinin-releasing activity, but after acidification released 20 ng-bradykinin equivalents/min/g wet wt. This is much less than the kininogenase activity of colon (2,860 ng-bradykinin equivalents/min/g wet wt.), pancreas (45,000 ng-bradykinin equivalents/min/g wet wt.), submandibular glands 150,000 ng-bradykinin equivalents/min/ml.[6] Whether this activity in kidney homogenates is due to intrarenal kallikrein or contamination by plasma kallikreins or other enzymes remains to be established.

Table 1. Characterisation of cat pancreatic kallikrein (CPK), cat urinary kallikrein (CUK), cat renal esterase (CRE) and cat pancreatic trypsin (CPT)

	CPK	CUK	CRE	CPT
Molecular weight	41,200	34,300	59,000	18,800
pI (25°C)	4.75	4.35	4.91	–
		4.45		
		4.70		
pH optimum	9.15	9.15	7.24	7.24
Kinin-releasing activity (μg-BK/min/A_{280})	91.9	328	–	1.18
ELISA (CSK-antiserum)	+	+	–	–

CPK comprised a single form of pI 4.75 by preparative isoelectric-focusing, which was similar to CUK that comprised three forms (pI 4.35-4.70). These values are similar to those observed for CSK (pI 4.15-4.76) and CCK (pI 4.08-4.61). CPT was not tested in our system, but since it was not bound to DEAE-Sephacel in 0.05 M-Tris/HCl buffer, pH 8.0, containing 1.0 mM-$CaCl_2$, it may be concluded that under these conditions CPT is uncharged or carries a net positive charge and is likely, therefore, to have a pI of greater than 8.0.

In common with CSK and CCK,[6] CPK and CUK hydrolysed Cbz-Lys-SBzl, D-Val-Leu-Arg-pNa, Bz-Arg-OEt and Tos-Arg-OMe, with Bz-Arg-OEt being hydrolysed the most rapidly by each enzyme. Furthermore, the ratios of rates of hydrolysis of Cbz-Lys-SBzl/Bz-Arg/OEt, D-Val-Leu-Arg-pNa/Bz-Arg-OEt and Bz-Arg-OEt/Tos-Arg-OMe obtained for CPK and CUK (Table 2) were very similar to those previously obtained for CSK (0.59, 0.11 and 2.26) and CCK (0.86, 0.126 and 1.78) respectively.[6] CPT hydrolysed the same group of substrates, but in this case Cbz-Lys-SBzl was the most rapidly hydrolysed, with markedly different relative rates of hydrolysis between substrates to those found for the kallikreins. CPT hydrolysed Bz-DL-Arg-Na 22-fold faster than Cbz-Lys-SBzl, an observation discriminating trypsin from kallikreins since we could not detect any hydrolysis of this substrate by either CPK or CUK or by CSK and CCK.[6] The substrate specificity of CRE was distinct from either the cat tissue kallikreins or CPT, with Cbz-Lys-SBzl, D-Val-Leu-Arg-pNa, Bz-Arg-OEt and Tos-Arg-OMe each being hydrolysed at least 100-fold slower by CRE than by the kallikreins and at different relative rates.

Kinetically, CPK and CUK were similar to CSK and CCK[6] in terms of the K_m values obtained for hydrolysis of Cbz-Lys-SBzl and D-Val-Leu-Arg-pNa. For these kallikreins, D-Val-Leu-Arg-pNa was the better substrate with K_m values of 14-33 µM compared to 76-140 µM for Cbz-Lys-SBzl. CPT and CRE davoured hydrolysis of Cbz-Lys-SBzl to D-Val-Leu-Arg-pNa, with K_m values

Table 2. Substrate specificity of cat pancreatic kallikrein (CPK), cat urinary kallikrein (CUK), cat renal esterase (CRE) and cat pancreatic trypsin (CPT)

	CPK	CUK	CRE	CPT
Relative rates of hydrolysis:				
Cbz-Lys-SBzl/Bz-Arg-OEt	0.59	0.71	1.08	1.90
D-Val-Leu-Arg-pNa/Bz-Arg-OEt	0.106	0.084	0.0088	0.57
Bz-Arg-OEt/Tos-Arg-OMe	1.81	2.31	12.0	0.66
K_m (µM):				
Cbz-Lys-SBzl	91.0	139	83.3	62.5
D-Val-Leu-Arg-pNa	13.7	30.3	100	125

of 62 µM and 125 µM respectively for CPT and 83.3 µM and 100 µM respectively for CRE. While it is difficult to distinguish a cat trypsin from a cat tissue kallikrein with certainty by determination of K_m for hydrolysis of Cbz-Lys-SBzl, the K_m values obtained for hydrolysis of the "tissue kallikrein substrate" D-Val-Leu-Arg-pNa by these two groups of enzymes are markedly different and allow this distinction to be made.

Whilst CPT was inhibited by all protease inhibitors tested, with the exception of chymostatin and t-AMCHA (Table 3), CPK and CUK were more specific in their inhibition profiles and were also unaffected by lima-bean and egg-white trypsin inhibitors and EDTA. CPK was only weakly inhibited by aprotinin and CUK was unaffected. These observations are all similar to the behaviour of CSK and CCK with various protease inhibitors reported previously.[6] CRE was very selective in its inhibition profile, being weakly affected by all inhibitors tested with the exception of diisopropylfluorophosphate, which partially inhibited the enzyme, suggesting its serine protease nature.

Table 3. Effects of various protease inhibitors on the hydrolysis of 0.1 mM-Cbz-Lys-SBzl by cat pancreatic kallikrein (CPK), cat urinary kallikrein (CUK), cat pancreatic trypsin (CPT) and cat renal esterase (CRE) in 0.1 M-Tris/HCl buffer, pH 8.0, at 37°C. See the Materials and Methods section for experimental details

Inhibitor	Inhibitor amount	% Inhibition			
		CPK*	CUK+	CPT‡§	CRE‖
Aprotinin	100 KIU	22	N.D.¶	100	8
Soya-bean trypsin inhibitor	2.5 mg	43	35	99	N.D.
Lima-b an trypsin inhibitor	2.5 mg	N.D.	N.D.	100	N.D.
Egg-white trypsin inhibitor	2.5 mg	N.D.	N.D.	100	N.D.
Leupeptin	0.5 mg	74	51	96	19
Chymostatin	0.5 mg	N.D.	5	1	8
Pepstatin	0.5 mg	11	16	76	N.D.
Antipain	0.5 mg	22	40	93	8
Tos-Lys-CH$_2$Cl	1.0 mM	N.D.	28	77	13
Diisopropylfluorophosphate	5.0 mM	48	72	66	41
EDTA	5.0 mM	9	2	30	N.D.
t-AMCHA	0.5 mg	N.D.	N.D.	N.D.	N.D.

* 4.5 units/ml (Cbz-Lys-SBzl units)

+ 4.0 munits/ml (Cbz-Lys-SBzl units)

‡ 32.0 munits/ml (Cbz-Lys-SBzl units)

§ 1.0 mM-CaCl$_2$ added to buffer

‖ 9.0 munits/ml (Cbz-Lys-SBzl units)

¶ Non-detectable

Double diffusion analysis of CPK, CUK, CCK and CSK using antibodies raised against CSK demonstrated their immunological similarity with single sharp precipitin lines that fused in reactions of complete identity (Figure 2). Precipitin lines were not detected with either CPT or CRE. Similar results were found by ELISA, where CUK was approximately 7-fold less reactive to CSK-antiserum than CSK, and CPK was approximately 40-fold less reactive than CSK.

These studies demonstrate the existence of typical tissue kallikreins in the pancreas and urine of the cat. The biological, chemical and immunological properties of CPK and CUK are very similar to those previously reported for CCK and CSK[6] and suggest that they are very similar enzymes, as is the case in other mammals, including man, pig and rat.[4] The properties of these cat kallikreins are significantly different from those of a trypsin isolated from cat pancreas.

We were unable to isolate any cat renal kallikrein. A serine protease (CRE) was isolated from cat kidney cortex, but this enzyme did not behave in an identical manner to cat tissue kallikreins and had few properties in common with either this group of enzymes or with CPT. It should be noted that following acidification of cat kidney cortex homogenates, some weak kininogenase activity was detected, but this could result from contamination of the extract by plasma kallikrein rather than from the presence of a true renal kallikrein. Furthermore, we were unable to detect any immunoreactivity towards CSK-antiserum with kidney homogenates by ELISA.[6] It has long been held that urinary kallikrein arises from synthesis of kallikrein in the kidney tubules.[2,11,15,19] It has recently been suggested that renal synthesis may account for only part of the kallikrein content of urine and that renal filtration of blood-borne tissue kallikreins contributes to the urinary kallikrein content.[5] This hypothesis is supported by evidence that immunoreactive tissue kallikreins, possibly of pancreatic or salivary origin, are present in both human[8,22] and rat plasmas.[10,18] These observations support the hypothesis that renal filtration may be a major source of urinary kallikreins. Our ability to isolate a kallikrein from cat urine but our failure to do so from kidney, suggests a non-renal origin of urinary kallikrein in the cat.

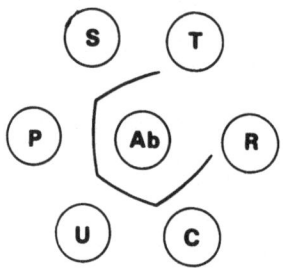

Figure 2. Double immunodiffusion of cat pancreatic (CPK), urinary (CUK), colon (CCK) and submandibular gland kallikreins (CSK), cat pancreatic trypsin (CPT) and cat renal esterase (CRE).

For conditions, see the text. Well S, 3.8×10^{-4} A_{280} units CSK; Well P, 1.1×10^{-4} A_{280} units CPK; Well U, 4.6×10^{-4} A_{280} units CUK; Well C, 1.1×10^{-4} A_{280} units CCK; Well R, 2.6×10^{-2} A_{280} units CRE: Well T, 5.2×10^{-4} A_{280} units CPT: Well Ab, 20% (v/v) antiserum to CSK.

ACKNOWLEDGEMENTS

We thank the Medical Research Council of Canada, the Alberta Heart Foundation and the Alberta Heritage Foundation for Medical Research for research grants.

REFERENCES

1. O. A. Carretero, & A. G. Scicli, Renal kallikrein; its localization and possible role in renal function, Fed. Proc., 35:194-198, (1976).
2. O. A. Carretero, & A. G. Scicli, The renal kallikrein-kinin system, Amer. J. Physiol., 238:F247-F255, (1980).
3. E. G. Erdös, & K. Yamada, Prekallikrein, kallikrein and renin in membrane fractions of rat kidney, Clin. Exp. Hypertens. A. Theor., 4: 2083-2096, (1982).
4. F. Fiedler, Enzymology of glandular kallikreins, in: Bradykinin, kallidin and kallikrein ed. by E. G. Erdös, Handb. Exp. Pharmacol., 25 Suppl., Springer-Verlag, Berlin, pp. 103-161, (1979).
5. F. Fiedler, & W. Gebhard, Isolation and characterization of native single-chain porcine pancreatic kallikrein, another possible precursor of urinary kallikrein, Hoppe-Seyler's Z. Physiol. Chem., 361:1661-1671, (1980).
6. H. Fujimori, P. R. Levison, & M. Schachter, Purification and partial characterisation of cat colon and submandibular gland kallikreins, Adv. Exp. Med. Biol., (in press, 1985).
7. Y. Fukuoka, Y. Hojima, S. Miyaura, & C. Moriwaki, Purification of cat submaxillary kallikrein, J. Biochem., 85:549-557, (1979).
8. R. Geiger, B. Clausnitzer, E. Fink, & H. Fritz, Isolation of an enzymatically active glandular kallikrein from human plasma by immunoaffinity chromatography, Hoppe-Seyler's Z. Physiol. Chem., 361:1795-1803, (1980).
9. D. J. Holdstock, A. P. Mathias, & M. Schachter, A comparative study of kinin, kallidin and bradykinin, Brit. J. Pharmacol. Chemother., 12:149-158, (1957).
10. W. J. Lawton, D. Proud, M. E. Frech, J. V. Pierce, H. R. Keiser, & J. J. Pisano, Characterization and origin of immunoreactive glandular kallikrein in rat plasma, Biochem. Pharmacol., 30:1731-1737, (1981).
11. H. S. Margolius, The kallikrein-kinin system and the kidney, Ann. Rev. Physiol., 46:309-326, (1984).
12. Y. Matsuda, K. Miyazaki, H. Moriya, & Y. Fujimoto, Human renal kallikrein: Purification and some properties, Chem. Pharm. Bull., 29: 2106-2108, (1981).
13. C. Moriwaki, K. Miyazaki, Y. Matsuda, H. Moriya, Y. Fujimoto, & H. Ueki, Dog renal kallikrein: Purification and some properties, J. Biochem., 80:1277-1285, (1976).
14. A. Nagamatsu, K. Abe, & S. Soeda, Purification and some properties of hog renal kallikrein, Chem. Pharm. Bull., 29:1981-1985, (1981).
15. L. Obika, Recent developments in urinary kallikrein research, Life Sci., 23:764-775, (1978).
16. G. S. Pinkus, O. Ole-Moi Yoi, K. F. Austen, & J. Spragg, Antigenic separation of a nonkinin-generating TAMe esterase from human urinary kallikrein and immunohistochemical comparison of their localization in the kidney, J. Histochem. Cytochem., 29:38-44, (1981).
17. J. L. Prado, Proteolytic enzymes as kininogenases, Handb. Exp. Pharmacol., 25:156-192, (1970).

18. S. F. Rabito, A. G. Scicli, V. Kher, & O. A. Carretero, Immunoreactive glandular kallikrein in rat plasma: a radioimmunoassay for its determination, Amer. J. Physiol., 242:H602–H610, (1982).

19. M. Schachter, Kallikreins (kininogenases) – a group of serine proteases with bioregulatory actions, Pharmacol. Rev., 31:1–17, (1980).

20. M. Schachter, M. W. Peret, C. Moriwaki, & J. A. A. Rodrigues, Localization of kallikrein in submandibular gland of cat, guinea pig, dog and man by the immunoperoxidase method, J. Histochem. Cytochem., 28:1295–1300, (1980).

21. D. D. Schroeder, & E. Shaw, Chromatography of trypsin and its derivatives. Characterization of a new active form of bovine trypsin, J. Biol. Chem., 243: 2943–2949, (1968).

22. K. Shimamoto, R. K. Mayfield, H. S. Margolius, J. Chao, W. Stroud, & A. P. Kaplan, Immunoreactive tissue kallikrein in human serum, J. Lab. Clin. Med., 103: 731–738, (1984).

THE LIVER IS THE MAIN ORGAN TO CLEAR PLASMA AND TISSUE KALLIKREINS FROM

RAT PLASMA, IN VIVO

Durval Borges,[1] Claudio Sampaio,[2] Pedro de la Llosa[3] and
José Leal Prado[2]

Departments of Medicine,[1] Biochemistry,[2] Escola Paulista de
Medicina, São Paulo, SP, Brazil and Laboratoire des Hormones
Polypeptidiques,[3] CNRS, Gif-sur-Yvette, France

SUMMARY

We report observations regarding the in vivo distribution of labelled
kallikreins in plasma, liver and some other organs, twenty minutes following their intravenous injection in the rat. The kallikreins used were:
tritiated homogeneous human plasma (HuPK) and horse urinary (HoUK) as well
as highly purified iodinated rat plasma kallikrein (RPK). The main findings were: a) the liver cleared 15% of HuPK, 38% of RPK and 69% HoUK;
b) with both types (plasma and tissue) of native kallikreins the liver was
the main clearing organ.

INTRODUCTION

We reported recently that perfused rat liver in situ is able to remove
and inactivate recirculating rat plasma kallikrein; the hepatocytes seem
to recognize RPK by a specific mechanism and the enzyme is then bound and
inactivated.[1,2,3] The present paper describes in vivo experiments with
labelled kallikreins in which we estimate rat liver participation in this
clearance. Initially a highly purified preparation of RPK, labelled with
radioactive iodine, was used; subsequently we measured the distribution,
between blood plasma and liver, of homogeneous preparations of native human
plasma and horse urinary kallikreins labelled with tritium. It will be
seen that the liver plays the major role in clearing these kallikreins from
circulation; differences in the clearing rates were observed for the urinary
and the plasma kallikreins. Although both the urinary and plasma kallikreins are able to release kinins from natural substrates, their chemical
properties are different.

A long term aim of these studies is to contribute to the understanding
of how the chemical composition of these glycoproteins affects their recognition by the liver.

MATERIALS AND METHODS

Kallikreins

a) Rat plasma kallikrein was purified 3900 x fold (22% yield) by a
four step purification method which involved affinity chromatography on
soybean-trypsin-inhibitor-Sepharose; its specific activity was 82 U/mg
protein on Pro-Phe-Arg-p-nitroanilide (S2302).[4] In spite of its high
purification, the stable enzyme preparation showed some impurity when 30
µg of protein were submitted to SDS-polyacrilamide gel electrophoresis.
^{125}I-RPK was obtained as follows: 72 µg of protein were incubated during
15 seconds with chloramine T (1.2 mM) and 0.5 mCi of Na ^{125}I; after addition of sodium metabisulfite (3.3 mM) the mixture was chromatographed on a
Sephadex G-25 column. The labelled RPK (1 µCi/µg protein) retained its
enzymatic activity and its radioactivity was 97% precipitated by 10% phos-
photungstic acid. The mild labelling conditions used preserved also the
RPK property of being cleared by the exsanguinated and perfused rat liver
(data not shown).

b) Human plasma kallikrein was prepared by affinity chromatography
in soybean-trypsin-inhibitor-Sepharose;[5] the enzyme, homogeneous by SDS-
electrophoresis, had a specific activity of 130 U/mg on Pro-Phe-Arg-p-nitroanilide.

c) Horse urinary kallikrein. Homogeneous HoUK was prepared[6] and had
a specific activity of 118 ± 5 Tos-Arg-OMe U/mg of protein.

d) Tritiated kallikreins. HoUK and HuPK were submitted to reductive
methylation with tritiated NaBH$_4$.[7] Tritiated HoUK had 56% of its lysine
residues methylated and a specific radioactivity of 19 Ci/mmol. Its enzymatic activity measured on Val-Leu-Arg-p-NA was unaffected by the reductive
methylation. HuPK had 68% of its lysine residues methylated and a specific
radioactivity of 190 Ci/mmol. Its enzymatic activity was 9 U/mg. As benzamidine, used to stabilize HuPK, was removed several days before tritiation,
we supposed that the large loss of its enzymatic activity was due to auto-
lysis. It is significant, however, that in the isolated and perfused rat
liver we observed (data not shown) that radioactivity and enzymatic activity
were cleared simultaneously.

Distribution Experiments

Male adult (200-250 g) albino rats, from the Department of Pharmacology
rat colony, were homogeneous, with many years of inbreeding. Under nembutal
anesthesia one heparinized rat would receive through a plastic catheter in
the femoral vein a single dose of one kallikrein; later, at chosen time
intervals the distribution of the kallikrein radioactivity was measured in
plasma (collected on contralateral side) and some organs (see Tables 1 and
2). These organs were removed from the killed rats, weighed and homogenized in three volumes of 0.25 M saccharose solution. The two rats injected
each with about 6 µg of ^{125}I-RPK, were thyroidectomized.

RESULTS

Table 1 shows that the liver was the main organ to remove from circulation the three kallikreins tested. But it is evident that HoUK was
the most effectively cleared.

Examining individual experiments in Table 2 (which includes one
further experiment with HuPK and one with HoUK where only plasma and liver
radioactivities were measured) it is possible to draw some conclusions:

Table 1. Distribution of kallikreins radioactivity injected intravenously in the rat

Kallikrein injected	Number of experiments	Average percent distribution[1]					
		Plasma	Liver	Kidneys	Lungs	Spleen	Total
Tritiated HuPK	3	61^2	15	4	1	1	82
^{125}I-RPK	2^3	41^2	38	9	ND^4	ND^4	88
Tritiated HoUK	2	14	69	4	0.6	0.6	88

[1]Measured 20 minutes following intravenous injection.
[2]From these values of tritiated HuPK and ^{125}I-RPK, 85% and 93% respectively could be precipitated in 12.5% TCA.
[3]In 2 preliminary experiments with ^{131}I-RPK lungs and spleen contained less than 2% of the radioactivity.
[4]Not determined.

Table 2. Plasma clearance and distribution in plasma and liver of tritiated human plasma or horse urinary kallikreins radioactivity (individual experiments)

Kallikrein injected	Plasma clearance ng.kg.min	Total plasma radioactivity, cpm x 10^{-6} [1]		Total liver radioactivity at 20 min, cpm x 10^{-6} [2]
		min	20 min	
			%	%
HuPK	34	1.2	0.8(67)	0.2(17)
	178	4.2	2.4(57)	0.8(19)
	322	7.6	5.2(68)	0.9(12)
	472	14.0	9.4(67)	1.8(13)
			(65 ± 5)	(15 ± 3)
HoUK	160	0.5	0.06(12)	0.4(80)
	406	1.7	0.3(17)	1.3(76)
	468	1.9	0.2(10)	1.2(63)
			(13 ± 4)	(73 ± 9)

[1]Total plasma radioactivity measured 2 min following i.v. injection of increasing doses (0.6, 2.1, 3.8 and 7.0 µg HuPK; 0.7, 2.4, and 2.7 µg of HoUK) of kallikrein in each rat was taken as 100%; at 100%; at 20 min they decreased to the values shown.
[2]Measured 20 min following kallikrein injection and given in absolute and percent (in brackets) values.

there exists a correlation between plasma clearances and respectives total plasma radioactivities measured at 2 minutes; the r (correlation coefficient) values 0.98 and 0.99 were calculated for HuPK and $\overline{\text{Ho}}$UK respectively; threshold plasma clearance rates were, thus, probably not reached.

DISCUSSION

Our distribution experiments in the rat show that the liver is the main organ to clear both plasma and tissue kallikreins from circulation. These native enzymes behave thus as several glycoproteins which were desialylated through neuraminidase pre-treatment in vitro.[8]

We have shown previously that prekallikrein accumulates in rat livers perfusates while plasma kallikrein itself is cleared.[9] We have also evidences[3] that specific carbohydrate residues, probably exposed in native rat plasma kallikrein, determine their liver clearance in the rat. Horse urinary kallikrein has a carbohydrate content of 16.8%[6] and we are unaware of published results on the carbohydrate composition of human plasma kallikrein, although it is known that its zymogen has a similarly high carbohydrate content.[10] Based solely on the described in vivo experiments one cannot determine how much of the injected kallikrein is being cleared via hepatocytic receptor compared to the clearance by the liver reticulo-endothelial-system of a possible complex kallikrein-plasma inhibitor.

It is clear however that the liver plays a major role in the homeostasis of these glycoproteins.

ACKNOWLEDGEMENTS

Research supported by FINEP (B76/80/002/00/000) and FAPESP (81/1054-5; 83-1270-4). J. L. Prado has a Research Fellowship from CNPq. Travel grants from CNPq (D. R. Borges and C. A. M. Sampaio) and FAPESP (J. L. Prado) are also acknowledged.

REFERENCES

1. D. R. Borges, A. H. Gordon, J. A. Guimarães, and J. L. Prado, Recognition and catabolism of plasma kallikrein by perfused rat liver, An. Acad. Brasil. Cienc. 53:846-847 (1981).
2. D. R. Borges, A. H. Gordon, J. A. Guimarães, and J. L. Prado, Recognition and catabolism of plasma kallikrein by perfused rat liver, in: "Recent Progress on Kinins," H. Fritz, G. Dietze, F. Fiedler, and G. L. Haberland, eds., Birkhäuser Verlag, Basel, Boston, Stuttgart (1982).
3. D. R. Borges, A. H. Gordon, J. A. Guimarães, and J. L. Prado, Rat plasma kallikrein clearance by perfused rat liver, Brazilian J. Med. Biol. Res. (In press).
4. M. Kouyoumdjian, D. R. Borges, J. A. Guimaraes, C. A. M. Sampaio, and J. L. Prado, Rat plasma kallikrein. Purification by affinity chromatography, activity towards synthetic and natural substrates and interactions with inhibitors (Manuscript in preparation).
5. M. L. Oliva, D. Grisolia, M. U. Sampaio, and C. A. M. Sampaio, Properties of highly purified human plasma kallikrein, in: "Recent Progress on Kinins," H. Fritz, G. Dietze, F. Fiedler, and G. L. Haberland, eds., Birkhäuser Verlag, Basel, Boston, Stuttgart (1982).

6. E. S. Prado, C. A. M. Sampaio, M. S. Araújo-Viel, and R. C. R. Stella, Characterization of horse urinary kallikrein, in: "Recent Progress on Kinins," H. Fritz, G. Dietze, F. Fiedler, and G. L. Haberland, Birkhäuser Verlag, Basel, Boston, Stuttgart (1982).

7. P. De la Llosa, P. Marche, J. L. Morgat, and M. P. De la Llosa-Hermier, A new procedure for labelling luteinizing hormone with tritium, FEBBS Lett. 45:162-165 (1974).

8. A. G. Morell, G. Gregoriadis, I. H. Scheinberg, J. Hickman, and G. Ashwell, The role of sialic acid in determining the survival of glycoproteins in the circulation, J. Biol. Chem. 246:1461-1467 (1971).

9. D. R. Borges, M. E. Webster, J. A. Guimarães, and J. L. Prado, Synthesis of prekallikrein and metabolism of plasma kallikrein by perfused rat liver, Biochem. Pharmacol. 30:1065-1069 (1981).

10. R. L. Heimark and E. W. Davie, Bovine and human plasma prekallikrein, in: "Methods in Enzymology," Sidney O. Colowick and Nathan O. Kaplan, eds., Academic Press (1981).

RECEPTOR-MEDIATED CLEARANCE OF TISSUE KALLIREINS BY RAT LIVER

Durval R. Borges,[1] Maria Kouyoumdjian,[2] Eline S. Prado[2] and
José Leal Prado[2]

Departments of Medicine[1] and Biochemistry,[2] Escola Paulista
de Medicina, Caixa Postal 20239, São Paulo, SP, Brazil

SUMMARY

The exsanguinated, isolated and perfused rat liver clears from the
perfusate, at comparable rates, some native tissue kallikreins: human and
horse urinary as well as hog pancreatic; the clearance rates were dependent
on the initial enzyme concentration in the perfusing fluid. Contrarywise,
rat urinary kallikrein was cleared at negligible rates. Neuraminidase pre-
treatment of these four kallikreins did not alter their clearance rates.

Horse urinary kallikrein binding to isolated prefixed hepatocytes was
calcium-dependent and inhibited by asialofetuin (but not by fetuin) and
some sugars; these characteristics are compatible with the interpretation
that this native tissue kallikrein is recognized by the hepatocyte asialoglycoprotein-receptor. It was calculated that there are about 300,000 receptor sites per cell either using perfusion experiments at 4°C or isolated
hepatocytes.

INTRODUCTION

We have shown that perfused rat liver in situ synthesizes prekallikrein
and metabolizes plasma kallikrein;[1] some characteristics of the receptor-
mediated clearance and posterior lysosomal degradation of plasma kallikrein
by the perfused rat liver have been studies.[2,3] We have also shown that
in vivo, the liver is the main organ to clear, from the circulation, not
only plasma but tissue kallikreins as well.[4] The mechanism(s) by which
the liver clears tissue kallikreins from circulation probably includes its
recognition by hepatic receptors and/or clearance, by the liver reticulo-
endothelial-system, of a possible complex kallikrein-plasma inhibitor. In
this paper we report that: a) native tissue kallikreins are cleared by
the perfused and exsanguinated rat liver; b) the clearance is dependent on
the initial concentration of the enzyme in the perfusion fluid but it is
not affected by previous treatment of the enzymes with neuraminidase; and
c) horse urinary kallikrein binds to the hepatocytic asialoglycoprotein-receptor. This receptor,[5] whose physiological role remains elusive,[6] is
known to recognize various ex-vivo pre-treated (sialic acid removal) glycoproteins.

MATERIALS AND METHODS

Kallikreins

Homogeneous horse urinary kallikrein (HoUK) with a specific activity
of 118 ± 5 Tos-Arg-OMe U/mg of protein was tritiated as described;[4] hog
pancreatic kallikrein (1168 KU/mg) was from Bayer Werk Elberfeld, lot SMU
2564 II; partially purified human urinary (0.65 S2266 U/A_{280}) and rat urinary
(4.2 Tos-Arg-Ome U/A_{280}) kallikreins were a gift from D. R. Stella and A.
Voos respectively. Fetuin (type III Sigma) and kallikreins were treated
with neuraminidase (Worthington Biochemical Corporation) as described.[3]
Ac-Phe-Arg-p-nitroalinide was a gift from D. L. Juliano, Dept. Biophysics,
Escola Paulista de Medicina.

Liver Perfusion Experiments

The isolated and exsanguinated rat liver was perfused at 37°C as previously described;[3] for estimation of exposed receptors, tritiated HoUK
(38 nM) was recirculated at pH 7.4 and 4°C, conditions under which bound
ligand is not internalized. After perfusing for 60 min, bound HoUK was
dissociated from the hepatocyte receptors by lowering the pH perfusion
medium to 4.25 by adding acetate buffer pH 3.6.[7] The perfusion continued
for 20 additional minutes at pH 4.25. The number of receptors per hepatocyte was calculated using 1.38×10^8 hepatocytes/g wet weight of liver and
assuming a 1:1 interaction for the ligand-receptor complex.[7]

Isolated Hepatocytes Binding-Receptor

For the binding experiments prefixed hepatocytes were obtained after
perfusion of the exsanguinated rat liver with 0.7% glutaraldehyde as described;[8] 80 ng of tritiated HoUK were incubated with 1×10^6 hepatocytes
in calcium (3 mM) containing buffer pH 7.4 at 4°C, in the absence or
presence of 0.18 μM fetuin, 0.18 μM asialofetuin or 5 mM sugars (lactose,
mellibiose, mannose, galactose and glucose). After 60 min at slow giration
(6 revolutions per minute) the bound HoUK was separated from medium and
unbound ligand by centrifugation through dibutylphthalate and the pellet
radioactivity was counted.

RESULTS

It is shown on Table 1 that human and horse urinary as well as hog
pancreatic kallikreins were cleared at comparable rates and that these rates
depended on the initial concentration of the enzymes in the perfusion
fluid. Rat urinary kallikrein, however, was cleared at negligible rates.
The clearance rates of these four kallikreins were unaffected by previous
treatment with neuraminidase: the clearance rate of the untreated kallikreins was first determined and then compared with an almost consecutive
determination in the same liver, with the neuraminidase-treated kallikreins.

Table 2 shows that the binding of HoUK to isolated prefixed hepatocytes is calcium-dependent, unaffected by fetuin being inhibited by asialofetuin and, in various degrees, by some sugars.

From the perfusion experiments with HoUK made at 4°C and the respective binding experiments on isolated hepatocytes we calculated that there
are about 300,000 receptor sites per cell.

Table 1. Clearances rates (mean ± standards error) of tissue kallikreins by perfused rat liver, at 37°C

Kallikrein	n	Initial Concentration mU/ml[(a)]	Clearance rate[(b)] mU/min/g liver
Human urinary	3	2	0.16 ± 0.05
Horse urinary	4	2	0.20 ± 0.07
	5	8	1.10 ± 0.10
	1	32	1.60
Hog pancreatic	1	3	0.20
	1	9	0.50
	5	17	1.50 ± 0.10
Rat urinary	6	3	0.04 ± 0.04

[(a)] Human urinary and hog pancreatic amidolytic activities were measured on Ac-Phe-Arg-p-nitroanilide; horse and rat urinary activities, on S2266 (Kabi).
[(b)] Calculated after 20 min of perfusion.

Table 2. Binding characteristics of tritiated horse urinary kallikrein on isolated prefixed rat hepatocytes

Modifications of suspending medium[(a)]	Percent Inhibition of Binding
1. Calcium free medium	93
2. Fetuin 0.18 μM	0
3. Asialofetuin 0.18 μM	57
4. Lactose 5 mM	59
5. Mellibiose 5 mM	49
6. Mannose 5 mM	43
7. Galactose 5 mM	20
8. Glucose 5 mM	0

[(a)] Substances 2-9 were dissolved in a pH 7.4 balanced salt solution containing 3 mM $CaCl_2$.

DISCUSSION

The isolated, exsanguinated and perfused rat liver is able to clear from the perfusate three native tissue kallikreins; the clearance rates were dependent on the initial concentration of the enzyme in the perfusion fluid (as occurred with rat plasma kallikrein[3]) and was also a two phase phenomenum: a rapid one followed by a slow exponential phase (data not shown). Surprisingly, rat urinary kallikrein was not cleared by the liver preparation at significant rates; pre-treatment of RUK with neuraminidase, which may possibly expose some sugar residues, did not alter this behavior. The neuraminidase treatment used was effective in removing sialic acid residues from fetuin and is known[9] to remove all sialic acid residues from both forms (α and β) of RUK. The fact that RUK is poorly cleared by the exsanguinated rat liver does not exclude, however, the possibility that, in vivo a complex RUK-plasma inhibitor may be cleared by the liver reticulo-endothelial-system. RUK in fact has important differences with other tissue kallikreins, as far as substrate specificity is concerned.[10]

Horse urinary kallikrein (which could be obtained in homogeneous form and successfully tritiated) binds to isolated hepatocytes. The binding of this native glycoprotein has characteristics (inhibition patterns, calcium-dependence, number of receptor sites per cell) which are compatible with the idea of this enzyme being recognized by the asialoglycoprotein-receptor of the hepatocytes.[6] Each mol of the used kallikrein has 13 moles of glucosamine, 5.7 moles of galactosamine, 4.6 moles of galactose, 3.1 moles of mannose, 1.3 moles of fucose[11] and only 2.5 moles of sialic acid. This means that HoUK must have terminal sugars, not masked by sialic acid residues, that may be recognized by the asialoglycoprotein-receptor.[6] In fact neuraminidase treatment of HoUK neither released sialic acid residues (data not shown) from the enzyme nor altered its clearance behaviour. All the other glycoproteins that are known to bind to the asialoglycoprotein-receptor, bind only after in vitro pre-treatment, where they are desialylated by incubation with neuraminidase.[5] Any possible physiopathological role of this receptor in the homeostasis of circulating native (untreated) tissue kallikreins remains to be determined.

REFERENCES

1. D. R. Borges, M. E. Webster, J. A. Guimarães, and J. L. Prado, Synthesis of prekallikrein and metabolism of plasma kallikrein by perfused rat liver, Biochem. Pharmacol. 30:1065–1069 (1981).
2. D. R. Borges, A. H. Gordon, J. A. Guimarães, and J. L. Prado, Recognition and catabolism of plasma kallikrein by perfused rat liver, in: "Recent Progress on Kinins," H. Fritz, G. Dietze, F. Fiedler, and G. L. Haberland, eds., Birhäuser Verlag, Basel, Boston, Stuttgart (1982).
3. D. R. Borges, A. H. Gordon, J. A. Guimarães, and J. L. Prado, Rat plasma kallikrein clearance by perfused rat liver, Brazilian J. Med. Biol. Res. (In press, 1984).
4. D. R. Borges, C. Sampaio, P. De la Llosa, and J. L. Prado, The liver is the main organ to clear plasma and tissue kallikreins from rat plasma, in vivo, (Accompanying paper, 1985).
5. G. Ashwell and J. Harford, Carbohydrate-specific receptors of the liver, Ann. Rev. Biochem. 51:531–534 (1982).
6. R. J. Stockert and A. G. Morell, Hepatic binding protein: the galactose-specific receptor of mammalian hepatocytes, Hepatology 3:750–757 (1983).

7. W. A. Dunn and A. L. Hubbard, Receptor-mediated endocytosis of epidermal growth factor by hepatocytes in the perfused rat liver: ligand and receptor dynamics, J. Cell Biol. 98:2148-2159 (1984).

8. S. Matsuura, H. Nakala, T. Sawamura, and Y. Tashiro, Distribution of an asialoglycoprotein receptor on rat hepatocyte cell surface, J. Cell Biol. 95:864-875 (1982).

9. H. Tunes, E. Silva, and M. Mares-Guia, Alpha- and beta-rat urinary kallikreins: chemical and physiocochemical properties, Brazilian J. Med. Biol. Res. 16:193-202 (1983).

10. E. S. Prado, L. Juliano, M. Araújo-Viel, and M. A. Juliano, Characterization of kallikreins by model oligopeptides (In these proceedings, 1985).

11. E. S. Prado, C. A. M. Sampaio, M. S. Araújo-Viel, and R. C. R. Stella, Characterization of horse urinary kallikrein, in: "Recent Progress on Kinins," H. Fritz, G. Dietze, F. Fiedler, and G. L. Haberland, eds., Birhäuser Verlag, Basel, Boston, Stuttgart (1982).

TISSUE KALLIKREINS AND RELATED ENZYMES: CHARACTERIZATION BY MODEL OLIGOPEPTIDES

Eline S. Prado,[1] Luis Juliano,[2] Mariana S. Araújo-Viel[1] and Maria A. Juliano

Departments of Biochemistry[1] and Biophysics,[2] Escola Paulista de Medicina, C. P. 20372, São Paulo, SP. Brasil

SUMMARY

The first purpose of this work was to obtain direct evidence that tissue kallikreins cleave arginyl bonds when the leaving group is Arg-Val, and on the contrary, do not split them when it is Arg-Pro; the second aim was to ascertain whether this specificity could be used as a criterion, for characterizing tissue kallikreins.

Two tetrapeptides A) Ac-Phe-Arg-Arg-Val-NH_2 and B) Ac-Phe-Arg-Arg-Pro-NH_2 were synthesized by the solid phase method and purified to homogeneity. They were used as substrates for homogeneous preparations of tissue and plasma kallikreins, as well as for some related serine proteases. Products identification and kinetic analyses were made by HPLC.

The hindering effect of the P_2 Pro residue in the hydrolysis by tissue kallikreins was unequivocally demonstrated. Results showed also that enzymes which cleave the Arg-Arg bond in peptide A but do not hydrolyze peptide B, may be classified as tissue kallikreins.

INTRODUCTION

Kallikdin liberation from kininogen has been the usual criterion for characterizing tissue kallikreins; in the kininogen sequence --Phe-Met-Lys-Arg-Pro-- these serine proteases cleave the Met-Lys bond instead of the Lys-Arg link which, in contrast, is split by bradykinin releasing enzymes. The resistance of the Lys-Arg bond in the kininogen sequence to tissue kallikreins was attributed by Prado et al.[1] to the proline residue in position P_2 (Schechter and Berg nomenclature).[2] This explanation was based on the following indirect evidence: a) the demonstration that the Arg-Arg bond in the sequence --Phe-Met-Arg-Arg-Val-- in the enkephalin derivative BAM 22P, then used as substrate, was highly susceptible to tissue kallikreins[1] b) the resistance of Ac-Phe-Arg-Arg-Pro-NH_2 to hydrolysis by porcine pancreatic kallikrein described by Fiedler.[3] Simultaneously, Chen and Bode[4] reported that the x-ray structure of the complex porcine pancreatic kallikrein A-bovine pancreatic trypsin inhibitor indicated that the proline residue would not interact favorably with the enzyme subsite S_2.

In the present workdirect evidence for the hindering effect of a Pro residue in the position P_2 was obtained; we used as substrates the tetrapeptide Ac-Phe-Arg-Arg-X-NH$_2$ (X = Pro or Val) to study their hydrolysis by three tissue kallikreins. We verified also that these peptides could be used for characterizing tissue kallikreins as well as other serine proteinases.

MATERIALS AND METHODS

Peptides

The solid phase method was used for the synthesis of Ac-Phe-Arg-Arg-Pro-NH$_2$ and Arg-Pro-NH$_2$; the other peptides (Ac-Phe-Arg-Arg-Val-NH$_2$; Ac-Phe-Arg-Arg; Ac-Phe-Arg and Arg-Val-NH$_2$) were synthesized in solution by standard procedures. Purification of the peptides was obtained by ion exchange chromatography on carboxymethylcellulose and gel-filtration on Bio-Gel P-2. Homogeneity of the peptides was demonstrated by aminoacid analysis and high voltage paper electrophoresis. High pressure liquid chromatography (under the conditions described in Methods) revealed that the tetrapeptides contained less than 1% impurities which were shown not to interfere with our work. The concentration of the peptide solutions was determined by aminoacid analysis; for the tetrapeptides they were confirmed by HPLC determination of Ac-Phe-Arg formed on total enzymatic hydrolysis.

Enzymes

Bovine trypsin (2x crystallized) from Worthington Biochem. Co.; plasmin from Sigma (1.4 U/mg protein; substrate D-Val-Leu-Lys-pNA); porcine pancreatic kallikrein (1374 KU/mg) from Bayer AG, FRG (a gift from Dr. E. Fink). The specific activities (U/mg protein measured on either D-Val-Leu-Arg-pNA or D-Pro-Phe-Arg-pNA) of the kallikreins prepared in this Department (method referred) were: horse urinary 2.87,[5] human urinary 6.9,[6] human plasma 6.1,[7] rat plasma 82.0; rat urinary kallikrein 13.6. Rat plasma kallikrein was purified 3900-fold by a four step purification method which involved affinity chromatography on soybean-trypsin-inhibitor-Sepharose.[8] Rat urinary kallikrein was purified by DEAE-cellulose chromatography[9] and further purified by affinity chromatography on trasylol-Sepharose.[10] All the enzyme preparations were shown to be homogeneous by acrylamide gel electrophoresis.

Identification of the Tetrapeptides Hydrolysis Products

The peptides, in 0.1 mM concentration, were incubated with 2 µg/ml of trypsin or tissue kallikreins, 10 µg/ml of plasma kallikreins and 200 µg/ml of plasmin. Incubations were carried out at 30°C in 0.05 M ammonium acetate buffer pH 8.0 for trypsin, plasmin and plasma kallikreins and pH 9.0 for tissue kallikreins. Aliquots were taken at different time intervals, and the reaction interrupted by dilution with the HPLC mobile phase (pH 2.2). Separation of the tetrapeptides and their hydrolysis products was achieved by high performance liquid chromatography (HPLC) using a 0.39 x 30 cm reverse phase column µBondapack C$_{18}$ from Waters Associates. The conditions used are described in Fig. 1-A, which shows the chromatography pattern of a mixture of Ac-Phe-Arg-Arg-Val-NH$_2$, Ac-Phe-Arg-Arg, Val-NH$_2$, Ac-Phe-Arg and Arg-Val-NH$_2$.

Kinetic Analyses

The initial hydrolysis rates were determined from the amounts of Ac-Phe-Arg formed at different time intervals, measured by HPLC. When Ac-Phe-Arg-Arg-Pro-NH$_2$ was the substrate, HPLC conditions used were those

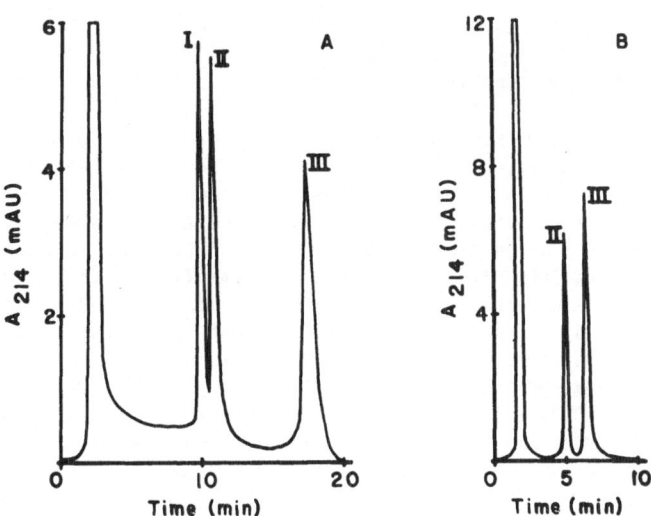

Fig. 1.   Separation of standard peptides by HPLC. The peptide solution (0.5
          nmol of each peptide in 200 µl of the mobile phase) was injected
          at zero time into the column (µBondapack C_{18}). The isocratic elution
          was monitored at 214 nm.
          A - HPLC of a mixture of Ac-Phe-Arg-Arg-Val-NH_2 and its synthetic
              fragments. The mobile phase, for isocratic elution at a flow
              rate of 1.5 ml/min, was 8.5% acetonitrile - 0.04 M phosphoric
              acid (pH 2.2). I = Ac-Phe-Arg-Arg; II = Ac-Phe-Arg; III =
              Ac-Phe-Arg-Arg-Val-NH_2. The C-terminal fragments, Arg-Val-
              NH_2 and Val-NH_2, were eluted at the void volume.
          B - HPLC of Ac-Phe-ARg-Arg-Val-NH_2 plus Ac-Phe-ARg and Arg-Val-
              NH_2. The mobile phase was 12% acetonitrile - 0.04 M phosphoric
              acid (pH 2.2) and the elution flow rate 2.5 ml/min. II = Ac-
              Phe-Arg; III = Ac-Phe-Arg-Arg-Val-NH_2; Arg-Val-NH_2 was eluted
              to V_o.

described in Fi. 1-A under which, there was a good separation of Ac-Phe-
Arg from the tetrapeptide (retention time 17 min). For the peptide Ac-
Phe-Arg-Arg-Val-NH_2 the conditions in Fig. 1-B, which decreased the retention
times, could be used.

     Active site titration was used for the determination of the molar con-
centration of horse urinary[11] and human plasma kallikreins[12] solutions.
The   kinetic parameters K_m and V_2 were calculated by a weighed least squares
program according to Wilkinson.[13]

RESULTS

Hydrolysis of Ac-Phe-Arg-Arg-Val-NH_2

     Analysis of tryptic hydrolysates by HPLC revealed the presence of two
N-terminal fragments, identified as Ac-Phe-Arg-Arg and Ac-Phe-Arg; this
result indicated that both arginyl bonds were cleaved by trypsin. In contrast, Ac-Phe-Arg ws the only N-terminal product formed by horse, human
and rat urinary kallikreins and by porcine pancreatic as well as by human
and rat plasma kallikreins. On total hydrolysis by these different kallikreins, Ac-Phe-Arg was recovered in stechiometric amounts. No traces of
Ac-Phe-Arg were detected in the incubate with plasmin, in spite of the high
enzyme concentration (200 µg) and 2 hour incubation time. Kinetic constants

for the hydrolysis by three kallikreins are presented in Table 1.

Hydrolysis of Ac-Phe-Arg-Arg-Pro-NH$_2$

a) Trypsin: as expected, it clealved only the Arg-Arg bond. b) Tissue kallikreins: no hydrolysis of this peptide by porcine pancreatic and the urinary kallikreins (horse and human) was detected even after 60 min incubation. Under the same conditions (see Methods) total hydrolysis of Ac-Phe-Arg-Arg-Val-NH$_2$ was reached within 10 min. When the concentration of Ac-Phe-Arg-Arg-Pro-NH$_2$ was increased to 4.0 mM (which is three orders of magnitude higher than the K_m for the hydrolysis of Ac-Phe-ARg-Arg-Val-NH$_2$ by horse urinary kallikrein) the rate of hydrolysis was still only 0.08 μmol.min^{-1}.mg^{-1}. This rate is 150-fold lower than the V_{max} obtained with Ac-Phe-Arg-Arg-Val-NH$_2$ (See Table 1). c) Rat urinary kallikreins: as shown on Table 1, both tetrapeptides were hydrolyzed with similar parameters. d) Both plasma kallikreins tested hydrolyzed the peptide; the k_{cat}/K_m value for human plasma kallikrein was about 5-fold lower for Ac-Phe-Arg-Arg-Pro-NH$_2$ (Table 1). e) This peptide was also not hydrolyzed by plasmin.

DISCUSSION

The tetrapeptide Ac-Phe-Arg-Arg-Val-NH$_2$ was shown to be a substrate for all the serine proteases used in this work, but plasmin. While trypsin hydrolyzed both arginyl bonds, tissue and plasma kallikreins cleaved only the Arg-Arg bond. This preference is due to the known secondary specificity of tissue[14] and plasma kallikreins[15] for hydrophobic residues at the position P$_2$. It is thus possible to use this peptide as a substrate to distinguish trypsin from plasmin and both enzymes from tissue and plasma kallikreins.

Table 1. Kinetic Parameters ($\pm$ sd) for the Hydrolysis of the Tetrapeptides by Kallikreins (30°C; pH 9.0 for the Urinary and pH 8.0 for the Plasma Enzymes)

SUB-STRATES		$\begin{array}{cccc} P_2 & P_1 & P_1' & P_2' \end{array}$ Ac-Phe-Arg-Arg-X*NH$_2$ (X = Val or Pro)			
KALLI-KREINS (a)	P$_2'$	K_m μM	V μmol.min^{-1}.mg^{-1}	k_{cat} sec^{-1}	k_{cat}/k_m sec^{-1}.mM^{-1}
HoUK	Val	4.3 ± 0.4	12 ± 0.6	5.3 ± 0.3	1225
	Pro	hardly hydrolyzed (b)			
RUK	Val	31 ± 3.0	27 ± 0.7	nd	
	Pro	28 ± 6.0	44 ± 4.0	nd	
HuPK	Val	255 ± 40	22 ± 2.0	33.0 ± 3.0	132
	Pro	626 ± 20	11 ± 0.1	1.7 ± 0.4	27

(a)HoUK = horse urinary; RUK = rat urinary; HuPK = human plasma.

(b)For [S] = 4 mM, V = 0.08 μmol.min^{-1}.mg^{-1} of protein.

Kinetic data showed that Ac-Phe-Arg-Arg-Val-NH$_2$ is a good substrate for horse urinary kallikrein; the k_{cat}/K_m value (Table 1) was similar to that found for horse HMW kininogen and 20-fold higher than that for D-Val-Leu-Arg-pNA.[16] This tetrapeptide and BAM 22P[1] are, up to now, the only good substrates described for the Arg-Arg bond cleavage by tissue kallikreins. Although we demonstrated seventeen years ago that horse urinary kallikrein was able to hydrolyze polyarginine,[17] the kinetics of this hydrolysis was not studied.

Porcine pancreatic kallikrein hardly hydrolyzes Ac-Phe-Arg-Arg-Pro-NH$_2$; this observation by Fiedler[3] was now extended to the well characterized kallikreins from horse[18] and human urine.[19] The striking difference between the susceptibility of Ac-Phe-Arg-Arg-Val-NH$_2$ and resistance of Ac-Phe-Arg-Arg-Pro-NH$_2$ to these three kallikreins demonstrates clearly the hindering effect of the P'_2 proline residue.

The observed hydrolysis of Ac-Phe-Arg-Arg-Pro-NH$_2$ by plasma kallikreins was expected since these enzymes cleave the Lys-ARg bond in kininogens. However, we have no explanation for the higher susceptibility of the Arg-Arg bond when Val is the residue in the position P'_2. The low k_{cat}/K_m values for both peptides may be due to the lack of a proline residue in the position P_3, whivch was shown to be important for the hydrolysis of peptidyl-arginine esters by human plasma kallikrein.[15]

Rat urinary kallikrein, unlike tissue but similarly to plasma kallikreins, hydrolyzed the peptide with Pro residue in the position P'_2. The K_m and V for both substrates were very similar. These data are consistent with the finding of Alhenc-Gelas et al.[20] that rat urine liberates bradykinin from kininogens of different animal species.

The above results indicate that the peptide Ac-Phe-Arg-Arg-Pro-NH$_2$ distinguises tissue kallikreins from bradykinin-releasing enzymes; plasmin does not hydrolyze it but, in addition, does not hydrolyze Ac-Phe-Arg-Arg-Pro-NH$_2$.

Concluding, tissue kallikreins are enzymes that cleave the Arg-Arg bond in Ac-Phe-Arg-Arg-Val-NH$_2$ but do not, in Ac-Phe-Arg-Arg-Pro-NH$_2$.

ACKNOWLEDGEMENTS

We wish to acknowledge the very helpful discussions with Dr. J. L. Prado in the preparation of this manuscript. Our thanks are also due to Dr. C. A. M. Sampaio for the human plasma kallikrein preparation and the aminoacid analyses, Dr. R. C. R. STella for the rat and human urinary kallikreins and M. Kouyoumdjian for the rat plasma kallikrein preparation. Research supported by FINEP (B76/80/002/00/000). E. S. Prado, L. Juliano and M. Araújo-Viel have a Research Fellowship from CNPq. Travel grant from CNPq (E. S. Prado) is also acknowledged.

REFERENCES

1. E. S. Prado, L. Prado de Carvalho, M. S. Araújo-Viel, N. Ling, and J. Rossier, A Met-enkephalin-containing-peptide, BAM 22P, as a novel substrate for glandular kallikreins, Biochem. Biophys. Res. Commun. 112:366-371 (1983).
2. I. Schechter and A. Berger, On the size of the active site in proteases 1: Papain: specific inhibitor of papain, Biochem. Biophys. Res. Commun., 27:157-162 (1967).

3. F. Fiedler, Enzymology of porcine tissue kallikreins, <u>Adv. Exp. Med. Biol.</u>, 156A:261-274 (1983).

4. Z. Chen and W. Bode, Refined 2.5 A x-ray crystal structure of the complex formed by porcine kallikrein A and the bovine pancreatic trypsin inhibitor, <u>J. Mol. Biol.</u>, 164:283-311 (1983).

5. E. P. Giusti, C. A. M. Sampaio, and E. S. Prado, Purification of horse urinary kallikrein by affinity chromatography, <u>Agents & Actions</u>, 8:164 (1978).

6. R. Geiger, U. Stuckstedte, and H. Fritz, Isolation and characterization of human urinary kallikrein, <u>Hoppe-Seyler's Z. Physiol. Chem.</u>, 361: 1003-1016 (1980).

7. M. L. Oliva, D. Grisolia, M. U. Sampaio, and C. A. M. Sampaio, Properties of highly purified human plasma kallikrein, <u>Agents & Actions</u>, 9:52-57 (1982).

8. M. Kouyoumdjian, D. R. Borges, J. A. Guimarães, C. A. M. Sampaio, and J. L., Prado, Manuscript in preparation.

9. J. Chao and H. S. Margolius, Isoenzymes of rat urinary kallikrein, <u>Biochem. Pharmacol.</u>, 28:2071-2079 (1979).

10. R. C. R. Stella, To be published.

11. C. A. M. Sampaio, M. U. Sampaio, and E. S. Prado, Active-site titration of horse urinary kallikrein, <u>Hoppe-Seyler's Z. Physiol. Chem.</u>, 365: 297-302 (1984).

12. C. A. M. Sampaio, S. C. Wong, and E. Shaw, Human plasma kallikrein. Purification and preliminary characterization, <u>Arch. Biochem. Biophys.</u>, 165:133-139 (1974).

13. G. N. Wilkinson, Statistical estimations in enzyme kinetics, <u>Biochim. J.</u>, 80:324-332 (1961).

14. F. Fiedler, Substrate specificity of porcine pancreatic kallikrein, <u>Adv. Exp. Med. Biol.</u>, 120A:261-271 (1979).

15. P. R. Levison and G. Tomalin, The kinetics of hydrolysis of some extended N-aminoacyl-L-arginine methyl esters by human plasma kallikrein, <u>Biochem. J.</u>, 203:149-153 (1982).

16. E. S. Prado, C. A. M. Sampaio, M. S. Araújo-Viel, and R. C. R. Stella, Characterization of horse urinary kallikrein, <u>Agents & Actions</u>, 9:162-166 (1982).

17. E. S. Prado, R. C. R. Stella, M. J. Roncada, and J. L. Prado, Action of horse urinary kallikrein on arginine and lysine-peptides, <u>in</u>: "International Symposium on Vaso-Active Polypeptides; Bradykinin and Related Kinins," M. Rocha e Silva and H. A. Rothschild, eds., EDART, São Paulo (1967).

18. E. S. Prado, M. E. Webster, and J. L. Prado, Kallidin (lysyl-bradykinin) the kinin formed from horse plasma by horse urinary kallikrein, <u>Biochem. Pharmacol.</u>, 20:2009-2015 (1971).

19. J. V. Pierce and M. E. Webster, Human plasma kallikdins. Isolation and chemical studies, <u>Biochem. Biophys. Res. Commun.</u>, 5:353-357 (1961).

20. F. Alhenc-Gelas, J. Marchetti, J. Allegrini, P. Corvol, and J. Menard, Measurement of urinary kallikrein activity. Species differences in kinin production, <u>Biochem. Biophys. Acta.</u>, 677:477-488 (1981).

RELEASE OF KALLIKREIN AND TONIN FROM THE RAT SUBMANDIBULAR GLAND

Subir R. Maitra, Sara F. Rabito and Oscar A. Carretero

Hypertension Research Division, Henry Ford Hospital
2799 W. Grand Blvd., Detroit, MI 48202

ABSTRACT

The interaction of neurotransmitters and hormones with specific receptors on the plasma membranes of cells results in enzyme secretion from exocrine glands. However, the effects of agonists on the release of kallikrein and tonin from the rat submandibular gland have not yet been evaluated systematically. The purpose of the present study was to investigate the effects of norepinephrine, isoproterenol, methacholine, and cholecystokinin on the simultaneous release of kallikrein and tonin from the rat submandibular gland. Submandibular gland slices were incubated in vitro at 37° C in a modified Krebs-Ringer medium containing 0.2% each of glucose and bovine serum albumin and bubbled with a gas mixture of 95% O_2 and 5% CO_2. Glandular kallikrein and tonin secreted into the incubation medium were determined by specific radioimmunoassays. Norepinephrine at 10^{-5}M concentration increased kallikrein secretion from a control value of 7.7 ± 1.5 to 114.7 ± 26.9 ng/min/mg tissues ($p<.01$), and at 10^{-4}M concentration kallikrein secretion increased to 265.9 ± 58.3 ng/min/mg tissue ($p<.01$). Similarly, norepinephrine at 10^{-5}M enhanced the release of tonin from a basal rate of 4.4 ± 0.6 to 57 ± 14.4 ng/min/mg tissue ($p<.05$), and at 10^{-4}M the rate increased to 91.3 ± 20.0 ng/min/mg tissue ($p<.01$). In contrast, isoproterenol, methacholine, and cholecystokinin did not increase the secretion of kallikrein or tonin. We conclude that the secretion of kallikrein and tonin from rat submandibular glands upon sympathetic stimulation is mediated through stimulation of α-adrenoceptors only.

INTRODUCTION

Activation of α- and β-adrenergic and cholinergic receptors initiates the process of exocrine secretion in the salivary glands. Kallikrein and tonin are serine proteases located in granules in the convoluted granular tubules of the rat submandibular gland.[1,2,3] The secretion of these two proteases appears to be regulated by different receptors: kallikrein is secreted after stimulation of the α receptor[4,5,6], while tonin is released upon stimulation of the β receptor.[7,8,9,10] However, this discrepancy recently has been challenged by Izumi's study showing that the secretion of kallikrein-like esterase and tonin from the rat submandibular gland is mediated only by stimulation of α-receptors.[11]

In addition to studies on the role of the autonomic nervous system on kallikrein and tonin release, attempts have been made to determine how humoral factors participate in the regulation of salivary secretion. Mann et al.[12] examined the effect of cholecystokinin and pentagastrin on parotid kallikrein secretion in humans and found that cholecystokinin increased kallikrein secretion into saliva, but pentagastrin did not.

To obtain more information on the mechanisms involved in the secretion of kallikrein and tonin from the submandibular gland, we measured the release of these two proteases after stimulation with norepinephrine, isoproterenol, methacholine or cholecystokinin-octapeptide.

METHODS

Male Sprague-Dawley rats, weighing 250-300 g and fasted for 16 hours (with water ad libitum), were anesthetized with sodium pentobarbital (5 mg/100 g body weight, i.p.). Under anesthesia, both submandibular glands were rapidly removed and chilled over a Petri dish containing ice. After each gland was cut in half, three slices, each about 0.5 mm thick, were prepared from each portion with a Stadie Riggs microtome.

The resulting 12 slices were placed in stoppered flasks (two slices per flash) containing 5 ml of incubation medium. The incubation medium was composed of 125 mM NaCl, 4 mM KCl, 19 mM $NaHCO_3$, 2.6 mM $CaCl_2$, 1.2 mM NaH_2PO_4, 0.2 mM $MgSO_4$ and 0.2 g/100 ml each of glucose and bovine serum albumin. After five minutes of preincubation, the slices were transferred to separate flasks that contained fresh medium and were covered with aluminum foil. The slices were incubated for 30 minutes at 37°C in an atmosphere saturated with 95% O_2-5% CO_2. At 10, 20, and 30 minutes 0.5 ml samples of incubation medium were withdrawn for immunoreactive glandular kallikrein and tonin determinations. To study the dose-response curve for norepinephrine, isoproterenol, methacholine, and cholecystokinin, the drugs or vehicle were added to the incubation medium at 20 minutes, immediately after the withdrawal of the second control sample. Kallikrein and tonin secretion rates were calculated as the increment in the total amount of kallikrein or tonin during the 20- to 30-minute interval. During the experiments with norepinephrine and isoproterenol, Na-ascorbate 10^{-5}M was added to the incubation medium. At the end of the experiment the slices were removed and weighed.

The experiments were carried out in dim light, and the solutions were prepared in containers covered with aluminum foil to protect them. All solutions were freshly prepared, and the agents were used at concentrations as indicated below. Norepinephrine, isoproterenol, methacholine, and Na-ascorbate were purchased from Sigma Chemical. Cholecystokinin-octapeptide was obtained from E. R. Squibb & Sons, Inc. and bovine serum albumin from Miles Laboratories. All other reagents used were the highest grade commercially available.

The concentration of immunoreactive glandular kallikrein and tonin in the incubation medium were measured by radioimmunoassay as previously described.[13,14] Kallikrein and tonin secretion rates are expressed in ng/min/mg tissue.

The results are expressed as mean ± S.E. The Bonferroni test was used to assess the significance of the difference between means. A p value of less than 0.05 was considered statistically significant.

RESULTS

Table 1 contains the secretion rates for kallikrein after the four agonists were added in concentrations from 10^{-9}M to 10^{-3}M. Table 2 contains the secretion rates for tonin.

The rate of basal kallikrein secretion from rat submandibular gland slices was 7.7 ± 1.5 ng/min/mg tissue while tonin was released at the basal rate of 4.4 ± 0.6 ng/min/mg tissue. Adding norepinephrine to the incubation medium produced a dose-related increase in kallikrein release. Norepinephrine (10^{-5}M) increased the kallikrein secretion from a control value of 7.7 ± 1.5 to 114.7 ± 26.9 ng/min/mg tissue (p<.01), and at 10^{-4}M it increased the kallikrein secretion from the control value of 265.9 ± 58.3 ng/min/mg tissue (<0.01). Similarly, norepinephrine at 10^{-5}M significantly increased tonin release from the control value of 4.4 ± 0.6 to 57.4 ± 14.4 ng/min/mg tissue (p<.05). At 10^{-4}M concentration norepinephrine further enhanced the release of tonin to 91.3 ± 20.0 ng/min/mg tissue (p<.01).

Isoproterenol in the dose range of 10^{-11}M to 10^{-3}M did not significantly change the rate of either kallikrein or tonin secretion. Similarly, methacholine in doses of 10^{-6}M to 10^{-3}M and cholecystokinin at 10^{-9}M to 10^{-6}M had no effect on basal kallikrein or tonin secretion.

DISCUSSION

The present work studied the release of kallikrein and tonin from rat submandibular gland slices in vitro. Since Hokin et al.[15] first showed that exportable enzyme release could be induced in gland tissue incubated in vitro, the secretion of enzymes has been studied in many tissues by employing this system. In our study basal kallikrein release from submandibular gland slices was quite steady and reproducible, indicating the viability of the preparation. Moreover, since it has been reported that renin secretion from kidney cortex slices and tonin secretion from submandibular gland slices is temperature dependent,[16,9] the submandibular glands we used were rapidly removed and chilled, and the slices were prepared in the cold to avoid excess loss of kallikrein.

Sympathetic stimulation effects kallikrein release from the rat submandibular gland. Alpha-adrenergic stimulation has been shown to be 40 and 1500 fold more effective in releasing kallikrein into saliva than β-adrenergic and parasympathomimetic stimulation, respectively.[4] Previously our laboratory demonstrated that sympathetic nervous stimulation of the rat submandibular gland increases the release of immunoreactive kallikrein into the circulation through the stimulation of α_1-adrenoceptors.[5,6] This finding was confirmed by another study in which the infusion of norepinephrine increased kallikrein release from the perfused rat submandibular gland into the perfusate.[17] Studies with guinea pig submandibular gland slices have also suggested that norepinephrine induced kallikrein secretion.[18] In our present in vitro study, using a radioimmunoassay for the determination of immunoreactive glandular kallikrein, we have shown that norepinephrine significantly increased kallikrein secretion from the submandibular gland in a dose-related manner (Table 1).

By contrast, adding isoproterenol or methacholine to the incubation medium did not produce any significant change in kallikrein release. Others found that infusing isoproterenol into the rat submandibular gland increased kallikrein release into the venous effluent of the gland,[17] while studies with guinea pig submandibular gland slices indicated that acetylcholine induced release of kallikrein.[18] Although the reasons for the discrepancy between these two studies and our present results are not clear, both of these studies measured esterase activity to indicate kallikrein concentration. Since the submandibular gland is known to contain esterases other than kallikrein,[19] their results may be based on an erroneous measurement.

Mann et al.[12] reported that cholecystokinin stimulates the secretion of kallikrein from the human parotid gland. However, our in vitro study suggests that cholecystokinin, a gut hormone, has no effect on the secretion of kallikrein from the rat submandibular gland. Since the rat submandibular gland is developmentally quite distinct from the parotid gland,[20,21] we can expect that their response to neurotransmitter and/or hormones will be different.

In summary, our study indicates that norepinephrine induced the secretion of both kallikrein and tonin from the rat submandibular gland by stimulation of α-adrenoceptors only, since the rate of secretion of these two proteases did not change after stimulation of ∞-adrenoceptors with isoproterenol. These results confirm Izumi's recent work[11] showing that kallikrein-like esterase and tonin are released from dispersed submandibular gland cells only through stimulation of α-receptors. This author was concerned that the lack of response to other secretagogues could be due to perturbation of the receptor by proteolytic digestion during the preparation of the cell suspension. However, in our preparation of submandibular gland slices, since proteolytic digestion did not take place, the lack of secretory response to isoproterenol and methacholine cannot be attributed to receptor damage.

ACKNOWLEDGEMENTS

This work was supported in part by NIH grant HL 28982. Send reprint requests to Dr. Sara F. Rabito.

Table 1. Kallikrein Secretion (ng/min/mg tissue)

	Agonist Concentration (M)								
	0	10^{-11}	10^{-9}	10^{-8}	10^{-7}	10^{-6}	10^{-5}	10^{-4}	10^{-3}
Norepinephrine (n=5)	7.7 ± 1.5	-	-	7.9 ± 2.1	9.1 ± 1.9	11.6 ± 1.7	114.7** ± 26.9	265.9** ± 58.3	-
Isoproterenol (n=5)	8.8 ± 2.8	13.9 ± 2.7	16.1 ± 5.4	-	12.7 ± 2.6		8.3 ± 2.0	-	23.5 ± 10.8
Methacholine (n=4)	10.6 ± 3.3	-	-	-	-	12.5 ± 2.6	13.1 ± 4.7	34.2 ± 6.2	36.6 ± 15.4
Cholecystokinin (n=4)	8.33 ± 3.1	-	7.7 ± 2.4	5.9 ± 0.8	6.5 ± 2.3	7.4 ± 1.2	-	-	-

** $p < .01$

Table 2. Tonin Secretion (ng/min/mg tissue)

	Agonist Concentration (M)								
	0	10^{-11}	10^{-9}	10^{-8}	10^{-7}	10^{-6}	10^{-5}	10^{-4}	10^{-3}
Norepinephrine (n=5)	4.4 ± 0.6	-	-	6.5 ± 1.5	5.1 ± 1.70	5.7 ± 0.7	57.4* ± 16.61	91.3** ± 20.0	-
Isoproterenol (n=4)	7.2 ± 3.0	12.7 ± 7.0	9.4 ± 3.1	-	10.9 ± 3.5	-	12.2 ± 6.9	-	20.9 ± 9.2
Methacholine (n=4)	7.9 ± 3.7	-		-	-	17.1 ± 4.7	19.0 ± 8.6	17.6 ± 10.4	14.6 ± 6.8
Cholecystokinin (n=4)	3.05 ± 1.3	-	8.2 ± 2.1	4.4 ± 2.7	6.5 ± 2.8	10.0 ± 4.1	-	-	-

* $p < .05$;   ** $p < .01$

REFERENCES

1. E. G. Erdos, L. L. Tague, and I. Miwa, Kallikrein in granules of the submaxillary gland, Biochem. Pharmac., 17, 667 674, (1968).
2. T. B. Orstavik, P. Brandtsaeg, K. Nustad, and K. M. Halvorsen, Cellular localization of kallikreins in rat submandibular and sublingual glands, Acta. Histochem., 54, 183-192, (1975).
3. J. A. V. Simson, S. S. Spicer, J. Chao, L. Grim, and H. S. Margolius, Kallikrein localization in rodent salivary glands and kidney with the immunoglobulin-enzyme bridge technique, J. Histochem. Cytochem., 27, 1567-1576, (1979).
4. T. B. Orstavik and K. M. Gautvik, Regulation of salivary kallikrein secretion in the rat submandibular gland, Acta. Physiol. Scand., 100, 33-44, (1977).
5. S. F. Rabito, A. G. Scicli, T. B. Orstavik, O. A. Garretero, Role of the autonomic nervous system in the release of rat submandibular gland kallikrein and tonin into the circulation, Fed. Proc., 41, 1472, (1982).
6. S. F. Rabito, T. B. Orstavik, A. G. Scicli, A. Schork, and O. A. Carretero, Role of autonomic nervous system in the release of rat submandibular gland kallikrein into the circulation, Circ. Res., 52, 635-641, (1983).
7. R. Garcia, R. Boucher, and J. Genest, Tonin activity in rat saliva: Effect of sympathomimetic and parasympathomimetic drugs, Can. J. Physiol. Pharmac., 54, 443-445, (1976).
8. R. Garcia, K. Kondo, B. Scholkens, R. Boucher, and J. Genest, Effect in vivo of β-adrenergic stimulation, angiotensin II, dibutyryl cyclic AMP, and theophyline on tonin concentration in rat saliva and submaxillary gland, Can. J. Physiol. Pharmac., 55, 983-989, (1977).
9. K. Kondo, Release of tonin by rat submandibular gland slices in vitro, Jap. Circul. J., 43, 837-842, (1979).
10. J. Gutkowska, M. Lis, M. Cantin, and J. Genest, Solid-phase radio-immunoassay of tonin in extracts of submandibular glands of rats treated chronically with isoproterenol, Proc. Soc. Exp. Biol. Med., 170, 165-171, (1982).
11. H. Izumi, Release of kallikrein-like esterase and tonin from dispersed cells of the rat submandibular gland, Br. J. Pharmac., 82, 175-182, (1984).
12. K. Mann, J. Richter, and H. J. Karl, The influence of cholecystokinin and gastrin on human parotid kallikrein secretion, International Conference on Kallikreins - Kinins - Kininogens - Kininases, Abstract E.P.L., Munich (1981).
13. S. F. Rabito, A. G. Scicli, V. Kher, and O. A. Carretero, Immuno-reactive glandular kallikrein in rat plasma: A radioimmunoassay for its determination, Am. J. Physiol., 242, H602-H610, (1982).
14. S. Seto, S. F. Rabito, A. G. Scicli, and O. A. Carretero, Lack of evidence for the participation of tonin in the pathogenesis of one-kidney, one-clip renovascular hypertension, Circ. Res., 55, 580-584, (1984).
15. L. E. Hokin and A. L. Sherwin, Protein secretion and phosphate turnover in the phospholipids in salivary glands in vitro, J. Physiol. (Lond), 135, 18-29, (1957).
16. K. Yamamoto, H. Tanaka, K. Horiuchi, and J. Ueda, Release of renin from dog kidney cortex slices in vitro, Jap. J. Pharmc., 17, 685-686, (1967).

17. R. Garcia, G. Thibault, J. Gutkowska, and J. Genest, Release of tonin and of kallikrein by perfused rat submaxillary gland, Am. J. Physiol., 244, R228-R234, (1983).

18. K. D. Bhoola, P. F. Heap, and M. J. C. Lemon, The regulation of kallikrein secretion from isolated submandibular gland slices by neurotransmitters, cyclic neuleotides and calcium, Adv. Expt. Med. Biol., 70, 59-64, (1976).

19. M. Khullar, A. G. Scicli, O. A. Carretero, Purification and characterization of a new serine protease from rat submandibular gland, Fed. Proc., 43, 2067, (1984).

20. F. Jacoby and C. R. Leeson, The postnatal development of the rat submaxillary gland, J. Anat., 93, 201-216, (1959).

21. R. S. Redman and L. M. Sreebny, Morphologic and biochemical observations on the development of the rat parotid gland, Dev. Biol., 25, 248-279, (1979).

EFFECT OF SODIUM RESTRICTION AND CORTICOSTEROIDS ON GLANDULAR KALLIKREIN

IN PLASMA AND IN THE SUBMANDIBULAR GLAND

Shinji Seto, Sara F. Rabito, Subir R. Maitra, Jonathan N. Wu, and Oscar A. Carretero

Hypertension Research Division, Henry Ford Hospital, 2799 W. Grand Blvd., Detroit, MI 48202

SUMMARY

We investigated whether sodium restriction or mineralocorticoid in-fluence the release of submandibulary kallikrein into the blood and/or the concentration of kallikrein in glandular tissue. For this we measured sub-mandibular gland blood flow, arterial and submandibular gland venous kalli-krein, and kallikrein in glandular homogenates of male Sprague-Dawley rats after one week of either low sodium or deoxycorticosterone acetate (DOCA) treatment. We also studied the effect of dexamethasone on the concentration of kallikrein in gland tissue and peripheral plasma. Kallikrein in plasma and in homogenates was measured by radioimmunoassay. Blood flow was deter-mined by timed collections of venous outflow. Kallikrein release was calcu-lated as the arteriovenous difference in kallikrein times the rate of subman-dibular gland plasma flow. The concentration of kallikrein in arterial plasma, the basal submandibular kallikrein release into blood, and the concentration of kallikrein in submandibular gland tissue were all higher during low sodium than during normal sodium intake (20.1 ± 3.6 ng/ml vs 10.7 ± 0.5, $p < 0.05$; 0.40 ± 0.09 ng/min/100 g bw vs 0.18 ± 0.02, $p < 0.05$, and 81.6 ± 5.5 µg/mg protein vs 65.1 ± 4.0, $p < 0.05$, respectively). In contrast, DOCA treatment did not affect the concentration of kallikrein in arterial plasma, the basal release of kallikrein from the submandibular gland into blood, or the concentration of kallikrein in the gland. Dexa-methasone in doses that did not affect the normal growth of the animals had no significant effect on the concentration of kallikrein either in sub-mandibular gland tissue or in peripheral plasma. We concluded that sodium restriction increases the kallikrein content of the submandibular gland and its release into blood, but this effect is probably not caused by in-creases in mineralocorticoid levels. The increased release of submandibular gland kallikrein into blood may explain, in part, the increased plasma levels of kallikrein observed during sodium restriction.

INTRODUCTION

Glandular kallikreins are serine proteases which release the potent vasodilator decapeptide lysyl-bradykinin (kallidin) from kininogens. Glan-dular kallikreins are present in salivary and sweat glands, the digestive tract, pancreas, kidney, and in the exocrine secretion of these organs.[1] In addition, previous studies in our laboratory and in others have demonstrated that immunoreactive glandular kallikrein is also present in rat and human plasma.[2-5]

While the sources of circulating glandular kallikrein are not fully delineated, we have found that submandibular gland venous blood has a higher concentration of kallikrein than arterial blood and that removal of the submandibular glands significantly decreases the concentration of kallikrein in peripheral blood.[6] These findings indicate that part of the glandular kallikrein present in plasma derives from the submandibular gland. Moreover, we also observed that the release of glandular kallikrein into the vascular compartment increases about 60 times after sympathetic stimulation of the submandibular gland.[7]

Since glandular kallikrein may participate in the regulation of local blood flow in the organs where it is synthetized,[8-12] it is important to understand the factors that regulate the endocrine release of glandular kallikrein from the submandibular gland. In this study, we investigated the secretion rate from, and the content of glandular kallikrein in the rat submandibular gland in two different sets of experimental conditions: low sodium intake and administration of deoxycorticosterone acetate (DOCA). In addition, we studied the effect of dexamethasone treatment on the concentration of kallikrein in the gland and in peripheral plasma. We chose these experimental conditions because low sodium intake and mineralocorticoid treatment are known to increase the excretion of kallikrein into urine and saliva.[13,14] Furthermore, sodium restriction increases the concentration of kallikrein in plasma,[15] and glucocorticoids affect the excretion rate of kallikrein into urine and the concentration of kallikrein in renal and submandibular gland tissue.[16-20]

MATERIAL AND METHODS

Effects of Sodium Restriction and Deoxycorticosterone Acetate

We used male, Sprague-Dawley rats weighing 350-450 g in this study. Food was withheld for 24 hours before the experiment, but the naimals were allowed to drink water ad libitum. On the day of the experiment, the rats were anesthetized with pentobarbital (50 mg/kg, ip) and tracheotomized. Polyethylene catheters (PE-50) were placed in both femoral arteries and veins. The arterial catheters were used to sample arterial blood and to record mean arterial blood pressure continuously. The left venous catheter was used for blood replacement and the right venous catheter to return the uncollected submandiublar venous outflow to the rat. Then, the right submandibular gland was exposed, and the naimal was heparinized (1,000 U/kg). All tributaries joining the right submandibular gland vein were tied off, and a catheter (PE-60) was positioned to collect only submandibular gland venous blood. Timed collections of submandibular gland venous outflow (approximately 500 µl) were made into preweighed plastic tubes to measure blood flow and immunoreactive glandular kallikrein concentration. An equivalent volume of blood obtained 24 hours after nephrectomy from a donor rat was given to the rat after each blood withdrawal. Mean arterial blood pressure was recorded on a Gould Brush 440 recorder.

At the end of the experiment, the contralateral gland was removed, cleaned of adhering connective tissue, and kept at -20°C until homogenized. Four experimental groups were studied.

Low sodium group: 12 rats were fed a sodium-deficient diet (ICN Nutritional Biochemicals, Cleveland, OH), containing 0.05% of sodium for seven days. Control group: 10 rats received the same diet as the previous group for seven days, but with sodium added at the concentration of 0.48%. Both groups were allowed to drink tap water ad libitum.

DOCA group: 6 rats had one strip of DOCA-silicone rubber (100 mg of DOCA/kg bw) implanted subcutaneously 7 days before the experiment. Control group: 9 rats had one strip of silicone rubber, without DOCA, implanted 7 days before the study. Both groups were fed the same normal rat chow (Rodent Laboratory Chow #5001, Ralston Purina Co) and were allowed to drink tap water ad libitum. The implants of DOCA (Sigma) were prepared by mixing DOCA with silicone rubber (Dow Corning 3110 RTV) in a ratio of one part of DOCA to two parts of silicone.[21] The implants were approximately 1 mm thick.

Effect of Dexamethasone

We used male Sprague-Dawley rats, weighing 250-300 g, in this experiment. Six groups were used.

Group 1: 6 normal rats received daily subcutaneous injections of 0.1 ml of 0.9% sodium chloride. Group 2: 6 normal rats received daily subcutaneous injections of 100 µg/kg of dexamethasone (DEX). Group 3: 5 normal rats were injected subcutaneously with 1,000 µg/kg of DEX daily. Group 4: 7 adrenalectomized (ADX) rats received daily subcutaneous injections of 0.1 ml of 0.9% sodium chloride. Group 5: 7 ADX rats were injected subcutaneously with 10 µg/kg of DEX daily. Group 6: 7 ADX rats received daily injections of 100 µg/kg of DEX.

Adrenalectomy had been performed bilaterally through lumbar incisions two weeks before the experiment. All animals were fed normal rat chow. Normal rats received tap water ad libitum while adrenalectomized animals were maintained on 0.9% sodium chloride as drinking fluid. Dexamethasone sodium phosphate (Hexadrol; Organon Inc, NJ) was dissolved in 0.9% sodium chloride.

Before and at the end of the first and second week of treatment, the animals were weighed, and blood (500-600 µl) was withdrawn by cardiopuncture into heparinized syringes. Plasma was separated by centrifugation and kept at -20°C until used. At the end of the experiment, both submandibular glands were removed and kept at -20°C until homogenized. All surgical procedures and blood withdrawal were performe dunder ether anesthesia.

Analytical Procedures

The submandibular glands were minced and homogenized for 40 seconds in 6 ml of buffer solution (0.05 M Tris-HCl, pH 8.0 containing 0.05% Triton X-100) at 4°C with a Polytron (Brinkmann Homogenizer PT10/35, Brinkmann Instruments Co., Westbury, NY). Homogenates were centrifuged at 2,000 g for 60 minutes. Supernatants were saved and stored at -20°C until assayed for glandular kallikrein and protein content.

Immunoreactive glandular kallikrein in plasma and gland homogenates was determined by radioimmunoassay as described[6] and expressed in ng/ml of plasma and µg/mg of protein. Submandibular gland blood flow was estimated gravimetrically and transformed into volume units by using 1.054 as specific gravity for blood.[22] Plasma flow was calculated from values of blood flow and hematocrit. The glandular kallikrein secretion rate was calculated according to the following equation: KSR = (V-A) x PF, where KSR is the kallikrein secretion rate, V is the concentration of immunoreactive glandular kallikrein in submandibular gland vein plasma, A is the concentration of immunoreactive glandular kallikrein in arterial plasma, and PF is the submandibular gland plasma flow. Protein concentration in gland homogenates was determined by the Lowry's method[23] standardized against bovine serum albumin.

All results are expressed as mean ± SEM. Statistical evaluations were performed by Student's paired and unpaired t-tests, analysis of variance and the Bonferroni's test. A p value of less than 0.05 was considered statistically significant.

RESULTS

As shown in Fig. 1, low sodium intake for one week significantly increased the concentration of glandular kallikrein in peripheral plasma from 10.7 ± 0.5 ng/ml in the normal sodium group to 20 ± 3.6 ng/ml in the low sodium group ($p < 0.03$). Sodium restriction increased the kallikrein secretion rate by 120% from 0.18 ± 0.02 ng/min/100 g bw in the group with a normal sodium intake to 0.40 ± 0.09 ng/min/100 g bw in the low sodium group ($p < 0.05$). This increase in kallikrein release was associated with an increase in the concentration of kallikrein in submandibular gland tissue from 65.1 ± 4.0 µg/mg of protein in the normal sodium group to 81.6 ± 5.5 µg/mg protein in the low sodium group ($p < 0.05$).

To determine whether the effects of low sodium intake are mediated through increases in mineralocorticoid levels, we studied the effect of DOCA on submandibular gland kallikrein in a second protocol. DOCA in a dose of 100 mg/kg in one week had no significant effect on the concentration of kallikrein in peripheral plasma (15.0 ± 1.0 vs 13.0 ± 1.6 ng/ml in

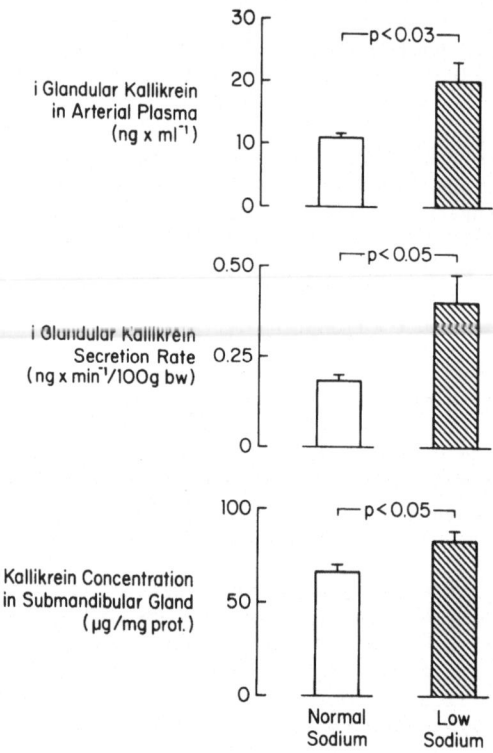

Fig. 1.   Effect of sodium restriction for one week on the concentration of glandular kallikrein in arterial plasma, the kallikrein secretion rate from the submandibular gland into blood, and the concentration of kallikrein in the gland.

controls), on the release of kallikrein into blood from the submandibular gland (0.25 ± 0.09 vs 0.22 ± 0.05 ng/min/100 g bw in controls), or on the concentration of kallikrein in submandibular gland tissue (93.6 ± 3.1 vs 86.9 ± 4.2 μg/mg protein in controls). The dose of DOCA used in this experiment (100 mg/kg bw) effectively increases urinary kallikrein excretion.[15]

In normal rats, dexamethasone in the dose of 1000 μg/kg/day significantly increased the concentration of kallikrein in peripheral plasma (Table 1). This effect was associated with a reduction in the concentration of kallikrein in submandibular gland tissue (Table 2) and a marked decrease in body weight (Table 3). No changes in the concentration of kallikrein in plasma and in the submandibular gland were observed when lower doses of dexamethasone were used.

DISCUSSION

The mechanisms that regulate the synthesis and release of kallikrein in the submandibular gland are not completely understood. Numerous observations support the concept that the secretion of proteins from the salivary glands is predominantly under neural control, and attempts have also been made to determine whether other humoral factors participate in the regulation of salivary secretion. When Mann, et al.[24] examined the role of cholecystokinin and pentagastrin on parotid kallikrein secretion in humans, they found that cholecystokinin increased both kallikrein and amylase release while pentagastrin stimulated amylase secretion only. Horwitz, et al.[14] reported that during sodium restriction human parotid saliva had a higher concentration of kallikrein in parotid saliva, they concluded that the increase in salivary kallikrein observed during sodium restriction was mediated by increased levels of mineralocorticoids. This observation agrees with previous reports showing that aldosterone is involved in the regulation of the ionic composition of parotid saliva in the rat and that the striated ducts, where kallikrein is located, are the site of action of aldosterone in the parotid gland.[25] In the submandibular gland, most of the kallikrein is located within granules in the convoluted granular tubules.[26-28]

We evaluated the synthesis of submandibular gland kallikrein during sodium restriction and DOCA treatment by measuring the concentration of

Table 1. Effect of Dexamethasone on Glandular Kallikrein in Plasma

	Glandular Kallikrein in Plasma (ng/ml)		
	Before	1 Week	2 Weeks
NL + SALINE	18.6 ± 0.7	20.6 ± 0.9	19.7 ± 0.8
NL + DEX 100 μg/kg/day	19.5 ± 0.4	19.9 ± 1.1	19.5 ± 0.9
NL + DEX 1000 μg/kg/day	18.0 ± 0.6	22.6 ± 1.0**	23.1 ± 1.1**
ADX + SALINE	19.9 ± 1.1	20.1 ± 0.9	20.9 ± 1.4
ADX + DEX 10 μg/kg/day	20.3 ° 1.4	18.3 ± 0.8	17.4 ± 0.5
ADX + DEX 100 μg/kg/day	18.2 ± 1.1	20.4 ± 1.1	20.4 ± 1.3

** $p < 0.01$ when compared to before treatment.
NL = normal, ADX = adrenalectomized, DEX = dexamethasone.

Table 2. Effect of Dexamethasone on Submandibular Gland Kallikrein

	Submandibular Gland Kallikrein µg/mg protein
NL + SALINE	66.8 ± 8.2
NL + DEX 100 µg/kg/day	47.6 ± 7.0
NL + DEX 1000 µg/kg/day	37.3 ± 1.7**
ADX + SALINE (n = 7)	63.8 ± 9.4
ADX + DEX 10 µg/kg/day (n = 7)	51.8 ± 3.7
ADX + DEX 100 µg/kg/day (n = 7)	67.7 ± 7.1

** $p < 0.01$ when compared to control group
NL = normal, ADX = adrenalectomized, DEX = dexamethasone

kallikrein in the gland and the release of kallikrein into the circulation. With this procedure, we demonstrated that sodium restriction for one week increased the content of kallikrein in th gland as well as the release of kallikrein into the circulation. Sodium restriction also increased the concentration of kallikrein in peripheral arterial plasma. A similar effect of sodium restriction on glandular kallikrein in plasma has been reported.[29]

DOCA treatment for one week did not affect the concentration of kalli-krein in the gland, the basal release of kallikrein into the circulation or the concentration of kallikrein in arterial plasma. The increased output of kallikrein into the vascular compartment during sodium restriction is probably caused by adrenergic stimulation,[7] since low sodium intake can augment sympathetic activity.[30,31] The mechanism by which sodium restriction increased the synthesis of kallikrein may also involve activation of an adrenoceptor. Besides eliciting secretion, adrenergic stimulation can also enhance growth[32-34] and increase the level of protein synthesis in submandi-bular gland cells through stimulation of either α or β receptors.[35] In addition, β adrenergic stimulation might stimulate the synthesis of kalli-

Table 3. Effect of Dexamethasone on Body Weight of Male Sprague-Dawley Rats

	Body Weight (g)		
	Before	1 Week	2 Weeks
NL + SALINE	246 ± 3	294 ± 5	323 ± 7
NL + DEX 100 µg/kg/day	248 ± 5	252 ± 1**	266 ± 6**
NL + DEX 1000 µg/kg/day	257 ± 2	216 ± 7**	203 ± 3**
ADX + SALINE	290 ± 16	328 ± 20	340 ± 28
ADX + DEX 10 µg/kg/day	273 ± 12	295 ± 13	308 ± 12
ADX + DEX 100 µg/kg/day	268 ± 16	271 ± 13	277 ± 11**

** $p < 0.001$ when compared to control group
NL = normal, ADX = adrenalelctomized, DEX = dexamethasone

krein in the rat submandibular gland.[36] These effects of dietary sodium restriction on the synthesis of submandibular gland kallikrein have not been seen when more chronic changes in sodium intake were examined.[36]

Contrary to the report of Chao and Margolius[20] that the activity and content of kallikrein increased in the rat submandibular gland after the administration of cortisol, we did not observe changes in immunoreactive kallikrein after treatment with dexamethasone at a dose that did not affect the animals' normal growth. In addition, no significant changes in the concentration of kallikrein in the submandibular gland were observed after adrenalectomy. The effects of glucocorticoids in other kallikrein-producing tissues, such as the kidney, are also controversial.[16-20]

In summary, our data show that neither mineralo- nor glucocorticoids participate in the regulation of kallikrein synthesis in or its release from the rat submandibular gland. Sodium restriction for one week increased both kallikrein synthesis in this salivary gland and the release of kallikrein into the vascular compartment. These effects of sodium restriction on submandibular gland kallikrein are probably caused by adrenergic stimulation.

ACKNOWLEDGEMENT

This work was supported in part by NIH grant HL 28982. Send reprint request to Dr. Sara F. Rabito.

REFERENCES

1. K. Bhoola, M. Lemon, and R. Matthews, Kallikrein in exocrine glands, in: "Handbook of Experimental Pharmacology," E. G. Erdos, ed., Springer (1979).
2. S. F. Rabito, V. Amin, A. G. Scicli, and O. A. Carretero, Glandular kallikrein in plasma and urine: Evaluation of a direct RIA for its determination, in: "Kinins II: Biochemistry, Pathophysiology, and Clinical Aspects," S. Fujii, H. Moriya, and T. Suzuki, eds., Plenum Press, Vol. 120A (1979).
3. K. Nustad, K. Gautvik, and T. B. Orstavik, Radioimmunoassay of rat submandibular gland kallikrein and the detection of immunoreactive antigen in blood, in: "Kinins II: Biochemistry, Pathophysiology and Clinical Aspects," S. Fujii, H. Moriya, and T. Suzuki, eds., Plenum Press, Vol. 120A (1979).
4. S. F. Rabito, A. G. Scicli, and O. A. Carretero, Immunoreactive glandular kallikrein in plasma, in: "Enzymatic Release of Vasoactive Peptides," F. Gross and G. Vogel, eds., Raven Press (1980).
5. W. J. Lawton, D. Proud, M. E. Frech, J. V. Pierce, H. R. Keiser, and J. J. Pisano, Characterization and origin of immunoreactive glandular kallikrein in rat plasma, Biochem. Pharmacol., 30:1731-1737 (1981).
6. S. F. Rabito, A. G. Scicli, V. Kher, and O. A. Carretero, Immunoreactive glandular kallikrein in rat plasma: A radioimmunoassay for its determination, Am. J. Physiol., 242:H602-H610 (1982).
7. S. F. Rabito, T. B. Orstavik, A. G. Scicli, A. Shork, and O. A. Carretero, Role of the autonomic nervous system in the release of rat submandibular gland kallikrein into the circulation, Circ. Res., 52:635-641 (1983).
8. S. M. Hilton and G. P. Lewis, The relationship between activity, bradykinin formation and functional vasodilatation in the submandibular salivary gland, J. Physiol., (London), 134:471-483 (1956).

9. S. M. Hilton and M. Jones, The role of the plasma kinins in functional vasodilatation in the pancreas, J. Physiol., (London), 195:521-533 (1968).

10. K. Gautvik, Parasympathetic neuro-effector transmission and functional vasodilatation in the submandibular salivary gland of cats, Acta. Physiol. Scand., 79:204-215 (1970).

11. K. Gautvik, Studies on kinin formation in functional vasodilatation of the submandibular salivary gland in cats, Acta. Physiol. Scand., 79:174-187 (1970).

12. T. B. Orstavik, O. A. Carretero, and A. G. Scicli, Kallikrein-kinin system in regulation of submandibular gland blood flow, Am. J. Physiol., 242:H1010-H1014 (1982).

13. R. G. Geller, H. S. Margolius, J. J. Pisano, and H. R. Keiser, Effects of mineralocorticoids, altered sodium intake, and adrenalectomy on urinary kallikrein in rats, Clin. Res., 31:857-861 (1972).

14. D. Horwitz, D. Proud, W. J. Lawton, K. N. Yates, P. Highet, J. J. Pisano, and H. R. Keiser, Effects of restriction of sodium or administration of fludrocortisone on parotid salivary kallikrein in man, J. Lab. Clin. Med., 100:146-154 (1982).

15. S. F. Rabito, A. G. Scicli, and O. A. Carretero, Immunoreactive glandular kallikrein in plasma during alterations of urinary kallikrein excretion, Hypertension, 5:V153-V157 (1983).

16. J. Colina-Chourio, J. C. McGiff, and A. Nasjletti, Effects of cortico-steroids on urinary kallikrein excretion, Clin. Res., 22:596 (Abstract) (1974).

17. C. P. Vio, J. S. Roblero, and H. R. Croxatto, Dexamethasone, aldosterone and kallikrein release by isolated rat kidney, Clin. Sci., 61:241-243 (1981).

18. Y. Noda, K. Yamada, R. Igic, and E. G. Erdos, Regulation of rat urinary and renal kallikrein and prekallikrein by corticosteroids, Proc. Natl. Acad. Sci., 80:3059-3063 (1983).

19. J. M. Lopez, E. Arteaga, J. A. Rodriguez, and H. Croxatto, Increased excretion of kallikrein during dexamethasone administration in normal man on low and normal salt intake, Clin. Sci., 65:487-490 (1983).

20. J. Chao and H. S. Margolius, Differential effects of testosterone, thy-roxine, and cortisol on rat submandibular gland versus renal kalli-krein, Endocrinology, 113:2221-2225 (1983).

21. H. S. Ormsbee and C. F. Ryan, Production of hypertension with desoxycor-ticosterone acetate-impregnated silicone rubber implants, J. Pharma-ceut. Sci., 62:255 (1973).

22. P. L. Altman and D. S. Dittmer, Blood and other body fluids. Biological Handbooks, Bethesda, MD. Federation of American Societies for Experi-mental Biology.

23. O. H. Lowry, N. J. Rosenbrough, A. C. Farr, and R. J. Randall, Protein measurement with the Folin reagent, J. Biol. Chem., 193:265-275 (1951).

24. K. Mann, J. Richter, and H. J. Karl, The influence of cholecystokinin and gastrin on human parotid kallikrein secretion. International Conference on Kallikreins - Kinisn - Kininogens - Kininases, Abstract E.P.L., Munich (1981).

25. J. A. Mangos and N. R. McSherry, Micropuncture study of sodium and potassium excretion in rat parotid saliva: Role of aldosterone, Proc. Soc. Exptl. Biol. Med., 132:797-801 (1969).

26. E. G. Erdos, L. L. Tague, and I. Miwa, Kallikrein in granules of the submaxillary gland, Biochem. Pharmac., 17:667-674 (1968).

27. J. A. V. Simson, S. S. Spicer, J. Chao, L. Grim, and H. S. Margolius, Kallikrein localization in rodent salivary glands and kidney with the immunoglobulin-enzyme bridge technique, J. Histochem. Cytochem., 27:1567-1576 (1979).

28. T. B. Orstavik, P. Brandtzaeg, K. Nustad, and K. M. Halvorsen, Cellular localization of kallikreins in rat submandibular and sublingual glands, Acta. Histochem., 54:183-192 (1975).

29. S. Tanaka, J. Chao, and H. S. Margolius, A direct radioimmunoassay for immunoreactive glandular kallikrein in rat serum, Fed. Proc., 41:1473 (Abstract) (1982).

30. M. G. Nicholls, W. Kiowski, A. J. Zweifler, S. Julius, M. A. Schork, and J. Greenhouse, Plasma norepinephrine variations with dietary sodium intake, Hypertension, 2:29-32 (1980).

31. L. J. Kaufman and R. R. Vollmer, Low sodium diet augments plasma and tissue catecholamine levels in pithed rats, Clin. Exp.-Theory and Practice, A6:1543-1558 (1984).

32. W. Selye, R. Veilleux, and M. Cantin, Excessive stimulation of salivary gland growth by isoproterenol, Science, 133:44 (1961).

33. R. Baserga, T. Sasaki, and J. P. Whitlock, Isoproterenol stimulated DNA synthesis in rat salivary glands, in: "Biochemistry of Cell Division," R. Baserga, ed., Thomas (1969).

34. T. C. Muir and D. Templeton, The role of 3',5'-adenosine monophosphate (cyclic AMP) in the ability of sympathetic nerve stimulation to enhance growth and secretion in rat salivary glands in vivo, J. Physiol., 259:47-61 (1976).

35. R. Garcia, G. Thibault, J. Gutkowska, and J. Genest, Release of tonin and kallikrein by perfused rat submaxillary gland, Am. J. Physiol., 244:R228-R234 (1983).

36. D. H. Miller, J. Chao, and H. S. Margolius, Tissue kallikrein synthesis and its modification by testosterone or low dietary sodium, Biochem. J., 218:37-43 (1984).

KALLIKREIN AND KININS INDEPENDENTLY STIMULATE RENIN RELEASE FROM ISOLATED

RAT GLOMERULI

William H. Beierwaltes and Oscar A. Carretero

Division of Hypertension Research
Henry Ford Hospital
Detroit, Michigan

SUMMARY

We studied the interaction between kallikrein, kinins, and renin release in isolated rat renal glomeruli and their attendant arterioles. Purified hog kallikrein (170 mEU/ml) significantly stimulated renin release 86% (p <0.025) above control. Inactivation of kallikrein by PMSF or inhibition with aprotinin blocked kallikrein stimulation of renin release. Partially purified rat submandibular gland kallikrein (160 mEU/ml) also increased renin by 87% (p <0.025). Superfusion of glomeruli with bradykinin (10^{-5} M) significantly increased renin release by 108% (p <0.025), and lys-bradykinin (10^{-5} M) similarly increased renin by 155% (p <0.025). Neither of the kinin analogues, des-arg[9] bradykinin or tyr[8] bradykinin (at 10^{-5} M), were able to alter renin released from isolated glomeruli. The vasodilator acetylcholine (10^{-5} M) had no effect upon renin release from glomeruli. No kininogen could be detected in glomeruli. Kallikrein superfusion did not result in any measurable kinin generation. We could not detect inactive renin in superfusate or glomeruli after renin activation with either kallikrein or trypsin. These results suggest that kallikrein stimulates renin release independent of kininogenase activity and that this stimulation does not appear to be due to activation of inactive renin. Further, we find that kinins can directly stimulate renin release.

INTRODUCTION

The kallikrein-kinin system and the renin-angiotensin system may be functionally interrelated. Angiotensin-converting enzyme (kininase II) is a component of both systems,[1] and both prorenin and prekallikrein can be activated by Hageman factor.[2] It has been suggested that kallikrein is an endogenous activator of inactive renin.[3] It has also been proposed that kallikrein in vitro stimulates renin,[4,5] but this has also been and discounted.[6] Various studies have suggested that renin and kinins interact to modify renal resistance,[7,8] and bradykinin infusion has been shown to transiently increase renin secretion,[9] although bradykinin has not been shown to affect renin in vitro.[5]

We have used an in vitro preparation of rat isolated renal glomeruli and their attendant arterioles[10] as a model to study the intraction of kallikrein and kinin with renin release. Using this model, which is free of exogenous hemodynamic, neural and humoral influences, we found that both kallikrein and kinins may stimulate renin release and that the effect of kallikrein is independent of its kininogenase activity.

METHODS

We performed experiments on glomeruli harvested from the kidneys of male Sprague Dawley rats, using a passive sieving technique as previously described.[10,11] Superfusion studies were carried out using equal aliquots of glomeruli (40-50 mg, wet weight) placed in enclosed chambers[10] and superfused with Krebs buffer, pH 7.4, containing 0.1% heat inactivated bovine serum albumin (BSA, Difco Laboratories, Detroit, MI) at a rate of 300 µl/min. Ten to twelve chambers were superfused in parallel by using a multiple channel monostat casette pump (Monostat Corp., New York, NY). After an initial 50-minute wash period of superfusion, two consecutive 10-minute collections of the chamber effluent were obtained. The first period served as a buffer control period, while the second period was either a second buffer (time) control, or the superfusate was modified for one of the experimental procedures outlined below. Three sets of superfusion experiments were carried out: those with various forms of kallikrein, those with kinins and kinin analogues, and a set with the vasodilator acetylcholine.

Kallikrein Superfusion

We ran buffer time controls (n=15) simultaneously with all kallikrein experiments. Purified hog pancreatic kallikrein with an esterase activity of 170 mEU/ml (3.0 µg/ml) was added to the superfusate during the second period, after the initial buffer control period (n=11). We carried out similar experiments using 3.0 µg/ml of purified hog kallikrein which had been inactivated (0 mEU/ml) with phenylmethylsulphonyl fluoride (PMSF, n=5). In another set of superfusion experiments, the buffer in both periods was further modified to contain 500 Kunitz-inhibitory units/ml (KIU/ml) of aprotinin. In the second period, the superfusate contained 170 mEU/ml of hog kallikrein (n=4). Finally, to address the problem of species specificity, and because previous reports have employed rat kallikrein,[4,5,6] we carried out studies in which the buffer in the second period contained 160 mEU/ml of semi-purified rat submandibular gland kallikrein (n=6).

Kinin Superfusion

We ran another set of buffer time controls (n=12) simultaneously with the kinin superfusion experiments. One of four different forms of kinin at 10^{-5} M were added to the buffer during the second period: bradykinin (n=5), lys-bradykinin (kallidin, n=5), and the kinin analogues des-arg[9] bradykinin (n=5), and tyr[8] bradykinin (n=5), all obtained from Bachem Pharmaceuticals, Torrance, CA.

Vasodilator Superfusion

Because bradykinin is a potent vasodilator, we wished to test whether vasodilation would stimulate renin release in isolated glomeruli. We compared renin release in the presence of the vasodilator acetylcholine (Sigma, St. Louis, MO) to our renin results in which kinins were used. Also, to induce vascular tone in the arterioles, we tested the effect of the vasodilator in the presence of the vasoconstrictor norepinephrine (Sigma, St. Louis, MO). We used concentrations derived from the work of Edwards,[12] who described in vitro vasodilation and vasoconstriction in microdissected arterioles attached to glomeruli. We ran another set of buffer time controls (n=11) simultaneously with all acetylcholine superfusion experiments. We ran the acetylcholine experiments at 10^{-5} M (n=11) by adding it to the superfusate during the second period. Additional studies were run by adding acetylcholine to superfusate that contained the vasoconstrictor norepinephrine at 10^{-7} M (n=8). Another set of experiments measured renin release, while norepinephrine alone was added to the superfusate (n=6) in the second period.

Inactive Renin

Measurement of inactive renin in our preparation was based on the technique of Sealey, et al.[13] Aliquots of 100-150 mg (wet weight) of glomeruli were suspended in distilled water (2 ml/50 mg), then homogenized or sonicated for 10 seconds, and the cellular debris was then removed by centrifuging. From the supernatant, 300 μl aliquots were equilibrated to -4°C for one hour. Then, either trypsin or purified hog kallikrein was added to each sample in titered amounts equaling 0, 50, 100, 500, 1000, or 2000 μg/ml in order to activate inactive renin. After the mixture was incubated at -4°C for one hour, and the incubation terminated by adding 5 μl of PMSF and titered to pH 5.7 with malic acid, it was then frozen for later determination of renin concentration. Inactive renin was calculated as the difference between renin concentration in untreated samples and renin in trypsin- or kallikrein-treated samples. We carried out similar experiments on glomerular superfusion samples from control experiments (basal renin release) and from glomeruli superfused with 1.8×10^{-4} M Isoproterenol (Elkins-Sinn, Inc., Cherry Hill, NJ) for stimulated renin release.[10]

Analytical Methods

We determined renin concentration after the method of Carretero, et al.[14] Samples were incubated with 48-hour nephrectomized rat plasma as renin substrate in quantities sufficient to generate 1000 ng of angiotensin I (AI). The generation of AI was measured by radioimmunoassay after the method of Haber, et al.[15] We calculated renin release as ng AI generated per hour of incubation per ml of superfusate per minute of superfusion per 50 mg of glomeruli (wet weight), hereafter abbreviated as ng AI/min. The enzymatic activity of kallikrein was determined by measuring its esterolytic activity.[16] We tested for endogenous kinin formation by measuring kininogen concentration in glomerular tissue after the method of Fasciolo, et al.[17] Kinin concentration was measured by radioimmunoassay.[18] The BSA was heat-inactivated by incubating it for three hours at 58°C, and we found that it contained neither kininogenase activity nor measurable kinins.[19]

All values are presented as the arithmetic mean ± one standard error, or as a % change from period 1 to 2. We evaluated changes in renin release from period 1 to 2 using the student's paired t-test, while we made other comparisons using unpaired analysis. Changes were considered significant when a p-value of less than 0.05 was obtained.

RESULTS

Results from superfusion with kallikrein are illustrated in Figure 1. Basal renin release over two consecutive time control periods decreased by 5%, from 16.0 ± 2.8 to 15.2 ± 3.0 ng AI/min. When glomeruli were superfused with 170 mEU of hog kallikrein, renin release was significantly increased by 86%, from 13.0 ± 1.8 to 24.3 ± 4.8 ng AI/min (p <0.025). When hog kallikrein was inactivated with PMSF, renin release was not significantly changed and decreased 4% from period 1. Similarly, when the

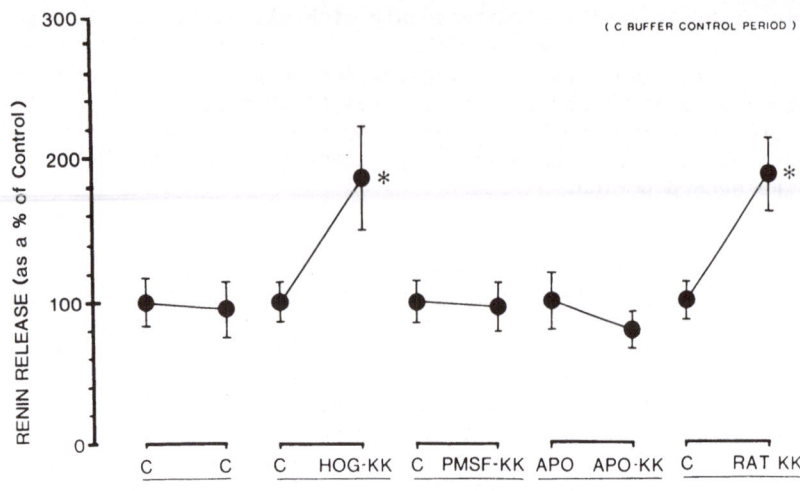

Fig. 1. Renin release presented as a percent of control, in response to
Krebs buffer time control (C), 170 mEU/ml of purified hog kallikrein (KK), PMSF-inactivated hog kallikrein (0 mEU/ml), 170 mEU/ml
hog kallikrein in the presence of 500 KIU Aprotinin (APO), and
160 mEU/ml semipurified rat kallikrein. Asterisks represent a
significant change from control with a p-value of <0.025.

superfusion media was altered by adding the protease inhibitor aprotinin,
renin release was unchanged by kallikrein and decreased 20% from the aprotinin control period. When rat glomeruli were superfused with rat kallikrein, renin release increased significantly by 87% (p <0.025) over the
control period.

Results from superfusion with different kinins are illustrated in
Figure 2. As with kallikrein experiments, basal renin release over consecutive time control periods decreased slightly 3%. Superfusion of 10^{-5} M
bradykinin significantly increased renin release by 108%, from 5.3 ± 0.8
to 11.0 ± 0.7 ng AI/min (p <0.025). Similarly, lys-bradykinin significantly increased renin release by 155%, from 5.8 ± 1.1 to 14.5 ± 2.6 ng AI/min
(p <0.025). This response did not differ from that elicited by bradykinin.
Neither of the bradykinin analogues, des-arg^9 bradykinin or tyr^8 bradykinin, had any significant effect upon renin release.

Superfusion with the vasodilator acetylcholine or the vasoconstrictor
norepinephrine had no apparent effect upon basal renin release; nor did
either result in stimulation. Paired buffer time controls declined from
6.8 ± 0.7 to 4.5 ± 0.5 ng AI/min. With acetylcholine, renin release declined 9% from 5.9 ± 0.5 to 5.4 ± 1.3 ng AI/min. When acetylcholine was
added to norepinephrine-treated glomeruli, there was no effect, as renin
declined from 5.8 ± 0.7 to 4.7 ± 0.5 ng AI/min. Norepinephrine also had
no effect, as renin decreased 2% from 4.8 ± 0.6 to 4.7 ± 0.5 ng AI/min.

Experiments to measure inactive renin with activation by trypsin or
with purified hog kallikrein from glomerular renin, basal or isoproterenol-
stimulated superfusate renin were inconclusive. We were unable to detect

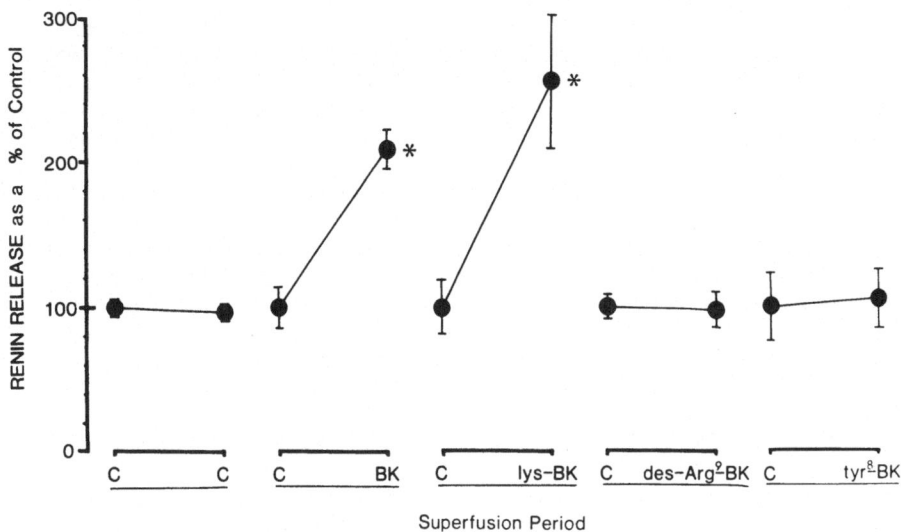

Fig. 2.   Renin release, presented as a percent of control, in response to
Krebs buffer time control (C) or superfusion with 10^{-5} M bradykinin (BK), lys-bradykinin, des-arg[9] bradykinin, or tyr[8] bradykinin. Asterisks represent a significant change from control with
a p-value of <0.025.

any measurable inactive renin in any of our studies.

We were unable to detect any kininogen in glomeruli. Furthermore,
when kallikrein was superfused and renin released from glomeruli, there was
no measurable kinin found in these samples.

DISCUSSION

Our studies show that both kallikrein and kinins can stimulate renin
release from a preparation of isolated glomeruli with their attendant arterioles, and that the effect of kallikrein is independent of its kininogenase activity.

We have shown that both hog and rat kallikrein can stimulate renin as
a function of enzymatic activity, since when we inhibited kallikrein activity
by either PMSF inactivation or inhibitory concentration of aprotinin, the
effect upon renin was eliminated. Further, we were unable to detect any
kininogen in our preparation, and we were unable to measure endogenous kinin
formation associated with kallikrein superfusion; these results suggest that
the action of kallikrein in this preparation was independent of kinin formation.

Suzuki, et al.[5] similarly reported that rat urinary kallikrein as well
as rat urinary esterase A2 could stimulate renin release from superfused
kidney slices. However, in a later study, they re-evaluated their results[6]
and suggested that increased renin was an artifact of media protein exerting
a protective effect upon renin in their samples. However, we showed that
renin was stimulated in the presence of media protein, and, further, we
eliminated this effect by blocking enzymatic activity without altering the
protein concentration.

The mechanism or the significance of the action of kallikrein upon renin is not clear. Although, it has been suggested that kallikrein may activate inactive renin,[3] we found no support for this hypothesis, since we were unable to find inactive renin in our preparation when we used either kallikrein or trypsin. Kallikrein has been reported to stimulate prostacyclin production in vascular endothelial cells,[20] and prostacyclin is the primary prostaglandin responsible for renin release in isolated glomeruli.[21] Renal kallikrein production has been localized in the connecting tubule,[22] and an anatomical association of this tubular region and the afferent arteriole has been reported.[23] Further, possible functional interrelationships between these anatomical sites have been suggested.[24] However, it is also possible that kallikrein in this preparation may only be mimicking some other endogenous serine protease. The exact nature of the kallikrein-renin interaction and its significance remain to be clarified.

We found that the biologically active kinins (bradykinin and kallidin) can stimulate renin release from isolated glomeruli. This is a concentration-dependent phenomenon,[11] and the inactive analogues, des-arg[9] bradykinin and tyr[8] bradykinin, do not affect renin release. Previously, Flamenbaum, et al.[9] reported that bradykinin transiently increased renin secretion in vivo, whereas Suzuki, et al.[5] using kidney slices, were unable to show any affect of bradykinin. However, kidney slices contain proximal tubules which are rich in kininase activity.[24] We have found that kidney slices rapidly degrade exogenous kinins, while isolated glomeruli are relatively free of kininase activity,[11,12] a difference which could account for our positive results.

The mechanism of the action of kinin upon renin release is unclear. It appears that it is not related to its vasodilatory properties, since we were unable to increase renin release by vasodilation alone, using acetylcholine, or by vasodilating after superimposing tone with norepinephrine.[12] Edwards[12] has observed that in vitro the afferent arterioles are vasodilated, suggesting that kinins acted upon a relaxed vessel in our preparation.

Bradykinin has been shown to be a potent activator of phospholipase A2, thereby increasing prostaglandin synthesis. Since endogenous prostacyclin synthesis has been shown to stimulate renin release in isolated glomeruli,[21] the action of kinin may be mediated by prostaglandin formation. However, Flamenbaum, et al.[9] found that bradykinin stimulation of renin in vivo was at least partially independent of prostaglandins. Thus the role of prostaglandins as a possible mediator of the kinin-renin interaction has yet to be defined.

The concentrations of bradykinin (10^{-5} to 10^{-6} M) used to stimulate renin in vitro[11] and in vivo[9] are significantly greater than the range of 10-11 to $\overline{10\text{-}12}$ M found in the circulation.[26] Whether results using such pharmacological levels of kinin reflect physiologic interactions is questionable. It is clear, however, that in the absence of endogenous kinases, kinins are capable of stimulating renin release from the afferent arterioles attached to isolated glomeruli.

In conclusion, we have shown that kallikrein can stimulate renin release from isolated glomeruli as a function of its enzymatic activity. This response is apparently not due to any activation of existent inactive renin. Further, we have found that the biologically active kinins also stimulate renin release from isolated glomeruli, apparently as a direct action not mediated by bradykinin-induced vasodilation. We have found that the action of kallikrein is not a function of its formation of endogenous kinins in this in vitro system, but rather both components of the kallikrein-kinin system are capable of independently stimulating the release of renin from isolated glomeruli.

ACKNOWLEDGEMENTS

The authors wish to thank Dr. G. L. Haberland, Beyer, Wuppertal 1, FDR, for the gift of purified hog pancreatic kallikrein and aprotinin. The partially purified rat submandibular gland kallikrein was supplied as a gift of Dr. A. G. Scicli of our institution. The authors acknowledge the contributions of Dr. Jorge Prada and of Ms. Donna Zobel, and the editorial assistance of Dr. Patricia Cornett.

This work was supported in part by N.I.H. grants HL-15839 and HL-28982. W. H. Beierwaltes is an Established Investigator of the American Heart Association.

REFERENCES

1. H. Yang, E. Erdos, and Y. Levin, A dipeptidyl carboxypeptidase that converts angiotensin I and inactivates bradykinin, Biochem. Biophys. Acta, 214:374-376 (1970).
2. F. Derkx, B. Bouma, M. Schalekamp, and M. Schalekamp, An intrinsic factor XII-prekallikrein-dependent pathway activates the human plasma renin-angiotensin system, Nature, 280:315-316 (1979).
3. J. E. Sealey, S. A. Atlas, and J. H. Laragh, Linking the kallikrein and renin systems via activation of inactive renin, Am. J. Med., 65:994-1000 (1978).
4. S. Suzuki, R. Franco-Saenz, S. Y. Tan, and P. J. Mulrow, Direct action of rat urinary kallikrein on rat kidney to release renin, J. Clin. Invest., 66:757-762 (1980).
5. S. Suzuki, R. Franco-Saenz, S. Y. Tan, and P. J. Mulrow, Direct action of kallikrein and other proteases on the renin-angiotensin system, Hypertension, 3(sp.1):I-13-17 (1981).
6. Y. Doi, A. Hinko, R. Franco-Saenz, and P. J. Mulrow, Reexamination of the effect of urinary kallikrein on renin release: Evidence that kallikrein does not release renin but protects renin from destruction, Endo., 113:114-118 (1983).
7. M. Rocha e Silva, Angiotensin and bradykinin: A study in contrasts, Can. Med. Assoc. J., 90:307-311 (1964).
8. P. A. Johnston, N. S. Perrin, D. B. Bernard, and N. G. Levinski, Control of rat renal vascular resistance at reduced perfusion pressure, Circ. Res., 48:734-739 (1981).
9. W. Flamenbaum, J. Gagnon, and P. Ramwell, Bradykinin-induced renal hemodynamic alterations: Renin and prostaglandin relationships, Am. J. Physiol., 237:F433-F440 (1979).
10. W. H. Beierwaltes, S. Schryver, P. Olson, and J. Romero, Interaction of the prostaglandin and renin-angiotensin systems in isolated rat glomeruli, Am. J. Physiol., 239:F602-F608 (1980).
11. W. H. Beierwaltes, J. Prada, and O. A. Carretero, Kinin stimulation of renin release in isolated rat glomeruli, Am. J. Physiol., (In press) (1985).
12. R. M. Edwards, Segmental effects of norepinephrine and angiotensin II on isolated renal microvessels, Am. J. Physiol., 244:F526-F534 (1983).
13. J. E. Sealey, S. A. Atlas, J. A. Laragh, N. B. Oza, and J. W. Ryan, Activation of a prorenin-like substance in human plasma by trypsin and by urinary kallikrein, Hypertension, 1:179-189 (1979).

14. O. A. Carretero, G. Enzmann, C. Polomski, N. B. Oza, and A. Schork, Role of the adrenal glands in the development of severe hypertension, Circ. Res., 33:516-520 (1973).

15. E. Haber, D. Loerner, L. B. Page, B. Kliman, and A. Purnode, Application of a radioimmunoassay for angiotensin I to the physiologic measurements of plasma renin activity in normal human subjects, J. Clin. Endocrinol., 29:1329-1355 (1969).

16. V. H. Beaven, J. V. Pierce, and J. J. Pisano, A sensitive isotopic procedure for the assay of esterase activity: Measurement of human urinary kallikrein, Clin. Chim. Acta., 32:67-73 (1971).

17. J. C. Fasciolo, J. Espada, and O. A. Carretero, The estimation of bradykinin content of the plasma, Acta. Phys. Lat. Am., 13:215-220 (1963).

18. O. A. Carretero, N. B. Oza, A. Piwonska, T. Ocholik, and A. G. Scicli, Measurement of urinary kallikrein activity by kinin radioimmunoassay, Biochem. Pharm., 25:599-606 (1976).

19. W. H. Beierwaltes, J. Prada, and O. A. Carretero, Effect of glandular kallikrein on renin release in isolated rat glomeruli, Hypertension, 7 (In press) (1985).

20. I. Morita, T. Kanayasu, and S. Murota, Kallikrein stimulates prostacyclin production in bovine vascular endothelial cells, Biochim. Biophys. Acta, 792:304-309 (1984).

21. W. H. Beierwaltes, S. Schryver, E. Sanders, J. Strand, and J. C. Romero, Renin release selectively stimulated by prostaglandin I2 in isolated rat glomeruli, Am. J. Physiol., 243:F276-F283 (1982).

22. K. Omata, O. A. Carretero, A. G. Scicli, and B. A. Jackson, Localization of active and inactive kallikrein (kininogenase activity) in the microdissected rabbit nephron, Kidney Int., 22:602-607 (1982).

23. L. Barajas, and K. Powers, The structure of the juxtaglomerular apparatus (JGA) and the control of renin secretion: An update. J. Hypertension, 2(sp.1):3-12 (1984).

24. O. A. Carretero and W. H. Beierwaltes, Effect of glandular kallikrein, kinins and aprotinin (a serine protease inhibitor) on renin release, J. Hypertension, 2:125-130 (1984).

25. P. E. Ward, R. C. Schultz, R. C. Reynolds, and E. G. Erdos, Metabolism of kinins and angiotensins in the isolated glomerulus and brush border of rat kidney, Lab. Invest., 36:599-606 (1977).

26. A. G. Scicli, T. Mindroiu, G. Scicli, and O. A. Carretero, Blood kinins, their concentration in normal subjects and in patients with congenital deficiency in plasma prekallikrein and kininogen, J. Lab. Clin. Med., 100:81-93 (1982).

REGULATION OF PAROTID KALLIKREIN SECRETION-ROLE OF THE $ALPHA_2$- AND BETA-ADRENERGIC SYSTEM

Arnold Röckel, Adolf Preissler, and August Heidland

Deutsche Klinik Für Diagnostik, Wiesbaden Med. Univ. Hosp. Würzburg, FRG

SUMMARY

The effects of pharmacologically induced alterations of $alpha_1$, $alpha_2$ and beta-adrenergic system on kallikrein secretion - measured as amidolytic activity - in rat parotid gland were tested in vivo. Beta and $alpha_{1/2}$-adrenergic stimulation (Orciprenaline, alpha-methylnorepinephrine) caused a comparably significant increase of parotid kallikrein secretion. $Alpha_2$-receptor blockade (yohimbine) but not the $alpha_1$-antagonist prazosin, partly abolished the effect of alpha-methylnorepinephrine. The effects of the $alpha_1$-adreno-receptor agonist norfenephrine on kallikrein secretion were significantly lower compared to $alpha_{1/2}$-adreno-receptor-stimulation.

Parotid kallikrein secretion is preferentially dependent on beta- and $alpha_2$-adrenergic activity.

INTRODUCTION

Glandular kallikreins are serine proteinases which convert kininogen to kallidin (lys-bradykinin). Mechanisms of renal kallikrein secretion are not fully understood. There are some hints that the urinary excretion is partly influenced by sodium and potassium balance, by mineralocorticoids[1,2] and by sympathetic activity.[3,4]

To get further insights into the mechanism of kallikrein secretion, in vivo studies in non-renal tissues are of interest. The parotid seems to be an appropriate test model since this gland contains large amounts of kallikrein in apical portions of the duct cells, which is secreted into the saliva.[3]

In rat[3] and in cat[5] submandibular gland the most efficient kallikrein secretion followed alplha-adrenergic stimulation. The kallikrein release after beta-adrenergic stimulation was significantly lower. In the guinea-pig submandibular gland, however, a comparable beta-adrenergically induced kallikrein release was observed.[6]

The aim of this study was to test the effects of stimulation and block-ade of $alpha_1$, $alpha_2$ and beta-adrenergic receptors in rat parotid kallikrein secretion under in vivo conditions.

METHODS

Animal Preparation

Non-fasting male wistar rats were anesthetized with Inactin[R] (100-120 mg/kg, i.p.) and maintained at 37°C. All animals were routinely tracheostomized and the femoral artery and vein cannulated. Blood pressure was monitored continuously. Pilocarpine (7.5 mg/kg, i.p.) evoked rat parotid saliva was obtained as previously described.[7] The kallikrein concentration (amidolytic activity) in parotid saliva (pKC) was measured using the method of Amundsen et al.[8] Studies were discontinued after a drop in mean arterial blood pressure >50 mm Hg, blood loss >0.4 ml, preparation time >45 minutes, and a salivary flow rate <10 ul/min.

Drugs

All drugs were dissolved in a warmed (37°C) Ringer's solution which was also used as placebo. Orciprenaline (14 µg/kg/min.), propanolol (11 µg/kg/min.), alpha-methylnorepinephrine (20 µg/kg/min.), norfenephrine (24 and 48 µg/kg/min.), prazosin (3 µg/kg/min.) and yohimbine (125 µg/kg/min.) were infused intravenously over 90 minutes. After start of infusion of the different drugs or placebo, saliva was collected for 9 consecutive periods of 10 minutes ech. Because of the dependence of pKC, pNa^+ C and pK^+ C on salivary flow rte, placebo and drug groups were compared in a flow rate range of 25-35 µl/min. using the drug periods 2-9. Correlation coefficients and significances were calculated using covariance analysis. Data are expresed as means ± sem.

RESULTS

Under <u>basal conditions</u> (pilocarpine 7.5 mg/kg/min i.p.; 0.5 ml Ringer's solution/45 min.) pNa^+ C decreased significantly (-12%, p <0.001) during the experiment. Flow rate (FR), mean arterial blood pressure (MAP), pKC, kallikrein secretion rate (KSR) and pK^+ C remained constant during the entire experiment.

There is an inverse correlation between kallikrein (R = 0.64) or potassium concentration (R = 0.61) and the flow rate and a direct one between sodium concentration and flow rate (R = 0.64). In Table 1 mean arterial blood pressure (MAP) and flow rate dependent (FR range 25-35 µl/min.) concentrations of electrolytes and kallikrein before and after drug administration are given.

Beta-adrenergic stimulation (orciprenaline) and $alpha_{1/2}$-adrenergic stimulation (alpha-methylnorepinephrine) caused a comparably significant increase of kallikrein and potassium concentration. Selective $alpha_2$-receptor blockade (yohimbine), but not the $alpha_1$-blocker prazosin, partly abolished the effect of alpha-methylnorepinephrine.

Compared to $alpha_{1/2}$-receptor stimulation (alpha-methylnorepinephrine) the effects of $alpha_1$-receptor stimulation (norfenephrine) on kallikrein and potassium handling were significantly lower.

DISCUSSION

   Salivary glands of mammals are parasympathetically and sympathetically innervated. Under parasympathetical stimulation a high flow rate but a slight increase of kallikrein concentration was observed.[5] Sympathetical stimulation caused a significant kallirkein release and only a slight in-

Table 1

Drugs	Dose (µg/kg x min)	MAP (mm Hg)		Flow Rate (µl/min)		PKC (U/l)		PK$^+$C (mval/l)		PNa$^+$C (mval/l)	
		pre	post	pre	post	pre	post	pre	post	pre	post
Orciprenaline	14	133.6±2.9	92.5±2.4	31.0±1.2	29.0±1.4	25.2±3.0	94.3±10.3	12.4±0.6	14.0±0.5	107.9±4.8	105.0±3.7
Propranolol	11	131.1±2.7	118.8±3.3	30.6±1.2	30.7±1.7	30.2±3.8	17.0±6.1	10.5±0.4	9.7±0.2	113.0±2.5	110.3±2.3
Alpha - MNA	20	121.4±3.5	146.3±2.5	30.5±1.5	29.0±1.0	28.6±1.6	72.9±5.8	11.0±0.4	14.0±0.7	105.0±3.2	104.3±2.1
Yohimbin + Alpha MNA	125 +20	79.8±4.3	77.3±2.8	27.5±1.2	26.0±1.0	27.3±3.0	56.2±4.4	11.1±0.3	11.9±0.3	108.8±2.6	109.2±1.7
Prazosin Alpha MNA	3 +20	78.1±2.5	86.8±2.8	31.1±1.1	30.0±2.1	29.6±2.3	74.6±6.7	10.9±0.2	13.5±0.9	111.4±2.4	106.7±2.2
Yohimbin	125	124.3±2.7	79.8±4.3	30.0±1.0	29.5±1.2	26.3±4.4	27.3±3.0	11.6±0.3	11.1±0.3	116.1±2.4	108.8±2.6
Prazosin	3	132.5±2.4	78.1±2.5	31.1±1.1	31.1±1.1	24.2±1.8	29.6±2.3	11.8±0.2	10.9±0.2	116.0±2.8	111.4±2.4
Norfenephrine	48	132.1±4.1	145.9±4.4	32.1±1.3	32.3±1.4	21.8±3.0	47.0±4.5	11.6±0.4	12.7±0.4	114.5±1.1	115.2±1.2
	24	121.6±3.7	129.8±2.7	31.3±1.7	29.3±1.2	26.3±3.3	30.7±2.1	11.3±0.5	11.5±0.6	117.1±1.4	116.4±1.2

crease of flow rate.[3] According to Batzri and Selinger[9] preferentially beta-adrenergic stimulation led to an enzyme release, whereas alpha-drenergic stimulation increases potasium secretion. Emmelin[10] and Orstavik et al.[3] however showed a significantly stronger enzyme secretion after alpha-adrenergic stimulation.

In rats and rabbits[11] and in guinea pigs[12,13] a comparable enzyme secretion was established after alpha- and beta-adrenergic stimulation. According with these results a significant increase of kallikrein secretion after beta- and $alpha_{1/2}$-adrenergic stimulation was observed. Thus, in contrast to the rat submandibular gland, the rat parotid seems to have a comparable number of alpha- and beta-adrenergic receptors. The importance of the beta-adrenergic system of the rat parotid gland is stressed by the results under beta-receptor blockade. Whereas $alpha_1$- and $alpha_2$-receptor blockade did not influence the pilocarpine-induced kallikrein secretion, propanolol caused a significant decrease.

$Alpha_{1/2}$-receptor stimulation (alpha-methylnorepinephrine) caused a significantly stronger enzyme release compared to the $alpha_1$-receptor agonist norfenephrine. Accordingly $alpha_2$-adrenergic blockade (yohimbine) - but not the $alpha_1$-receptor antagonist prazosin - could decrease the alpha-methyl-norepinephrine-induced kallikrein release. These results suggest that the kallikrein secretion in the parotid ductal system is preferentially $alpha_2$-adrenergically mediated.

REFERENCES

1. R. G. Geller, H. S. Margolius, J. J. Pisano, and H. R. Keiser , Effects of mineralocorticoids, altered sodium intake and adrenalectomy on urinary kallikrein in rats, Circulation Res., 31:857-861 (1972).
2. H. S. Margolius, D. Horwitz, R. G. Geller, R. W. Alexander, J. R. Gill, Jr., J. J. Pisano, and H. R. Keiser, Urinary kallikrein excretion in normal man. Relationships to sodium intake and sodium retaining steroids, Circulation Res., 35:812-819 (1974).
3. T. B. Orstavik and K. M. Gautvik, Regulation of salivary kallikrein secretion in the rat submandibular gland, Acta Physiol. Scand., 100:33-44 (1977).
4. R. L. Katz and I. D. Mandel, Action and interaction of isoproterenol and alpha and beta-adrenergic blocker on parotid and submaxillary secretion in man, Proc. Soc. Exp. Biol. Med., 128:1140-1145 (1968).
5. K. M. Gautvik, M. Kritz, K. Lund-Larsen, and K. Nustad, Control of kallikrein secretion from salivary glands, in: "Secretory Mechanisms of Exocrine Glands," Thorn and Petersen, eds., Munksgaard, Copenhagen (1974).
6. K. D. Bhoola and M. J. C. Lemon, Studies on enzyme secretion and cyclic AMP in the submaxillary gland and pancreas, J. Physiol., 245:121-122 (1975).
7. F. O. Stählin, G. Schmid, K. Hempel, and A. Heidland, Technique of continuous collection of parotid saliva in the rat, Res.,Exp. Med., 172:247-253 (1978).
8. E. Amundsen, M. J. Gallimore, A. O. Aasen, M. Larsbraaten, and K. Lyngaas, Activation of human plasma prekallikrein: Influence of activators, activation time and inhibitors, Thromb. Res., 13:625-636 (1978).
9. S. Batzri and Z. Selinger, Enzyme secretion mediated by the epinephrine receptor in rat parotid slices. Factor governing efficiency of the process, J. Biol. Chem., 248:356-360 (1973).
10. N. Emmelin, Sympatholytic agents used to separate secretory and vascular effects of sympathetic stimulation on the submaxillary gland, Acta Physiol. Scand., 34:29-371 (1955).

11. N. Emmelin, J. Holmberg, and P. Ohlin, Receptors for catecholamines in the submaxillary gland of rats, <u>Brit. J. Pharmac. Chemother.</u> 25:134-138 (1965).

12. J. Albano, K. D. Bhoola, P. F. Heap, and M. J. C. Lemon, Stimulus-secretion coupling: Role of cyclic AMP, cyclic GMP and ccalcium in mediating enzyme (kallikrein) secretion in the submandibular gland, <u>J. Physiol.</u>, 258:631-658 (1976).

13. T. Hayashi, T. Kudo, J. Takezawa, R. Inoki, and I. Yamamoto, Effects of adrenergic agents on secretion of salivary kallikrein in the submandibular gland of the dog, <u>Folia. Pharmacol. Jap.</u>, 71: 527-538 (1975).

EFFECT OF FUROSEMIDE ON THE RAT SUBMANDIBULAR GLAND KALLIKREIN SECRETION

O.L. Catanzaro, S.B. Vila, A. Zuccolo, and A.M. Seeber

Anatomia Comparada y Fisiologia Humana, Dep. Ciencias
Biologicas
Facultad de Farmacia y Bioquimica—UBA
Buenos Aires — Argentina

SUMMARY

The effects of furosemide and Captopril were studied in normals and
nephrectomized rats. Different doses of furosemide (5 to 50 mg/kg) increased the saliva kallikrein activity of submaxillary gland perfused with
pilocarpine. Rats injected with captopril (10 mg) increased the blood flow
of the gland, but did not modify the blood pressure. After furosemide
(50 mg/kg) and captopril (10 mg), a decrease in arterial blood pressure was
observed. The results suggest a release of glandular kallikrein which is
secreted from the gland directly into the vascular compartment. On the
other hand, rats sialodectomized showed no alterations in blood pressure in
response to both drugs. These data suggest that submaxillary gland kallikrein play a role in regulating blood flow of the gland and blood pressure,
at least in our experimental conditions.

INTRODUCTION

The submaxillary gland is an organ rich in kallikrein[1]. Significant
amounts of the gland enzyme are released into the circulation after sympathetic stimulation[2]. According to Hilton and Lewis[3], glandular kallikrein-
kinin system in salivary glands regulates local vasodilatation with a
significant effect on plasma substrate kininogen. Release of glandular
kallikrein into the circulation increases the generation of kinin in blood[4].
Experimental observations showed that furosemide increases renal blood flow
and urinary kallikrein[5]. The present study shows the effects of furosemide
and captopril on submaxillary gland.

METHODS

Male WISTAR rats weighing 300–400 g were used. To eliminate the effect
of captopril on renin-angiotensin renal system, bilateral nephrectomy was
performed 48 h before the experiments. Rats were anesthetized with urethane
(1 g/kg) and a catheter was placed in the jugular vein for drug injection.
In one group mean arterial pressure was recorded on a polygraph by a catheter
implanted in the carotid artery with heparin saline solution (100 U/ml) and
connected to a pressure transducer (Statham P 23 Db). In another group

submandibular blood flow was measured from venous outflow of the gland through a catheter (PE-10) inserted into the submandibular gland vein. Blood samples were collected at time intervals in preweighed plastic tubes and the volume of each sample was estimated by reweighing tubes. To restore the volume an equal volume of blood was given intravenously. Blood flow and mean arterial pressure in both groups were measured before and after the drugs administration. Rats were treated in one of the following ways:

a) Captopril: 10 mg in 0.5 ml saline solution administered intravenously.
b) Furosemide: 5, 10, 25 and 50 mg/kg in 0.5 ml saline solution administered intravenously.
c) Furosemide plus captopril administered intravenously in similar doses.
d) Sialodectomized rats with a similar treatment.

When both drugs were injected, captopril was injected 5 min. after furosemide.

Saliva secretion was induced with pilocarpine-HCl (5 mg/kg) and saliva samples were collected at time intervals in glass microsample tubes. Protease like kallikrein was determined with α-N-Tosyl-arginine-methyl-ester HCl (TAME)[6].

Statistical Analysis. To compare changes induced by drugs among groups, a two way analysis of variance was used, according to Snedecor and Cochram[7]. The 5% probability level was used as a criterion for significance.

RESULTS

Venous flow from submandibular glands: Blood flow showed no significant changes before or after furosemide (65-1; 55 $\pm$ 5 ul/min/g w Wt) respectively. Rats injected with captopril showed a significant increase of the blood flow (102 $\pm$ 1; $P < 0.01$). Table 1 shows that association of both drugs increased the blood flow significantly. Mean arterial pressure: After furosemide or captopril no significant changes were observed. Before treatment (mmHg) 112 $\pm$ 6; furosemide: 110 $\pm$ 7; captopril: 86 $\pm$ 6. On the other hand, after furosemide and captopril the mean arterial pressure decreased significantly (Table 1, Fig. I). Rats sialodectomized showed no significant differences in blood pressure in response to both drugs (Table I). It is interesting to point out that captopril was injected 5 or 6 min. after furosemide and the decrease of mean arterial pressure was detected seconds after captopril.

TABLE 1. Mean blood pressure and blood flow of submandibular gland.

Treatment	None Before (8)	Furosemide $\pm$ Captopril After (8)
BP (mmHg)	112 $\pm$ 6	49 $\pm$ 6*
BF (ul/min/g w. Wt)	65 $\pm$ 1	141 $\pm$ 9*
SIALODECTOMY		
BP (mmHg)	97 $\pm$ 4	83 $\pm$ 6 (ns)

Results shown as mean value $\pm$ SE* $P < 0.01$ by comparing before and after. ns: not significant, BP: blood pressure, BF: blood flow ul g gland wet weight. ( ) number of animals.

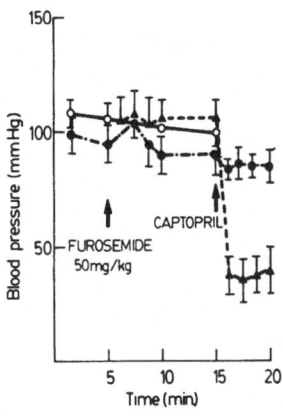

Figure 1. Effects of Furosemide and Captopril
on Mean Arterial Blood Pressure.

The values are the mean + SEM. Control (o----o); Furosemide (●----●)
Furosemide +Captopril (▲---▲).

Table 2 shows the effects of different doses of furosemide on salivary
flow and kallikrein activity stimulated by pilocarpine. After 10, 25 and
50 mg/kg of furosemide salivary flow decreased. On the other hand kallikrein activity started to increase with 25 and 50 mg/Kg of the drug.

Table 2. Effect of furosemide on salivary flow and kallikrein activity

Treatment	Salivary Flow (ul/min/g gland min)	Kallikrein EU/100 mg	Activity w.t./min
Control (8)	39.5 ± 1.5	22 ± 7	(n.s.)
Furosemide (6) mg/kg			
5 (n=6)	37.1 ± 3.9 (n.s.)	18 ± 3	(n.s.)
10 (n=6)	29.2 ± 1.8 (n.s.)	24 ± 5	(n.s.)
25 (n=7)	23.1 ± 3.7*	238 ± 88*	
50 (n=7)	21.5 ± 4.3*	222 ± 31*	

Results show a mean value ± S.E. (n.s.) not significant, * P < 0.01 by
comparing with the control.

DISCUSSION

It has been suggested that glandular kallikrein could regulate blood
flow through the formation of kallikrein (Lysil-bradykinin) in organs rich
in glandular kallikrein[8]. Arterial pressure could be regulated by release
of kinin from plasma kininogen. In addition, kallikrein secreted from
submaxillary gland, pancreas and intestine could play an important role in
regulating blood flow of the organs, and in some experimental conditions
regulates the systemic pressure. In the present study we have shown the
effect of furosemide and captopril in regulating blood flow of the gland
and systemic arterial pressure. On the other hand, an interesting effect
of furosemide on saliva kallikrein was observed. The observations of greater
changes in saliva kallikrein after furosemide and, also, after captopril
in glandular blood flow and arterial blood pressure, suggest that glandular

kallikrein after reaching vascular compartment release kinin from plasma kininogen. Since nephrectomy has been demonstrated to increase plasma kininogen concentration, probably kallikrein release after furosemide and captopril could act on kininogen to increase the circulating kinin. The increase of local blood flow of the gland after captopril could suggest a rapid formation of kinin in the local circulation, with a consequent vaso-dilatation. In sialodectomized rats the effects of drugs was absolutely absent, this effect could suggest that the origin of the glandular kalli-krein is the submaxillary gland. Thus, it is reasonable to assume that the hypotensive effect observed with captopril and furosemide administration probably is due to a decrease of peripheral resistance, since it was ac-companied by an increased submandibular blood flow. However, we cannot exclude the possibility of releasing other different substances after the drugs.

ACKNOWLEDGEMENTS

This work was supported by the Consejo Nacional de Investigaciones Cientificas y Tecnicas – Argentina and Lucio Cherny Foundation.

REFERENCES

1. Orstavik, T.B. J. Histochem. Cytochem. 28: 881 (1980).
2. Orstavik, T.B., Carretero, O.A. and Scicli, A.G. Amer. J. Physiol. 242: H1010 (1983).
3. Hilton, S.M. and Lewis, G.P. J. Physiol. (Lond) 134: 471 (1956).
4. Scicli, A.G., Orstavik, T.B., Rabito, S.F., Murray, R.D. and Carrertero, O.A. Hypertension Supp. 15: 101 (1983).
5. Bonner, G., Beck, D., Deeg, M., Marin-Grez, M. and Gross, F. Clin. Sci. 63: 447 (1982).
6. Nustad, K. and Pierce, J.V. Biochemistry 13: 2312 (1974).
7. Snedecor, G.W. and Cochram, W.G. Statistical Methods (Iowa State Unive. Press. Amer.) pp. 149 (1980).
8. Rabito, S.F., Scicli, A.G., Kher, V. and Carretero, O.A. Amer. J. Physiol. 242: H602 (1982).

INDIVIDUAL REACTION STEPS IN THE RELEASE OF KALLIDIN FROM KININOGEN BY TISSUE KALLIKREIN

Franz Fiedler, Heide Hinz and Friedrich Lottspeich*

Abteilung für Klinische Chemie und Klinische Biochemie in der Chirurgischen Klinik Innenstadt der Universität München, Nussbaumstr. 20, D-8000 München 2; *Max-Planck-Institut für Biochemie, D-8033 Martinsried

SUMMARY

At low pH values (around 6), porcine pancreatic β-kallikrein B attacks at first the C-terminal ARg bond of the kinin moiety in bovine HMW kininogen. Arg-cleaved kininogen accumulates as an intermediate in the solution. Kallidin is released by cleavage of the aminoterminal Met-Lys bond in a second step. At pH values between 7.6 and 9, however, Arg-cleaved kininogen does not occur as a free intermediate. The participation as a (free, not only enzyme-bound) intermediate of Arg-cleaved kininogen in a short-lived especially reactive conformation or of Met-cleaved kininogen is also unlikely. Probably, both the Met and the Arg bonds are hydrolyzed in one enzyme-substrate complex which does not dissociate between these two events.

Kinetic constants for the release of kallidin from native single-chain HMW kininogen and from Arg-cleaved kininogen (even if this Arg residue is removed) remarkably have the same values. Evidently, the rate of the reaction is determined by steps leading to the hydrolysis of the Met bond. As the state of the C-terminal Arg residue has no influence, the efficient cleavage of the Met bond by tissue kallirkein is probably not due to some strain in the kininogen molecule in the region of this bond. As modification of Arg residues of kininogen prevents cleavage also of the Met bond, some Arg residue(s) appear(s) to play a crucial role in this process. k_{cat}/K_m (1.4×10^6 M^{-1} sec^{-1} at pH 9, 25° C) is very high for a proteolytic reaction, mainly because of the low value of K_m (0.6 µM). k_{cat}/K_m for the hydrolysis of the Met bond in kininogen is 3 500 times higher than in the peptide Ser-Leu-Met-Lys-brady-kinin with a partial kininogen sequence. Important interactions with the enzyme thus occur in regions of the kininogen molecule outside this sequence. K_{cat}/K_m for the hydrolysis of the Arg bond in the kininogen peptide Pro-Phe-Arg-Ser-Val-Gln is also 14 times lower than this constant for the release of kallidin from kininogen, but k_{cat} is 6 times higher. This can explain why cleavage of the Arg bond is not reflected in the kinetic constants of single-chain kininogen.

INTRODUCTION

For the characteristic release of kallidin by tissue kallikrein (EC 3.4.21.35) two bonds have to be hydrolyzed, an Arg-Ser bond and a Met-Lys bond in bovine kininogen.[1,2] Previous studies with model substrates have demonstrated a high specificity of porcine pancreatic kallikrein for the Phe-Arg sequence at the Arg cleavage site in kininogen.[3,4] As a first step towards the elucidation of the causes of the strange hydrolysis of a Met bond in kininogen, the order of cleavage by porcine pancreatic kallikrein of the two bonds in bovine HMW kininogen and the respective kinetic constants were investigated.

MATERIALS AND METHODS

Porcine pancreatic -kallikrein B was further purified by ion exchange chromatography[5] from purified preparations generously supplied by Dr. Schmidt-Kastner, Bayer AG.[6] Native single-chain bovine HMW kininogen was isolated in a similar way as described in the literature,[7,8] using repeated chromatography on CM-Sephadex as the final step. Preparations typically contained only 3% (SDS-electrophoresis) of nicked kininogen. A mixture of Arg-cleaved and of des-Arg-kininogen was obtained as side component during the purification of bovine HMW kininogen. It was treated with endoproteinase Arg-C (Boehringer) to cleave all singlel-chain kininogen present and rechromatographed on CM-Sephadex. Des-Arg-kininogen was prepared from Arg-cleaved kininogen (obtained by the action of endoproteinase Arg-C on HMW kininogen) by treatment with carboxypeptidase B and rechromatography on CM-Sephadex.

Reversed-phase HPLC was used for the quantification of kinins (4 x 200 mm column, M & N, Nucleosil 5C8; 0.1 M Na-phosphate pH 3 + 16 vol % aceto-nitrile, isocratic, 1 ml/min). Absorbance was monitored at 200 nm and the procedure calibrated with a kallidin solution standardized by quantitative amino acid analysis. The molar absorbance of des-(Arg-10)-kallidin was taken as 90% of that of kallidin. Retention times: kallidin, 7 min; brady-kinin, 10-)-kallidin, 12 min.

RESULTS AND DISCUSSION

Does a Free Intermediate, Kininogen with a Single Bond Cleaved, Occur in the Reaction?

Kallidin released from native single-chain bovine HMW kininogen by porcine pancreatic β- kallikrein B was monitored by HPLC and the formation of cleaved kininogen (the sum of kinin-free kininogen and of possible forms with a single bond split) by SDS-electrophoresis.

At pH 8 (as well as 9), the rates of kallidin release and of formation of cleaved kininogen are similar (Fig. 1). There is no rapid accumulation of free intermediate, kininogen with a single bond hydrolyzed. This finding resembles data reported for the hydrolysis of human HMW kininogen by porcine pancreatic kallikrein,[10] whereas with human salivary kallikrein the latter substrate was cleaved prior to kinin release.[11] Whether a minor amount of a free intermediate exists in our system cannot be safely decided because of the limited accuracy of the experiment. If the release of kallidin occurs in two consecutive steps, cleavage of the first bond must be the rate-determining, slow step.

At pH 5.3 (and 6.2), however, kininogen cleavage was more rapid than kallidin release. An intermediate accumulated. Amino-terminal sequence analysis after removal of kallidin by dialysis revealed only the sequence Ser-Val-Gln-Val- in the expected amounts. These amino acids follow the kinin moiety in bovine kininogen.[1] The free intermediate appearing at low pH is thus Arg-cleaved kininogen. The Met bond is hydrolyzed under these conditions in a second, slower step.

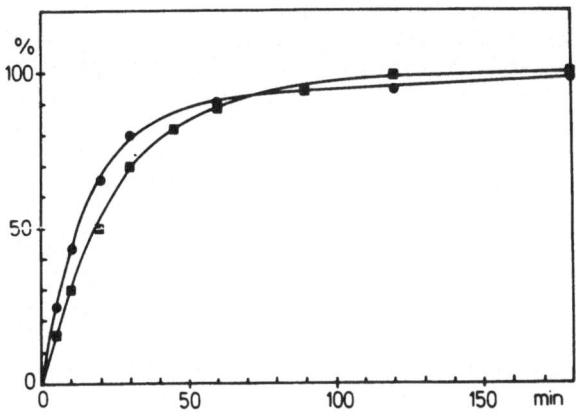

Fig. 1. Release of kallidin (■) from native single-chain bovine HMW
kininogen and formation of cleaved kininogen (●) by porcine pancreatic β-kallikrein B at pH 8. 20 nmolls kininogen were incubated at
25° C in 0.20 ml 0.1 M Tris/HCll, pH 8.0, 0.1 mM EDTA, 0.2 M NaCl
with 0.2 μg pancreatic kallikrein. Samples of 5 μl were withdrawn
at the times indicated. They were added either to 120 μl 0.1 N
HCl, and kallidin was determined by HPLC, or to 100 μl phosphate
buffer containing 8 M urea, 2% SDS and 2% dithioerythritol and
immediately heated to 100° C for 5 min. Aliquots were then subjected to SDS gel electrophoresis.[9] Gels were stained with
Coomassie Blue and scanned in a densitometer.

Is Arg-Cleaved Kininogen Also Intermediate at Physiological pH Values?

Low concentrations of an intermediate would not have been recognized
in the experiments at pH 8 or 9. In order to detect small amounts of Arg-
cleaved kininogen as a possible free intermediate, des-Arg-kininogen (Arg-
cleaved kininogen devoid of the C-terminal ARg residue) was used as a
"trapping reagent".

The method is based on the observation that release of kallidin by
porcine pancreatic kallikrein from Arg-cleaved kininogen strictly parallels
the release of des-(Arg-10)-kallidin from des-Arg-kininogen in a mixture of
these two kininogen derivatives. This result indicates a close similarity
of the kinetic constants for the hydrolysis of the Met bond inb oth nicked
kininogens. In a mixture of single-chain kininogen and des-Arg-kininogen,
Arg-cleaved kininogen generated from single-chain kininogen as a free intermediate would mix with the large pool of des-Arg-kininogen. This mixture
would release on cleavage of the Met bond mainly des-(Arg-10)-kallidin in
the earlier phases of the reaction. This is, however, definitely not the
case at pH 9 as well as pH 7.6: the release of kallidin (from single-chain
kininogen) by porcine pancreatic kallikrein strictly parallels the release
of des-(Arg-10)-kallidin already from the onset of the reaction.

These observations rule out the formation of even a low concentration
of free (not enzyme-bound) Arg-cleaved kininogen as an intermediate of
kallidin release at these pH values. (At pH 6.2, where Arg-cleaved and des-
Arg-kininogens are also hydrolyzed at the same rates, formation of this
intermediate could be demonstrated by the present method.)

The experiments further indicate that the kinetic constants for the
release of kallidin from single-chain kininogen (requiring cleavage of the
Met and the Arg bonds) and from Arg-cleaved kininogen (cleavage only of the
Met bond) are remarkably similar.

There remains the possibility that on cleavage of the Arg bond kininogen is released in an especially reactive conformation which is different from the conformation of isolated Arg-cleaved kininogen attained only after some time. This special conformation might be based e.g. on the cis/trans isomerism of the proline residues in the kinin moiety. However, in this case the identity of the values of the kinetic constants for kallidin release from isolated Arg-cleaved kininogen (cleavage of the Met bond) and from single-chain kininogen (rate-limiting cleavage of the Arg bond according to the presently discussed mechanism) would appear as a ver strange coincidence.

Is Met-Cleaved Kininogen a (Free) Intermediate in the Reaction?

In a first experiment, native single-chain kininogen was treated with pancreatic kallikrein, until 1/3 of the m ximal amount of kallidin was released. Kallidin was removed by dialysis. The only aminoterminal sequence detected in the partially cleaved kininogen was Ser-Val-Gln-. The sequence resulting from cleavage of the Met bond, Lys-Arg-Pro-, was present, if at all, in amounts below the detection limit, which was in this experiment about 20% of the cleaved or 10% of the uncleaved kininogen present at the termination of the enzymatic reaction.

If the release of kallidin from native kininogen involved the two consecutive steps

$$\text{single-chain kininogen } (S_1) \xrightarrow[K_{m1}]{k_{cat1}} \text{ Met-cleaved kininogen } (S_2) \xrightarrow[K_{m2}]{k_{cat2}}$$

kallidin + kinin-free kininogen, v_1 (rate of cleavage of the Met-bond) =

$$\frac{k_{cat1} \dfrac{[S_1]}{K_{m1}} [E]o}{1 + \dfrac{[S_1]}{K_{m1}} + \dfrac{[S_2]}{K_{m2}}} \text{ , and } v_2 \text{ (rate of cleavage of} = \frac{k_{cat2} \dfrac{[S_2]}{K_{m2}} [E]o}{1 + \dfrac{[S_1]}{K_{m1}} + \dfrac{[S_2]}{K_{m2}}} .$$
the Arg-bond)

When the middle phase of the reaction is treated to a first approximation as a steady state,

$$v_1 = v_2, \text{ whence } \frac{k_{cat2}}{K_{m2}} \bigg/ \frac{k_{cat1}}{K_{m1}} = \frac{[S_1]}{[S_2]} .$$

As the experiment shows that $[S_1] \gtrsim 10 [S_2]$, $k_{cat2}/K_{m2} \gtrsim 10 k_{cat1}/K_{m1}$. k_{cat1}/K_{m1}, the specificity constant for the cleavage of the Met bond in single-chain kininogen, must be at least as high as the constant for the release of kallidin, which is 1.4×10^6 M^{-1}sec^{-1} (see below). So k_{cat2}/K_{m2} for the cleavage of the Arg bond in Met-cleaved kininogen would have to be $\gtrsim 1.4 \times 10^{-7}$ M^{-1}sec^{-1}, a value appearing implausibly high. This makes the participation of Met-cleaved kininogen as a free intermediate in the reaction not very likely, especially if further more sensitive experiments can still increase the lower limit for k_{cat2}/K_{m2}.

If neither Arg-cleaved nor Met-cleaved kininogen is a free (not exclusively enzyme-bound) intermediate in the release of kallidin by porcine

286

pancreatic β- kallikrein from bovine single-chain HMW kininogen at physiological pH values, the cleavage of both the Arg and the Met bond must take place in one enzyme-substrate complex which does not dissociate between these two events, a surprising and hitherto unique reaction.

Kinetic Constants for the Release of Kinin From Native and From Nicked Kininogen

Until now, we have determined kinetic constants for the release of kallidin by porcine pancreatic β- kallikrein from single-chain bovine HMW kininogen and of des-(Arg-10)-kallidin from des-Arg-kininogen (Table 1). Initial rates were obtained at several substrate concentrations (0.5-5 μM) by following the rate of kinin release by quantitative HPLC.

The relatively high errors are due to the unfavourable working conditions forced by the low values of K_m. With this restriction, also the release of kallidin from single-chain kininogen (cleavage of two bonds) followed Michaelis-Menten kinetics. The process is very efficient: k_{cat}/K_m is very high for a proteolytic reaction, mainly because of the low K_m value. The kinetic constants are similar to those determined for horse urinary kallikrein/horse LMW kininogen,[12] whereas K_m for human urinary kallikrein/human HMW kininogen is about tenfold higher.[13,14]

The data demonstrate directly the identity of the kinetic constants for the cleavage of single-chain and of des-Arg-kininogen, as inferred already (also for Arg-cleaved kininogen) from the results on kininogen mixtures. The additional hydrolysis of the Arg bond of single-chain kininogen is not reflected in the kinetic constants, which evidently are determined only by steps leading to cleavage of the Met bond of kininogen.

The state of the C-terminal ARg residue of the kinin moiety (whether the Arg bond is cleaved or the residue even is absent) is of no concern for the rate of kinin release. Thus, the rapid hydrolysis of the Met bond in kininogen is presumably not caused by some strain in the kininogen molecule around this bond. Such a strain would be expected to be relieved if the carboxy terminus of the kinin moiety is free to move. The Arg residue in question is not necessary for aiding the correct interaction of kininogen with tissue kallikrein required for cleavage of the Met bond.

Table 1.   Kinetic Constants for the Hydrolysis of Kininogen and Kininogen Peptides by Porcine Pancreatic β-Kallikrein B (pH 9, 25° C)

	k_{cat} (sec^{-1})	K_m (μM)	k_{cat}/K_m (mM^{-1}sec^{-1})
Single-chain bovine HMW kininogen	0.87	0.60(± 13%)	1 450
Bovine HMW des-Arg-kininogen	0.75	0.55(± 14%)	1 360
Pro-Phe-Arg+Ser-Val-Gln (3)	5.7	57	100
Ser-Leu-Met+Lys-bradykinin (4)			0.4

k_{cat}/K_m for cleavage of the Met bond in kininogen is 3 500 times higher than in the peptide Ser-Leu-Met-Lys-bradykinin with a partial kininogen sequence (Table 1). Interactions essential for the efficient hydrolysis of the Met bond in kininogen thus occur with parts of the substrate molecule outside this sequence. Presumably, these interactions are somewhat analogous to those observed in protein inhibitor-serine proteinase complexes.

k_{cat}/K_m for the release of kallidin from single-chain kininogen is also 14 times higher than in the peptide Pro-Phe-Arg-Ser-Val-Gln with the sequence around the crucial ARg bond in kininogen, indicating additional interactions in the cleavage of this bond, too. k_{cat} for the peptide, however, is 6 times higher than the rate of kallidin release. This high value achieved already by favourable interactions of the hexapeptide with the primary and adjacent secondary specificity sites of the enzyme allows to understand why cleavage of the Arg bond is not reflected in the kinetic constants of single-chain kininogen.

Modification of Arg-Residues of Kininogen

In an attempt to prepare Met-cleaved kininogen, single-chain kininogen was treated with bisacetyl/borate to reversibly modify Arg residues and thus to block cleavage of the Arg bond. However, this modification prevented also hydrolysis of the Met bond, as seen on SDS electrophoresis. Kininogen had not been irreversibly damaged, as kallidin could be released again after deblocking of Arg.

The experiment points out the importance of some Arg residue(s) of kininogen for a successful attack of tissue kallikrein at the Met bond. However, it does not allow to decide whether one of the Arg residues of the kinin moiety is involved or whether Arg in other parts of the kininogen molecule is of importance for the formation of the enzyme-substrate complex.

REFERENCES

1. E. Habermann, Strukturaufklärung kininliefernder Peptide aus Rinderserum-Kininogen, Arch. Exp. Path. Pharmak., 253:474-483 (1966).
2. Y. N. Han, H. Kato, S. Iwanaga, and T. Suzuki, Bovine plasma high molecular weight kininogen: The amino acid sequence of fragment 1 (glycopeptide) released by the action of plasma kallikrein and its location in the precursor protein, FEBS Lett., 63:197-200 (1976).
3. F. Fiedler and G. Leysath, Substrate specificity of porcine pancreatic kallikrein, Adv. Exp. Med. Biol., 120A:261-271 (1979).
4. F. Fiedler, Enzymology of porcine tissue kallikrein, Adv. Exp. Med. Biol., 156A:263-274 (1983).
5. F. Fiedler, E. Fink, H. Tschesche, and H. Fritz, Porcine glandular kallikreins, Methods Enzymol., 80:493-532 (1981).
6. C. Kutzbach and G. Schmidt-Kastner, Kallikrein from pig pancreas: Purification, separation of components A and B, and crystallization, Hoppe-Seyler's Z. Physiol. Chem., 353:1099-1106 (1972).
7. M. Komiya, H. Kato, and T. Suzuki, Bovine plasma kininogens. I. Further purification of high molecular weight kininogen and its physiocochemical properties, J. Biochem. (Tokyo), 76:811-822 (1974).
8. T. Shimada, T. Sugo, H. Kato, and S. Iwanaga, A method for preparation of a single chain high-molecular-weight (HMW) kininogen from bovine plasma, J. Biochem. (Tokyo), 92:679-688 (1982).
9. K. Weber and M. Osborn, The reliability of molecular weight determinations by dodecyl sulfate-polyacrylamide gel electrophoresis, J. Biol. Chem., 244:4406-4412 (1969).

10. W. Müller-Esterl, G. Rauth, H. Fritz, F. Lottspeich, and A. Henschen, Human kininogens, in: "Kininogenases-Kallikrein 6," G. L. Haberland, J. W. Rohen, H. Fritz, and P. Huber, eds., F. K. Schattauer Verlag (1983).
11. K. Mori, W. Sakamoto, and S. Nagasawa, Studies on human high molecular weight (HMW) kininogen. III. Cleavage of HMW kininogen by the action of human salivary kallikrein, J. Biochem. (Tokyo), 90:503-509 (1981).
12. E. S. Prado, C. A. M. Sampaio, M. S. Araujo-Viel, and R. C. R. Stella, Characterization of horse urinary kallikrein, in: "Recent Progress on Kinins (Agents and Actions Supplements 9)," H. Fritz, G. Dietze, F. Fiedler, and G. L. Haberland, eds., Birkhäuser Verlag (1982).
13. J. V. Pierce and J. A. Guimaraes, Further characterization of highly purified human plasma kininogens, in: "Chemistry and Biology of the Kallikrein-Kinin System in Health and Disease," J. J. Pisano and K. F. Austen, eds., U. S. Government Printing Office, without year (1976).
14. M. Maier, K. F. Austen, and J. Spragg, Kinetic analysis of the interaction of human tissue kallikrein with single-chain human high and low molecular weight kininogens, Biochemistry, 80:3928-3932 (1983).

THE TISSUE KALLIKREIN-KININ SYSTEM IN HUMAN SEMINAL PLASMA -

BIOCHEMICAL AND FUNCTIONAL ASPECTS

Edwin Fink, Wolf-Bernhard Schill*, Franz Fiedler,
Kazuaki Shimamoto**, Franz Krassnigg*, and Julian Frick+

Abteilung für Klinische Chemie und Klinische Biochemie in
der Chirurgischen Klinik Innenstadt der Universität
München, FRG. *Dermatologische Klinik und Poliklinik der
Ludwig-Maximilians Universität München, FRG   **The Second
Department of Internal Medicine, Sapporo Medical College,
Japan. +Urologische Abteilung, Landeskrankenhaus Salzburg,
Austria

SUMMARY

At least three species of tissue kallikrein-like antigens are present in human seminal plasma which differ in their molecular masses and
enzymatic activities. At least one of these species is a genuine tissue
kallikrein as judged by the criteria of molecular mass, immunoreactivity,
inhibition by aprotinin and non-inhibition by soybean trypsin inhibitor,
and the ability to release kallidin from kininogen. The prostatic gland
was identified as the origin of the seminal fluid tissue kallikrein first
by indirect studies and then by demonstrating the presence of immunoreactive
tissue kallikrein both in prostatic tissue and secretion.

INTRODUCTION

During the past ten years evidence has accumulated indicating the involvement of a kallikrein-kinin system in the regulation of sperm number
and sperm motility (reviewed in 1,2). The occurrence of kininogens, the
kininogenase acrosin and kininases in human seminal fluid has been described by Palm et al.[3] Later on, the presence of immunoreactive tissue kallikrein was detected by radioimmunoassays in porcine and human seminal
plasma[4,5].

METHODS

Radioimmunoassays

Human tissue kallikrein was determined by a direct radioimmunoassay
for human urinary kallikrein. The assay conditions were identical to
those described in[6]. The radioummunoassay for kinins was similar to that
described in [7].

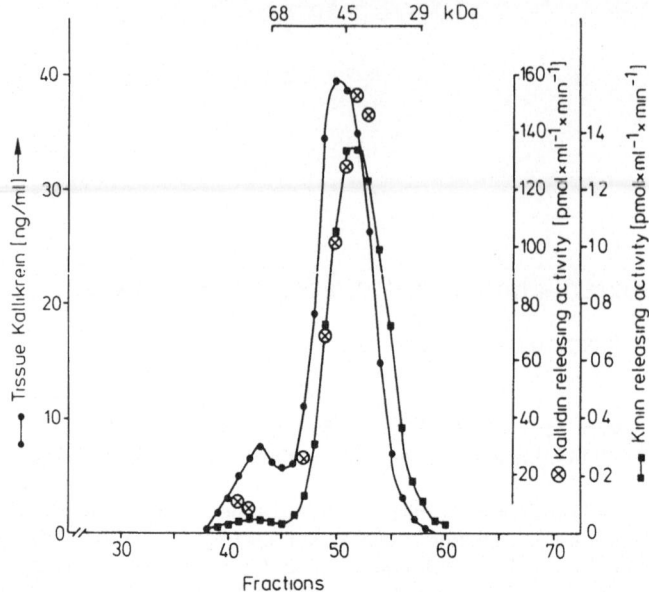

Fig. 1   Gel filtration of a sample of human seminal plasma.   The
fractions were analyzed for immunoreactive tissue kallikrein
and kininogenase activity (by methods A and B.).

Gel Filtration

Samples of seminal plasma were subjected to gel filtration on Ultro-
gel AcA 44 (LKB-Instruments) as described previously[8,9,10].   The eluted
fractions were analyzed for immunoreactive tissue kallikrein by the direct
radioimmunoassay and for kininogenase activity.

Kininogenase Activity

Kininogenase activity was determined by two methods.   Method A.:   The
sample was incubated with dog kininogen[11] in 0.1 M NaH_2PO_4, 0.003 M o-
phenanthroline, 0.03 M EDTA, pH 8.5 for 30 min at 37°C.   After ethanol

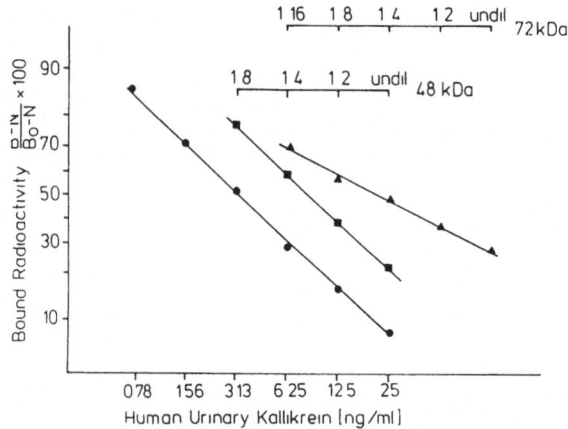

Fig. 2   Radioimmunoassay standard curve with human urinary kallikrein and
dose-response curves of the 48 and 72-80 kDa peaks (Fig. 1) of
immunoreactive tissue kallikrein of human seminal plasma.

extraction the released kinin was determined by radioimmunoassay.
Method B: The sample was incubated with highly purified bovine high molecular mass kininogen and the released kinin was identified and quantified by reversed phase high performance liquid chromatography[12].

Specimen Collection

Samples of semen and split ejaculates were obtained as described in (8,9,10). Specimens of prostatic tissue were obtained during surgery for hypertrophy or carcinoma of the prostate. The tissue was homogenized in 0.9% saline (2 ml per 1 g wet tissue) for 60 sec and centrifuged for 60 min at 1500 g. The supernatant was analyzed by the direct radioimmunoassay for human urinary kallikrein.

RESULTS

Characterization of Tissue Kallikrein in Seminal Plasma

When samples of seminal plasma were subjected to gel filtration (Fig. 1) and the eluted fractions analyzed by a radioimmunoassay for human urinary kallikrein, two peaks of immunoreactive tissue kallikrein were detected. The elution positions of these peaks corresponded to molecular masses of 48 and 72 - 80 kDa. Judged by these molecular masses the 48 kDa peak should represent free tissue kallikrein, whereas the second peak might be the complex of tissue kallikrein with α 1-proteinase inhibitor or another tissue kallikrein-binding protein.

The two forms of immunoreactive tissue kallikrein behave differently in the radioimmunoassay. Dose-response curves of the 48 kDa form parellel the calibration curve obtained with human urinary kallikrein as standard, whereas dose-response curves of the form with 72 - 80 kDa have a significantly different slope (Fig. 2). This finding might explain the often observed incomplete parallelity of dose-response curves of seminal plasma[8,9] since seminal plasma samples contain both forms in varying ratios.

Fractions 26 - 70 (Fig. 1) were analyzed for kininogenase activity by method A. Only about four percent of the total eluted activity were found in the 72-80 kDa peak. Whether this activity is intrinsic or due to dissociation of the (assumed) complex is unclear at present.

The elution position of the main peak of kininogenase activity is slightly but clearly different from that of the main peak of immunoreactivity: the maximum of the kininogenase peak corresponds to about 44 kDa. This finding indicates that the 48 kDa peak contains at least two different forms of the enzyme which differ in their specific activities and in their apparent molecular masses. Possibly the peak contains prokallikrein or a complex of tissue kallikrein with a low molecular mass inhibitor in addition to active tissue kallikrein. Attempts to activate the assumed inactive form by trypsin treatment were not successful.

The kininogenase activity could not be inhibited by soybean trypsin inhibitor, but was abolished by aprotinin.

The kininogenase activity of single, selected fractions was also determined by method B (Fig. 1). The released kinin was identified as kallidin which is typical for most tissue kallikreins.

Origin of Seminal Plasma Tissue Kallikrein

Our first approach to identify the origin of the tissue kallikrein in seminal plasma was by the split ejaculate technique[8,9,10]. When ejaculate is collected in two fractions, the first fraction contains mainly the secretions of the epididymides and the prostate gland, the second fraction mainly the secretion of the seminal vesicle. Extending our earlier studies[8], we investigated eleven split ejaculates. The first fraction contained 69.6 $\pm$ 2.1%, the second fraction 30.4 $\pm$ 2.1% (mean $\pm$ SEM) of the total tissue kallikrein in both fractions. Therefore, at least most of the tissue kallikrein should be secreted by the prostate gland or the epididymides or by both.

Table 1. Concentration of Immunoreactive Tissue Kallikrein in Human Seminal Plasma before and after Vasectomy (n = 13).

	Before vasectomy	After vasectomy
Mean $\pm$ SEM	113 $\pm$ 30 ng/ml	107 $\pm$ 23 ng/ml
Range	16 -344 ng/ml	12 - 293 ng/ml

To distinguish between these possibilities we also studied seminal plasma samples of men who underwent vasectomy. If the tissue kallikrein originated mainly from the epididymides the tissue kallikrein concentration should be significantly lower after vasectomy. The concentration of immunoreactive tissue kallikrein was determined in the seminal plasma of thirteen men before and several weeks after vasectomy. No significant decrease of the tissue kallikrein concentration was found after vasectomy (Table 1) indicating that the epididymides do not contribute a significant amount - if any at all - to the tissue kallikrein in seminal plasma. Thus, taking into account the study by the split ejaculate technique, this result suggests strongly that the prostate gland is the origin of the seminal plasma tissue kallikrein.

This conclusion was confirmed by a more direct approach. The tissue kallikrein concentrations in samples of prostatic tissue and of prostatic secretion were determined by radioimmunoassay (Tab. 2). In both kinds of samples the tissue kallikrein concentrations varied in a wide range. However, the results clearly demonstrate that the prostate contains and secretes tissue kallikrein.

Table 2. Concentrations of Immunoreactive Tissue Kallikrein in Human Prostate Tissue and Secretion.

	Tissue	Secretion
Number	12	15
Mean $\pm$ SEM	57 $\pm$ 13 ng/g	609 $\pm$ 136 ng/ml
Range	6 -135 ng/g	50 -2779 ng/ml

DISCUSSION

The first evidence for a kallikrein-like enzyme in male reproductive organs was presented by Bhoola et al.[13]. The authors found a potent kininogenase particularly in the coagulation gland, but also in the prostate gland of the guinea pig. In contrast, they could not detect kininogenase activity in the coagulation gland of the rat and the prostate gland of rat, rabbit, dog and man. The presence of a kininogenase in human seminal plasma was suggested by Suominen[14,15]. The author demonstrated the presence of an arginine esterase in human seminal plasma which - like kallikreins - increased vascular permeability when injected intracutaneously. However, contrary to other tissue kallikreins and to our results, this arginine esterase was inhibited by soybean trypsin inhibitor[15].

Recently immunoreactive tissue kallikrein has been detected by direct radioimmunoassays in porcine[4] and human[5] seminal plasma. Subsequently, a preparation of an active enzyme was isolated from human seminal plasma by immunoaffinity chromatography with antibodies to human urinary kallikrein[16]. The properties of this enzyme were similar to those of human urinary kallikrein.

By employing a radioimmunoassay for human urinary kallikrein the concentration of immunoreactive tissue kallikrein in 156 seminal plasma samples of ejaculates with different semen quality was estimated[8,9]. The mean concentration was 62 ng/ml and the range 9 - 380 ng/ml, for samples of normozoospermic ejaculates (n = 20) the mean concentration was 43 ng/ml and the range 14 - 145 ng/ml.

The studies presented here demonstrate that several species of immunoreactive tissue kallikrein are present in seminal plasma. One of these species is an active tissue kallikrein as judged by immunoreactivity, molecular mass, kallidin-releasing activity and by the fact that the activity can be inhibited by aprotinin but not by soybean trypsin inhibitor. The other form(s) of immunoreactive tissue kallikrein in the 48 kDa peak (Fig. 1) may represent immunologically crossreacting protein(s) different from tissue kallikrein or the complex of tissue kallikrein with a low molecular mass inhibitor or the zymogen of tissue kallikrein.

The tissue kallikrein present in seminal plasma may originate from the epididymides, the prostate gland or the seminal vesicles. Our first studies on the origin by the ejaculate technique[9] indicated that the epididymides or/and the prostate gland secrete the tissue kallikrein. The additional studies in men who underwent vasectomy and the more direct approach to determine the tissue kallikrein concentration in prostate tissue and prostate tissue and prostate secretion show beyond doubt that the prostate gland contains and secretes (immunoreactive) tissue kallikrein.

Considering the concentrations of tissue kallikrein in seminal plasma [8,9] and in prostatic secretion, and taking into account that prostatic secretion is in the ejaculate about fivefold diluted, it seems highly probable that all the immunoreactive seminal plasma tissue kallikrein originates from the prostate gland.

The prostatic origin of the human seminal plasma tissue kallikrein is in agreement with the recent finding that the dog prostate synthesizes a proteolytic enzyme with arginine-esterase activity which belongs to the kallikrein family[18].

ACKNOWLEGEMENTS

This research was supported by the Deutsche Forschungsgemeinschaft, SFB 0207, LP 19 and LP 20. The skillful technical assistance of Mrs. G. Godec and Mrs. C. Hirschauer is particularly acknowledged.

REFERENCES

1. Johnson, A.R.: Effects of kinins on organ systems. In: Handbook of Exp. Pharmacol., Vol. 25 Suppl., Ed. by E.G. Erdos. Springer-Verlag pp. 357-399 (1979).
2. Schill, W.-B.: Kinin-releasing pancreatic proteinase kallikrein. In: Treatment of Male Infertility, ed. by J. Bain, W.-B. Schill and L. Schwarzstein. Springer-Verlag pp. 125-142 (1982).
3. Palm, S., Schill, W.-B. Wallner, O., Prinzen, R. and Fritz, H.: Occurrence of components of the kallikrein-kinin system in human genital tract secretions and their possible function in stimulation of sperm motility and migration. In: Kinins. Pharmacodynamics and Biological Roles, ed. by F. Sicuteri, N. Back and G.L. Haberland. Plenum Press pp. 271-279 (1976).
4. Fink, E., Seifert, J., Geiger, R. and Güttel, C.: Studies on the physiological function of glandular kallikrein by radioimmunoassay. In: Current Concepts in Kinin Research, ed. by G.L. Haberland and U. Hamberg. Pergamon Press pp. 111-119 (1979).
5. Mann, K., Göring, W., Lipp, W., Keipert, B., Karl, H.J., Geiger, R., Fink, E.: Radioimmunoassay of human urinary kallikrein. J. Clin. Chem. Clin. Biochem. 18: 395-401 (1980).
6. Fink, E., and Güttel, C.: Development of a radioimmunoassay for pig pancreatic kallikrein. J. Clin. Chem. Clin. Biochem. 16: 381-385 (1978).
7. Shimamoto, K., Ando, T., Tanaka, S., Nakahashi, Y., Nishitani, T., Hosoda, S., Ishida, H., and Iimura, O.: An improved method for the determination of human blood kinin levels by sensitive kinin radio-immunoassay. Endocrinol. Japon. 29: 487-494, (1982).
8. Fink, E. and Schill, W.-B.: Tissue kallikrein in human seminal plasma. In: Kinins III, ed. by H. Fritz, N. Back, G. Dietze and G.L. Haberland. Plenum Press pp. 1175-1180 (1983).
9. Fink, E. and Schill, W.-B.: Studies on tissue kallikrein in human seminal plasma. In: Kininogenases. Kallikrein. Vol. 6, ed. by G.L. Haberland, J.W. Rohen, H. Fritz, and P. Huber. Schattauer Verlag pp. 147-154 (1983).
10. Fink, E., Schill, W.-B. and Fiedler, F.: Tissue kallikrein in human seminal fluid. In: Protides of the Biological Fluids. XXXIInd Colloquium, ed. by H. Peeters. Pergamon Press, in press.
11. Marin-Grez, M. and Carretero, O.A.: A method for measurement of urinary kallikrein. J. Appl. Physiol. 32: 428-431 (1972).
12. Fiedler, F., Hinz, H. and Lottspeich, F.: Individual reaction steps in the release of kallidin from kininogen by tissue kallikrein. (This volume).
13. Bhoola, K.D., May May Yi, R., Morley, J. and Schachter, M.: Release of kinin by an enzyme in the accessory sex glands of the guinea-pig. J. Physiol. 163: 269-280 (1962).
14. Suominen, J.J.O. and Niemi, M.: Influence of human seminal proteases on vascular permeability. Nature New Biol. 232: 90-91 (1971).
15. Suominen, J.J.O.: Properties of kallikrein-like enzyme and plasminogen activators of human seminal plasma. In: Conference Proc. VI Mott Center Symposium. Techniques of Human Andrology. Ed. by E.S.E. Hafez. Elsevier, Amsterdam, abstract 20 (1976).
16. Geiger, R. and Clausnitzer, B.: Isolation of enzymatically active tissue kallikrein from human seminal plasma by immunoaffinity

chromatography. Hoppe-Seyler's Z. Physiol. Chem. 362: 1279-1283 (1981).

17. Schill, W.-B., Krassnigg, F., Müller-Esterl, W. and Fink, E.: Quantitative determination of different proteins in normal and pathological semen. In: Protides of the Biological Fluids, ed. by H. Peeters. Pergamon Press, in press.

18. Lazure, C., Leduc, R., Seidah, N.G., Chretien, M., Dube, J.Y., Chapdelaine, P., Frenette, G., Paquin, R. and Tremblay, R.R.: The major androgen-dependent protease in dog prostate belongs to the kallikrein family: confirmation by partial amino acid seqencing. FEBS Letters 175: 1-7 (1984).

NEW SYNTHETIC SUBSTRATE FOR KALLIKREIN AND ITS APPLICATION

Setsuro Fujii*, Yuji Hitomi*, Kenjiro Kimura**, Masao Ishii**,
Masateru Kurumi*** and Takuo Aoyama***

*Division of Reguration of Macromolecular Function, Inst.
 for Protein Res., Osaka Univ., Suita, Osaka, Japan
**Second Dep. of Internal Med., Faculty of Medicine, Tokyo
 University, Tokyo, Japan
***Research Labs., Torii & Co., Ltd., Ichikawa, Chiba,
 Japan

SUMMARY

We developed a new synthetic substrate, Pro-Phe-Arg-α-naphthyl ester,
for kallikrein. We found that this substrate had higher specificity and
sensitivity for kallikrein and was applied for the preparation of zymogram
and for the histochemical demonstration.

With Pro-Phe-Arg-α-NE as substrate, the minimum detectable concentration of human urinary kallikrein was about 0.001 KU and then
kallikrein could be determined with 25 ul of human urine.

We also found the possibility that occurring of abnormalities during
pregnancy were predicted by the determination of urinary kallikrein of
pregnants.

Zymograms were prepared for various kinds of kallikrein using this
substrate.

The localization of kallikrein-like enzyme in rat kidneys was defined by the application this substrate for histochemistry.

Moreover, cytochemical demonstrations of leucocytes in human blood
were done using Ts-Lys-α-NE and Ac-Tyr-α-NE.

INTRODUCTION

In recent years, many synthetic oligopeptide substrates have been
developed by many researchers.[1] These substrates can be constructed to
simulate the active site directed fragments of the natural substrates.
When a sufficient degree of specificity toward an enzyme is built into a
synthetic substrate with a detector moiety attached and the amount of
synthetic substrate greatly exceeds the amount of the natural substrate, numerous proteases can be measured with specificity and accuracy.
However, use of most of these synthetic substrates is accompanied by

difficulties in qualitative analyses of proteases such as zymogram preparation, histochemical application and so on.

In this paper, we will report on new synthetic substrate L-prolyl-L-phenylalanyl-L-arginine- α-naphthyl ester for kallikrein and its application to sensitive colorimetric assay for human urinary kallikrein, zymogram preparation of kallikrein, histochemical demonstration of localization of kallikrein-like enzymes in rat kidneys and so on.

Furthermore, we will also report on the application of new - naphthyl ester substrates.

MATERIALS AND METHODS

Pro-Phe-Arg-α-naphthyl ester (Pro-Phe-Arg-α-NE), acetyl-Tyr-α-naphthyl ester (Ac-Tyr-α-NE) and tosyl-Lys-α-naphthyl ester (Ts-Lys-α-NE) were prepared in Research labs., Toril & Company, Lts., Tokyo, Japan. Various p-nitroanilide type substrates were purchased from KABI AB, Sweden. Leupeptin, chymostatin and tosyl arginine methyl ester (TAMe) were purchased from Protein Research Foundation, Osaka, Japan. Fast Violet B salt, Fast Red ITR salt, Fast Garnet GBC salt were purchased from Sigma Chemical Company, St. Louis, USA. Ampholine was purchased from LKB. Highly purified bovine α-thrombin and factor Xa were kindly provided by Dr. Iwanaga. Highly purified human plasmin and urokinase were prepared as described previously. Highly purified porcine plasma and pancreatic kallikreins were kindly supplied by Research Labs., Ono Pharmaceutical Co., Osaka, Japan. Highly purified human urinary kallikrein was kindly provided by Dr. Kato.

Enzyme assays: The incubation mixture consisted of substrate solution (0.1 ml) containing Pro-Phe-Arg-α-NE (1 mM), enzyme solution (0.1 ml) and buffer solution (50 mM sodium phosphate, pH 7.0) (0.8 ml) in a final volume of 1 ml. Incubation were carried out at 25° C for 30 min. The blank test was done by incubating a mixture of the buffer solution (0.9 ml) and substrate solution (0.1 ml). After incubation, 1% Fast Violet B salt (0.1 ml) was added to the mixture. The mixture was allowed to stand at 0°C for 30 min. Then, glacial acetic acid (1.0 ml) was added to it. Absorbance of the wine-color developed by the diazo-coupling reaction was measured at 515 nm.

Determination of human urinary kallikrein: The incubation mixture consisted of urine sample (0.1 ml) and buffer solution (50 mM sodium phosphate containing 0.03% SDS, pH 7.0) (1.0 ml). After incubation at 37°C for 5 min., the substrate solution (0.1 ml) containing Pro-Phe-Arg-α-NE (2 mM) was added to the mixture and the resulting mixture was incubated at 37°C for 30 min. The sample blank test was done by incubating a mixture of urine (0.1 ml), buffer solution (1.0 ml) and water (0.1 ml), and the reagent blank test was done by incubating a mixture of water (0.1 ml), buffer solution (1.0 ml) and substrate solution (0.1 ml). After incubation, 1% Fast Red ITR salt solution in 30% acetic acid (0.1 ml) was added to the mixture. The mixture was allowed to stand at 37°C for 5 min. Then, glacial acetic acid (1.0 ml) was added to it. Absorbance of color developed by diazo-coupling reaction was measured at 475 nm. Absorbance depending on urinary kallikrein was obtained as the difference between the complete system and corresponding blank tests. Urinary kallikrein activity was calculated from calibration curve depending on the absorbance.

Zymogram preparation: Polyacrylamide disc gel isoelectrophoresis
was carried out using ampholine of pH 3.5-5 at final concentration of 2%.
The electrodes were soaked in 0.1 M sodium hydrozide (cathode) and 0.1 M
phosphoric acid (anode). Samples of each 50 μl were applied to each disc
gel and isoelectrophoresis was carried out at 200 V for 4 hr. After
electrophoresis, each gel was washed in distilled water and equilibrated
with 0.25 M sodium phosphate buffer (pH 7.0) (12 ml) at 37°C for 5 min.
Then it was soaked in substrate buffer solution containing Pro-Phe-Arg-
α-NE (0.2 nM) and 0.1% Fast Violet B salt in 0.25 M sodium phosphate
buffer (pH 7.0) at 25° C for 30 min. Bands stained gradually during the
incubation.

Histochemical demonstration: After decaptation of rats, the kidneys
were immediately removed and cut sagitally to a thickness of about 2 mm.
The sections were embedded in OCT-compound and then were frozen rapidly
in dry-ice acetone. The sections were sliced to 6 microns thick by a
cryostat at -15°C. After a few minutes of fixation in cold acetone, the
sections were placed in the reaction mixture containing Pro-Phe-Arg-α-NE
(0.1 mg/ml), Fast Garnet GBC (0.6 mg/ml) and 0.2 M tris-HCl buffer solution (pH 6.8). After the reaction was completed, the sections were
washed in distilled water and mounted in glycerine jelly for microscopic
examination.

Cytochemical assays: Blood smears were air-dried for 60 min., and
then fixed in formalin vapor for 30 min. The fixed smears were washed in
water and incubated in substrate buffer solution containing 0.5 mM substrate and 0.1% Fast Violet B salt in 0.25 M sodium phosphate buffer
solution (pH 7.0) (100 ml). When the inhibitions were tested, they were
added into substrate buffer solution. During incubation at room
temperature for 60 min., the blood smears gradually became wine-color.
After incubation, the smears were washed in water and counter-stained with
1% methyl green in 50 mM acetate buffer (pH 4.0) at room temperature for
10 min. Non-specific esterase activities in human monocytes were demonstrated by using -naphthyl butyrate as substrate.

RESULTS

Hydrolysis of Pro-Phe-Arg-α-NE by Various Proteases: Hydrolysis
of Pro-Phe-Arg-α-NE by thrombin, factor XA, plasmin, three kinds of
kallikrein and urokinase were presented in Table 1. Among these
enzymes, three kinds of kallikrein showed higher specificities than the
other enzymes for this substrate.

Relative sensitivities of various substrates toward kallikreins:
The relative sensitivities of various substrates toward three kinds
of kallikrein were presented in Table 2. Hydrolytic activities of
enzymes on TAMe were determined by the hydroxamate method and pNA substrates were determined by the method of Svendsen et al. As results,
pNA substrates were about ten to twenty times more sensitive than TAMe
for three kinds of kallikrein. Furthermore, α-naphthyl ester was found
to be much more sensitive than pNA substrates for these kallikreins.

Effects of SDS on spontaneous hydrolysis of Pro-Phe-Arg-α-NE: Pro-
Phe-Arg-α-NE was rather unstable and hydrolyzed spontaneously above 30°C
or in weak alkali. The presence of SDS reduced this spontaneous
hydrolysis considerably. As shown in Figure 1, with increase of the
concentration of SDS, spontaneous hydrolysis decreased, but inhibition

Table 1. Hydrolysis of Pro-Phe-Arg-α-NE by Various Proteases

Δ O.D.

| Thrombin | Factor Xa | Plasmin | Kallikrein | | | Urokinase |
			Plasma	Pancreas	Urine	
0.30	0.05	0.23	0.80	0.70	0.75	N.D.

Enzyme: 2 x 10^{-9} M, N.D.: Not detectable

of the enzyme activity increased. Therefore, the enzyme assay was
carried out at final concentration of 0.03% SDS, which reduced spontaneous
hydrolysis considerably but did not inhibit the enzyme activity appreciably.

Hydrolysis of Pro-Phe-Arg-α-NE by Human Urinary Kallikrein: The
hydrolysis of Pro-Phe-Arg-α-NE by purified human urinary kallikrein and
human urine samples at various concentrations was presented in Figure 2.
These assays were done in the presence of SDS. Activities of human
urinary kallikrein and human urine could be measured with as little as
0.001 KU and 25 μl of urine, respectively.

Relationship Between Urinary Kallikrein Level and Abnormalities
During Pregnancy: Urinary kallikrein excretion in pregnants was presented

Table 2. Relative Sensitivities of Various Substrates Toward Three Kinds
of Kallikrein

| Substrates | Relative sensitivities of kallikrein | | |
	Plasma	Pancreas	Urine
Tos-Arg-methylester	1.0	1.0	1.0
D-Pro-Phe-Arg-pNA	19.5	12.6	10.4
D-Val-Leu-Arg-pNA	0.7	12.4	11.3
Pro-Phe-Arg-α-NE	118.6	101.1	109.4

Tos-Arg-methylester: Hydroxamate method

pNA substrates: Method by Svendsen et al.

302

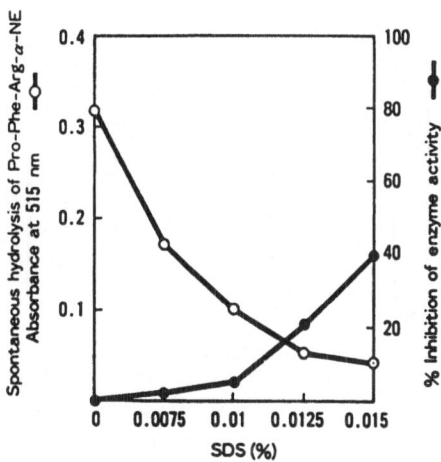

Figure 1. Effects of SDS on Spontaneous Hydrolysis of Pro-Phe-Arg-α-NE
and Kallikrein Activity

in Figure 3. In general, pregnants maintained high level excretion of
urinary kallikrein. As shown in Figure 3, the initial stage of
pregnancy, weeks 8-24, the urinary kallikrein level was high and
gradually decreased as pregnancy weeks passed. In Table 3, the data
obtained in 610 subjects who had normal blood pressure in the diagnosis
made at weeks 12-30 of pregnancy is shown. Among these 610 subjects,
however, 60 subjects were found to show low level excretion of urinary
kallikrein. In other words, these 60 subjects had normal blood
pressure and low level excretion of urinary kallikrein. And, thus, these
60 pregnants were further subjected to the follow-up study.

Other than 610 pregnants shown in Figure 3, there were 20 pregnants
who showed hypertension or gestosis already in the diagnosis made at
weeks 12-30 of pregnancy. In these pregnants, the urinary kallikrein
excretion was found to be low as shown in Table 3.

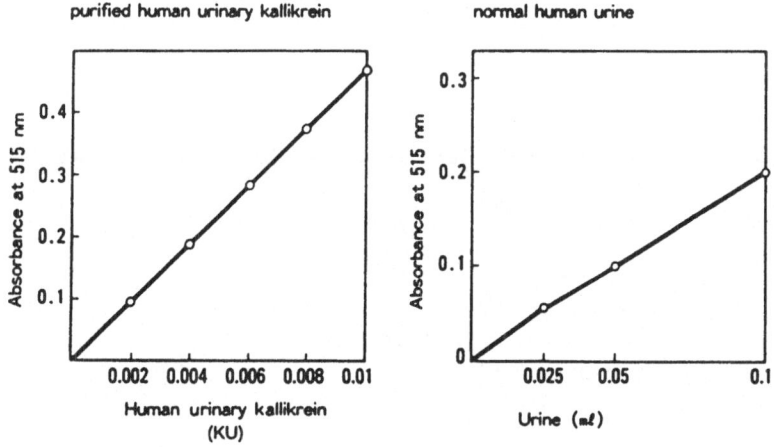

Figure 2. Hydrolysis of Pro-Phe-Arg-α-NE by Purified Human Urinary
Kallikrein and Normal Human Urine

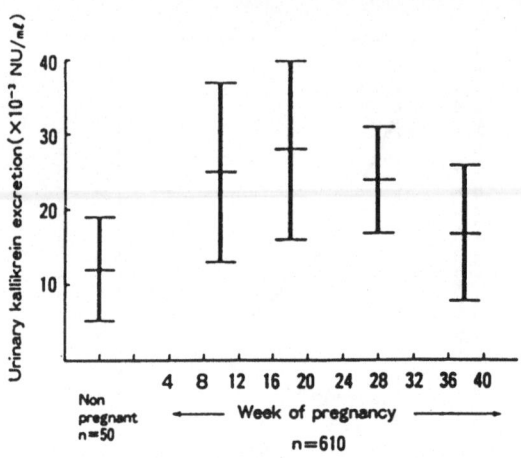

Figure 3. Urinary Kallikrein Excretion in Pregnants
(M. Seito et al., Hirosaki University)

As mentioned, these 610 normotensive pregnants were divided into 2 groups, that is 550 pregnants having normal blood pressure and high level of urinary kallikrein excretion, and 60 pregnants having normal blood pressure but low excretion of urinary kallikrein. Among these 60 pregnants, in the diagnosis made at week 12-30 of pregnancy, 44 pregnants were found to have or have had some abnormalities such as hereditary hypertensive diathesis, anemia, threatening abortion, premature labor and so on. The remaining 16 pregnants were found to be normal.

Prognosis of these 60 subjects after week 32 are shown in Table 4 on the right. Gestosis, anemia and premature labor occurred at high rate in these 60 subjects, particularly in 16 pregnants.

Zymogram Preparation: Zymogram preparation was done using Pro-Phe-Arg-α-NE as a substrate on polyacrylamide disc gel isoelectrophresis As the result, in the case of human urinary kallikrein, there are 6 kinds of multiform, in the case of hog pancreatic kallikrein, three bands and in the case of hog plasma kallikrein, 7 bands.

Table 3. Urinary Kallikrein (UK) Level and Blood Pressure at Week 16-32 of Pregnancy

	n	Blood Pressure (mmHg)	UK level $(x\ 10^{-3}\ NU/ml)$
Pregnants with Gestosis	20	≥140 (systolic > 90 (diastolic)	9.6 4.5
Normo-tensive pregnants	610	──	28.0 12.0 (w 13-24) 24.0 6.7 (w 25-32)

Table 4. Follow-up Study: 610 Normotensive Pregnants

n	at W 16-32			Follow-up after W 32
	UK level (X 10^{-3} NU/ml)	Diagnosis and Anamnesis		
550	>10.0	NO abnormality		———
60	<10.0	Hereditary hypertensive diathesis	16	Gestosis 11(5):18% (31%)
		Anemia	11	Anemia 11(5):18% (31%)
		Threatened abortion and premature labor	10	Premature labor 6(1):10% (6%)
		Diabetes mellitus	5	—————————————
		Heart disease	5	( ): among 16 pregnants without abnormality in diagnosis at W 16-32
		Others	12	
		—————————————		
		No abnormality	16	

(M. Saito, et al., Hirosaki University)

Histochemical Demonstration of Kallikrein-like Enzyme in Rat Kidneys: The localization of kallikrein-like enzyme in rat kidneys was demonstrated. The results are shown in Figure 4. The enzyme activity was located in the cytoplasm of the renal tubles and frequently increased in the liminal part of the cells. No definite identification of the different tubular segments was possible in histochemical sections.

Cytochemical Demonstration of Proteases in Human Blood Cells: The cytochemical demonstration of proteases in human peripheral blood cells was tried by use of new α-naphthyl ester substrates. A summary of cytochemical studies was shown in Table 5.

With both substrates, Ts-Lys-α-NE and Ac-Tyr-α-NE, neutrophils strongly stained a wine-color, while other cells stained not at all or weakly. It was not clear whether the cytoplasm or granules in the cells were staining. With α-naphthyl butyrate as substrate for nonspecific esterase, only monocytes were stained.

Incidentially, we also examined the effects of protease inhibitors on cytochemical demonstration of proteases in neutrophils with Ts-Lys-α-NE or Ac-Tyr-α-NE or Ac-Try-α-NE as substrates. As a result, Ts-Lys-α-NE and Ac-Try-α-NE hydrolytic activities of neutrophils were completely inhibited by DFP and chymostatin, but not by leupeptin or iodoacetate as shown in Table 6.

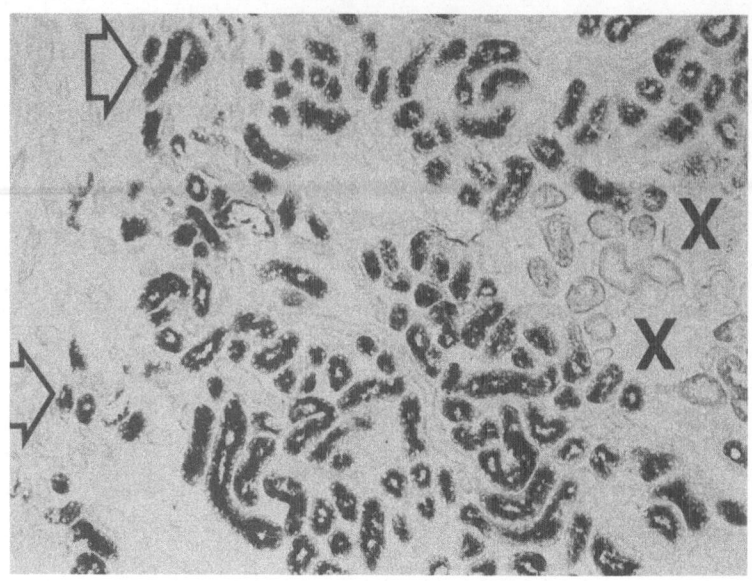

Figure 4. "X" indicates juxtamedullary glomeruli and open arrows indicate the lower boundary of enzyme activity.

DISCUSSION

In Table 7, the main synthetic substrates for kallikrein are summarized. p-Nitroanilide type substrates were developed by Svendsen et al. in 1972. By using these substrates, absorbance at 405 nm of p-nitroaniline liberated from enzyme-substrate reaction was determined. MCA and AIE type substrates were assayed fluorometrically. For these substrates, pNA substrates showed moderate sensitivity and MCA and AIE substrates showed high sensitivity.

Table 5. Cytochemical Demonstrations of Protease in Human Peripheral Blood Cells by use of New α–naphthyl Ester Substrates

Cell population	Substrate		
	Tos–Lys–α–NE	Ac–Try–α–NE	α–Naphthyl-butyrate
Lumphocytes	–	–	–
Eosinophilic granu-locytes	–	–	–
Neutrophilic granu-locytes	+++	+++	–
Basophilic granulocytes	±∿+	±∿+	–
Monocytes	±∿+	±∿+	+++

Key: –: no activity; ±:questionable; +:weak, ++:moderate, +++:strong

Table 6. Effects of Various Inhibitors on Cytochemical Demonstration of Normal Human Neutrophilic Granulocytes

Inhibitor	Substrate	
	TLNE	ATNE
DFP	+	+
Leupeptin	−	−
Chymostatin	+	+
Iodoacetate	−	−

Key: + = inhibition, − = not inhibition

Pro-Phe-Arg-α-NE was developed by us as a new synthetic substrate for kallikrein.[2] Colorization of this substrate is based upon the diazo-coupling reaction of -naphthol released from the substrate by enzyme reaction with diazonium salt. Advantages of this substrate are easy preparation of zymogram and sensitive colorimetric assay of enzymes.[3]

Recently, we studied development of the human urinary kallikrein assay set, the so-called Naphtest UK, using Pro-Phe-Arg-α-NE as a substrate.

Table 7. Synthetic Substrates for Kallikrein and Their Properties

Substrate	Principle of assay method	Sensitivity	Zymogram and Histochemical application
D-Val-Leu-Arg-pNA	Colorimetric assay		
D-Pro-Phe-Arg-pNA		Moderate	Difficult
Bz-Pro-Phe-Arg-pNA	O.D. 405 nm		
Pro-Phe-Arg-MCA	Fluorometric assay		
Z-Phe-Arg-MCA		High	Difficult
Bz-Ser-Pro-Phe-Arg-AIE	Ex: 380 nm; Ex. 335 nm; Em. 460 nm Em. 430 nm		
Pro-Phe-Arg-α-NE	Colorimetric assay O.D. 515nm + FVB or (+AcOH) FRITR	High	Easy

At present, this set is subjected to a study of relationship between high blood pressure and urinary kallikrein level.[4] As one of studies, very interesting finding has been so far obtained on abnormal pregnancy, particularly, gestosis and lowered excretion of urinary kallikrein. The results are shown in Tables 3 and 4, and indicate that measurement of urinary kallikrein is quite worthwhile as the diagnosis for prediction of abnormality such as gestosis, anemia and premature labor at pregnancy, especially in the later stages.

Applications of this substrate for zymogram preparation and histochemical demonstration were studied. Preparation of zymogram was easily done as described above. Histochemical demonstration using this substrate was applied to a study of localization of kallikrein-like enzyme in rat kidneys.[5] As can be seen in Figure 4, it was defined that this substrate could be applied for histochemical field.

The cytochemical differentiation of human blood cells by the demonstration of proteases was studied with Ts-Lys-α-NE and Ac-Tyr-α-NE as substrates.[6] Neutrophils stained strongly with both substrates as shown in Table 5, and their hydrolytic activities were inhibited completely by DFP and chymostatin as shown in Table 6. Chymostatin is a strong inhibitor of chymotrypsin-like proteases, as shown by Umezawa et al. However, neutrophils were not stained with α-naphthyl butyrate, a substrate for non-specific esterase as shown in Table 5. These facts suggest that chymotrypsin-like enzyme(s) exist in neutrophils.

From the results of these studies, new α-naphthyl ester derivatives were found to be very useful synthetic substrates for biochemical, histochemical, cytochemical and clinical studies for kallikrein and other proteases. And we are presently studying the application of these substrates for diagnosis.

REFERENCES

1. R. M. Houseby and R. E. Smith, Synthetic oligopeptide substrates: Their diagnostic application in blood coagulation, fibrinolysis, and other pathologic state, Semi. Thrombo. Haemo., 6, 175-314,(1980).
2. Y. Hitomi, M. Niinobe, and S. Fujii, A sensitive colorimetric assay for human urinary kallikrein, Clin. Chim. Acta, 100, 275-283, (1980).
3. M. Niinobe, Y. Hitomi, and S. Fujii, A sensitive colorimetric assay for various proteases using naphthyl ester derivatives as substrates, J. Biochem., 87, 779-783, (1980).
4. M. Saito, S. Munakata, I. Sada, Y. Nishimura, Y. Nakamura, Y. Nomura, and N. Shinagawa, Changes of urinary kallikrein levels during pregnancy, Sanfujinka no Sekai (in Japanese), 36, 173-176, (1983).
5. K. Kimura, M. Takagi, T. Igari, M. Ishii, T. Ikeda, T. Takeda, and S. Murano, Histochemical localization of kallikrein-like Pro-Phe-Arg-naphthyl ester esterase activity in the rat kidney, Histochem., 75, 91-98, (1982).
6. T. Honda, Y. Hitomi, M. Niinobe, and S. Fujii, Cytochemical demonstrations of protease in human peripheral blood cells by use of new α-naphthyl ester derivatives, Histochem., 77, 299-302, (1983).

PLASMA HALF-LIFE AND ORGAN UPTAKE RATIO OF RADIOLABELED GLANDULAR KALLIKREIN

IN CONTROL AND NEPHRECTOMIZED RATS

Kazutaka Nishimura, Takeru Iwata and Tatsuo Kokubu

The 2nd Department of Internal Medicine, Ehime University
School of Medicine, Shigenobu, Ehime 791-02, Japan

SUMMARY

The purified rat urinary kallikrein was radiolabeled by lactoperoxidase method and by chloramine T method. Plasma half-life of radiolabeled kallikrein was 5.06 ± 0.59 (n=5) min in control rats and 5.24 ± 0.42 (n=5) min in nephrectomized rats. There was no difference between two groups. From autoradiogram, main metabolic organs of radiolabeled kallikrein were liver, kidney and spleen. Total uptake of radiolabeled kallikrein in ech organ was the highest in liver (73.2%). The uptake per g tissue of radiolabeled kallikrein in each organ was high in liver (33.0%), kidney (31.4%) and spleen (21.1%). These results suggest that the active kallikrein is metabolized mainly in the liver, and kidney is not so an important organ to metabolize or to eliminate the active kallikrein in plasma.

In order to clarify the mode of existence of active kallikrein in plasma, the following experiment was done by using disc gel eclectrophoresis. Radioactive profile of radiolabeled kallikrein showed one peak (Rf=1.0), but radiolabeled kallikrein mixed with rat plasma showed two peaks, that is small peak (Rf=1.0), and main peak (RF=0.5). The most of radiolabeled kallikrein was bound to plasma protein and only five per cent was in free form. Furthermore, the binding of radiolabeled kallikrein to plasma protein was interfered by the addition of active kallikrein. These results suggest the possibility of existence of kallikrein binding protein in plasma.

INTRODUCTION

Glandular kallikrein exists in some tissues, such as kidney, pancreas, salivary gland, intestine, etc.[1-3] It is an enzyme that liberates a kinin from kininogen and is suggested to control electrolyte balance in situ, and also, to regulate the local blood flow.[4]

Roblero et al.[5] reported that renal kallikrein is secreted into the bloodstream. Ferreira and Smaje[6] also reported salivary glandular kallikrein is secreted into the bloodstream. These reports suggest that the glandular kallikrein-kinin system in plasma may participate in controlling the systemic blood pressure.

We[7] and Geiger et al.[8] reported the existence of active glandular kalli-krein in plasma. For the investigation of the physiological importance of active kallikrein in plasma, it is necessry to know the fte of glandular kallikrein in plasma. In this report, we mesured plasma half-life and organ uptake ratio of radiolabeled glandular kallikrein in control and nephrecto-mized rats.

MATERIALS

Na ^{125}I was purchased from New England Nuclear (Boston). Enzymobead reagent which consists of immobilized preparation of lactoperoxidase was obtained from Bio-Rad Laboratories (California). Chloramine T and carboxy-methyl cellulose were from Nakarai Chemicals Ltd. (Kyoto, Japan).

METHODS

Radiolabeling of Rat Urinary Kallikrein

(a) Lactoperoxidase method: The rat urinary kallikrein was labeled according to the modified method of Miyachi et al.[9] Five microliters (1.5 µg of the purified rat urinary kallikrein in 0.01 M citrated phosphate buffer, pH 5.0) was mixed with 50 µl of enzymobead reagent in 0.4 M sodium acetate buffer, pH 5.6 and 2 µl (0.2 mCi) of Na ^{125}I. Ten microliters of 0.3% H_2O_2 was added and incubated for 2 min at room temperature. Then, the reaction ws stopped by the addition of 100 µl of 1% NaN_3 and 100 µl of 1% bovine serum albumin in 0.01 M phosphate buffered saline was added. The labeled protein was separated from free iodine by Sephadex G-25 column (1 x 16 cm) and excluded dimer using Ultragel AcA 44 column chromatography (1.6 x 82 cm). Total counts were 9.3 µCi and the specific activity of the labeled protein ws 12.4 µCi per µg.

(b) Chloramine T method: The rat urinary kallikrein was labeled ac-cording to the modified method of Hunter and Greenwood.[10] The labeled protein was separated with the same methods described above. The specific activity of the labeled protein was 15.0 µCi per µg.

Experimental Protocol

Wister male rats were anesthetized with sodium pentobarbital (40 mg per kg) and two catheters were implanted in the inferior vena cava and left carotid artery. Heparin (100 units) was injected through the inferior vena cava catheter. A pulse injection of radiolabeled kallikrein in lactoperoxi-dase method was given into the inferior vena cava and blood sample (0.1-0.3 ml) was withdrawn from the carotid artery at 0, 3, 6, 10, 20 min for measurement of radiolabeled kallikrein in blood. At the end of the experi-ment, each organ (liver, kidney, spleen, lung, heart) was removed and weighed. 0.5-1 g of tissue was cut off from each organ and its radioactivity was counted. The experiment was done, using control and nephrectomized rats.

Autoradiography

The radiolabeled kallikrein in chloramine T method (6.0 x 10[7] cpm per ml in PBS) was injected into the inferior vena cava. The rat was killed after 20 min by anesthetizing with sodium pentobarbital, embedding in a mixture of carboxymethyl cellulose and water and freezing in acetone cooled with solid CO_2. The embedded rat was sectioned in a microtome according to the method of Ullberg.[11] A series of 20 m thick whole-body sagittal sections were taken and the contents of radioactivity were analyzed by autoradiography,. The sections were attached to X-ray film (Industrex C Kodak) under light pressure. The exposure time was 1 month.

RESULTS AND DISCUSSION

(a) Half-life of radiolabeled kallikrein in blood.

Fig. 1 shows disappearance of radiolabeled kallikrein from blood after injection. Half-life of radiolabeled kallikrein in control rats was 5.06 ± 0.59 (n=5) and that in nephrectomized rats was 5.24 ± 0.42 (n=5), shown in Table 1. There is no difference of half-life between control and nephrectomized rats.

(b) Autoradiogram

A high radioactivity was present in liver, kidney and spleen, shown in Fig. 2.

(c) Uptake ratio of radiolabeled kallikrein in each organ.

Uptake ratio (%) of liver, lung, spleen, heart, kidney and urine in lactoperoxidase method was 73.2 ± 1.0, 2.6 ± 0.6, 2.8 ± 0.4, 1.0 ± 0.3, 15.2 ± 2.2 and 5.3 ± 1.5 (n=5), respectively. Uptake ratio per g tissue weight (%) of liver, lung, spleen, heart and kidney was 33.0 ± 0.9, 9.2 ± 1.8, 21.1 ± 1.5, 5.5 ± 2.0, 31.4 ± 4.0 (n=5), respectively.

(d) Analysis of radiolabeled kallikrein in plasma by disc gel electro-phoresis.

Fig. 3 shows radioactive profile of radiolabeled kallikrein. The most of radiolabeled kallikrein bounds to plasma protein and only five per cent was in free form. The binding of radiolabeled kallikrein to plasma protein was interfered by the addition of active non-labeled kallikrein. Our results show that the kidney is not the important organ to metabolize or to eliminate the kallikrein in plasma. Main metabolic organ of radiolabeled kallikrein was liver. Also, electrophoretic analysis of kallikrein in plasma shows

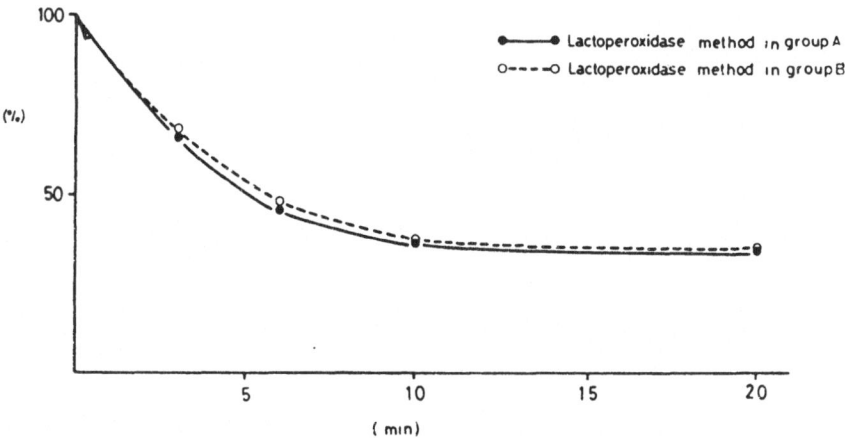

Fig. 1. Disappearance of radiolabeled kallikrein from blood. Group A: control rat, Group B: nephrectomized rat.

Table 1. Half-Life of Radiolabeled Kallikrein in Blood. Values are
Expressed in Minutes. Group A: Control Rat, Group B: Nephrectomized Rat.

Experiment	Exp. 1	Exp. 2	Exp. 3	Exp. 4	Exp. 5	mean ± SE
Group A	4.6	7.4	4.5	4.3	4.5	5.06 ± 0.59
Group B	4.7	6.0	6.5	4.5	4.5	5.24 ± 0.42

a high possibility of the existence of kallikrein specific binding protein
in plasma.

It is very important to point out that the glandular kallikrein exists
in plasma, has a short turnover and also, there is the kallikrein binding
protein in plasma. These suggest that the glandular kallikrein-kinin system
in blood may play an important role to control the systemic blood pressure,
coworking with renin-angiotensin system.

ACKNOWLEDGEMENT

We are very grateful to Mr. Morishige Tanaka and Miss Takako Miyoshi
for their excellent technical assistance.

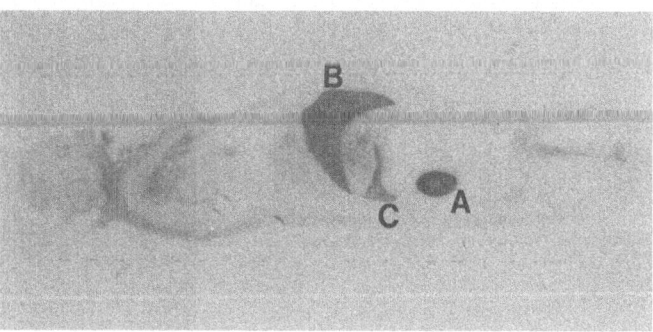

Fig. 2. Autoradiogram of radiolabeled kallikrein in chlormine T method
(6.0×10^7 cpm). A: kidney, B: liver, C: spleen.

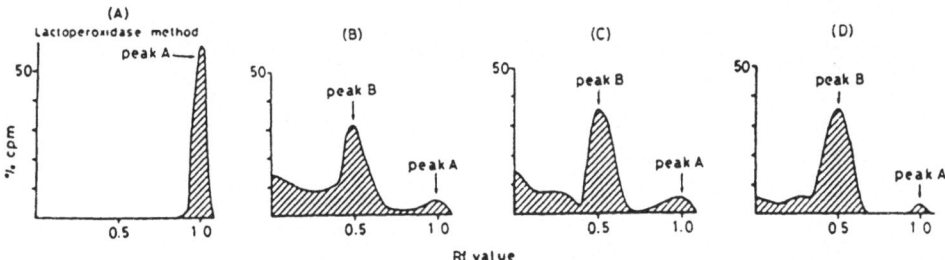

Fig. 3. Analysis of radiolabeled kallikrein in plasma by disc gel electrophoresis. (A) Radiolabeled kallikrein, (B) Radiolabeled kallikrein
mixed with rat plasma at 0°C, (C) Plasma at 0 time after injection
of radiolabeled kallikrein, (D) Plasma at 6 min after injection.

REFERENCES

1. Fiedler, Enzymology of glandular kallikreins, in: "Bradykinin, Kallikrein
    and Kallidin," E. G. Erdös, ed., Springer-Verlag, Berlin-Heiderberg-
    New York (1979).
2. E. R. Hare and J. A. Verpoorte, The purification and partial characteri-
    zation of human salivry kallikrein, Biochem. Biophys. Acta, 709:65-
    72 (1982).
3. I. J. Zeitlin, Y. N. Singh, F. Lembeck, and M. Theiler, The molecular
    weights of plasma and intestinal kallikreins in rats, Arch.
    Pharmacol., 293:159-161 (1976).
4. I. H. Mills, N. A. A. MacFarlane, P. E. Ward, and L. F. O. Obika, The
    renal kallikrein-kinin system and the regulation of salt and water
    excretion, Fed. Proc., 35:181-188 (1976).
5. J. Roblero, H. R. Croxatto, R. Garcia, J. Corthorn, E. De Vito, Kalli-
    krein-like activity of perfusates and urine of isolated rat kidneys,
    Am. J. Physiol., 231:1383-1389 (1976).
6. S. H. Ferreira and L. H. Smaje, Bradykinin and functional vasodilatation
    in the salivary gland, Br. J. Pharmacol., 58:201-209 (1976).
7. K. Nishimura, H. Shimizu, and T. Kokubu, Existence of prokallikrein
    in the kidney: its biochemical properties compared to three active
    glandular kallikreins from the kidney, serum and urine of the rat,
    Hypertension, 5:205-210 (1983).
8. R. Geiger, B. Clausnitzer, E. Fink, and H. Fritz, Isolation of an
    enzymatically active glandular kallikrein from human plasma by immuno-
    affinity chromatography, Hoppe Seylers Z Physiol. Chem., 361:1795-
    1803 (1980).
9. Y. Miyachi, J. L. Vaitukaitis, E. Nieschlag, and M. B. Lipsett, Enzymatic
    radioiodination of gonadotropins, J. Clin. Endocrinol., 34:23-28
    (1972).
10. W. M. Hunter and F. C. Greenwood, Preparation of iodine-131 labeled
    human growth hormone of high specific activity, Nature, 194:495-
    496 (1962).
11. S. Ullberg and G. Bengtsson, Autoradiographic distribution studies with
    natural oestrogens, Acta Endocrinol., 43:75-86 (1963).

HORMONAL REGULATION OF GLANDULAR KALLIKREIN ACTIVITY AND ITS INHIBITOR

IN HUMAN PLASMA

Hideki Koh*, Kagehiro Uchida**, Seiki Nambu*, and Masao Ikeda*

Division of Atherosclerosis and Metabolism*, Department of
Internal Medicine, and the Department of Clinical
Laboratory**, National Cardiovascular Center, 5-7
Fujishiro-dai, Suita, Osaka, 565 Japan

SUMMARY

Plasma glandular kallikrein (GK) activity, serum 3,5,3'-triiodothyronine (T_3), thyroxine (T_4), reverse T_3, thyroid-stimulating hormone, plasma $alpha_2$ macroglobulin ($\alpha_2 M$) and $alpha_1$ antitrypsin ($\alpha_1 AT$) levels were determined in twenty-nine non-diabetic female subjects given normal ad-lib diet or one of several kinds of caloric composition for more than 7 days after an overnight fast.

Positive exponential correlation was found between serum T_3 level and plasma GK activity (r=0.54), and there was positive linear correlation between serum T_3 level and plasma $_2 M$ level (r=0.51). Positive natural logarithmic correlation was found between plasma GK activity and plasma $\alpha_2 M$ level (r=0.47). There was no correlation between plasma GK activity and plasma $\alpha_1 AT$ level, and between serum T_3 level and plasma $\alpha_1 AT$ level. No correlation was found between serum T_4 level and plasma GK activity, and between serum T_4 level and plasma $\alpha_2 M$ level. There was no correlation between serum T_4 and T_3 level, but positive exponential correlation was found between serum T_4 and reverse T_3 level (r=0.82).

These data suggest that T_3 responds to dietary carbohydrate through Kallikrein-Kinin system, and T_3 regulates both GK activity and its inhibitor ($\alpha_2 M$) in human plasma.

INTRODUCTION

It is well-known that caloric restriction is associated with low serum 3,4,3'-triiodothyronine (T_3) levels in man. Hypocaloric diet consisting of only carbohydrate, however, was reported to exhibit no change in serum T_3 level.[1]   Recently, we reported changes of glandular kallikrein (GK) activity in human plasma following glucose ingestion and suggested that active GK was utilized during glucose uptake at peripheral tissues.[2] Furthermore, the presence of GK in rat thyroid gland has been described.[3] This study was conducted in order to clarify the relationship between serum T_3 level and plasma GK activity in human.

MATERIALS

L-prolyl-L-phenylalanyl-L-arginine-4-methyl-coumaryl-7-amide (Pro-Phe-Arg-MCA) were purchased from Protein Research Foundation, Osaka, Japan. Soybean trypsin inhibitor was obtained from Sigma Chemical Co., USA. M-Partigen®-alpha$_2$ macroglobulin and M-Partigen®-alpha$_1$ antitrypsin were purchased from Behringwerke AG, Marburg, W. Germany.

SUBJECTS AND METHODS

1. Study Design

Twenty-nine non-diabetic female subjects were studied. Nineteen were normal volunteers, aged 24.3 ± 0.72 yr (mean $\pm$ SEM) and ten were in-patients, aged 53.7 ± 2.82 yr. Volunteers were not given any instructions concerning diet before study and in-patients were given one of several kinds of caloric composition (Table 1) for more than 7 days. After an overnight fast, venous samples were withdrawn to determine plasma GK activity, plasma alpha$_2$ macroglobulin (α_2M) and alpha$_1$ antitrypsin (α_1AT) levels, serum T_3, tyroxine (T_4), reverse T_3 and thyroid-stimulating hormone (TSH) levels.

TABLE 1: Nutrient composition of each diet

Diet (kcal/day)	Protein(g)	Fat(g)	Carbohydrate(g)
2012.0 ± 17.20	81.0 ± 1.13	49.0 ± 2.08	299.0 ± 3.40
1508.0 ± 11.53	81.0 ± 1.13	41.0 ± 1.13	188.0 ± 1.70
1397.0 ± 11.53	78.0 ± 1.13	39.0 ± 1.13	168.0 ± 1.70
1156.0 ± 11.53	70.0 ± 1.13	39.0 ± 1.13	139.0 ± 1.70

mean±SEM.　n=28 days

2. Assay of GK activity in plasma

GK activity in human plasma was measured as the hydrolyzing activity of synthetic fluorogenic substrate (Pro-Phe-Arg-MCA) using our recently-developed assay system.[4] One unit (U) of GK activity in plasma is defined as the amount of enzyme which hydrolyzes 1 n mol of synthetic substrate per min per ml of plasma.

3. Assay of plasma α_2M and α_1AT levels

Plasma α_2M and α_1AT were measured by single radial immunodiffusion method.

4. Assay of serum T_3, T_4, reverse T_3 and TSH levels

Serum T_3, T_4, reverse T_3 and TSH were determined by radio-immunoassay.[5,6,7,8]

5. Analysis of Results

The data were analyzed using linear and nonlinear regression analysis. All the mean values are given with the standard error of the mean (SEM).

RESULTS

Mean serum TSH levels in volunteers were $3.2 \pm 0.43 \mu U/ml$ and those in in-patients were 3.8 ± 0.54 U/ml. Mean serum T_4 levels in volunteers were $8.4 \pm 0.31 \mu g/dl$ and those in in-patients were $9.0 \pm 0.66 \mu g/dl$. Positive exponential correlation was found between serum T_3 level and plasma GK activity (r=0.54, n=29) as shown in Figure 1.

Positive linear correlation was found between serum T_3 level and plasma $_2M$ level (r=0.51, n=29) as shown in Figure 2. Furthermore, there was positive natural logarithmic correlation between plasma GK activity and plasma α_2M level (r=0.47, n=29) as shown in Figure 3. However, there was no correlation between plasma GK activity and plasma α_1AT level as shown in Figure 4, and there was also no correlation between serum T_3 level and plasma α_1AT level as shown in Figure 5. No correlation was found between serum T_4 level and plasma GK activity, and between serum T_4 level and plasma α_2M level. There was also no correlation between serum reverse T_3 level and plasma GK activity, and between serum reverse T_3 level and plasma α_2M level. No correlation was found between serum T_4 and T_3 level, but there was positive exponential correlation between serum T_4 and reserve T_3 level (r=0.82, n=29) as shown in Figure 6.

DISCUSSION

In human, to obtain low T_3 levels in peripheral circulation physiologically, restriction of carbohydrate quantity in the diet along with that of total calorie seems to be a most appropriate method because it does not increase serum TSH level,[9] and this was also confirmed in the

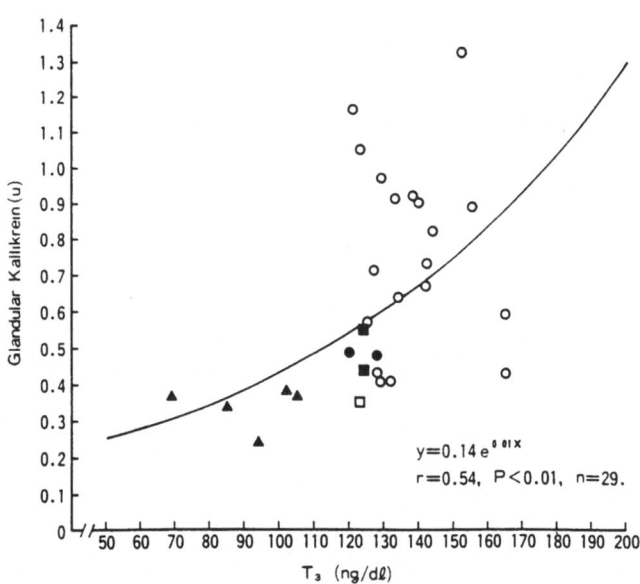

Figure 1. Correlation between T_3 and GK activity in normal volunteers and in-patients given each diet for more than 7 days.
0 : normal ad-lib diet   ● :2012 kcal diet
■ : 1508 kcal diet   □ :1397 kcal diet
△ : 1156 kcal diet

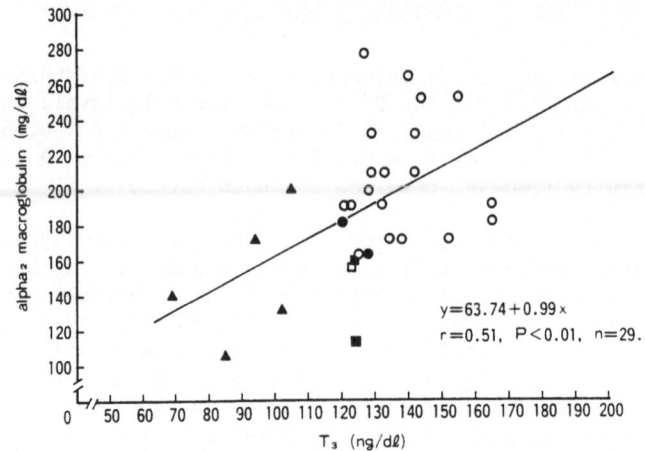

Figure 2.   Correlation between T3 and   α2M in normal volunteers and
            in-patients given each diet for more than 7 days.
            0 : normal ad-lib diet   ● : 2012 kcal diet
            ● : 1508 kcal diet   □ : 1397 kcal diet
            ▲ : 1156 kcal diet

present study.   Taking it into consideration, we could c rify that there
was positive exponential correlation between serum T3 level and plasma
GK activity in human.

    Recently, we reported that plasma GK activities decreased initially
from mean base line level and then returned to baseline level with the
lapse of time after oral glucose load[2]: the first decrement suggested
that active GK was utilized during glucose uptake at peripheral tissues,
and the latter increment suggested that GK secretion and GK activation
were stimulated by humoral factors.

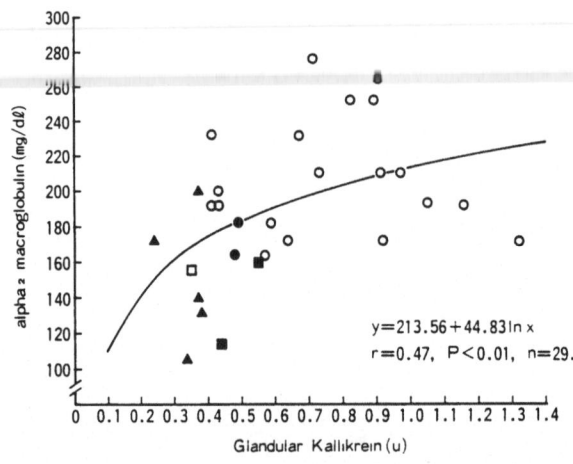

Figure 3.   Correlation between GK activity and   α2M in normal
            volunteers and in-patients given each diet for more than 7
            days.
            0 : normal ad-lib diet   ● : 2012 kcal diet
            ■ : 1508 kcal diet   □ : 1397 kcal diet
            ▲ : 1156 kcal diet

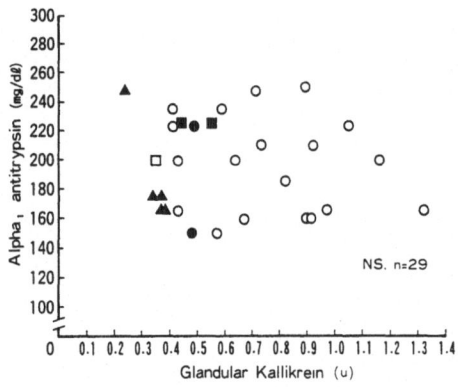

Figure 4.   Correlation between GK activity and α_1 AT in normal volunteers
and in-patients given each diet for more than 7 days.
NS: not significant   0 : normal ad-lib diet
●: 2012 kcal diet   ■ : 1508 kcal diet
□: 1397 kcal diet   ▲ : 1156 kcal diet

    Therefore, T_3 could be one of humoral factors which stimulate the
secretion and biosynthesis of GK, and this could be supported by the
presence of GK in rat thyroid gland.[3]   On the other hand, there was
positive linear correlation between serum T_3 level and plasma α_2 M
level: as it was considered that there was little difference in protein
intake among subjects in this study, it could be suggested that within
physiological ranges, T_3 regulates plasma α_2 M levels by the stimulation
of hepatic protein synthesis.

    Furthermore, there was positive natural logarithmic correlation
between plasma GK activity and plasma α_2 M level: close correlation was

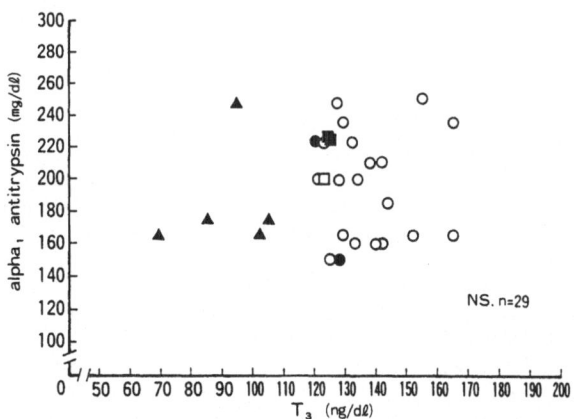

Figure 5.   Correlation between T_3 and α_1 AT in normal volunteers and
in in-patients given each diet for more than 7 days.
NS: not significant   0 : normal ad-lib diet
●: 2012 kcal diet   ■ : 1508 kcal diet
□: 1397 kcal diet   ▲ : 1156 kcal diet

319

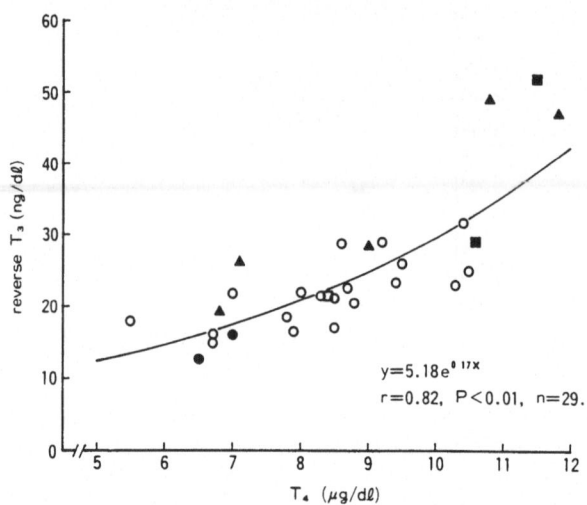

Figure 6. Correlation between T_4 and reverse T_3 in normal volunteers
and in-patients given each diet for more than 7 days.
0 : normal ad-lib diet   ● : 2012 kcal diet
■ : 1508 kcal diet   □ : 1397 kcal diet
▲ : 1156 kcal diet

found when plasma GK activities were not so high, but the correlation was
weak when GK activities at higher levels. Therefore, it was suggested
that plasma $\alpha_2 M$ levels should necessarily have been low when plasma GK
activities were at higher levels because of the rapid clearance of
$\alpha_2 M$–GK complexes from the circulation by reticuloendothelial system.[10]

The clinical significance of this study is that T_3 plays an important
and physiological role in carbohydrate metabolism, and it responds to
dietary carbohydrate through Kallikrein-Kinin system. Furthermore, it is
important to note that T_3 regulates both GK activity and its inhibitor
($\alpha_2 M$) in human plasma, although its precise mechanism awaits further investigation.

REFERENCES:

1. S. W. Spaulding, I. J. Chopra, R. S. Sherwin, and S. S. Lyall: Effect
   of caloric restriction and dietary composition on serum T_3 and
   reverse T_3 in man, J. Clin. Endocrinol. Metab., 42:197-200, (1976).
2. H. Koh, K. Uchida, S. Nambu, M. Tsushima, Y. Nishioheda, K. Murakami,
   and M. Ikeda, Changes of glandular kallikrein activity in human
   plasma following glucose ingestion, Arzneim.-Forsch., 32(II):1564-
   1566, (1982).
3. K. Uchida, H. Kushiro, J. Kodama, Y. Hitomi, M. Niinobe, and S. Fujii,
   Rat thyroid kallikrein: its purification and properties, Agents
   and Actions (Suppl.), 9:167-172, (1982).
4. K. Uchida, H. Koh, S. Yoshimura, K. Okuma, H. Kushiro, S. Nambu,
   J. Kodama, and S. Fujii, Estimation of plasma and glandular
   kallikrein activity using fluorogenic substrates and its clinical
   application, Agents and Actions (Suppl.), 9:91-96, (1982).

5. I. J. Chopra, R. S. Ho, and R. Lam, An improved radioimmunoassay of triiodothyronine in serum: its application to clinical and physiological studies, J. Lab. Clin. Med., 80:729–739, (1972).

6. I. J. Chopra, A radioimmunoassay for measurement of thyroxine in unextracted serum, J. Clin. Endocrinol. Metab., 34:938–947, (1972).

7. I. J. Chopra, A radioimmunoassay for measurement of 3,3',5'-triiodothyronine (reverse T3), J. Clin. Invest., 54:583–592, (1974).

8. W. D. Odell, J. F. Wilber, and W. E. Paul, Radioimmunoassay of thyrotropin in human serum, J. Clin. Endocr., 25:1179–1188, (1965).

9. R. Pasquali, L. Mattioli, M. Capelli, M. Parenti, M. Gallo, and N. Melchionelra, Effect of dietary calorie and carbohydrate levels on thyroid hormone concentrations in obese subjects, in: Proceeding of the Serono Symposia, ed. by G. Enzi, G. Crepaldi, G. Pozza, and A. E. Renold, Academic Press, Volume 28, pp. 215–223, (1981).

10. K. Ohlsson, Elimination of ^{125}I-trypsin α-macroglobulin complexes from blood by reticuloendothelial cells in dog, Acta Physiol. Scand., 81:269–272, (1971).

A COMPARATIVE STUDY OF PROKALLIKREINS AND KALLIKREINS FROM RAT PANCREATIC TISSUE AND JUICE

A. A. Jaffa, M. Hussain, Z. Rashid and G. S. Bailey

Department of Chemistry
University of Essex
Colchester, UK

SUMMARY

Two zymogens, designated prokallikreins A and B, were isolated from homogenates of rat pancreatic tissue. The two forms of prokallikrein were found to be very similar in size and charge properties. They gave rise to very similar kallikreins on activation with exogeneous trypsin. Differences in carbohydrate content of the two zymogens were probably responsible for differences seen in their behaviour on ion-exchange chromatography and immunoelectrophoresis.

In contrast, only one form of prokallikrein was isolated from rat pancreatic juice. It showed almost identical behaviour on ion-exchange chromatography and identical mobility on electrophoresis to prokallikrein A. Thus it can be tentatively suggested that it is prokallikrein A which is secreted into the pancreatic juice and represents the physiologically important zymogen.

INTRODUCTION

Prokallikrein exists in two different forms in both rat and pig pancreatic tissue.[1,2] However, it is not known which form is secreted into the pancreatic juice. The present paper compares some of the properties of the prokallikreins isolated from rat pancreatic tissue. As an extension of that comparative study, it was deemed necessary to isolate the prokallikrein or kallikrein present in rat pancreatic juice in order to characterize what is, presumably, the physiologically important molecule.

METHODS

Prokallikreins A and B were isolated from homogenates of rat pancreatic tissue by sequential anion-exchange, gel filtration and immunoaffinity chromatographies.[1,3] The amounts of neutral hexoses present in the zymogens were estimated by the method of Roe.[4] All other methodology was performed as reported previously.[1,3] Pancreatic juice was collected from rats (300-350 g), anaesthetized with an intraperitoneal injection of sodium pentabarbitone (20 mg), with the aid of pancreozmyin which was administered intravenously by a syringe infusion pump at the rate of 15 Crick units/hour.

RESULTS AND DISCUSSION

Purification of Prokallikreins from Rat Pancreatic Tissue

The existence of two different forms of prokallikreins in rat pancreas can be shown by anion-exchange chromatography of homogenates of that tissue. Prokallikrein, identified on the basis of enzymatic and immunochemical properties, was separated into two fractions designated A and B which were eluted by 0.4M and 0.8M NaCl respectively (see Figure 1). Measurements by radioimmunoassay showed that B contained approximately twice as much prokallikrein as A. Pure samples of the zymogen were obtained from both fractions by gel filtration followed by immunoaffinity chromatography. Thus from 12 g of pancreatic tissue 200 μg of prokallirein A and 470 μg of prokallikrein B were obtained.

Properties of Tissue Prokallikreins A and B

It can be suggested, considering the physiochemical properties recorded in Table 1 that the small differences in size and isoelectric point recorded for prokallikreins A and B may be due to differences in carbohydrate content. A similar situation has been reported for porcine pancreatic kallikreins.[2]

Properties of Trypsin-Activated Prokallikreins A and B

Trypsin-activation of both prokallikreins resulted in a small decrease in size and isoelectric point [$Mr(SDS)$ 34000, pI 4.15 for kallikrein A, and $Mr(SDS)$ 35500, pI 4.20 for kallikrein B]. The active enzymes themselves were very similar in their catalytic properties, as shown in Table 2.

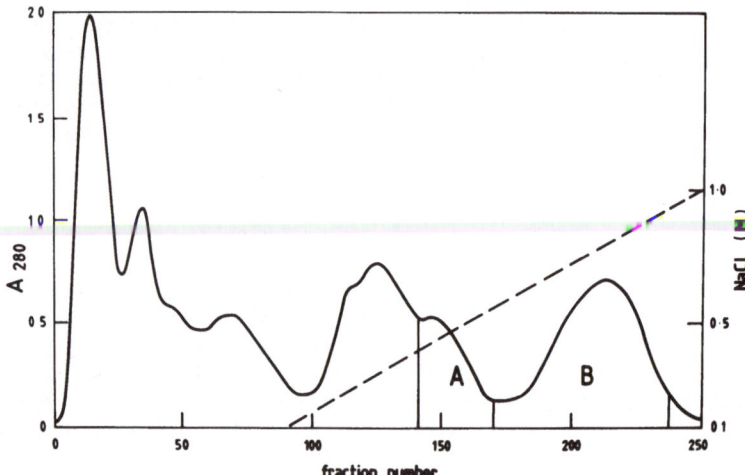

Fig. 1. Ion-exchange chromatography of rat pancreatic homogenate. Supernatant of crude homogenate of rat pancreatic tissue was chromatographed on DEAE Sephadex A-50 column (5x12 cm), equilibrated with 0.01M sodium phosphate/0.1M NaCl, pH 6.0. Column ws first washed with equilibrating buffer (600 ml) and then eluted with a linear gradient (1200 ml) 0.01M sodium phosphate/0.1M NaCl, pH 6.0, to 0.01M sodium phosphate/1.0M NaCl, pH 6.0. Flow rate was 45 ml/h and 7.5 ml fractions were collected.

Table 1. Properties of Pancreatic Tissue Prokallikreins A and B

	Mr(gf)	Mr(SDS)	pI	Hexose (% w/w)	N terminus
Prokallikrein A	35900	36500	4.25	6.5	Val
Prokallikrein B	37400	38400	4.35	12.0	Val

The Existence of Only One Form of Prokallikrein in Rat Pancreatic Juice

Pancreatic juice was collected from six rats and pooled. It showed
no activity against arginine esters and SBTI was added to suppress possible
autoactivation. A sample of the juice (1.80 ml, 288 mg protein, 403 μg
prokallikrein) was applied to a column (5 x 10 cm) of DEAE-Sephadex A-50
resin. The column was initially washed with 0.01M phosphate buffer, containing 0.1M NaCl and 0.3 mg/ml SBTI at a flow rate of 45 ml/hour, and collecting 7.5 ml fractions. Adsorbed material was removed by application of a
linear salt gradient (0.1M to 1.0M NaCl in phosphate pH 6.0 buffer, total
volume 1200 ml). analysis by titrimetric assay and radioimmunoassay of
individual fractions showed that significant prokallikrein was present only
in those tubes corresponding to area F3 on the elution profile (Figure 2).
However, after pooling and subsequent concentration of those fractions,
the resultant concentrated sample (25.2 mg protein, 320 μg kallikrein) was
found to contain fully-active kallikrein rather than its inactive zymogen
counterpart.

Purification of Prokallikrein from Rat Pancreatic Juice

Pancreatic juice (0.5 ml, 70 mg protein, 91 μg prokallikrein) was diluted with phosphate buffer pH 6.0 (1.5 ml). The sample was adjusted to
pH 7.4 with 1M NaOH and 0.5% (w/w) bovine serum albumin was added. It was
then allowed to interact for 20 hours at 4°C with immunoadsorbent resin
(2.0 ml), prepared by coupling the IgG fraction (14 mg) purified from a
fresh batch of antiserum to tissue prokallikrein B[1] to 0.8 g CNBr-activated
Sepharose 4B. A small column was packed and the first eluate (E_1, containing 14 g prokallikrein) was collected. The column was washed to give
eluate E_2 (10 μg prokallikrein) with 0.01M sodium phosphate buffer pH 7.4
(20 ml) containing 0.5M NaCl and 0.5% bovine serum albumin. The adsorbed
prokallikrein was removed in eluate E_3 (60 μg prokallikrein) by 0.1M sodium
acetate buffer pH 4.0 (20 ml) containing 0.5 NaCl and 0.5% bovine serum
albumin. The pH of E_3 was immediately brought to pH 7.4 with 2M K_2CO_3.

Table 2. Kinetic Constants of Pancreatic Tissue Kallikreins A and B

Substrate	Kallikrein A		Kallikrein B	
	Km (μm)	kcat (s^{-1})	Km (μm)	kcat (s^{-1})
Cbz-Arg-OMe	86	212	75	227
Bz-Arg-OEt	75	172	70	178
Tos-Arg-OMe	107	181	80	163

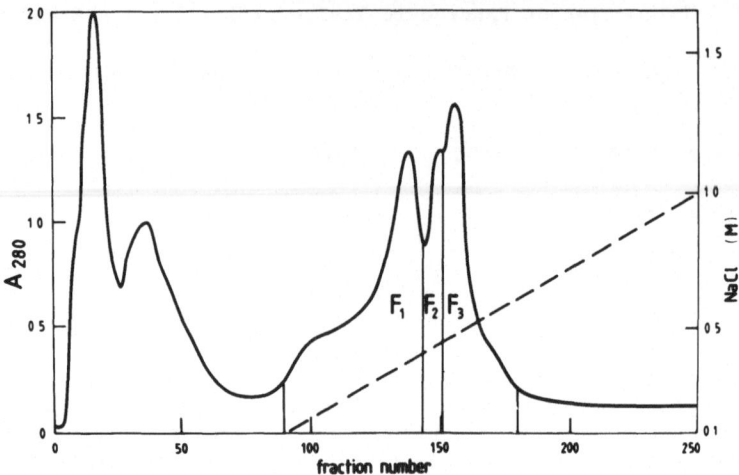

Fig. 2.   Ion-exchange chromatography of rat pancreatic juice.

E_3 was subjected to ultra-filtration to remove albumin and to give a concentrated sample of 52 µg prokallikrein. The sample was active against Bz-Arg-OMe only after activation with a catalytic amount of trypsin, giving a specific activity of 312 µmole/min/mg. It was homogeneous on disc and immunoelectrophoresis.

Comparison of Rat Pancreatic Juice and Tissue Prokallikreins

Prokallikrein of rat pancreatic juice was eluted at 0.45M NaCl from the anion-exchange resin, similar to tissue prokallikrein A (0.4M NaCl). Both zymogens showed the same mobility on immunoelectrophoresis and could thus be distinguished from tissue prokallikrein B (see Figure 3). Furthermore, the kallikreins produced by trypsin-activation of juice prokallikrein and tissue prokallikrein A had identical mobilities on immunoelectrophoresis and were in that respect different from activated prokallikrein B. Similar results were seen on disc electrophoresis on 16% polyacrylamide gels at pH 9.4; both juice prokallikrein and tissue prokallikrein A had an identical aodic mobility which was slightly greater than that of prokallikrein B.

CONCLUSION

Rat pancreatic tissue contains two forms of prokallikrein, A (minor) and B (major), which can be separated by anion-exchange chromatography. The two zymogens differ slightly in size and charge properties and those differences are manifest in electrophoresis. They are activated by trypsin to produce kallikreins of very similar enzymatic activity. The small differences in properties of the two zymogens are probably due to differences in carbohydrate content.

Anion-exchange chromatography was carried out on rat pancreatic juice in order to check in which form prokallikrein was secreted. Only one form of prokallikrein was detected. That zymogen was isolated by immunoadsorption chromatography of pancreatic juice. It was found to have identical electrophoretic mobility to that of prokallikrein A. Thus it would appear that it is the minor form of the tissue zuymogen which is present in rat pancreatic juice. That, in turn, raises the important question of the function of prokallikrein B. One possibility is that it is a storage form of the zymogen that is subsequently converted into prokallikrein A during secretion.

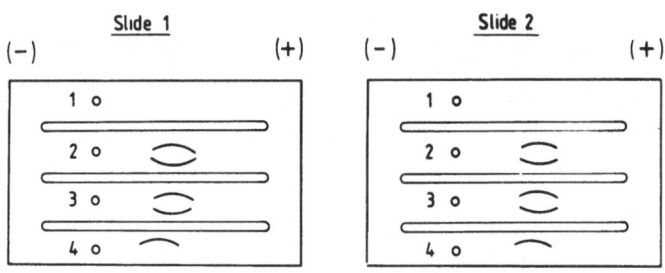

Fig. 3. Immunoelectrophoresis at pH 8.6.

Slide 2   Slide 2
Well 2 Rat pancreatic tis-   Well 2 Kallikrein A produced by
       sue prokallikrein A   trypsin-activation of pro-
                                        kallikrein A

Well 3 Rat pancreatic juice   Well 3 Kallikrein produced by
       prokallikrein   trypsin-activation of juice
                                        prokallikrein

Well 4 Rat pancreatic tis-   Well 4 Kallikrein B produced by
       sue prokallikrein B   trypsin-activation of pro-
                                        kallikrein B

Antiserum to rat pancreatic tissue prokallikrein B was added to
each channel of both slides.

Obviously further research is required to clarify the situation.

REFERENCES

1. M. Hussain and G. S. Bailey, Purification and some properties of a
    second prokallikrein from rat pancreas, Biochem. Int., 5:59-66
    (1982).
2. F. Fiedler and C. Hirschauer, On the various forms of the glandular
    kallikrein from autolyzed porcine pancreas, Hoppe Seyler's Z. Phy-
    siol. Chem., 362:1209-1218 (1981).
3. M. Hussain and G. S. Bailey, An improved method of isolation of rat
    pancreatic prokallikrein, Biochim. Biophys. Acta, 719:40-46 (1982).
4. J. H. Roe, The determination of sugar in blood and spinal fluid with
    anthrone reagent, J. Biol. Chem., 212:335-343 (1955).

AN INACTIVE FORM OF KALLIKREIN IN HUMAN URINE

Kazuyuki Kizuki, Yuuji Shimamoto, Masahiko Ikekita
and Hiroshi Moriya

Department of Biochemistry, Faculty of Pharmaceutical Sciences
Science University of Tokyo, 12, Ichigaya-Funakawara-machi
Shinjuku-ku, Tokyo 162, Japan

SUMMARY

An inactive form of human urinary kallikrein (inactive HUK) was highly purified from fresh urine collected from healthy men. Inactive HUK was separated from the active kallikrein (HUK) initially presents in the urine by affinity chromatography on a column of aprotinin immobilized on Sepharose 4B and further purified by gel filtration, ion-exchange chromatography and immunoaffinity chromatography on an anti-HUK antibody immobilized Sepharose 4B column.

Inactive HUK was rapidly actigvted by a trace amount of trypsin. While, plasmin, urokinase, thrombin and chymotrypsin caused no activation of inactive HUK.

The molecular weights of inactive HUK and HUK were estimated to be 4.8×10^4 and 4.5×10^4, respectively. The molecular weight of active HUK generated from inactive HUK by the action of trypsin (HUK") was almost the same as that of HUK.

The mobility of inactive HUK was slightly slower than that of HUK on both immunoelectrophoresis and polyacrylamide gel disc electrophoresis. On the other hand, the electrophoretic mobility of HUKK" was almost the same as that of HUK. These two types of active HUK had no significant difference in the Km values for H-Pro-Phe-Arg-MCA hydrolysis and inhibition profiles by various protease inhibitors and anti-HUK antibody.

Inactive HUK was unable to be measured by the direct radioimmunoassay (RIA) but HUK" generated by the action of trypsin could be measured by the RIA.

INTRODUCTION

Kallikrein excretion into urine is widely known to be related to certain physiological and/or pathological regulations of renal functions. However, the significance of urinary kallikrein excretion has not been understood well in many cases. Recently, existence of a large amount of inactive form of kallirkein in human urine (about 60-70% of the total kalli-

krein in the urine) klhas been recognized,[1,2] whether this inactive kallikrein is a proenzyme or the enzyme whose active site might be masked with
some materials has been unsolved. Thus, in order to elucidate the physiological and/or pathological meanings of human urinary kallikrein, isolation
and characterization of this inactive HUK must be very important problems.

The authors isolated this inactive HUK and compared the properties
of kallikrein generated from this inactive HUK by the action of trypsin
with those of HUK initially presents in urine.

MATERIALS AND METHODS

The activity of HUK towards H-Pro-Phe-ARg-MCA was measured fluorometrically as described by Iwanaga et al.[3] with minor modifications. The activity
was expressed as amidase unit (AU). One AU is the amount of enzyme that
can hydrolyze 1 μmole of H-Pro-Phe-Arg-MCA per min at 30°C and pH 8.0.
The amount of inactive HUK was determined in the following way. The sample
solution, 0.1 ml, was incubated with 0.1 ml of trypsin solution (0.5 mg/ml
in 0.1 M Tris-HCl uffer, pH 8.0) for 10 min at 30°C (activation of inactive
HUK). Next, 0.1 ml of SBTI solution (3 mg/ml in H_2O) was added to it (inhibition of trypsin) and the activity of this mixture was measured. The amount
of inactive HUK was expressed as AU (after the treatment with trypsin) minus
AU (before the treatment with trypsin).

Guanidinated aprotinin-Sepharose 4B[4] and trypsin-Sepharose 4B were
prepared in our laboratory.

The HUK preparation purified in our laboratory was used for the preparation of anti-HUK rabbit serum as antigen. The titer of the finally obtained
rabbit serum was 128 when determined by the interfacial ring test using
the solution of 1 mg/ml of antigen. The IgG fractions were isolated by
ammonium sulfate precipitation and DEAE-cellulose column chromatography.
The IgG fraction (386 A_{280} in 120 ml) was immobilized on Sepharose 4B gels
(100 ml). More than 95% of the proteins were bound to the gels.

The direct solid-phase radioimmunoassay (RIA) kit for HUK[5] was obtained
from the Green Cross Co., Japan.

RESULTS

Purification of Inactive HUK

Table 1 summarizes the purification of inactive HUK. Fresh urine collected from healthy men was dialyzed against running tap water for 14 hr
at room temperature. Then, the pH and the electric conductivity of the
dialysate were adjusted to 6.0 and 5 mmho/cm, respectively. After that,
DEAE-Sephadex A-50 gels which had been equilibrated with 5 mmho/cm of ammonium acetate, pH 6.0, were added to it and the mixture was stirred for 2 hr
at room temperature. The gels were collected and washed with 3-5 1 of the
same solution, and packed in a column. Next, the adsorbed materials were
eluted with 45 mmho/cm of ammonium acetate, pH 6.0. The inactive HUK fractions overlapping with active kallikrein were pooled and the following
chromatographies were performed.

Step 1 Guanidinated Aprotinin-Sepharose 4B Chromatography: Inactive
HUK solution obtained above (1.3 1) was concentrated to about 100 ml with
polyethylene glycol #20000. Then, it was dialyzed against 0.1 M Tris-HCl
buffer, pH 8.0 and then it was applied to the guanidinated aprotinin-Sepharose 4B column equilibrated with the same buffer. Active kallikrein was

Table 1. Summary of the Purification of Inactive HUK from Human Urine

Human urine (103 1)
↓
Dialysis against tap water (overnight, at room temperature)
↓
DEAE-Sephadex A-50 Chromatography (adsorbed fraction)
↓
Continued to the following Table

Chromatographies	Protein (A_{280})	Recovery (%)	Inactive HUK (AU)[a]	Recovery (%)	S.A.[c] (mAU/A_{280})	P.F.[d]
1. Guanidinated aprotinin-Sepharose 4B	2181.5	100	112.52(3.2%)[b]	100	52	1
2. Sephadex G-75	724.8	33.2	64.89 (15.6%)	57.7	90	1.7
3. DEAE-Sephadex A-50	128.8	5.9	42.39 (17.3%)	37.7	329	6.3
4. Anti-HUK IgG-Sepharose 4B	3.27	0.15	15.83 (25.3%)	14.1	4841	93

a) Assayed after treatment with trypsin.
b) Contents of the active form of kallikrein (AU,untreated/AU,treated with trypsin X 100).
c) Specific activety.
d) Purification factor.

331

adsorbed on the column, while inactive HUK passed through the column. So, the non-adsorbed fractions were pooled as an inactive HUK fraction. This fraction contained only 3.2% of the active kallikrein. The inactive HUK solution obtained here was dialyzed against distilled water and lyophilized. After redissolved in 30 ml of 0.05M Tris-HCl buffer, pH 8.0, it was divided into 2 portions and steps 2 and 3 were performed twice.

Step 2 Sephadex G-75 Gel Filtration: The inactive HUK solution (15 ml) was applied to a Sephadex G-75 column (2.6 X 92 cm) which had been equilibrated with 0.05 M Tris-HCl buffer, pH 8.0 and eluted with the same buffer. Fractions No. 76 to 99 were pooled (each fraction; 3.2 ml). The pooled inactive HUK solution contained 15.6% of the active form. This active kallikrein is probably kallikrein spontaneously generated from inactive HUK during or after the gel filtration, because we had pooled as the starting material for this process inactive HUK fractions which contained only 3.2% of the active form.

Step 3 DEAE-Sephadex A-50 Chromatography: Next, the inactive HUK solution was directly applied to a DEAE-Sephadex A-50 column (2.2 X 58 cm) equilibrated with 0.05 M Tris-HCl buffer, pH 8.0, containing 0.05 M NaCl, and the linear gradient elution with 0.05 to 0.6 M NaCl in the same buffer (total 1200 ml) was carried out. Fractions No. 71 to 86 (each fraction; 6.0 ml) in which small amount of active kallikrein was eluted overlapping with inactive HUK were pooled. Two pooled inactive HUK solutions from separate DEAE-Sephadex A-50 chromatographies were combined.

Step 4 Immunoaffinity Chromatography: Inactive HUK was further purified on an anti-HUK antibody immobilized Sepharose 4B column. As shown in Fig. 1, inactive HUK was purified very effectively on this column. The specific activity of the pooled inactive HUK preparation (fractions No. 165-174) was 4841 mAU/A_{280} (after treatment with trypsin). However, 25.3% of the active form of kallikrein was contaminated in this inactive HUK preparation. So, this inactive HUK preparation was again applied to a guanidinated-Sepharose 4B column to remove active HUK from the inactive HUK

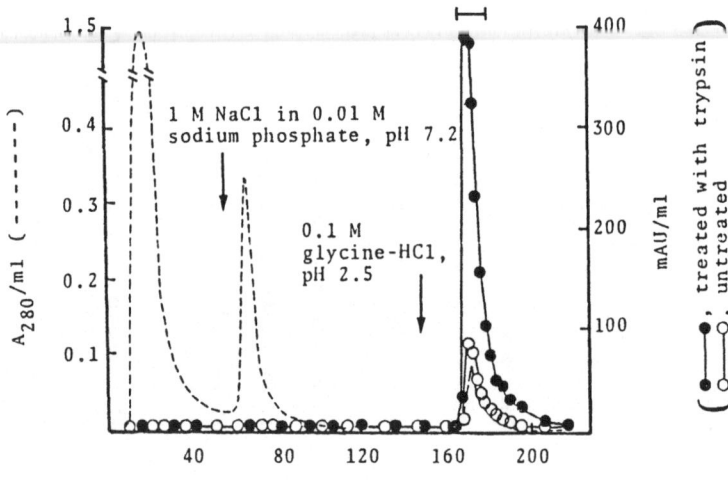

Fig. 1. Immunoaffinity chromatography of inactive HUK on an anti-HUK antibody immobilized Sepharose 4B column.

preparation. The non-adsorbed fractions which contained no active kallikrein were pooled and dialyzed against 2 mmho/cm of ammonium formate, pH 6.8 for 20 hr at 4°C. The dialysate, however, contained 16.3% of active kallirkein probably spontaneously generated during the dialysis. The specific activity of the dialysate was 1062.1 mAU/A_{280}. The reason why the specific activity decreased in this process was not clear, but the dialysate obtained here was stored at -25°C and mainly usd in the following experiments.

Polyacrylamide Gel Disc Electrophoresis

The final inactive HUK preparation gave almost a single but a broad protein band in 10% polyacrylamide gel disc electrophoresis (Fig. 2). The activity observed after the treatment with trypsin coincided with the position of this broad protein band.

Immunological Analyses

The final inactive HUK preparation formed one precipitin line against anti-HUK rabbit serum fused with those of concentrated human urine and purified HUK when it was analyzed by the double immunodiffusion analysis.

On the other hand, inactive HUK migrated more slowly than HUK on the immunoelectrophoresis (Fig. 3-A). The mobility of HUK" was almost the same as that of HUK (Fig. 3-B). The same relation of the electrophoretic mobilities among inactive HUK, HUK" and HUK was observed on the disc electrophoresis (Fig. 2).

(+)   (-)

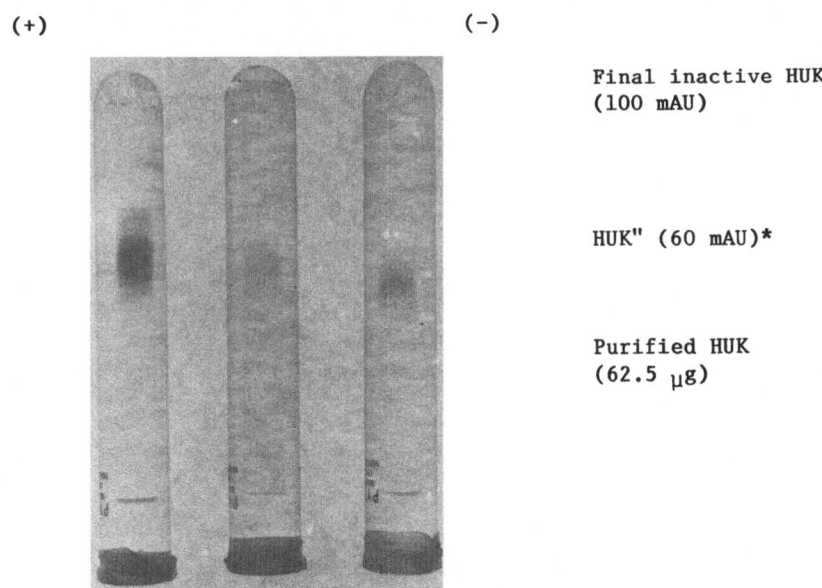

Final inactive HUK
(100 mAU)

HUK" (60 mAU)*

Purified HUK
(62.5 μg)

Fig. 2. Polyacrylamide gel disc electrophoresis of inactive HUK, HUK" and HUK.
   *: Inactive HUK was activated by trypsin immobilized on Sepharose 4B

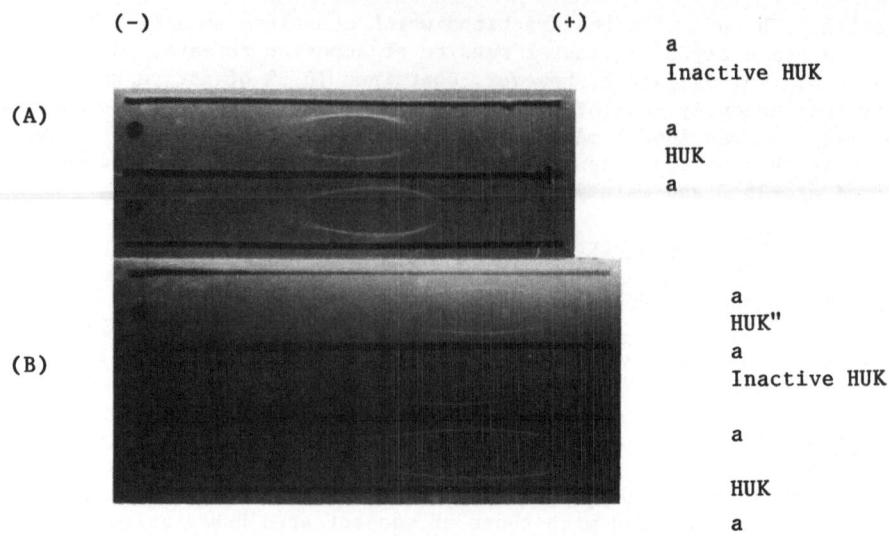

(−)   (+)

a
Inactive HUK

a
HUK
a

(A)

a
HUK"
a
Inactive HUK

a

HUK
a

(B)

Fig. 3.   Immunoelectrophoresis of inactive HUK, HUK and HUK".
a: Anti-HUK rabbit serum.

Effects of Trypsin, Plasmin, Thrombin, Urokinase and Chymotrypsin on Activation of Inactive HUK

The ability of some proteases to activate inactive HUK was investigated. As shown in Fig. 4, 0.65 EU/ml (final concentration) of trypsin gradually activated inactive HUK with the lapse of incubation time.   On the other hand, maximum activation was observed within 2 min by 13.65 EU/ml of trypsin. Plasmin, thrombin, urokinase and chymotrypsin caused no detectable activation of inactive HUK.

Activation of inactive HUK by trypsin was also confirmed by the vaso-dilative activity assay in dog.

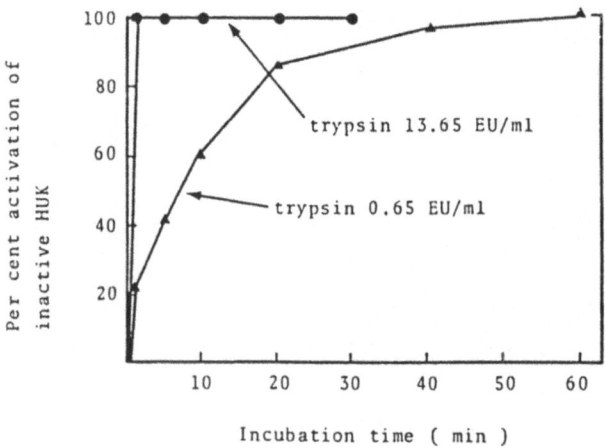

Fig. 4.   Activation of inactive HUK by trypsin.   EU: μmole BzARgOEt/min.

Molecular Weights of Inactive HUK, HUK" and HUK

The approximate molecular weights of inactive HUK and HUK determined by gel permeation chromatography on interconnected Shodex A-803 and A-804 columns (Showa Denko Co., Tokyo) were 4.8×10^4 and 4.5×10^4 respectively. The molecular weight of HUK" was almost the same as that of HUK.

Km Values of HUK" and HUK for H-Pro-Phe-Arg-MCA

The Km values of HUK" and HUK for H-Pro-Phe-Arg-MCA were calculated to be 3.8×10^{-5} and 3.2×10^{-5} M, respectively.

Effects of Anti-HUK Antibody and Some Protease Inhibitors on the Enzymatic Activities of HUK" and HUK

The profiles of the effects of anti-HUK antibody and various concentrations of aprotinin, SBTI, LBTI and EWTI on the enzymatic activities of HUK" and HUK were closely resembled each other and no significant difference was observed between HUK" and HUK.

Table 2. Contents of Inactive HUK in the HIghly Purified Inactive HUK Preparation, Urine and the Partially Purified HUK Preparation Assayed by Various Methods

Sample	Method	Active*	Total**	Inactive
Highly purified inactive HUK	MCA (mAU/ml)	5.24 ± 0.31 (n = 8)	32.04 ± 1.82 (n = 9)	26.80 (83.6%)***
	Dog (KU/ml)	0.54 ± 0.03 (n = 24)	1.95 ± 0.09 (n = 50)	1.41 (72.3%)
	RIA (μg/ml)	1.52 ± 0.07 (n = 3)	4.06 ± 0.40 (n = 2)	2.54 (62.6%)
Urine	MCA (mAU/ml)	0.457	2.136	1.679 (78.6%)
	RIA (μg/ml)	0.146	0.462	0.316 (68.4%)
Partially purified HUK****	MCA (mAU/ml)	17.63	67.11	49.48 (73.7%)
	Dog (KU/ml)	4.52 ± 0.23 (n = 13)	12.62 ± 0.85 (n = 13)	8.10 (64.2%)
	RIA (μg/ml)	3.12	10.71	7.59 (70.9%)

```
 * and **:  Before and after treatment with trypsin, respectively.
     ***:  % of the inactive kallikrein.
    ****:  The dialyzed human urine was applied to a DEAE-Sephadex A-50
           column and the adsorbed materials were eluted with 45 mmho/cm of
           ammonium acetate, pH 6.0.
```

Determination of Inactive HUK by Various Methods

Contents of inactive HUK and active HUK in the highly purified inactive HUK preparation were measured by the amidelytic activity assay, the vasodilative activity assay in dog[6] and the direct RIA. As shown in Table II, after the treatment with trypsin (generation of HUK"), the amounts of kallirkein measured by these 3 assays significantly increased. The same observation was obtained when the amounts of inactive HUK in urine and the partially purified HUK preparation were measured by these 3 assays. Namely, inactive HUK was unable to be measured by the RIA but HUK" generated by the action of trypsin could be measured by the RIA. The content of inactive HUK in human urine measured by the RIA was about 70%.

DISCUSSION

Inactive HUK was highly purified. The specific activity of the purified HUK is 4.3 AU/A_{280} (unpublished). The specific activity of the inactive HUK obtained from the immunoaffinity chromatography (step 4) was 4841 mAU/A_{280} . Judging from these values and the result of the polyacrylamide gel disc electrophoresis (Fig. 2), the purity of our inactive HUK preparation was considered to be extremely high. However, the specific activity of the non-adsorbed fractions of a guanidinated aprotinin-Sepharose 4B chromatography which was carried out after step 4 to remove active kallikrein contaminated in the inactive HUK preparation was calculated to be 1062 mAU/A_{280}. Whether this decrease of specific activity in this process is due to experimental error or other reasons is not clear as yet.

Whether this inactive HUK is a so-called proenzyme or an enzyme-inhibitor complex is the important problem. Concerning this point, the authors have no definite evidence now but this inactive HUK might be a proenzyme, because this inactive HUK was rapidly activated by low concentration of trypsin and the approximate molecular weight difference between this inactive HUK and HUK was observed to be only 3000. It is difficult to consider that this inactive kallikrein would be a complex with protease inhibitors ever reported, such as α_1-antitrypsin and other inhibitors, although Geiger et al.[7] reported a low molecular weight kallikrein-specific inhibitor in rat kidney which has the molecular weight of 4700. As mentioned above, the molecular weight of our inactive HUK was only about 3000 higher than that of active HUK. So, the possibility that this inactive kallikrein would be a complex with such a low molecular weight substance can not be denied absolutely. However, we could not recognize the existence of such a low molecular weight kallikrein inhibitor in urine or any other organs of man or any other animals.

The isoelectric poihnt of inactive HUK was considered to be slightly higher than that of HUK as judged from the result of immunoelectrophoresis, while the pI of HUK" was considered to be similar to that of HUK. Other properties of HUK" investigated in the present work were closely resembled to those of HUK.

Both purified inactive HUK and inactive HUK in urine were unable to be measured by the RIA. We observed only little difference between the molecular weights of inactive and active HUKKs. So, the reason why inactive HUK was unable to be measured by the RIA has been speculated to be the different cross-reactivity between inactive and active HUKs. Kallirkein generated from inactive kallikrein by the action of trypsin may have almost the same cross-reactivity as kallikrein initially presents in urine, may be due to the change of three-dimensional configuration or any other reasons.

Judging from above points, HUK" and HUK were considered to be closely similar or identical, although the problems that whether trypsin is the major activator of inactive HUK or not and the meanings of inactive kallikrein excretion into urine still remain to be elucidated.

REFERENCES

1. J. Corthorn, T. Imanari, H. Yoshida, T. Kaizu, J. V. Pierce, and J. J. Pisano, Isolation of prokallikrein from human urine, in: "Adv. Exp. Med. Biol; Kinin II," Vol. 120B, S. Fujii, H. Moriya, and T. Suzuki, eds., Plenum Press, New York (1979).

2. N. B. Oza, W. Lieberthal, D. B. Bernard, and N. G. Levinsky, Antibody that recognizes total human urinary kallirkein; radioimmunological determination of inactive kallikrein, J. Immunol. , 126:2361-2364 (1981).

3. S. Iwanaga, T. Morita, H. Kato, T. Harada, N. Adachi, T. Sugo, I. Matuyama, K. Takada, T. Kimura, and S. Sakakibara, Fluorogenic peptide substrates for proteases in blood coagulation, kallikrein-kinin and fibrinolysis systems, in: " Adv. Exp. Med. Biol.; Kinin II," Vol. 120A, S. Fujii, H. Moriya, and T. Suzuki, edfs., Plenum Press, New York (1979).

4. M. Lemon, F. Fiedler, B. Forg-Brey, C. Hirschauer, G. Leysath, and H. Fritz, The isolation and properties of pig submandibular kallikrein, Biochem. J., 177:159-168 (1979).

5. S. Morichi, E. Sako, M. Tsuda, Y. Iga, S. Kitagawa, M. Nishida, K. Kizuki, M. Ikekita, and H. Moriya, Determination of active and inactive kallikrein in human urine by direct solid phase-radioimmunoassay, J. Immunol., (Submitted).

6. H. Moriya, K. Yamazaki, and H. Fukushima, Biochemical studies on kallikreins and their related substances; I. Isolation and purification of human saliva kallikrein, J. Biochem., 58:201-207 (1965).

7. R. Geiger and K. Mann, A kallikrein-specific inhibitor in rat kidney tubules, Hoppe-Seyler's Z. Physiol. Chem., 357:553-558 (1976).

PURIFICATION OF INACTIVE KALLIKREIN FROM RAT URINE

Mansanori Takaoka, Hirofumi Okamura, Takahiro Iwamoto
and Shiro Morimoto

Department of Pharmacology, Osaka College of Pharmacy
2-10-65 Kawai, Matsubara, Osaka 580, Japan

SUMMARY

An inactive kallikrein was purified from rat urine, and some of the properties of this enzyme were examined, in comparison with those of rat urinary kallikrein (RUK). The purified inactive kallikrein reacted with the antiserum against RUK and migrated slightly more slowly than RUK, on the immunoelectrophoresis. The molecular weights of the inactive kallikrein and RUK were estimated to be 44,000 and 38,000 by gel filtration, respectively. These results indicate that the rat urinary inactive kallikrein is immunologically identical with RUK, but this inactive enzyme has biochemical properties different from those of RUK, with respect to molecular weight and electrophoretical mobility.

INTRODUCTION

Urinary kallikrein is a glandular kallikrein (EC 3.4.21.35) which is synthesized by the kidney and secreted into the tubuler lumen.[1-4] In recent years, it has been demonstrated that the inactive kallikrein, which is activated with trypsin, is present in human and rat urine.[5-7] There are a few data indicating that the inactive form of kallikrein is released from kidney slices or from the isolated and perfused kidney, as is the active form of kallikrein.[8-11] However, the intrinsic nature of rat urinary inactive kallikrein has not been reported. Described herein are some properties of the inactive kallikrein purified from rat urine.

MATERIALS AND METHODS

Chemicals

The chemicals obtained from commercial sources were: DEAE-cellulose (DE-52) from Whatman Ltd. (U.K.); Sephadex G-75, Sephadex G-100, phenyl-Sepharose CL-4B and molecular weight standards from Pharmacia Fine Chemical AB (Sweden); prolyl-phenylalanyl-arginine-4-methylcoumaryl-7-amide (Pro-Phe-Arg-MCA) and 7-amino-4-methylcoumarin from the Protein Research Foundation (Japan); trypsin (bovine pancreas, Type III) and ovomucoid (chicken egg white, Type III) from Sigma Co. (U.S.A.). Other chemicals used were of reagent grade.

Rat urine

Male Wistar rats weighing 250-300 g were kept in individual stainless-steel metabolic cages, and 24 h urine samples were collected into flasks containing toluene to prevent bacterial growth. After the exclusion of toluene, the urine was centrifuged to remove solid debris, dialyzed against distilled water at 4° C for 48 h, and stored at −20° C until required.

Measurement of inactive kallikrein

Inactive kallikrein was detected by measuring kallikrein amidolytic activity produced after activation with trypsin, as described previously.[7] A mixture of 0.1 ml each of enzyme sample and trypsin (50 µg/ml) in 0.1 M Tris-HCl buffer (pH 8.0) containing 0.15 M NaCl was incubated at 37° C for 15 minutes. The reaction was terminated by the addition of 0.1 ml of ovomucoid (500 µg/ml) in the same buffer. Then, the amidolytic activity of kallikrein generated in the reaction mixture was determined by the method of Morita et al.,[12] using Pro-Phe-Arg-MCA as the substrate. One unit of kallikrein amidolytic activity was defined as the amount of the enzyme which hydrolyzed 1 µmole of Pro-Phe-Arg-MCA at 37° C for min.

Amino acid analysis

The purified enzyme was hydrolyzed in evacuated, sealed tubes at 110° C with 5.7 N HCl for 24, 48, and 72 hours. The amino acid composition was determined with an amino acid analyzer (Irica Model A-300, Japan), according to the method of Spackman et al.[13]

Preparation of anti-rat urinary kallikrein serum

Rat urinary kallikrein (RUK, 13.77 units/mg of protein) which had been purified in our laboratory was used for the preparation of anti-RUK serum. The homogeneity of this enzyme was confirmed, as a single protein band on a 12.5% SDS-polyacrylamide gel. The purified RUK (0.5 mg/ml) was mixed with an equal volume of complete Freund's adjuvant, and this emulsion was injected weekly into the foot pads and the backs of a rabbit for 4-week period. The whole blood was collected one week after the last injection. The serum was obtained by centrifugation at 900 g for 15 min, and the ammonium sulfate precipitate formed between 0 and 50% saturation was collected by centrifugation at 10,000 g for 15 min. The precipitate was dissolved in 10 mM sodium phosphate buffer (pH 7.0) and then dialyzed against the same buffer. The dialysate was used as an anti-RUK serum.

Immunological analysis

Immunodiffusion analysis was performed by the double diffusion techniques of Ouchterlony.[14] The analysis was made in 1.0% agarose in 0.05 M Tris-HCl buffer (pH 7.2) containing 0.15 M NaCl. Ten µl each of antigens and antiserum was applied to a well (4 mm diameter). Immunoelectrophoresis of 10 µl samples was performed on 1.2% agarose gel in 0.05 M veronal buffer (pH 8.6) at a constant current of 3 mA/cm. Antiserum (100 µl) was then added to each channel, and diffusion allowed to take place during 24 h at room temperature. The purified RUK and inactive kallikrein (about 15 µg) were used as antigens against anti-RUK serum.

Estimation of molecular weight

Molecular weight of the purified enzyme was estimated by gel filtration on a Sephadex G-100 column[15], and SDS-polyacrylamide gel electrophoresis[16] as follows. A Sephadex G-100 column (2.0 x 90 cm) was previously equilibrated with 40 mM sodium phosphate buffer (pH 7.4) containing 0.1 M NaCl. The column was eluted with the same buffer at a flow rate of 8.0 ml/h, and 2.0 ml fractions were collected at 4° C. Void volume of the column was estimated by using blue dextran. Bovine serum albumin (Mr 67,000), ovalbumin (Mr 43,000), α-chymotrypsinogen A (Mr 25,000) and ribonuclease A (Mr 13,700) were used as molecular weight standards. SDS-Polyacrylamide gel electrophoresis was performed using 12.5% slab gel (140 x 150 mm, 1.0-mm thick) at pH 8.9. A portion of purified sample was treated with 2-mercaptoethanol at 100° C for 3 min, and then subjected to electrophoresis at 15 mA/gel using bromophenol blue as a tracking dye. After electrophoresis, the gel was stained with 0.25% Coomassie brilliant blue R-250 dissolved in 45% methanol and 10% acetic acid, then de-stained in 25% methanol and 10% acetic acid.

RESULTS

The analytical data, at each stage of purification, is presented in Table I. The inactive kallikrein preparation obtained by the last Sephadex G-75 gel filtration was confirmed to be essentially homogeneous by polyacrylamide gel electrophoresis, as reported elsewhere.[17] This preparation was used as the pure rat urinary inactive kallikrein, in the following experiments.

Table I. Summary of the purification of inactive kallikrein

Purification step	Total protein (mg)	Total activity (units)	Specific activity (units/mg)	Yield (%)
Rat urine (2.8 liters)	9968	230	0.023	100
1. 30-70% Ammonium sulfate precipitation	5940	215	0.036	93
2. 1st DEAE-cellulose	165	65.4	0.397	28
3. 2nd DEAE-cellulose	62.1	48.8	0.786	21
4. Sephadex G-100	27.5	30.1	1.10	13
5. Phenyl Sepharose CL-4B	6.76	18.7	2.76	8.1
6. 3rd DEAE-cellulose	4.78	15.8	3.31	6.9
7. Sepadex G-75	1.15	8.87	7.71	3.9

Table II shows the amino acid composition of the purified inactive kallikrein. The contents of glutamic acid, serine, glycine, aspartic acid and lysine were high, and those of methionine, arginine and histidine were low in the enzyme.

Table II. Amino acid composition of inactive kallikrein from rat urine

Amino Acid	Nearest Integer
Aspartic acid	30
Threonine	24
Serine	60
Glutamic acid	65
Proline	17
Glycine	58
Alanine	25
Valine	17
Methionine	4
Isoleucine	13
Leucine	22
Tyrosine	11
Phenylalanine	10
Lysine	31
Histidine	9
Arginine	6
Cysteine	n.d.
Tryptophan	n.d.

Values for threonine, serine and tyrosine were extrapolated to zero time
of hydrolysis. Values for valine and isoleucine were those obtained
after hydrolysis for 72 h.   n.d. - not determined.

        The results of double immunodiffusion analysis are shown in
Figure 1-A. The purified inactive kallikrein reacted with the antiserum
against RUK, and formed one precipitin line fused with that of the purified RUK. Figure 1-B shows the immunoelectrophoretic patterns of the
purified RUK and inactive kallikrein. The inactive kallikrein gave one
precipitin line, and migrated slightly more slowly than RUK.

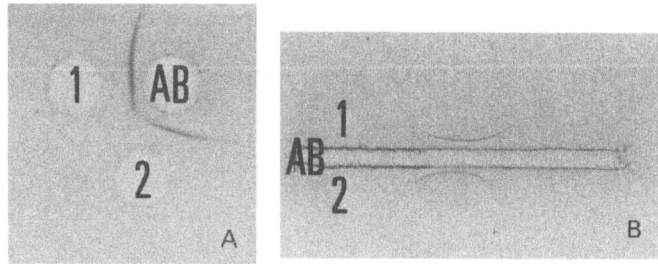

Figure 1. Immunological analysis of rat urinary kallikrein and inactive
           kallikrein.   AB: antiserum to pure rat urinary kallikrein;
           (1): pure rat urinary kallikrein; (2): pure rat urinary
           inactive kallikrein.

Two methods were used for the estimation of molecular weights of the purified RUK and inactive kallikrein. The results are summarized in Table III. The molecular weights of RUK and inactive kallikrein were estimated to be 39,000 and 41,000 by SDS-polyacrylamide gel electrophoresis, and to be 38,000 and 44,000 by gel filtration, respectively. In addition, the trypsin-activated form of inactive kallikrein was found by gel filtration, to have a molecular weight of 38,000.

TABLE III. Determination of the apparent molecular weight of rat urinary kallikrein and inactive kallikrein

	Rat urinary kallikrein	Inactive kallikrein	Trypsin-activated form of inactive kallikrein
SDS-polyacrylamide gel electrophoresis	39,000	41,000	n.d.
Gel filtration with Sephadex G-100	38,000	44,000	38,000

n.d.: not determined

DISCUSSION

The present study showed that the purified inactive kallikrein from rat urine is immunologically identical with RUK, but this inactive enzyme has biochemical properties different from those of RUK, with respect to molecular weight and electrophoretical mobility.

In the processes of purification of rat urinary inactive kallikrein, the first DEAE-cellulose chromatography decreased the yield of this enzyme to 28%. This suggests that a urinary enzyme which is activated with trypsin other than the inactive kallikrein may be present in the rat urine and be separable from the inactive kallikrein by the DEAE chromatography. These findings are supported by our observations[18] that rat urine contains an enzyme which is activated by trypsin treatment, and that this enzyme is eluted in the flow-through fraction of the DEAE-cellulose column. Therefore, when inactive kallikrein is isolated from rat urine, the separation of the other enzyme from the inactive enzyme by an ion-exchange chromatogrphy should first be taken into consideration.

In the present study, we examined the immunological properties of the inactive kallikrein purified from rat urine, and found that this enzyme reacted with antiserum against RUK (Figure 1). These results indicate that the inactive kallikrein is immunologically identical with RUK. On the other hand, the electrophoretic mobility of inactive kallikrein was slightly slower than that of RUK (Figure 1-B), indicating that the inactive enzyme may have a more basic isoelectric point than RUK. The above properties of rat urinary inactive kallikrein are consistent with those of porcine pancreatic prokallikrein A isolated by Kizuki et al.,[19] and may hold true for those of inactive glandular kallikreins which have not been isolated from various organs or urine, in various species.

343

From the amino acid analysis of the purified inactive kallikrein (Table II), the number of total amino acid residures was 411, and the molecular weight calculated according to the amino acid composition was about 42,500. However, it seems that the molecular weight of inactive kallikrein is in fact larger than that estimated by the amino acid composition, because cystein, tryptophan and carbohydrates were not determined in this work. Accordingly, the actual molecular weight of rat urinary inactive kallikrein is considered to be fairly close to the value of 44,000, as estimated by gel filtration (Table III). Here, the molecular weight of the purified inactive kallikrein was found to be reduced to 38,000 by trypsin treatment. As the molecular weight of RUK was also estimated to be 38,000 by the same method, in accordance with a previous report,[7] the present results show that the purified inactive kallikrein is converted to the active form with the release of small polypeptide fragment by trypsin treatment.

We recently reported that the purified inactive kallikrein is proteolytically activated by trypsin, but not by detergents or acidification known to dissociate the enzyme-inhibitor complex.[17] We suggested that the inactive form of kallikrein in rat urine had properties compatible with those of a precursor. This indicates that trypsin is useful as for the activation of urinary inactive kallikrein. However, it is unlikely that trypsin is an activator of the inactive form of kallikrein in the kidney, a possible origin of urinary inactive kallikrein.[20] To clarify the precise mechanism of activation of the inactive kallikrein, we are now isolating endogenous renal activator(s), by assessing the activation of the purified urinary inactive kallikrein.

ACKNOWLEDGEMENTS

We are grateful to Professor H. Matsubara and Dr. K. Wada, Department of Biology, Faculty of Science, Osaka University for providing facilities to measure amino acid composition of rat urinary inactive kallikrein, and to M. Ohara, Kyushu University, for reading the manuscript. This study was supported in part by a grant-in-aid for Encouragement of Young Scientists (59771765) from the Ministry of Education, Science and Culture of Japan.

REFERENCES

1. K. Nustad, The relationship between kidney and urinary kininogenase, Brit. J. Pharmacol. 39:73-86, (1970).
2. K. Nustad, K. Vaaje, and J. V. Pierce, Synthesis of kallikrein by rat kidney slices, Brit. J. Pharmacol. 53:229-234, (1975).
3. A. G. Scicli, O. A. Carretero, A. Hampton, P. Cortes, and N. Oza, Site of kininogenase secretion in the dog nephron, Am. J. Physiol. 230:533-536.
4. J. Roblero, H. Croxatto, R. Garcia, J. Corthorn, and E. De Vito, Kallikrein activity in perfusates and urine of isolated rat kidneys, Am. J. Physiol. 231:1383-1389.
5. J. J. Pisano, J. Corthorn, K. Yates, and J. V. Pierce, The kallikrein-kinin system in the kidney, Contr. Nephrol. 12:116-125, (1978).
6. J. Corthorn, T. Imanari, H. Yoshida, T. Kaizu, J. V. Pierce, and J. J. Pisano, Isolation of prokallikrein from human urine, Adv. Exp. Med. Biol. 120:575-579, (1979).

7. M. Takaoka, H. Akiyama, K. Ito, H. Okamura, and S. Morimoto, Isolation of inactive kallikrein from rat urine, Biochem. Biophys. Res. Commun. 109:841-847, (1982).

8. H. Nolly and M. C. Lama, Active and inactive kallikrein released by kidney slices from normotensive and hypertensive rats, Hypertension. 3 (Suppl):35-38, (1981).

9. J. Corthorn, L. Bio, and J. Roblero, Release of activatable kallikrein by isolated rat kidneys, Hypertension. 3 (Suppl):39-41, (1981).

10. J. Misumi, F. Alhenc-Gelas, M. Marre, J. Marchetti, P. Corvol, and J. Menard, Regulation of kallikrein and renin release by the isolated perfused rat kidney, Kidney Int. 24:58-65, (1983).

11. B. H. Van Leeuwen, S. M. Crinblat, and C. I. Johnston, Release of active and inactive kallikrein from the isolated perfused rat kidney, Clin. Sci. 66:207-215, (1984).

12. T. Morita, H. Kato, S. Iwanaga, K. Takada, T. Kimura, and S. Sakakibara, New fluoregenic substrates for α-thrombin, factor Xa, kallikrein, and urokinase, J. Biochem. 82:1495-1498, (1977).

13. D. H. Spackman, W. H. Stein, and S. Moore, Automatic recording apparatus for use in the chromatography of amino acids, Anal. Chem. 30:1190-1206, (1958).

14. O. Ouchterlony, Diffusion-in-gel methods for immunological analysis, in: Progress in allergy, vol. 5, ed. by P. Kallos and B. H. Waksman, Kargel, pp. 1-78, (1958).

15. P. Andrews, The gel filtration behavior of proteins related to their molecular weights over a wide range, Biochem. J. 96:595-606, (1965).

16. U. K. Laemmli, Cleavage of structual proteins during the assembly of the head of bacteriophage T4, Nature, 277:680-685, (1970).

17. M. Takaoka, H. Okamura, T. Iwamoto, C. Ikemoto, Y. Mimura, and S. Morimoto, Purification to apparent homogeneity of inactive kallikrein from rat urine, Biochem. Biophys. Res. Commun. 122: 1282-1288, (1984).

18. S. Morimoto, M. Nakajima, Y. Mizunoya, H. Okamura, H. Akiyama, and M. Takaoka, A kinin-generating amidase activated by trypsin in rat urine, Chem. Pharm. Bull. 32:4572-4579, (1984).

19. K. Kizuki, M. Kamada, M. Ikekita, and H. Moriya, Porcine pancreatic prokallikrein. II. Purification and some properties of pro-kallikrein A, Chem. Pharm. Bull. 30:3354-3361, (1982).

20. H. Okamura, M. Takaoka, T. Iwamoto, and S. Morimoto, Renal inactive kallikrein as the possible origin of urinary inactive kallikrein in the rat, J. Pharm. Dyn. 8:in press, (1985).

RELEASE OF TISSUE KALLIKREIN FROM THE ISOLATED PERFUSED KIDNEY

Namir Lâuar and Kanti Bhoola

Department of Pharmacology, Medical School, University of
Bristol, Bristol BS8 1TD, England

SUMMARY

Experiments were designed to determine the action of regulatory
peptides and potassium on the secretion of tissue kallikrein by the
isolated perfused rat kidney. Such experiments indicated that in spite
of the directly evoked release of kallikrein by arginine-vasopressin (AVP,
ADH), oxytocin and potassium from isolated renal cortical slices, the
secretion and clearance of active and total tissue kallikrein by the
isolated kidney was primarily sensitive to changes in the perfusion pressure.

INTRODUCTION

Previously, most of the information on the regulatory control
exercised by electrolytes, transmitters and peptide hormones on the secretion of renal kallikrein into urine was derived from studies performed
in anaesthetised animals. However, in order to define more clearly the
physiological importance of renal kallikrein it is necessary to examine
precisely the factors that regulate its release by using in vitro preparations.[1] Studies on isolated kidneys have provided useful information
about renal physiology. Such preparations offer advantages in that delivery and removal of administered drugs proceed through renal vascular
channels, without distribution to peripheral tissues. In addition, interference by non-renal factors are excluded. Furthermore, observed responses
are specific to the kidney so that interpretations of the data becomes
more precise. Because of such clear investigative advantages, we designed
experiments to evaluate on the isolated perfused rat kidney the action of
potassium, AVP and oxytocin, since they had evoked significant release of
kallikrein from renal cortical slices.[1]

METHODS

Perfusion Apparatus

The water jacketed, glass perfusion chamber (siliconized prior to
each experiment) is schematically illustrated in Figure 1. The perfusion

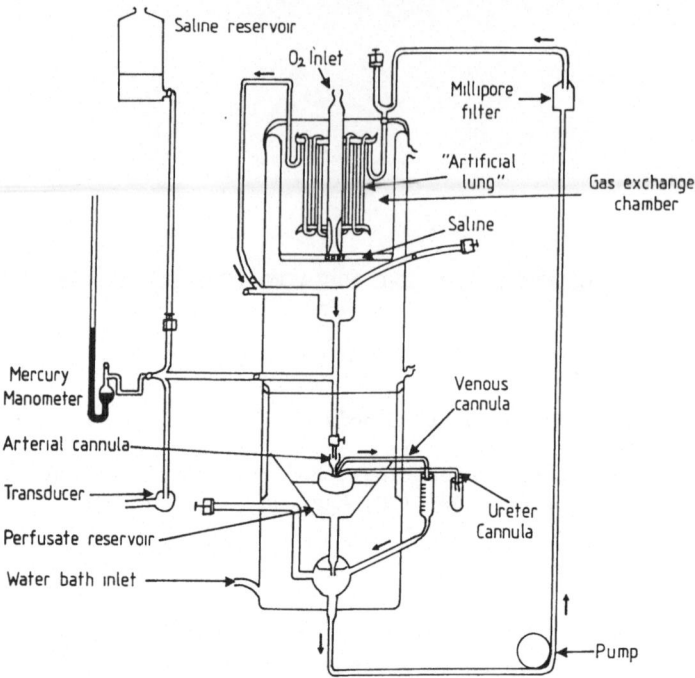

Figure 1. Schematic representation of the perfusion apparatus.

medium was either circulated (open system) or continuously re-circulated
(closed system) from a reservoir using a pulsatile pump (Watson-Marlow
Ltd). The perfusate was serated through an 'artificial lung' consisting
of 4 metres of silastic tubing (Dow Corning, U.S.A.), housed in a gas
exchanging chamber containing 95% O_2 - 5% CO_2. From the 'lung' the perfusate travelled in flexible tubing to the arterial cannula inserted into
the renal artery of the kidney. The enous effluent was returned to the
glass reservoir via a 2 ml graduated syringe (flow-meter). Perfusion
pressure was read on a mercury manometer and simultaneously monitored by
a pressure transducer (Elcomatic EM750), connected to a pen recorder
(Bryans). Such monitoring was necessary in order to achieve when required,
constant perfusion pressure by regulating the speed of the perfusion pump.
The connecting tubes to the water bath and all tubing external to the perfusion chamber were insulated.

Perfusion Medium

The perfusate consisted of a Krebs-buffer solution (m-mole/1:NaCl,
94.8; KCl, 4.7; Mg.SO_4 $7H_2$), 1.2; $CaCl_2$, 2.5; KH_2PO4, 1.2; $NaHCO_3$, 25.0;
Na-pyruvate, 4.9; Na-fumarate, 5.3; Na-glutamate, 4.9; glucose, 11.7),
containing 1% lyophilized, bovine serum albumin, 4% Ficoll and 0.2 mg/ml
creatinine. The solution was filtered through a Millipore filter (0.45
μm pore size) and equilibrated with 95% O_2 - 5% CO_2 mixture before and
throughout the experiment. The initial volume of the circulating
perfusate was 90 ml.

Operative Procedure

Male Wistar rates (350 - 450g) were used as kidney donors. The rats
were anaesthetized with urethane (1.75g/kg body weight), injected intraperitoneally. An operative technique for direct pulsatile perfusion of
the kidney through the renal artery[2] was used with minor modifications.
Immediately following completion of surgery, the kidney was perfused through

the arterial cannula with Krebs-buffer solution fed by gravity from a reservoir placed 130 cm above the organ; the distal end of the venous cannula was open, thereby permitting free flow of the perfusion medium. The kidney was next removed from the animal and connected inside the perfusion chamber. The initial venous effluent of 20 - 30ml was discarded and perfusion commenced with fresh Krebs-buffer solution. The temperature of the perfusion medium and the chamber was maintained at 37°C. In all experiments, the initial mean perfusion pressure was adjusted to ∿ 120 mmHg. The kidney was allowed to equilibrate for 60 min; the end of which was taken as zero time. To ensure comparable protocols no drugs were injected into the arterial line later than 30 min after zero time.

Collection of Samples and Preparation of Homogenate

Urine samples were collected in Eppendorf tubes kept on ice at 30 min intervals over a 2h period. Perfusate samples were collected from the venous line at the beginning and at the end of each urine collection period and stored on ice. Samples of urine and perfusate were centrifuged at 1,600g (MSE-Coolspin) for 20 min at 4°C and analysed within 24h of collection. At the end of each experiment, the perfused kidney was weighed (wet weight) and homogenised in saline (0.9%, 10 ml). The homogenate was centrifuged at 1,600g (MSE-Coolspin) for 20 min at 4°C; kallikrein activity was assayed in the supernatant.

Biochemical Measurements

Tissue kallikrein activity in urine, perfusate and homogenate samples was measured spectrophotometrically by following the rate of hydrolysis of the selective chromogenic substrate, H-D-Val-Leu-Arg-pNA (S2266, Kabi-Vitrum, Diagnostica). Assays were performed in the presence of soya bean trypsin inhibitor (SBTI), at a cuvette concentration of 0.8 mg/ml. Total (active + inactive) kallikrein was determined after activation with trypsin (100 µg/ml) with subsequent inactivation with 800 µg/ml SBTI. Tissue kallikrein activity was expressed as mU (10^{-3} pNA Units)/ml. The clearance of active and total kallikrein was calculated from the traditional formula:

$$\frac{\text{Urinary concentration (U) x Volume of urine (V)}}{\text{Perfusate concentration (P)}}$$

and expressed as µl/min.

Glomerular filtration was assessed by creatinine clearance and integrity of renal cells followed with lactate dehydrogenase.

RESULTS

Isolated kidneys perfused in a closed (Table 1) or open system at 120 ± 5 mmHg excrete and clear tissue kallikrein into the urine. Raising the perfusion pressure above 120 mmHg produces a pressure dependent increase in the excretion (Figure 2) and clearance (Figures 3, 4) of active and total kallikrein. The ratio of active to total changed from 2.0 (collection time, 30 min) and 2.5 (collection time, 120 min) at 120 mmHg to 3.0 and 5.9 respectively, when the perfusion pressure was raised above 195 mmHg.

Table 1. Time-course of parameters recorded during perfusion of the isolated rat kidney with the perfusate recycled. Perfusion pressure at 120 ± 5 mmHg (n=8).

Collection periods (min)	Perfusion flow rate (ml/min)	Perfusate LDH activity (B-B U/ml)	Urine flow (µl/min)	Creatinine clearance (µl/min)
0-30 (I)	14.7 ± 0.03	247.0 ± 52.0	19.0 ± 5.0	200.0 ± 50.0
30-60 (II)	14.3 ± 0.7	317.0 ± 56.0	16.5 ± 3.0	171.0 ± 37.0
60-90 (III)	13.7 ± 1.3	397.0 ± 84.0	15.0 ± 3.0	158.0 ± 30.0
90-120 (IV)	12.3 ± 2.0	510.0 ± 97.0	13.0 ± 4.0	141.0 ± 35.0
120-150 (V)	10.3 ± 2.0	670.0 ± 170.0	14.0 ± 4.0	148.0 ± 36.0

Collection periods (min)	Urinary kallikrein excretion (mU/min)		Kallikrein clearance (µl/min)	
	Active	Total	Active	Total
0-30 (I)	0.05 ± 0.02	0.18 ± 0.05	121.0 ± 24.0	60.0 ± 18.0
30-60 (II)	0.06 ± 0.01	0.19 ± 0.04	114.0 ± 24.0	54.4 ± 12.0
60-90 (III)	0.07 ± 0.02	0.22 ± 0.03	135.0 ± 29.0	66.0 ± 18.0
90-120 (IV)	0.08 ± 0.04	0.18 ± 0.04	137.0 ± 24.0	55.0 ± 20.0
120-150 (V)	0.09 ± 0.03	0.20 ± 0.05	129.0 ± 23.0	53.0 ± 22.0

In our previous experiments on kidney slices, we established that high K^+ and Ca^{++}, low Na^+ and Mg^{++}, AVP, Oxytocin and PGE_2 promoted the secretion of renal tissue kallikrein. In contrast, angiotensin II, lysine-vasopressin, substance P, vasoactive intestinal peptide, carbachol, noradrenaline and dopamine were relatively ineffective (see 1). We

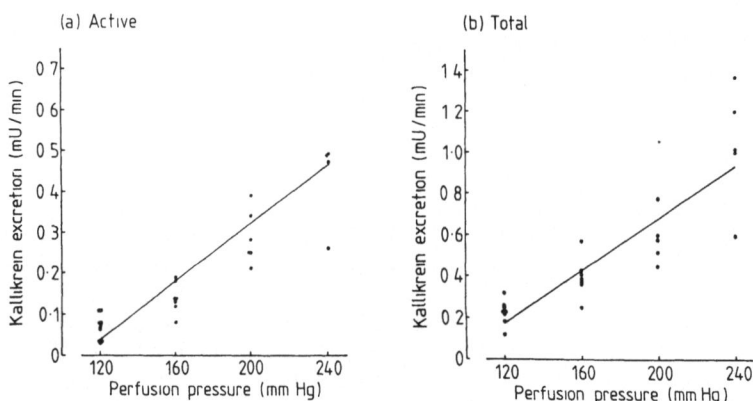

Figure 2. Relationship between perfusion pressure and excretion of active and total tissue kallikrein into urine produced by the isolated perfused kidney.
Perfusate recycled. r= 0.97   p < 0.01.

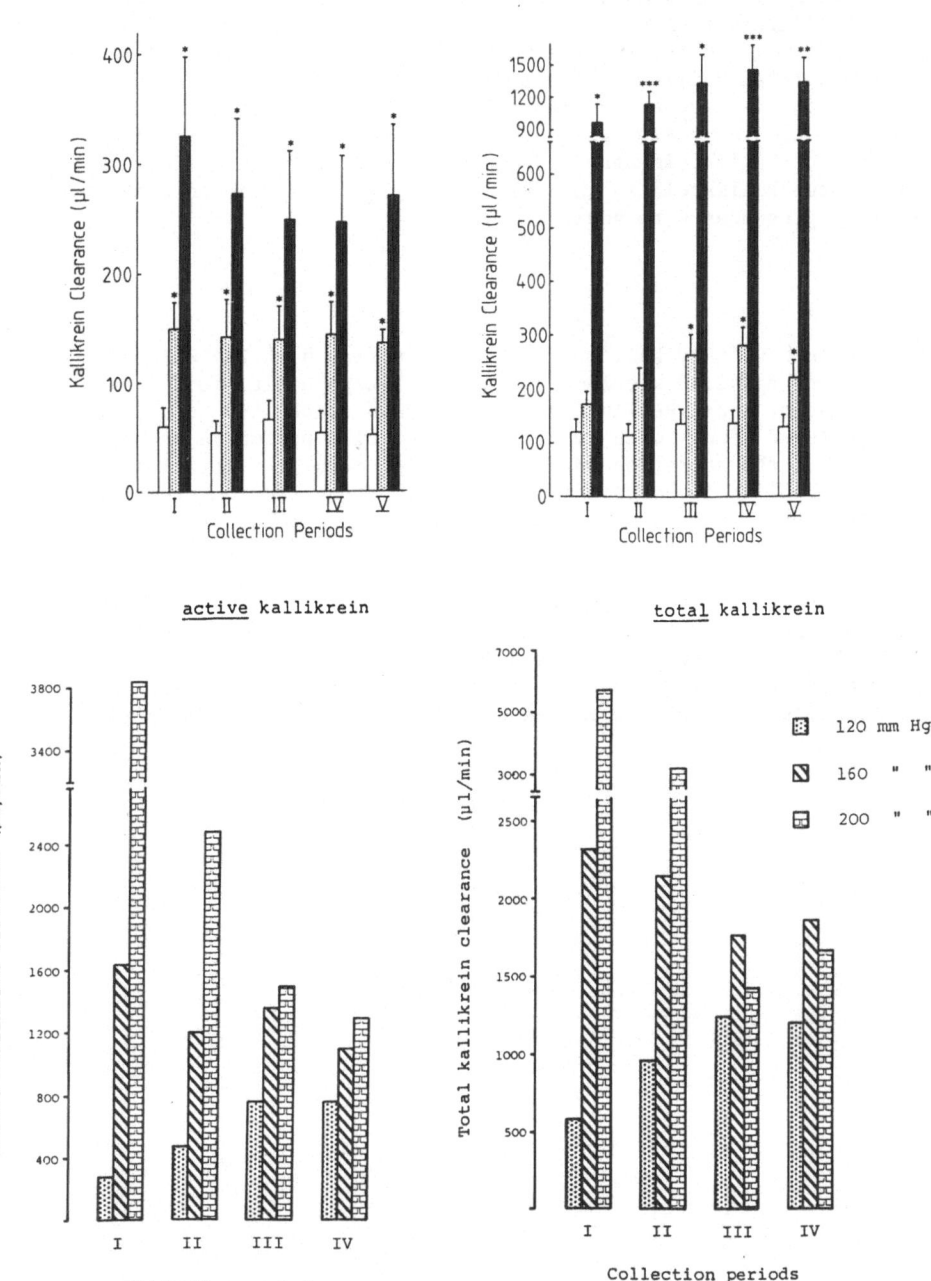

CLOSED SYSTEM – Figure 3   OPEN SYSTEM – Figure 4

Figures 3 and 4.   Effect of perfusion pressure on the clearance of active
                   and total kallikrein by the isolated perfused kidney –

n=8
          120 mmHg
n=2
                        n=6
                                  160 mmHg
                        n=2
                                            n=5
                                                      200 mmHg
                                            n=2

1 to V sequential 30 min collection periods.

*p<0.005, **p<0.02, ***p<0.01, ****p<0.001

therefore considered it worthwhile to evaluate on the isolated perfused kidney the action of some of the agents that caused a clear secretion of tissue kallikrein from the renal cortical slices. APV (4×10^{-10}M) and oxytocin (2×10^{-6}M) stimulated markedly the secretion and clearance of active and total kallikrein but only when the perfusion pressure was permitted to rise above 120 mmHg following injection of the drugs (See Figures 5, 6). Perfusion pressure dependent changes in the release and clearance of kallikrein were also observed with potassium (50 mM). Total renal tissue kallikrein in the perfused kidneys was reduced only when high perfusion pressures were achieved.

DISCUSSION

Although urinary kallikrein originates from both the kidney[3] and the circulation[4] detailed knowledge about the biosynthesis, mode of activation and release of renal kallikrein is still inadequate. By using the isolated perfused kidney with cycled and non-cycled perfusate we have demonstrated that the secretion and clearance (glomerular filtration) of active and total kallikrein correlated highly with the perfusion pressure. Two mechanisms may regulate kallikrein secretion: a direct effect of filtration pressure and a pressure sensitive local neuronal or humoral arc operative between the afferent arteriole and the distal connecting tubule cells. A positive secretory stimulus was also observed with AVP and oxytocin, but only when the perfusion pressure was permitted to rise above 120 mmHg.[5] The present experiments seem to indicate that an increase in the mean arterial pressure or in glomerular filtration rate is a primary pre-requisite for the increase in the excretion of tissue kallikrein

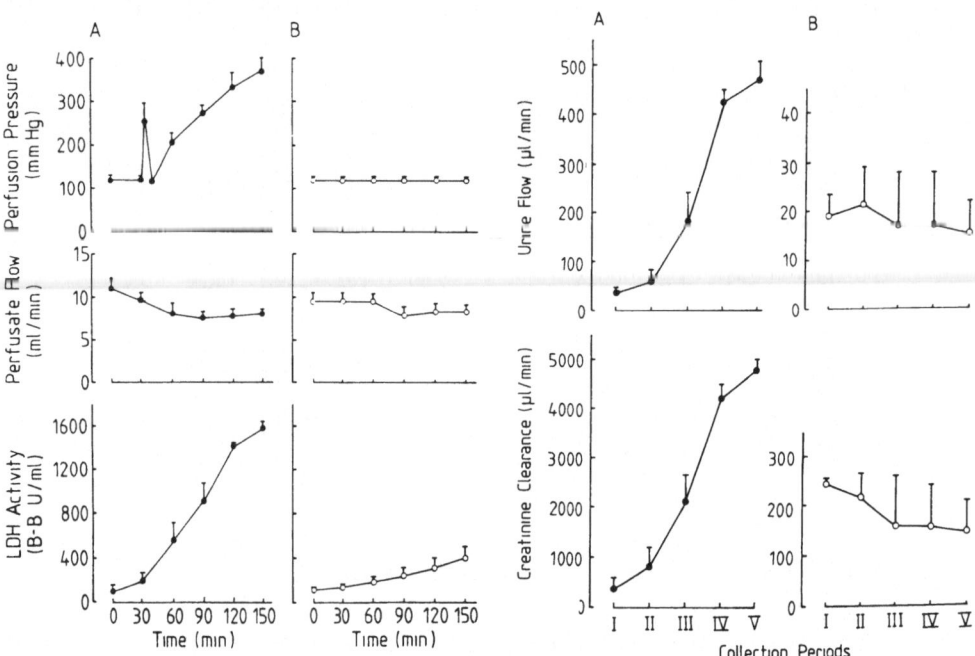

Figure 5. Effect of AVP (4×10^{-10}M) on perfusion pressure, perfusate flow, LDH activity, urine flow and creatinine clearance. Perfusate recycled.

A = perfusion pressure permitted change (●——●), B = perfusion pressure maintained at ∿120 mmHg (o——o). 1 to V = sequential 30 min collection periods. Bar = 1 S.E.M. (n=5).

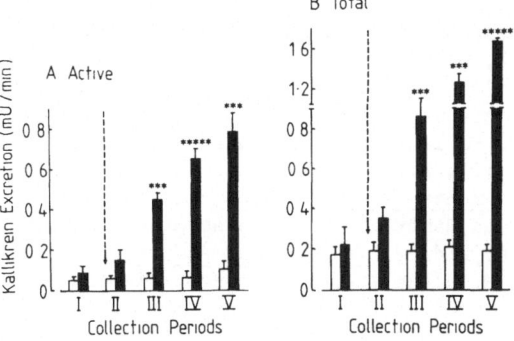

Figure 6. Effect of AVP (4×10^{-10}M) on the excretion of active and
total kallikrein into urine produced by the isolated perfused
kidney. Perfusate re-cycled. Dotted arrow = injection of AVP.

■ Perfusion pressure permitted to change

□ Perfusion pressure maintained at 120 mmHg.

1 to V = Sequential 30 min collection periods. Bar = 1 S.E.M.
(n=5)

***$p < 0.01$, ****$p < 0.001$ when compared to 1st collection period.

produced by AVP and oxytocin. However, in view of our positive results
with kidney cortical slices, an additional direct effect of these peptides
is not excluded. Vasopressin receptors have been located on the basolateral membrane cells of the terminal segment of the distal tubule and
of the collecting tubule. Kallikrein is considered to be released mainly
from the cells of the connecting tubule. This proximity favours possible
interactions between tissue kallikrein release and AVP (ADH).

Potassium also increased urinary excretion of kallikrein by the
isolated perfused kidney. Although this result was obtained with very
high concentrations of the ion (10 to 20 fold above the normal), values
close to these have been reported for the distal tubule fluid from
nephrons of rats submitted to a high potassium diet.[6] As the excretion
of urinary kallikrein in man varies directly with K^+ intake,[7] and leads
to a high potassium concentration in the distal tubule fluid, it is
tempting to suggest that a potassium load in the distal tubule may
directly by exchange or depolarization stimulate the secretion of renal
tissue kallikrein.

ACKNOWLEDGEMENTS

Namir Lâuar was a CAPES (Brazil) Fellow. Kanti Bhoola thanks the
Wellcome Trust for Research Grants.

REFERENCES

1. Namir Lâuar, Mary Shacklady, and K. D. Bhoola, Factors influencing
   the in vitro release of renal kallikrein, in: Recent Progress
   on Kinins, H. Fritz, G. Dietze, F. Fiedler and G. L. Haberland,
   eds., Birkhäuser, Agents and Actions Suppl., 9:545-552, (1982).

2. J. M. Nishiitustsuji-Umo, B. D. Ross and H. A. Krebs, Metabolic activities of the isolated perfused rat kidney, <u>Biochem. J.</u> 103:852-862, (1967).

3. K. Nustad, K. Vaaje and J. V. Pierce, Synthesis of kallikreins by rat kidney cortex slices, <u>Br. J. Pharmac.</u> 53:229-234, (1975).

4. E. Fink and M. Schleuning, Glomerular filtration of tissue kallikrein, <u>in</u>: Kinins III, H. Fritz, N. Back, G. Dietze and G. L. Haberland, eds., <u>Adv. in Exp. Med. and Biol.</u> 156B:939-947, (1983).

5. K. D. Bhoola and Namir Lâuar, Release of kallikrein by the isolated perfused rat kidney, <u>Br. J. Pharmac.</u> 80:690P.

6. G. Malnic, R. M. Kloze and G. Giebisch, Micropuncture study of renal potassium excretion in rat, <u>Am. J. Physiol.</u> 206:674-684, (1964).

7. D. Horwitz, H. S. Margolius and H. R. Keiser, Effects of potassium intake on urinary kallikrein and aldosterone excretion, <u>Clin. Res.</u> 23:221A, (1975).

ANALYTICAL STUDY OF KALLIKREIN AND KALLIKREIN-LIKE ESTERASE ACTIVITY IN
SUBFRACTIONS FROM RAT KIDNEY CORTEX MICROSOMES AND ISOLATED SUBCELLULAR
MEMBRANES

Knut-Jan Andersen and Jarle Ofstad

Medical Department A
University of Bergen
N-5016 Haukeland Sykehus
Bergen, Norway

SUMMARY

Heavy and light microsomal fractions were subfractioned using high
performance zonal rotors, and assayed for approtenin sensitive kallikrein-
like amidolytic activity (pH 8.2). The activity profiles for the various
substrates assayed show rather complex distribution pattern demonstrating
kallikrein-like amidolytic activity in plasma membranes, basolateral membranes, rough endoplasmic reticulum and membranes derived from the Golgi
complex.

INTRODUCTION

Kallikrein assays based on synthetic substrates like lysine and
arginine esters and amides[1] resembles classical biochemical assays currently used for marker enzymes in subcellular work and are much easier to
perform than the rather cumbersome bioassays. Although these assays have
been claimed to be of limited specificity,[2] most of the subcellular work
describing the localization of renal kallikrein in the distal tubular cells
are based on spectrophotometrically assays with D-Val-Leu-Arg-p-nitroanilide.

Recently, the histochemical localization of kallikrein-like Pro-Phe-
Arg-naphthylester esterase activity in the proximal tubular cells of human
and rat kidneys[3,4] have been reported. D-Pro-Phe-Arg-p-nitroanilide (pNa)
is the substrate commonly used for plasma kallikrein (S-2302, Kabi Diagnostica), while glandular kallikrein is assayed with D-Val-Leu-Arg-pNa
(S-2266, Kabi). Plasma kallikrein has low affinity with D-Val-Leu-Arg-pNa,
while glandular kallikrein shows similar activity with both substrates.[5]

The purpose of this study was therefore to compare the distribution
of D-Pro-Phe-Arg-pNa, D-Val-Leu-Arg-pNa, and other Arg- and Lys-amidolytic
activity with classical marker enzymes in rat kidney cortex microsomes
subfractioned using high performance zonal rotors.

ANALYTICAL TECHNIQUES

The kidney cortices from ten to twelve male rats (Wistar, 150-200 g), starved overnight, were homogenized in 0.25 M sucrose/5 mM Tris HCl, pH 7.4, and the nuclear (N)- and mitochondrial/lysosomal (ML)-fractions were pelleted as previously described.[6] The heavy microsomes (HMic) were sedimented at 18.000 rev/min for 10 min before the light microsomes (LMic) were pelleted at 43.000 rev/min for 60 min (Table 1).

The two microsomal fractions were further subfractioned by isopycnic banding. The heavy microsome were resuspended in 0.25 M sucrose/5 mM Tris HCl, pH 7.4, and loaded into a B-14 zonal rotor (MSE Scientific Instruments, UK) containing a linear sucrose gradient, 0.7M-2.3M sucrose. The rotor was then spun at 45.000 rev/min for approx. 16 h. The light microsomes were resuspended in 2 M sucrose and loaded into a Kontron TZT 48.650 zonal rotor (Kontron Analytical, Switzerland) at precisely the 2 M point of the gradient, 0.7M-2.3M. The rotor was spun at 45.000 rev/min overnight. Finally, 20 ml fractions were collected from both rotors for the various assays.

PROTEIN AND MARKER ENZYMES

N-acetyl-β-glucosaminidase, acid β-glycerophosphatase (lysosomes), glucose-6-phosphatase (endoplasmic reticulum), alkaline phosphatase and 5'-nucleotidase (brush border – plasma membrane) were assayed as described elsewhere,[6,7] while Na-K-ATP'ase (basolateral membrane) was assayed using assay procedure A described by Schwartz et al.[8]

The distribution of aprotenin sensitive (100 KIU/ml) amidolytic activity was assayed essentially as described by Amundsen et al.[9] at pH 8.2 (0.2M Tris-HCl) using the substrates listed in Table 2 at a final concentration of 1.5 mM. S-substrates were from Kabi Diagnostica, Stockholm, Sweden, while Pk-1 was obtained from Nyegaard Diagnostica, Oslo, Norway.

Table 1.

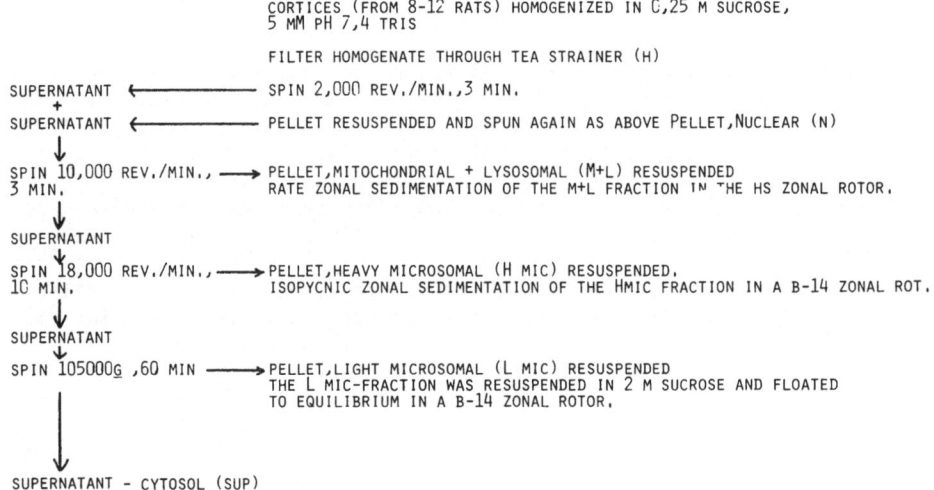

CORTICES (FROM 8-12 RATS) HOMOGENIZED IN 0,25 M SUCROSE, 5 MM PH 7,4 TRIS

FILTER HOMOGENATE THROUGH TEA STRAINER (H)

SUPERNATANT ⟵——————— SPIN 2,000 REV./MIN.,3 MIN.
+
SUPERNATANT ⟵——————— PELLET RESUSPENDED AND SPUN AGAIN AS ABOVE PELLET,NUCLEAR (N)

SPIN 10,000 REV./MIN., ⟶ PELLET,MITOCHONDRIAL + LYSOSOMAL (M+L) RESUSPENDED
3 MIN.   RATE ZONAL SEDIMENTATION OF THE M+L FRACTION IN THE HS ZONAL ROTOR.

SUPERNATANT

SPIN 18,000 REV./MIN., ⟶ PELLET,HEAVY MICROSOMAL (H MIC) RESUSPENDED.
10 MIN.   ISOPYCNIC ZONAL SEDIMENTATION OF THE HMIC FRACTION IN A B-14 ZONAL ROT.

SUPERNATANT

SPIN 105000G ,60 MIN ⟶ PELLET,LIGHT MICROSOMAL (L MIC) RESUSPENDED
    THE L MIC-FRACTION WAS RESUSPENDED IN 2 M SUCROSE AND FLOATED
    TO EQUILIBRIUM IN A B-14 ZONAL ROTOR.

SUPERNATANT - CYTOSOL (SUP)

Table 2. Substrates assayed

Name	Formula	Clinical Assay
S-2266	D-Val-Leu-Arg-pNa	Glandular kallikrein
S-2251	D-Val-Leu-Lys-pNa	Plasmin/plasminogen
S-2288	D-Ile-Pro-Arg-pNa	Serine proteases, plasminogen activator
S-2302	D-Pro-Phe-Arg-pNa	Plasma kallikrein
S-2314	D-Val-Ser-Arg-pNa	Complement factors
Pk-1	D-α-amino-butyric-acid-1-cyclohexyl-Ala-Arg-pNa	Plasma kallikrein

RESULTS AND DISCUSSION

Sedimentation of heavy microsomes gave isopycnic banding for all ami-dolytic substrates, 5'-nucleotidase, alkaline phosphatase and the major protein peak at a density of 1.18. In addition, both S-2288 and S-2302 showed a distinct, tailing shoulder together with a second, distinct peak of Pk-1 at a density of 1.15. The plasma membrane (PM) marker enzyme, 5'-nucleotidase, showed a very broad distribution (1.12-1.18 g/ml) suggest-ing the presence of rather heterogeneous populations of these membranes. However, the brush border marker, alkaline phosphatase, gave a more defined peak at density 1.18. The rather broad band obtained for glucose-6-phos-phatase (1.14-1.17 g/ml) marks the position of smooth endoplasmic reticulum (ER) with a distinct shoulder of the enzyme at higher densities (1.20 g/ml) attributable to rough ER vesicles as confirmed by the pattern of RNA. The basolateral membrane marker, Na-K-ATP'ase, banded at a density of 1.16 with a leading shoulder at density 1.18. The lysosomal markers, acid-β-glycero-phosphatase and N-actyl-β-glucosaminidase showed distribution profiles dif-ferent from the amidolytic activity, although some non-latent activity banded at densities 1.15-1.18, representing fragments of lysosomal membranes and "released" acid hydrolase activity trapped by smooth membrane vesicles. Although all approtenin sensitive amidolytic activity appear to have similar distributions among the heavy microsomal subfractions, the relative total activity per fraction for each substrate, banding at densities 1.15 and 1.18, are different. This is demonstrated in Table 3 where the activities are expressed as a percentage of the peak S-2266 activity.

While flotation of the light microsomes gave similar distribution pattern and identical densities for the marker enzymes, the distribution pattern for amidolytic activity was different from the heavy microsomes. All substrates showed a major peak banding at a density of 1.15. In addi-tion, both S-2266 and S-2251 showed a second peak banding together with a distinct leaning shoulder of S-2288, S-2302, S-2314 and Pk-1 activity at 1.18 g/ml. The relative total activity per fraction banding at densities 1.15 and 1.18 are shown in Table 4 where the activities for all substrates are expressed as a percentage of the peak fraction of S-2266 activity.

This study demonstrates the presence of membrane bound kallikrein-like amidolytic activity in both heavy and light microsomes from rat kidney cortex. The activity profiles for the various substrates show rather complex distribution pattern due to multi-membrane localization. The dis-

Table 3. Distribution of amidolytic activity in rat kidney cortex heavy microsomes. The activities are expressed as a percentage of peak S-2266 activity

Density	1.15	1.18
S-2266	17.1	100.0
S-2251	0	7.5
S-2288	20.5	49.7
S-2302	17.8	28.2
S-2314	6.7	21.1
Pk-1	13.4	20.5

tribution patterns confirm the presence of amidolytic activity in several populations of the PM and the basolateral membrane.[10] In addition, amidolytic activity was found to co-sediment with rough endoplasmic reticulum and membranes derived from the Golgi complex. These observations give evidence in support of the very elegant ultrastructural immunocytochemical studies of Dr. Vio and coworkers[11] demonstrating that kallikrein is synthesized in the kidney.

Table 4. Distribution of amidolytic activity in rat kidney cortex light microsomes. The activities are expressed as a percentage of peak S-2266 activity

Density	1.15	1.18
S-2266	100.0	76.7
S-2251	9.5	5.0
S-2288	75.7	32.6
S-2302	104.5	22.9
S-2314	16.9	6.3
Pk-1	97.1	16.3

REFERENCES

1. P. Friberger, Chromogenic peptide substrates. Their use for the assay of factors in the fibrinolytic and plasma kallikrein-kinin systems, Scand. J. Clin. Lab. Invest., 42(suppl. 162):11-37.
2. O. A. Carretero, A. G. Scicli, and A. Nasjletti, The glandular kallikrein-kinin system: Methodology for its measurement, in: "Hypertension Research - Methods and Models," F. M. Radzialowski, ed., Marcel Dekker (1982).
3. K. Kimura, Segmental localization of kallikrein-like pro-phe-arg-naphthylester in the rat nephron, Acta Path. Microbiol. Immunol. Scand., 91(Sect. A):35-42 (1983).

4. K. Kimura and H. Moriya, Enzyme- and immuno-histo-chemical localization of kallikrein. II. The human kidney, Histochemistry, 80:443-448 (1984).

5. Kabi Diagnostics (S-11287 Stockholm, Sweden), Products for diagnostic use and research (1983).

6. K-J. Andersen, H. J. Haga, and M. Dobrota, Heterogeneity of rat kidney-cortex lysosomes fractionated by gradient centrifugation in zonal rotors, Biochem. Soc. Trans., 8:5976-598 (1980).

7. K-J. Andersen, M. Dobrota, and H. J. Haga, The effect of sucrose on assaying enzymes and protein in the subcellular fractions of the rat kidney cortex, J. Biochem. Biophys. Methods, 1:309-311 (1979).

8. A. Schwartz, K. Nagano, M. Nakao, G. E. Lindenmayer, and J. C. Allen, The sodium- and potassium-activated adenosinetriphosphatase system, Meth. Pharmacol., 1:361-388 (1971).

9. E. Amundsen, J. Puter, P. Friberger, M. Knos, M. Larsbraten, and G. Claeson, Methods for the determination of glandulary kallikrein by means of a chromogenic tripeptide substrate, Adv. Exp. Med. Biol., 120A:83-95 (1979)

10. K. Yamada and E. Erdös, Isolation of two forms of kallikreins from rat kidney, Adv. Exp. Med. Biol., 156A:387-391 (1983).

11. C. P. Vio, C. D. Figueroa, and I. Caorsi, Renal kallikrein: Cellular localization and subcellular distribution by ultrastructural immunocytochemistry, This Proceedings.

ENDOGENOUS KALLIKREIN INHIBITOR IN RAT KIDNEY CORTEX-EFFECT OF

GLUCOCORTICOID ADMINISTRATION

Kodo Ito, Kenichi Yamada, Setsuko Yoshida, Keiji Hasunuma,
Yasushi Tamura and Sho Yoshida

The Second Department of Internal Medicine, Chiba University
School of Medicine, Chiba 280, Japan

SUMMARY

Kallikrein inhibiting proteins with two different molecular weight
($6-8 \times 10^4$, $8-9 \times 10^4$ respectively) were observed in adrenalectomized rat
kidney cortical soluble fraction. The larger one was observed in the
kidneys of the adrenalectomized rats only when they had received chronic
administration of excess amount of dexamethasone, and its kallikrein
inhibitory activity was not lost with treatment with trypsin. This protein
appears to be induced by chronic administration of glucocorticoid and might
participate in the process of glucocorticoid regulating renal kallikrein
kinin system.

INTRODUCTION

There are several reports that glucocorticoids participate in the
activation of renal and urinary kallikrein-kinin system.[1,2] On the process
of investigating the effects of glucocorticoids on renal kallikrein system,
we found that a protein characterized by the inhibition of kallikrein activity might be induced in renal cortical soluble fraction by the chronic administration of excess amount of dexamethasone. The aim of present study
was to report some characteristics of the inhibitory protein.

MATERIALS AND METHODS

Male Splague Dawley rats weighing 200 g to 250 g were anesthetized
with sodium pentobarbital 50 mg/kg intraperitoneally and adrenalectomized
bilaterally. They were fed with normal rat chow and 0.9% saline to drink
ad libitim. After adaptation to metabolism cage, daily doses of 250 µg of
dexamethasone diluted in ethanol and olive oil was injected intraperitoneally
for seven days. The same amount of olive oil was given to the vehicle administered rats as control. Kidneys were taken out after decapitation and
the cortex was minced and homogenized in 0.01 M Tris HCl buffer pH 7.4 containing 0.25 M sucrose (1:4 = W/V). The homogenate was centrifuged at
800 x g for 15 min. and the supernatant again at 105,000 x g for 60 min.
The supernatant (rat kidney cortical soluble fraction) was divided into
two and a half of them was applied on Sephadex G-100 column (2 x 100 cm)
and eluted with 0.05 M Tris HCl, 0.1 M NaCl buffer pH 7.4. After concen-

tration with PM10 ultrafiltration membrane (Amicon), these eluates were incubated with trypsin (250 μg/ml) at 37°C for 60 min. at pH 7.4, and then lima bean trypsin inhibitor (2.5 mg/ml) was added to terminate the reaction with trypsin. Endogenous kallikrein was absorbed by the method of double antibody using anti rat urinary kallikrein goat serum (anti-RUK) and anti goat IgG antibody. Endogenous kallikrein in each eluate was assayed and was confirmed to be negligible. Anti RUK antibody was completely removed by anti goat IgG and had no effect on the following procedure. Rat urine (0.025 ml = approximately 1000 pg bradykinin production/min. - as kallikrein standard) was incubated at 37°C for 60 min. in 0.1 M Tris HCl buffer pH 7.4 with these eluates which were treated with or without trypsin previously, and the kininogenase activities of these urine-eulate mixture were assayed to evaluate the effect of these eluates on urinary kallikrein activity.

The other half of the preparated soluble fraction was incubated with Sepharose-4B-bound trypsin prepared by previous method,[3] at room temperature in 0.05 M Tris HCL buffer pH 7.4 for 60 min. on a rotary mixing table, and the bound trypsin was then removed by brief centrifugation. Endogenous kallikrein in the supernatant was absorbed by the method of double antibody described above, and this soluble fraction was subjected to gel filtration through the same Sephadex G-100 column. Each eluates were incubated with 0.025 ml of rat urine for 60 min. at 37°C, pH 7.4, after concentration with PM10 ultrafiltration membrane and the kininogenase activities of the mixture were assayed to evaluate the effect of these eluates on the kininogenase activity of the rat urine.

Bovine serum albumin, commercial gel filtration standard (BIO-RAD, containing gamma globulin M.W. 158,000, Ov albumin M.W. 44,000, and myoglobin M.W. 17,000) were used as gel filtration standard protein. Kininogenase activity was assayed by determining the kinin released from heated dog plasma by radioimmunoassay.[3]

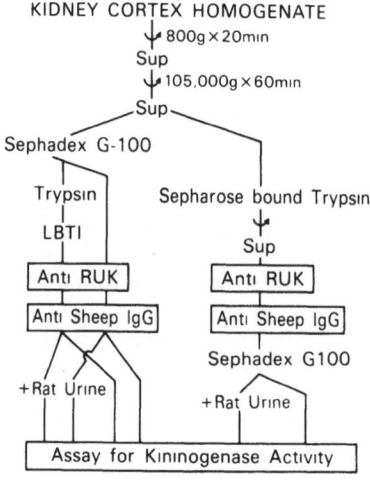

Fig. 1.

RESULTS

    Upper panel of the Fig. 2 shows the gel filtration profile of the
kallikrein inhibitory activity of the dexamethasone-treated rat kidney
cortical soluble fraction. Kininogenase activity of the rat urine was
markedly reduced by the non trypsin-treated eluates (closed circle) corresponding to the molecular weight of 6-8x10^4 on gel filtration. After treatment of each eluate with trypsin (open circle), reduction of kallikrein
activity was still found at the molecular weight of 8-9x10^4.

    The gel filtration profile of the kallikrein inhibitory activity of
kidney cortical soluble fraction prepared from vehicle-administered control
rats (Fig. 2, lower panel) was different from the one prepared from the
dexamethasone-administered rats. While non trypsin-treated eluates (closed
circle) inhibited kallikrein activity at the same molecular weight range,
however, after treatment with trypsin (open circle), no kallikrein inhibitory activities were observed in all of these eluates.

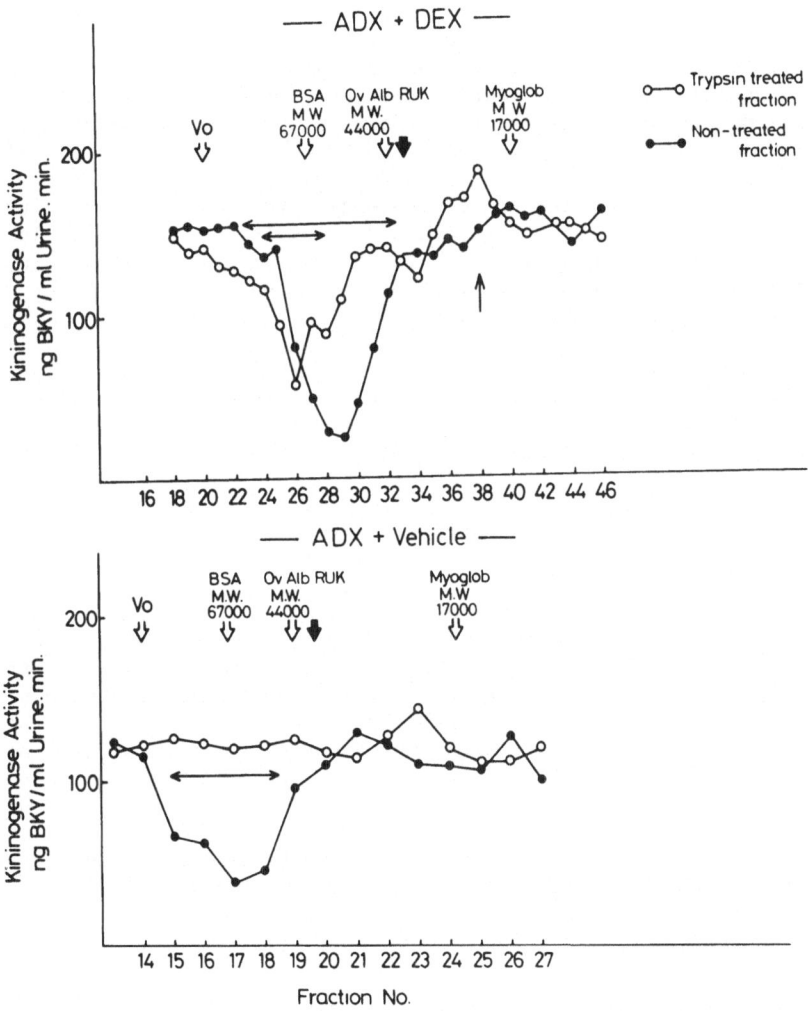

Fig. 2. Effect of gel-filtrated kidney cortical soluble fraction on
urinary kallikrein activity.

When the kidney cortical soluble fraction was treated with trypsin before gel filtration, no kallikrein inhibitory activities were detected in the gel-filtrated eluates both of the fraction prepared from dexamethasone administered and control rats.

DISCUSSION

It has been shown that chronic glucocorticoid treatment caused to decrease kallikrein excretion in rats[1,4,5] and reduced the ratio of active-to-total kallikrein in urine and also in renal cortical basolateral membrane[1,5]. Several explanations could be proposed; At first, glucocorticoid may induce kallikrein-inhibitor(s) in kidney, then, increase the synthesis of prekallikrein (inactive kallikrein), and thirdly inhibit the conversion of inactive to active kallikrein, directly or indirectly. At this time, we examined the first possibility whether kallikrein-inhibitor(s) was(were) induced in kidney by glucocorticoid. In our present study, it was suggested that two components characterized by the inhibition of kallikrein activity seemed to be separate from chronically dexamethasone-administered rat kidney soluble fraction, by using the method of gel filtration as shown in Fig. 1. The apparent molecular weight of large one was approximately $8-9 \times 10^4$, and that of small one, $6-8 \times 10^4$. Since the kallikrein-inhibitory activity of small component, corresponding to the M.W. of $6-8 \times 10^4$, was lost with trypsin-treatment, so it might be α_1-protease inhibitor (α_1-trypsin inhibitor), considering the evidences that α_1-protease inhibitor shows almost same molecular and glucocorticoids also increase the trypsin inhibitor in urine.[6,7]

However, the large component corresponding to the molecular weight of $8-9 \times 10^4$ was also showing the kallikrein-inhibitory activity and looked like to be different from α_1-protease inhibitor since it was not inactivated with trypsin-treatment, i.e., it neither made complex with nor was digested by an excess amount of trypsin.

Although data not shown here, Rf value of complex of this componen with purified ^{125}I-kallikrein showed difference from that of small one on polyacrylamide gel electrophoresis. Therefore it was suggested that new kallikrein-inhibitor was induced in the kidney by chronic administration of dexamethasone.

However, considering that no kallikrein-inhibitory activity was observed in each gel-filtration eluate of trypsin-pretreated kidney soluble fraction, it might be proposed that the moiety itself associated with kallikrein-inhibitory activity would be small, so that inhibitory activity was unable to detect in this gel-filtration system after trypsin treatment, suggesting that this large protein characterized by kallikrein-inhibitory activity might consist of small active moiety and its carrier protein. Although Geiger et al.[8] reported a kallikrein-specific inhibitor in kidney tubule, of which the molecular weight was about 4700, it remains to be determined whether our small fragment described here is the same as that or not.

Recently Rapp et al.[2] reported that dexamethasone increased the excretion of protein that bound to kallikrein, probably kallikrein-inhibitor. From the present study we cannot determine if this kallikrein inhibitor induced by chronic administration of glucocorticoid is excreted into urine or not.

It has been thought that kallikrein in the kidney is bound to plasma membrane[9] and basolateral membrane,[3,10] and different physical properties have been identified in the kidney.[9,10]

Therefore it appears that glucocorticoids play an important role to regulate the renal function, in part, by participating in the regulation of renal kallikrein activity with kallikrein inhibitor induced by glucocorticoids in kidney.

REFERENCES

1. Y. Noda, K. Yamada, R. Igic, and E. G. Erdös, Regulation of rat urinary and renal kallikrein and prekallikrein by corticosteroids, Proc. Natl. Acad. Sci. USA , 80:3059-3063 (1983).
2. J. P. Rapp, D. L. Sustarsic, R. P. McPartland, and C. L. Batten, Hormonal effects on kallikrein, esterase A2, and their inhibitors in rat urine, Endocrinology,, 114:951-956 (1984).
3. K. Yamada, W. W. Schulz, D. S. Page, and E. G. Erdös, Kallikrein and prekallikrein on the basolateral membrane of rat kidney tubules, Hypertension, 3(Suppl II):II-59-64 (1981).
4. G. Bönner, R. Authenrieth, M. Marin-Grez, W. Rasher, and F. Gross, Effects of sodium loading, desoxycorticosterone acetate, and corticosterone on urinary kallikrein excretion, Horm. Res., 14:87 (1981).
5. K. Yamada, K. Ito, M. Watanabe, Y. Tamura, A. Kumagai, N. Sagawa, and E. G. Erdös, Effect of glucocorticoid and mineralocorticoid on renal kallikrein and prostaglandin biosynthesis, Perspectives in Prostaglandin Research, Y. Shiokawa, M. Katori, and Y. Mizushima, Excerpta Medica, 202-205 (1983).
6. H. Fritz, I. Trautschold, and E. Werle, Protease inhibitors, in: "Methods of Enzymatic Analysis," Vol. 2, H. U. Bergmeyer, ed., Academic Press, Inc., Second English Edition, 1064-1080.
7. H. J. Faarvang, The influence of glucocorticoids and corticotropic hormone on output of human urinary trypsin inhibitor (and hyaluronidase inhibitor), Acta Pharmacol. Toxicol., 19:293 (1962).
8. R. Geiger and K. Mann, A kallikrein-specific inhibitor in rat kidney tubules, Hoppe-Seyler's Z. Physiol. Chem., 357:553-558 (1976).
9. K. Nishimura, P. E. Ward, and E. G. Erdös, Kallikrein and renin in the membrane fractions of the rat kidney, Hypertension, 2:538 (1980).
10. K. Yamada and E. G. Erdös, Kallikrein and prekallikrein of the isolated basolateral membrane of rat kidney, Kidney International, 22:331-337 (1982).

METABOLISM OF BRADYKININ IN ISOLATED PERFUSED RAT KIDNEY

MEASUREMENT OF KININASE ACTIVITY IN PERFUSATE AND URINE

Tohru Ogihara, Therese Dupin***, Haruyuki Nakane*, Yoko Nakane*,
Takao Saruta**, Jiro Misumi***, and Jöel Mènard***

Department of Internal Medicine, Hiratsuka City Hospital
Kanagawa, Japan
*Department of Internal Medicine, Urawa City Hospital
Saitama, Japan
**Department of Internal Medicine, Keio University School of
Medicine, Tokyo, Japan
***Inserm U36, Paris, France

SUMMARY

The effect of bradykinin and kininase on renal function and the
metabolism of bradykinin in the kidney were examined in isolated perfused
rat kidney. In this experimental system, exogenous bradykinin did not
affect the water and electrolyte handling by the kidney. Most of bradykinin and kininase in urine were derived from kidney but not from circulating medium. Kininase II may not have a major role in bradykinin
destruction by the kidney.

INTRODUCTION

It has been suggested that the renal kallikrein-kinin system plays
an important role in the regulation of blood pressure and water electrolyte balance.[1,2] The key product of this system is kinin, which activity
is influenced by many factors, such as kallikrein, kininogen, kininase and
kallikrein inhibitors.

In this presentation, the effect of bradykinin on renal function
was evaluated together with the simultaneous assessment of the renal
metabolism of bradykinin using the model of isolated rat kidney perfusion.
The origin of urinary kininase and the role of kininase II in the
degradation of bradykinin by the kidney were also examined.

METHODS

Kidney Perfusion

Male Wistar rats (300-400 g) maintained of a regular rat chow were
anesthetized with sodium pentobarbital (50 mg/kg, i.p.). The right
kidney was isolated and perfused in a closed recirculating perfusion

system as previously described.[3] Eighty ml of Krebs-Ringer bicarbonate buffer pH 7.4 containing 65 g/liter bovine serum albumin (Cohn's fraction V, Sigma) and 5.5 mM glucose, kept at $37^{\circ}C$ and continuously aerated with O_2 and CO_2 (95:5) were used as the perfusion medium. After 30 min equilibration period, kidneys were perfused at a constant perfusion pressure of 90 mmHg for 90 min. Following perfusions were performed (Figure 1).

Assays

1. Bradykinin assay - One ml of timed perfuase samples were collected in ice-cold tubes containing EDTA (10^{-3} M) and o-phenanthroline (10^{-3} M) as the kininase inhibitors and were immediately precipitated with 5 ml of 95% ethanol ($-30^{\circ}C$). After centrifugation, the supernatant was evaporated and the dry residue dissolved in RIA buffer and the BK was quantified by RIA.[4] Urine samples were collected every 30 min in ice-cold tubes containing EDTA (10^{-3} M) and o-phenanthroline (10^{-3} M) and the BK in urine was directly quantified by RIA. The antiserum used in this study cross-reacted less than 0.5% with des-Arg[1]-BK and less than 1.0% with des-Arg[9]-BK, and had negligible cross-reactivity with the possible products of degradated BK. This assay was capable of detecting 1.5 femtomole BK.

2. Kininase activity - Kininase activity in perfusate and urine was estimated by its BK degradating activity. In preliminary experiment, pH optimum for urinary kininase showed at pH 8.0 and that of perfusate showed between 7.5 and 8.5. Consequently all incubations for the estimation of kininase activity were performed at pH 8.0. The amount of BK as the substrate for kininase was chosen 8.4 pmol according to the preliminary results of approximately 50% degradation of BK after 90 min incubation with urine or perfusate.

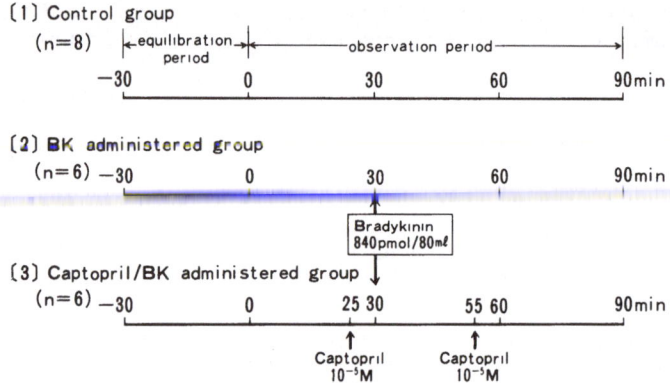

Figure 1. Perfusions
(1) Control perfusion (n=8): urine samples were collected every 15 min to measure kininase activity. Perfusate samples were taken at 0, 30, 60 and 90 min for the measurement of kininase activity. Urinary water and electrolytes excretion, renal flow and glomerular filtration rate were also measures. (2) Bradykinin (BK)-administered group (n=6): after an initial 30 min of perfusion, 840 pmol of synthetized BK (Sigma) was injected into the recirculating perfusate. During the next 60 min, the effect of BK on renal function, urinary excretion of BK and the metabolism of BK by the kidney were studied. (3) Captopril/Bk-administered group (n=6): 840 ml of BK was injected into perfusate at 30 min of observation period. At 25 and 55 min of observation period, captopril (10^{-5} M) was administered into perfusate. The metabolism of BK by the kidney were studied during the next 60 min.

Then, in this study, kininase activity was estimated as the following condition (Figure 2). Ten μl urine was incubated with 8.4 pmol BK at 37ºC for 90 min in 0.2 M Tris pH 8.0 containing 0.15 M NaCl, 1 g/liter lysozyme and 1000 U/ml aprotinin (Iniprol) in a final volume of 0.4 ml. Incubation was stopped by cooling and by adding EDTA (10^{-3} M). The amount of BK present after incubation was then quantified. BK degradated was corrected by subtracting the non-specific disappearance of BK during procedure. This was performed by incubating 10 μl 0.2 M Tris buffer instead of urine sample with 8.4 pmol BK under the same condition. To determine kininase activity in perfusate, 300 μl perfusate was incubated with 8.4 pmol BK at 37ºC for 90 min in 0.2 M Tris pH 8.0 containing 0.15 M NaCl, 1 g/liter lysozyme and 1000 U/ml aprotinin in a total volume of 0.6 ml. After stopping the incubation by cooling and by adding EDTA, BK was quantified.

Since the perfusion medium contained 6.5% Cohn's fraction V from bovine serum, there was a possibility that the fresh perfusate contains a certain peptidase activity as reported previously.[5] When fresh perfusate was incubated with BK under same condition as described above, 0.49±0.14 pmol BK was destroyed during 90 min incubation. Therefore, whenever perfusate kininase activity was determined, the kininase activity in fresh, non-circulated perfusate was also determined and the difference in the amount of BK degradated between experimental and fresh perfusate was taken as the perfusate kininase activity.

To evaluate the proportional amount of kininase II against total kininase activity, urine and perfusate sample were also incubated with BK in the presence of captopril (10^{-6} M) under the same condition as described above and BK degradating activity with and without captopril was compared.

Kininase activity in urine or perfusate was expressed as femtomole BK degradated per ml sample per minute incubation ($fmolBK \cdot ml^{-1} \cdot min^{-1}$).

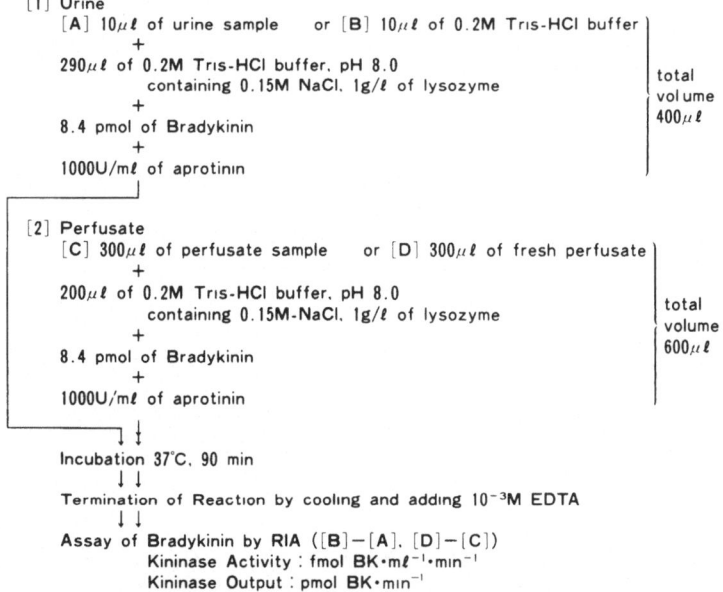

Figure 2. Assay of Kininase Activity

Urinary kininase secretion was calculated for each 15 min sample and expressed as pmol BK degradated per minute incubation by total enzyme present in urine (pmolBK·min^{-1}). Kininase secretion in perfusate was expressed as pmol BK degradated per minute incubation by total enzyme secreted into perfusate (pmolBK·min^{-1}).

3. Other Analysis – The glomerular filtration rate (GFR) was calculated by the clearance rate of ^{3}H-methoxy-insulin added to perfusate. Urine volume (UV) was determined gravimetrically. Sodium and potassium were measured by flame photometry (Klina, Beckman).

All results are expressed as means±SEM. Paired and non-paired Student's t-test were used for statistical analysis. Apparent half-life of BK was determined from least-squares regressions for the decrease with time of its perfusate levels.

RESULTS

Functional parameters of the isolated perfused kidney

Table 1 summarizes the functional parameters of perfused kidneys. Initial control period (0–30 min) and the period after BK injection (30–90 min) were compared. In both BK- and captopril/BK-injected groups, there was no significant difference in these parameters during the whole study. These results suggests that, in this experimental system, circulating exogenous bradykinin did not affect the water and electrolyte handling by the kidney.

Kininase activity secreted from the isolated perfused kidney

The relationship between the incubation time and kininase activity in perfusate or urine was linear till 120 min of incubation time when 300 µl of perfusate or 10 µl of urine was incubated with 8.4 pmol BK as the substrate. There was also a linear relationship between the volume of perfusate or urine sample and kininase activity when 8.4 pmol BK was incubated with sample at 37°C for 90 min. These findings suggest that in the present experimental condition, kininase inhibitors are not present in perfusate or urine.

Table 1. Functional Parameters of Control, Bradykinin Administered and Captopril/Bradykinin administered Perfusions

Period min	Group	RPF ml·min^{-1}	GFR ml·min^{-1}	UV µl·min^{-1}	UNaV µmol·min^{-1}	Na Reabsorption %
0–30	Control (n = 8)	13.5±0.2 NS	0.525±0.034 NS	49.29±6.95 NS	3.61±0.49 NS	95.0±0.7 NS
	BK (n = 6)	12.0±0.7 NS	0.431±0.039 NS	40.01±8.41 NS	3.14±0.75 NS	94.9±1.2 NS
	Captopril/BK (n = 6)	13.2±1.4	0.441±0.043	41.68±12.77	3.72±1.61	94.2±2.4
30–90	Control	14.7±0.2 NS	0.369±0.015 NS	72.57±5.06 NS	4.85±0.34 NS	91.0±0.6 NS
	BK	12.9±0.6 NS	0.319±0.021 NS	68.50±8.09 NS	4.94±0.72 NS	89.8±1.2 NS
	Captopril/BK	13.9±1.6	0.299±0.028	69.42±14.47	4.48±1.23	90.9±1.9

mean±SEM   Perfusion Pressure: 90 mmHg

Figure 3 shows perfusate and urinary kininase secretion for each 30 min in control group. Kininase secretion in urine during 90 min of control perfusion was three times greater than that in perfusate (20.9±3.1 pmolBK min^{-1}; 6.7±1.2 pmolBK·min^{-1}, respectively). And the kininase secretion in urine increased significantly in time course (p<0.005) whereas the kininase secretion in perfusate did not significantly.

When perfusate or urine sample was incubated with BK in the presence of captopril, kininase activity decreased slightly in both samples (not statistically significant).

Bradykinin metabolism in the isolated perfused rat kidney

Figure 4 shows the bradykinin output in urine. The administration of bradykinin in perfusate did not significantly affect the bradykinin excretion in urine.

Figure 5 shows the time course of the disappearance of injected BK from perfusate. The half-life of exogenous BK in perfusate during perfusion was 15.1±1.3 min, and 18.4±0.9 min under the existence of captopril. The difference of the half-life of BK in the absence and in the presence of captopril was not significant.

DISCUSSION

Our results showed that the isolated perfused kidney is a useful tool in studying the degradation and production of bradykinin by the kidney excluding the influence of extrarenal organs.

Kininase output in urine during 90 min of control perfusion was three times greater than that in perfusate. And the kininase output in urine increased significantly in time course whereas the kininase secretion in perfusate did not. These data indicate that the most of kininase in urine was derived from kidney but not from circulating medium.

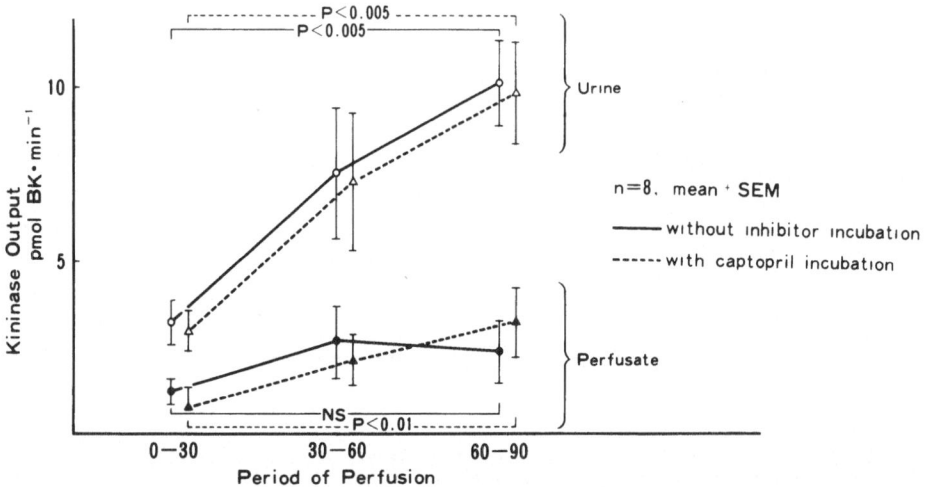

Figure 3. Kininase Output in Perfusate and Urine of Control Perfusions

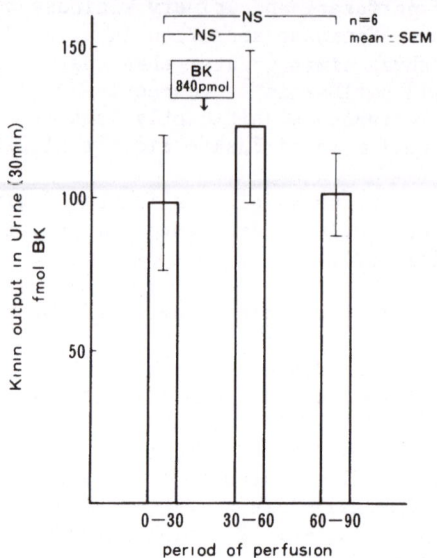

Figure 4. Kinin Output in Urine of Bradykinin Administered Perfusion (30 min)

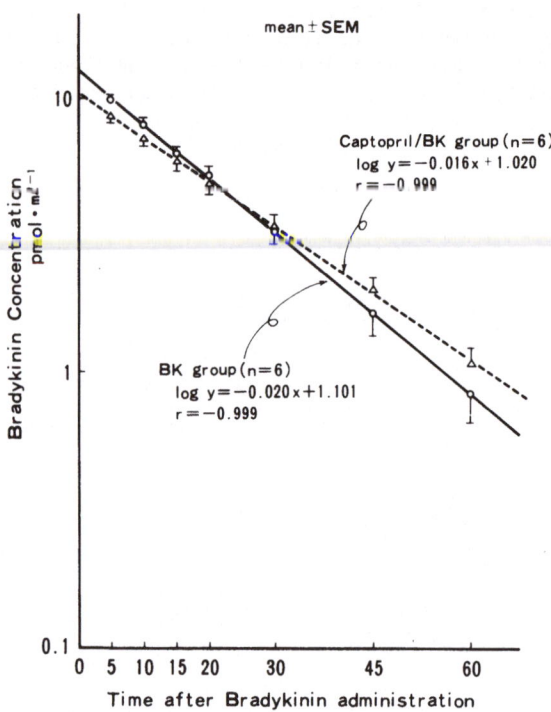

Figure 5. Effect of Captopril on the Degradation of Bradykinin in Isolated Perfused Rat Kidney

In our study, circulating exogenous bradykinin did not alter the water and electrolyte handling by the kidney. This may be related to the denervation of the kidney and lack of kininogen and renin substrate in perfusate.

The administration of bradykinin in perfusate did not increase the bradykinin excretion in urine, which suggests that the most of bradykinin in urine was produced and excreted by the kidney.

Bradykinin administered in the perfusate may be metabolized by the following ways: firstly, bradykinin can be metabolized by the kininase in renal vascular bed. Secondly, it can be metabolized by kininase in perfusate secreted from kidney. Finally, bradykinin in perfusate filtered in urine or bradykinin secreted in urine from kidney can be metabolized by the kininase in urine secreted from kidney. Among above possibilities, because the amount of kininase present in perfusate is too low to full account for the observed rapid kinin degradation, and because the filtration fraction was less then 4% in this experimental system, most of the bradykinin administered in perfusate is thought to be metabolized by the kininase in renal vascular bed.

The lack of significant difference in half-life of bradykinin in the absence and in the presence of captopril indicates that kininase II may not have a major role of bradykinin destruction by the kidney. Nevertheless, we cannot exclude the possibility that the intrarenal kininase II was not completely blocked by the captopril administered in perfusate.

REFERENCES

1. O. A. Carretero and A. G. Scicli, The renal kallikrein-kinin system, Am. J. Physiol., 238:F247–F255, (1980).
2. A. Nasjletti, J. Colina-Chourio, and J. C. McGiff, Disappearance of bradykinin in the renal circulation of dogs. Effects of kininase inhibition. Circ. Res., 37:59–65, (1975).
3. H. Nakane, Y. Nakane, G. Reach, F. Corvol, and J. Menard, Aldosterone metabolism in isolated perfused rat kidney, Am. J. Physiol., 234:E472–E479, (1978).
4. F. Alhenc-Gelas, J. Marchetti, J. Allegrini, P. Corvol, and J. Menard, Measurement of urinary kallikrein activity. Species differences in kinin production, Biochim. Biophys. Acta., 677:477–488, (1981).
5. J. Misumi, F. Alhenc-Gelas, M. Marre, J. Marchetti, P. Corvol, and J. Menard, Regulation of kallikrein and renin release by the isolated perfused rat kidney, Kidney Int., 24:58–65, (1983).

FUNCTIONAL SIGNIFICANCE OF THE SUBUNITS OF CARBOXYPEPTIDASE N (KININASE I)

Randal A. Skidgel*, Marleen S. Kawahara** and Tony E. Hugli**

*Department of Pharmacology, University of Texas Health
 Science Center, 5323 Harry Hines Boulevard, Dallas
 Texas 75235

**Department of Immunology, Scripps Clinic and Research
 Foundation, LaJolla, California 92037

SUMMARY

Carboxypeptidase N (kininase I; 280K) was purified to homogeneity from human plasma. The inactive 83K and active 48K subunits were separated by gel filtration after treatment of homogeneous 280K with guanidine. The two subunits differ in amino acid composition and immunological reactivity. The activities of the 280K and 48K enzymes with naturally occurring substrates were compared to determine whehther the 83K subunit affects enzymatic activity of the 48K. At 60 μM concentration, both the 280K and 48K enzymes cleaved (Lys6)-Met5)-enkephalin fastest followed by (Arg6)-enkephalin, anaphylatoxin C3a, (arg6)-(Leu5)-enkephalin, C3a octapeptide[1] and bradykinin. The activity ratios (280K/48K) were: (Arg6)-(Leu5)-enkephalin, 0.9; bradykinin, 1.0; (Lys6)-(Met5)-enkephalin, 1.1; (Arg6)-(Met5)-enkephalin, 1.2; and anaphylatoxin C3a, 1.7. Thus, while most substrates were cleaved at similar rates, assuming 2 active sites per 280K molecule, anaphylatoxin C3a was cleaved significantly faster by 280K than by 48K. The ratio of activity was similar (1.9) when the C-terminal octapeptide of C3a was the substrate. These results indicate that the larger, inactive 83K subunit may increase the efficiency of cleavage of some peptides by 48K.

INTRODUCTION

Human plasma carboxypeptidase N (EC 3.4.17.3) cleaves the C-terminal basic amino acid of kinins, anaphylatoxins, protamine fibrino-peptides, hexapeptide enkaphalins, and other peptide substrates.[1,2]

---

[1]The C3a octapeptide used here was an analogue of the C-terminal sequence of human anaphylatoxin C3a (See Figure 2).

Becuase of the variety of substrates it cleaves, it has been called kininase I, arginine carboxypeptidase, serum carboxypeptidase B, protaminase and anaphylatoxin inactivator.[1] The enzyme is a 280,000 dalton tetramer consisting of two active 48,000 or 55,000 dalton subunits (48K or 55K) and two inactive 83,000 dalton subunits (83K).[3,4] We have shown previously that the 83K subunit contains carbohydrate and stabilizes the activity of the 48K subunit at 37° or low pH.[4] We undertook the present study to determine whether the 83K subunit could enhance the hydrolysis of naturally occurring substrates by the 48K subunit.

METHODS

Carboxypeptidase N (280K) was purified to homogeneity from outdated human plasma by ion-exchange and affinity chromatography.[4] The subunits were dissociated with 3M guanidine and isolated by gel filtration.[4] Antisera to the 280K enzyme and the 48K and 83K subunits were raised in rabbits. Immunological cross reactivity of the subunits was tested by the "Western blot" procedure.[5,6] Briefly, carboxypeptidase N was run in three lanes of an SDS-polyacrylamide gel and electrophoretically blotted onto nitrocellulose paper. The paper was cut into three strips corresponding to the three lanes of the gel and incubated with antibody to either the 280K enzyme, the 83K subunit or the 48K subnit. The paper was then exposed to radiolabeled goat anti-rabbit IgG and the labeled protein bands visualized by autoradiography. Hydrolysis of hexapeptide enkephalins and bradykinin was measured by HPLC.[2] The release of arginine from anaphylatoxin C3a or the C3a octapeptide was measured in an amino acid analyzer.

RESULTS

Antisera raised in rabbits to carboxypeptidase N, the 83K and 48K subunits were used in the "Western blot" procedure to determine whether the subunits were immunologically distinct. As shown in Figure 1, antibody to the 48K subunit recognizes only the 48K subunit and antibody to the 83K subunit recognizes only the 83K subunit. Antibody to the 280K enzyme recognizes both subunits. In addition, a small amount of a 55K protein is recognized by the antibodies to the 48K subunit and also by antibodies to the 280K enzyme (Figure 1). The amount of 55K protein varies from preparation to preparation and is very rapidly converted to the 48K protein by limited proteolysis.[3,4] After treatment with guanidine and separation of the subunits by gel filtration, we obtained only the 48K subunit.[4] Further studies are required to determine the importance and function of the 55K protein.

Further evidence for the distinctly different nature of the 83K and 48K subnits was obtained by amino acid analysis. The two subunits differed significantly in amino acid composition, most notably in the hydrophobic and aromatic amino acids. The 83K subunit had more than twice the amount (on a mole % basis) of leucine and less than half the amount of tyrosine when compared with the 48K subunit.[7] In addition, the amino acid composition of the 48K subunit was quite different from that reported for the 34,000 dalton human pancreatic carboxypeptidase B.[7,8]

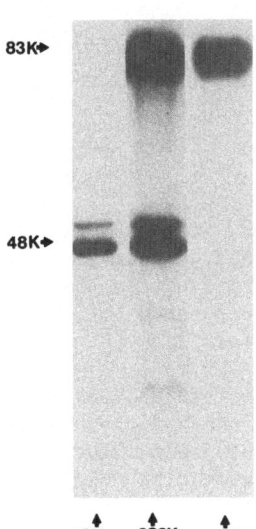

83K➤

48K➤

48K   280K   83K
Antiserum

Figure 1. "Western blot" of carboxypeptidase N (280K) using antisera to
the 280K enzyme, 83K or 38K subunit.

Because the 83K subnit stabilizes the 48K subunit,[4] we wondered
whether it might also enhance the ability of the 48K subunit to
hydrolyze the short or long naturally occurring peptide substrates
shown in Figure 2. The hydrolysis rates for the intact enzyme (280K)
and the 48K subunit with various peptides at 60 µM concentration are
shown in Table 1. Activities were calculated on the basis of µmol substrate cleaved per min per µmol active site, assuming 2 active sites
per 280K and one per 48K molecule. Of all substrates tested, (Lys6)-
(Met5)-enkephalin was hydrolyzed fastest by both enzymes followed by
(Arg6)-(Met5)-enkephalin, anaphylatoxin c3a, (Arg6)-(Leu5)-enkephalin,

Bradykinin	Arg-Pro-Pro-Gly-Phe-Ser-Pro-Phe-Arg
(Arg6)-(Met5)-enkephalin	Tyr-Gly-Gly-Phe-Met-Arg
(Arg6)-(Leu5)-enkephalin	Tyr-Gly-Gly-Phe-Leu-Arg
(Lys6)-(Met5)-enkephalin	Tyr-Gly-Gly=Phe-Met-Lys
Anaphylatoxin C3a (C-terminal sequence)	.....Ala-Ser-His-Leu-Gly-Leu-Ala-Arg
C3a Octapeptide	Ala-Ala-Ala-Leu-Gly-Leu-Ala-Arg

Figure 2. Amino acid sequence of naturally occurring peptide substrates of carboxypeptidase N.

C3a octapeptide and bradykinin. When the activity ratios (280K/48K) were calculated, the rates of hydrolysis were similar for most peptides, but anaphylatoxin C3a and its C-terminal octapeptide were cleaved significantly faster by the 280K enzyme.

DISCUSSION

This study gives further evidence that carboxypeptidase N consists of immunologically and structurally distinct subunits of different functions. The 83K subunit probably stabilizes the 48K active subnit in the circulation[4] and may function to enhance the activity of the 48K subunit with certain peptide substrates.

It was initially assumed that the 83K subunit may enhance the ability of the 48K subunit to attach and hydrolyze some large naturally occurring peptide substrates, as has been seen with other enzymes. For instance, intact plasma kallikrein cleaves high molecular weight kininogen 3.5 times faster than the isolated, active light chain.[9] This difference was not seen with a small synthetic peptide substrate.[9] We found the 280K enzyme to cleave the large, 9000 dalton anaphylatoxin C3a 1.7 times faster than the isolated 48K subunit. However, the 280K enzyme also cleaved the C-terminal octapeptide of anaphylatoxin C3a 1.9 times faster than the 48K subunit. This indicates that the difference in hydrolysis rates could not entirely be due to the size of the substrate but it may depend partially or completely on the C-terminal sequence of the peptide. It is known that the penultimate amino acid of a peptide substrate influences the rate of hydrolysis of the C-terminal basic amino acid by carboxypeptidase N. For example, CBZ-Ala-Arg is cleaved 32 times faster than CBZ-Gly-Arg.[10] Anaphylatoxin C3a (with a C-terminal Ala-Arg) is also cleaved faster than anaphylatoxins C4a or C5a which have C-terminal Gln-Arg or Gly-Arg.[7] Thus, alanine may fit in the substrate binding pocket better than other penultimate amino acids. One possible explanation for the more rapid hydrolysis of anaphylatoxin C3a and the C3a octepeptide by the 280K enzyme is that the isolated 48K subunit may have an altered conformation which cannot interact with the penultimate alanine as well as in its native conformation bound to the 83K subunit.

Of all the substrates tested, carboxypeptidase N cleaved (Lys6)-(Met5)-enkephalin fastest. In fact, bradykinin, the natural substrate first shown to be cleaved by carboxypeptidase N,[11] was cleaved much slower at the substrate concentration used (60 μM). This illustrates the confusion that can arise following the naming or renaming of an enzyme after a single substrate (e.g., kininase I, anaphylatoxin inactivator, enkephalin convertase, etc.). Carboxypeptidase N, therefore, is probably involved in many processes in vivo.

Some of the possible functions of a lysine/arginine carboxypeptidase are shown in Figure 3. Many peptide hormones are now known to be synthesized as larger precursor molecules. Processing at paired basic residues by a protease releases a peptide with an additional arginine or lysine which then can be removed by a carboxypeptidase to activate the mature peptide. Enkephalin-containing peptides can be released from the adrenal gland into the circulation[12] where carboxypeptidase N could then act to remove their C-terminal arginine or lysine. Another important function of carboxypeptidase N is the inactivation of peptide hormones such as kinins, anaphylatoxin C3a, fibrinopeptides, etc.[1]

In addition, carboxypeptidase N could modulate the action of peptide hormones (Figure 3). While removal of the C-terminal arginine on brady-kinin abolishes its activity in most tissues, the activity of des-(Arg9)-bradykinin on the rabbit aorta is 11-fold higher, indicating the presence of a "B1 receptor".[13]   Similarly, the potent anaphylatoxin C5a has both spasmogenic and chemotactic properties.[14] Removal of the C-terminal

I.   Processing of Peptide Hormones

(e.g., Enkephalins, Insulin, etc.)

Prohormone ----X-Arg-Lys--------X-Arg-Arg---------

⬇ Serine Protease or Catheptic Enzyme

--------X-Arg

⬇ Carboxypeptidase

Mature Peptide   --------X

II. Inactivation of Peptide Hormones

Removal of a C-terminal Basic Amino Acid Can Inactivate Peptides Such As: Kinins, Anaphylatoxin C3a, Fibrinopeptides, and others.

III. Modulation of Peptidase Hormone Action

	ACTIVITY	
PEPTIDE	NATIVE FORM	DES-ARG FORM
Bradykinin	Binds "B2" Receptors	Binds "B1" Receptors
Anaphylatoxin C5a	Spasmogenic and Chemotactic	Chemotactic
Enkephalin-(Arg/Lys)[6]	Binds "Kappa" Receptors	Binds "Delta" and "Mu" Receptors

Figure 3. Possible functions of lysine/arginine carboxypeptidases.

arginine from C5a results in a loss of spasmogenic and histamine-releasing activity while its chemotactic effectiveness is retained.[14] Thus, carboxypeptidase N could function in the processing of peptide hormones as well as in the inactivation or modulation of their activity.

ACKNOWLEDGEMENTS

We thank Richard Davis and Youngsook Kim for their expert assistance. This study was supported by Grants HL16411, HL16320, HL20594, and HL28813 from M.I.H. and by a Grant-In-Aid (82782) from the American Heart Association.

REFERENCES

1   E. G. Erdös, Kininases, in: Handbook of Experimental Pharmacology, Vol. 35, Suppl., ed. by E. G. Erdös, Springer-Verlag, pp. 427-487, (1979).

2. R. A. Skidgel, A. R. Johnson, and E. G. Erdös, Hydrolysis of opioid hexapeptides by carboxypeptidase N., Presence of carboxypeptidase in cell membranes, Biochem. Pharmacol. 33:3471-3478, (1984).

3. T. H. Plummer and M. Y. Hurwitz, Human plasma carboxypeptidase N, Isolation and characterization, J. Biol. Chem. 253:3907-3912, (1978).

4. Y. Levin, R. A. Skidgel, and E. G. Erdös, Isolation and characterization of the subunits of human plasma carboxypeptidase N (kininase I), Proc. Natl. Acad. Sci., USA 79:4618-4622, (1982).

5. W. N. Burnette, "Western Blotting"; Electrophoretic transfer of proteins from sodium dodecylsulfate-polyacrylamide gels to unmodified nitrocellulose, Anal. Biochem., 112:195-203, (1983).

6. R. A. Skidgel, R. M. Davis, and E. G. Erdös, Purification of a human urinary carboxypeptidase (kininase) district from carboxypeptidases A, B or N, Anal. Biochem., 140:520-531, (1984).

7. R. A. Skidgel, M. S. Kawahara, and T. E. Hugli, Hydrolysis of anaphylatoxins C3a, C4a and C5a by carboxypeptidase N and its isolated active subunit, To be submitted.

8. D. V. Marinkovic, J. N. Marinkovic, C. J. G. Robinson, and E. G. Erdös, Purification of two forms of carboxypeptidase B from human pancreas, Biochem. J., 163:253-260, (1977).

9. F. van der Graff, G. Tans, B. Bouma, and J. H. Griffin, Isolation and functional properties of the heavy and light chains of human plasma kallikrein, J. Biol. Chem., 257:14300-14305, (1982).

10. G. Oshima, J. Kato, and E. G. Erdös, Plasma carboxypeptidase N, subunits and characteristics, Arch. Biochem. Biophys., 170:132-138, (1975).

11. E. G. Erdös and E. M. Sloane, An enzyme in human blood plasma that inactivates bradykinin and kallidins, Biochem. Pharmacol., 11:585-592, (1962).

12. M. R. Boarder, E. Erdelyi, and J. D. Barchas, Opioid peptides in human plasma: Evidence for multiple forms, J. Clin. Endocr. Metab., 54:715-720, (1982).

13. D. Regoli and J. Barabe, Pharmacology of bradykinin and related kinins, Pharmac. Rev., 32:1-46, (1980).

14. T. E. Hugli, The structural basis for anaphylatoxin and chemotactic functions of C3a, C4a, and C5a, in: Critical Review of Immunology, Vol. 1, ed. by M. Z. Atassi, Chemical Rubber Co., pp. 321-366, (1981).

KININASE ONE-AN'-A-HALF: THE NEWEST MEMBER OF THE KININASE FAMILY

Randal A. Skidgel and Ervin G. Erdös

Departments of Pharmacology and Internal Medicine, The University of Texas Health Science Center at Dallas, 5323 Harry
Hines Boulevard, Dallas, Texas 75235

SUMMARY

A kininase I-like enzyme (carboxypeptidase) was purified to homogeneity
from human urine and compared to the 48,000 mol. wt. (48K) active subunit
of carboxypeptidase N. The urinary carboxypeptidase had a mol. wt. of 73,000
in gel filtration and 76,000 in SDS-polyacrylamide gel electrophoresis.
It had a pH optimum of 7.0 and differed from the 48K subunit in stability,
susceptibility to trypsin, and enzymatic activity. The urinary enzyme did
not cross-react with antibody to carboxypeptidase N in "Western blotting".
Urine from a patient genetically deficient in plasma carboxypeptidase N
(21% of normal) contained normal levels of urinary carboxypeptidase with
similar properties to that from pooled human urine.

Membrane fractions from several tissues contained a similar carboxypeptidase activity. The activity was highest in a microvillous membrane fraction from human placenta (65 nmol/min/mg with Bz-Gly-Lys as substrate).
High specific activities were also found in membrane fractions of human
kidney (18 nmol/min/mg) and lung (8 nmol/min/mg). The membrane-bound enzyme
was distinguished from lysosomal and catheptic carboxypeptidases as well
as "enkephalin convertase" by the use of specific inhibitors.

These results show that urine contains a carboxypeptidase capable of
cleaving arginine or lysine from the C-terminus of peptides. The enzyme
does not arise from plasma carboxypeptidase N, but may be released into
the urine from the renal brush border.

INTRODUCTION

Several enzymes are known under the collective misnomer of "kininases"
because they inactivate kinins. Their function, however, is not limited
to the inactivation of kinins as they can readily lhydrolyze a vareity of
other peptide substrates. Kininase I is carboxypeptidase N (EC 3.4.17.3).
In addition to releasing the C-terminal arginine of kinins, it cleaves anaphylatoxins, fibrinopeptides, protamine[1] and (Arg6)- or (Lys6)-enkepha-
lins.[2,3] Kininase II is the angiotensin I converting enzyme (1; EC 3.4.15.1)
but it hydrolyzes numerous other peptides, such as LHRH,[4] substance P,[5]
enkephalins,[6] and neurotensin.[5] Kininase to-an'-a-half is the "enkephalinase" or better known as neutral endopeptidase (7,8; EC 24.11) that cleaves

peptides at the amino side of hydrophobic amino acids, including bradykinin which it splits at the same site as kininase II.[9]

Plasma carboxypeptidase N is synthesized in the liver as a 280,000 mol. wt. protein complex containing two 83,000 mol. wt. and two 48,000 or 55,000 mol. wt. subunits.[10] Because the 48,000 mol. wt. (48K) subunit contains the active center of the enzyme, we investigated the possibility that some of the known kininase activity in urine[11] could be due to the excretion of this low mol. wt. subunit.

METHODS

A carboxypeptidase-type kininase was purified to homogeneity from human urine.[12] A four-hundred-fold purification was achieved after sequential steps of Affi-Gel Blue chromatography, Sepharose-arginine affinity chromatography and HPLC gel filtration on a TSK-G3000SW column. Carboxypeptidase N was purified to homogeneity from outdated human plasma and the 48K subunit isolated by gel filtration after treatment of the enzyme with 3 M guanidine.[10] Immunological crossreactivity was determined by the "Western blot" procedure as described.[12] Enzymatic activity was measured spectrophotometrically[10,12] using Bz-Ala-Lys, Bz-Gly-argininic acid, Bz-Phe-Lys, Bz-Gly-Lys and Bz-Gly-Arg as substrates. Hydrolysis of bradykinin was determined by HPLC analysis of the products released.[9,12]

RESULTS

The urinary carboxypeptidase (kininase one-an'-a-half) obtained was homogeneous as determined by polyacrylamide gel electrophoresis in the presence and absence of SDS. From the purification data, the concentration of the carboxypeptidase-type kininase (kininase one-an'-a-half) in normal human urine can be estimated to be about 109 µg/liter.

"Western blot" analysis of the urine (with antiserum to carboxypeptidase N) at various stages of purification revealed crossreacting bands which were removed during the final stage of purification. As shown in Figure 1, homogeneous urinary carboxypeptidase did not crossreact with antibody to carboxypeptidase N, indicating that the two proteins are immunologically distinct. The enzyme had a mol. wt. of 73,000 in gel filtration (Figure 2) and 76,000 in SDS-polyacrylamide gel electrophoresis.[12]

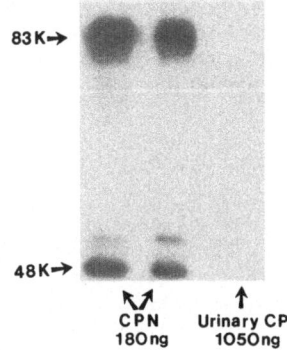

Fig. 1. Western bot with antisera to CPN. Antiserum to carboxypeptidase N (CPN) crossreacts with both the high and low mol. wt. subunits, but not with homogeneous urinary carboxypeptidase.

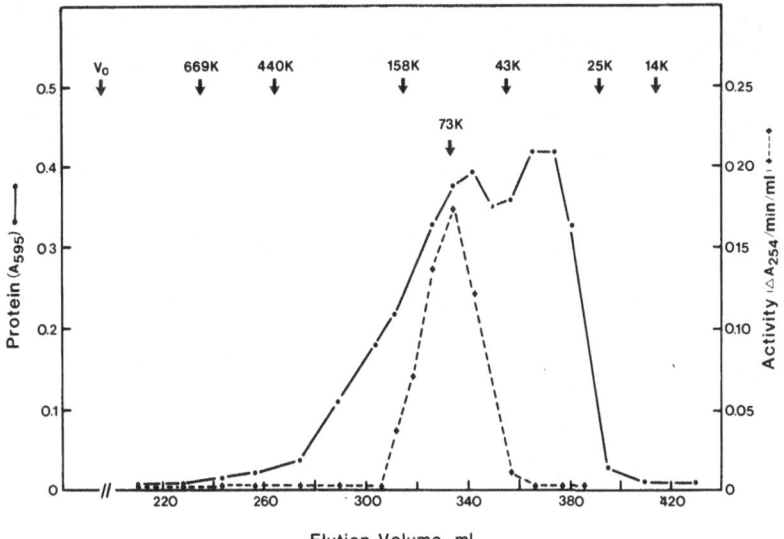

Fig. 2. Gel filtration of crude urinary carboxypeptidase on a Sephacryl
S-300 column. The molecular weight of the urinary carboxypeptidase
was 73,000 in gel filtration. Activity was determined with Bz-
Gly-argininic acid as substrate.

The urinary carboxypeptidase differed in many properties from the 48K
active subunit of carboxypeptidase N (Table 1). The urinary enzyme was less
active at pH 6 and more stable at 37° than the 48K subunit of carboxypeptidase
N. The ratio of the rates of substrate hydrolysis was also different from
that of carboxypeptidase N or B. The urinary carboxypeptidase cleaved the
ester substrate at a higher relative rate than the peptide substrates.
The Km of bradykinin in presence of $CoCl_2$ was 33 µM with the urinary enzyme.
When Bz-Gly-Lys was used as substrate $CoCl_2$ (1 mM) enhanced the activity
five-fold. Cadmium acetate, which inhibits the esterase activity of carboxypeptidase N and enhances that of carboxypeptidase B, did not affect the
esterase activity of the urinary carboxypeptidase.

With the cooperation of Dr. Kenneth Mathews at the University of Michigan, we obtained a 24-hour urine sample from a patient whohas a genetic
deficiency of plasma carboxypeptidase N with an activity of only 21% of
the normal value.[13] The carboxypeptidase activity of the urine of this
patient was 65% of the value found in normal pooled urine and the specific
activity (per mg protein) was about 70% of the normal value. Gel filtration
on a Sephacryl S-300 column showed the enzyme to have a molecular weight
similar to that from normal urine and the ratio of esterase (Bz-Gly-Argininic
acid) to peptidase (Bz-Ala-Lys) activity was 3.05, about the same as found
for the purified enzyme from normal urine (3.4). This is taken as additional
evidence which confirms that the urinary enzyme is unrelated to the plasma
enzyme.

Very likely, the urinary carboxypeptidase with a mol. wt. of 75,000
would not be filtered through the glomerulus and therefore it probably originates from the kidney. Thus, we investigated the presence of carboxypeptidase activity in subcellular fractions of homogenized kidney and other
tissues. We found a membrane-bound form of an arginine/lysine carboxypeptidase in plasma membrane enriched fractions of vrious tissues, some with
higher specific activities than plasma (16 nmol/min/mg protein with Bz-
Gly-Lys as substrate). The highest activity was found in the microvillous

383

Table 1. Properties of the Human Urinary Carboxypeptidase and the Active
48K Subunit of Human Plasma Carboxypeptidase N

PROPERTY	URINARY CARBOXYPEPTIDASE	CARBOXYPEPTIDASE N (48 K SUBUNIT)
STRUCTURE:		
Mol. Wt.	75 K	48 K
Trypsin Cleavage	–	+
Ab to Carboxy. N	Does not react	Crossreacts
STABILITY (Activity Remaining):		
@pH 4, 1 hr	42%	5%
@37°C, 2 hr	93%	25%
ACTIVITY:		
Peptidase @pH 6	40%	100%
Hip-Argininic Acid Bz-Ala-Lys	3.4 (activity ratio)	0.7
CdOAc (0.1 mM)	inhibits peptidase only	inhibits esterase & peptidase
Bradykinin Km:	46 µM	35 µM
Kcat:	32 min^{-1}	70 min

(brush border) fraction of human placenta (65 nmol/min/mg) followed by human
kidney (18 nmol) and lung (8 nmol). Cultured human endothelial cells or
fibroblasts had a low (1 to 2 nmol) activity.

The plasma membrane bound enzyme had a neutral pH optimum, was inhibited
by o-phenanthroline,2-mercaptomethyl-3-guanidinoethylthiopropanoic acid
(MGTA), a potent inhibitor of carboxypeptidase N,[14] and stimulated in the
presence of CoCl$_2$. The enzyme was distinct from lysosomal or cathectic
carboxypeptidases[15] including a recently described acid carboxypeptidase
("enkephalin convertase") found in bovine adrenal chromaffin granules and
rat brain.[16] In contrast to the membrane-bound enzyme, these enzymes have
acid pH optima, are inhibited by sulfhydryl reagents and heavy metals and
are stimulated by SH-compounds such as dithiothreitol.

Because placental microvillous membranes contain kappa opiate receptors[17] and (Lys6)- or (Arg6)-enkephalins bind to kappa receptors,[18] we investigated whether the carboxypeptidase in placental microvilli[19] could
convert(Lys6)-(Met5)-enkephalin to (Met5)-enkephalin. Indeed, when incubated
at pH 7.5 (37°C), the placental microvilli readily converted 0.1 mM (Lys6)-
(Met5)-enkephalin to (Met5)-enkephalin at a rate of 3.7 nmol/min/mg protein.

DISCUSSION

The very rapid and effective inactivation of kinins by pancreatic carboxypeptidase B in vitro, and after injecting the enzyme into animals in

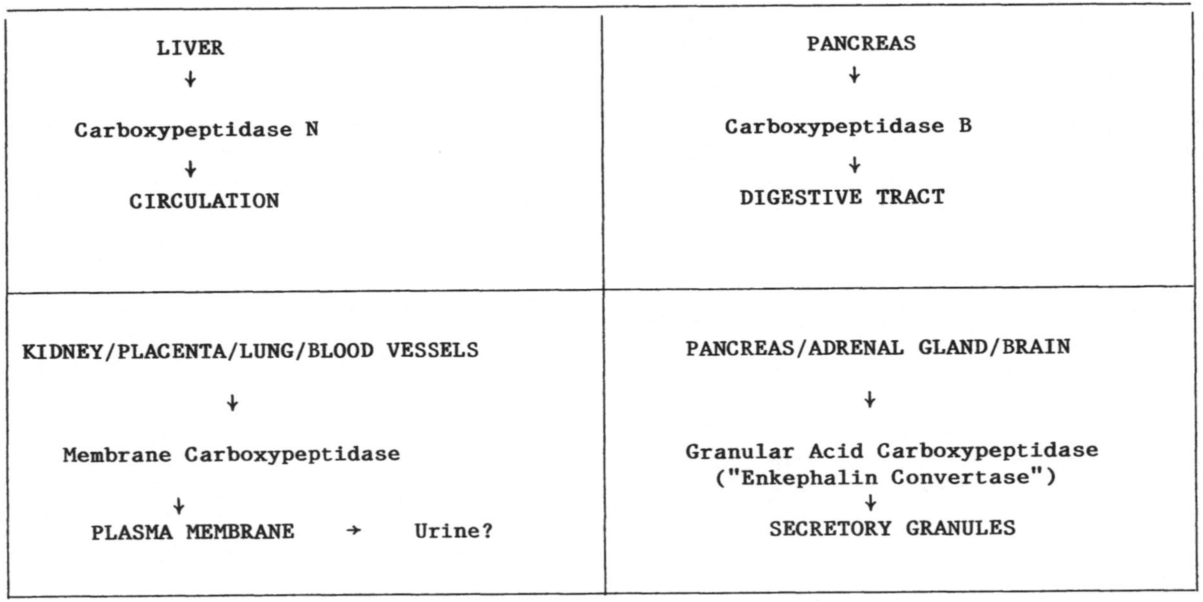

Fig. 3. Sources and probable sites of action of carboxypeptidase which cleave basic C-terminal amino acids.

Table 2. Properties of Arginine/Lysine Carboxypeptidases From Different Sources

	Carboxy. N*	Membrane Carboxy.	Granular Acid Carboxy.	Carboxy. B
OCCURRENCE:	Plasma	Kidney, Lung Placenta, Cultured Cells, Urine ?	Pancreas Adrenal Gland, Brain	Pancreas
MOL. WEIGHT:	280 Kd	75 Kd (urine)	50 Kd	34 Kd; 25 Kd
STRUCTURE:	2-48/55 Kd subunits 2-83 Kd subunits	1 chain (urine)	1 chain	1 chain
pH OPTIMUM:	7	7	5.6 - 6	7
ACTIVATORS:	Co^{++}	Co^{++}	Co^{++} & SH compounds	Co^{++}
INHIBITORS:	Chelators, MGTA, Cd^{++}	Chelators, MGTA, Cd^{++}	Chelators, PCMS MGTA, Cd^{++}	Chelators, MGTA, Cd^{++}

*Abbreviations: MGTA = 2-mercaptomethyl-3-guanidinoethylthiopropanoic adic; Kd = kilodalton; PCMS = p-chloromercuriphenylsulfonate; Carboxy. = carboxypeptidase.

vivo, was observed over two decades ago. About the same time, carboxypepti-dase N was discovered in blood plasma.[20,21] This enzyme was named kininase I to distinguish it from kininase Ii which is a peptidyldipeptidase that releases C-terminal Phe-Arg from bradykinin or His-Leu from angiotensin I.[22,23] It appears that there are several carboxypeptidases in tissues which are different from the plasma or pancreatic carboxypeptidase, although they all release C-terminal basic amino acids. The sources of these carboxy-peptidases are outlined in Figure 3 and their properties are compared in Table 2. Potentially, the urinary and the microvillous, membrane-bound carboxypeptidases can hydrolyze kinins, hence the tongue-in-cheek name, kininase one-an'-a-half. Clearly, the urinary carboxypeptidase can be dis-tinguished from plasma carboxypeptidase N, pancreatic carboxypeptidase B and the so-called "enkephalin convertase" or granular acid carboxypeptidase from adrenal chromaffin granules (Tables 1 and 2, Figure 3). We assume that the urinary enzyme originates from kidney, possibly from brush border, which is rich in peptidases. it is possible that the placental brush border carboxypeptidase is identical with the kidney or urinary enzyme however this requires further study.

The functions of these arginine/lysine carboxypeptidases extend beyond cleaving kinins. In addition to inactivating many other peptides (e.g., anaphylatoxin C3a, fibrinopeptides, etc.) these carboxypeptidases could be involved in the processing of peptide hormones. They may also modulate hormone action, as removal of a C-terminal basic amino acid has been shown to alter the receptor binding activities of bradykinin,[24,25] anaphylatoxin C5a[26] and (Arg6)- or (Lys6)-enkephalins.[18]

ACKNOWLEDGEMENTS

We thank Richard Davis for his expert assistance. These studies were supported by Grants HL 16320, HL 20594, and HL 28813 from the National Insti-tutes of Health and by a Grant-In-Aid (82782) from the American Heart Asso-ciation.

REFERENCES

1. E. G. Erdös, Kininases, in: "Handbook of Experimental Pharmacology," E. G. Erdös, ed., Vol. 25, Springer-Verlag (1979).
2. R. A. Skidgel, A. R. Johnson, and E. G. Erdös, Hydrolysis of opioid hexapeptides by carboxypeptidase N. Presence of carboxypeptidase in cell membranes, Biochem. Pharmacol., 33:3471-3478 (1984).
3. R. A. Skidgel, A. R. Johnson, and E. G. Erdös, Conversion of enkephalin hexapeptides to enkephalin by human plasma and tissue carboxypepti-dases, Fed. Proc., 43:651 (1984).
4. R. A. Skidgel and E. G. Erdös, Novel activity of human angiotensin I converting enzyme: Release of the N- and C-terminal tripeptides from the luteinizing hormone-releasing hormone, Proc. Natl. Acad. Sci. (In press).
5. R. A. Skidgel, S. Engelbrecht, A. R. Johnson, and E. G. Erdös, Hydrolysis of substance P and neurotensin by converting enzyme and neutral endo-peptidase, Peptides, 5:769-776 (1984).
6. E. G. Erdös, A. R. Johnson, and N. T. Boyden, Hydrolysis of enkephalin by cultured human endothelial cells and by purified peptidyl dipepti-dase, Biochem. Pharmacol., 27:843-848 (1978).
7. M. A. Kerr and a. J. Kenny, The purification and specificity of a neutral endopeptidase from rabbit kidney brush border, Biochem. J., 137:477-488 (1974).

8. R. Matsas, I. S. Fulcher, A. J. Kewnny, and A. J. Turner, Substance P and (Leu)enkephalin are hydrolyzed by an enzyme in pig caudate synaptic membranes that is identical with the endopeptidase of kidney microvilli, Proc. Natl. Acad. Sci. USA, 80:3111-3115 (1983).

9. J. T. Gafford, R. A. Skidgel, E. G. Erdös, and L. B. Hersh, Human kidney "enkephalinase", a neutral metalloendopeptidase that cleaves active peptides, Biochemistry, 22:3265-3271 (1983).

10. Y. Levin, R. A. Skidgel, and E. G. Erdös, Isolation and characterization of the subunits of human plasma carboxypeptidase N (kininase I), Proc. Natl. Acad. Sci. USA, 79:4618-4622 (1982).

11. E. Werle and E. G. Erdös, Uber eine neue blutdrucksenkende, darm- und uteruserregende Substanz im menschlichen Urin, Arch. Exper. Path. und Pharmakol., 223:234-243 (1954).

12. R. A. Skidgel, R. M. Davis, and E. G. Erdös, Purification of a human urinary carboxypeptidase(kinase) distinct from carboxypeptidases A, B or N. Anal. Biochem., 140:520-531 (1984).

13. K. P. Mathews, P. M. Pan, N. J. Gardner, and T. E. Hugli, Familial carboxypeptidase N deficiency, Ann. Intern. Med., 93:443-445 (1980).

14. T. H. Plummer and T. J. Ryan, A potent mercapto bi-product analogue inhibitor for human carboxypeptidase N, Biochem. Biophys. Res Commun., 98:448-454 (1981).

15. L. M. Greenbaum and R. Sherman, Studies on catheptic carboxypeptidase, J. Biol. Chem., 237:1082-1085 (1962).

16. L. D. Fricker and S. H. Snyder, Enkephalin convertase: Purification and characterization of a specific enkephalin-synthesizing carboxypeptidase localized to adrenal chromaffin granules, Proc. Natl. Acad. Sci. USA, 79:3886-3890 (1982).

17. G. Porthe, A. Valette, A. Moisand, M. Tafani, and J. Cros, Localization of human placental opiate binding sites on the syncitial brush border membrane, life Sci., 31:2647-2654 (1982).

18. J. Magnan, S. J. Paterson, and H. W. Kosterlitz, The interaction of (Met5)enkephalin and (Leu5)enkephalin sequences, extended at the C-terminus, with the μ-δ-and k-binding sites in the guinea pig brain, Life Sci., 31:1359-1361 (1982).

19. A. R. Johnson, R. A. Skidgel, J. T. Gafford, and E. G. Erdös, Enzymes in placental microvilli: Angiotensin I converting enzyme, angiotensinase A, carboxypeptidase, and neutral endopeptidase ("enkephalinase"), Peptides, 5:789-796 (1984).

20. E. G. Erdös, Enzymes that inactivate polypeptides, in: "Metabolic Factors Controlling Duration of Drug Action," B. B. Brodie and E. G. Erdös, eds., Pergamon Press (1962).

21. E. G. Erdös, A. G. Renfrew, E. M. Sloane, and J. R. Wohler, Enzymatic studies on bradykinin and similar peptides, Ann. N.Y. Acad. Sci., 104:222-234 (1963).

22. H. Y. T. Yang and E. G. Erdös, Second kininase in human blood plasma, Nature, 215:1402-1403 (1967).

23. H. Y. T. Yang, E. G. Erdös, and Y. Levin, A dipeptidyl carboxypeptidase that converts angiotensin I and inactivates bradykinin, Biochim. Biophys. Acta, 214:374-376 (1970).

24. C. E. Odya, P. Moreland, J. M. Steward, J. Barabé, and D. C. Regoli, Development of a radioimmunoassay for (des-Arg9)-bradykinin, Biochem. Pharmacol., 32:337-342 (1983).

25. D. Regoli and J. Barabé, Pharmacology of bradykinin and related kinins, Pharmac. Rev., 32:1-46 (1980).

26. T. E. Hugli, The structural basis for anaphylatoxin and chemotactic functions of C3a, C4a, and C5a, in: " Critical Reviews in Immunology, Vol. 1," M. Z. Atassi, ed., Chemical Rubber Co. (1981).

PARTIAL CHARACTERIZATION OF A LIVER SERINE-PEPTIDASE FROM DIFFERENT

SPECIES WHICH INACTIVATES BRADYKININ

Maria da Graca N. Mazzacoratti**, Misako U. Sampaio*,
Paula C. Duarte* and Claudio A. M. Sampaio*

*Departamento de Bioquimica, Escola Paulista de Medicina and
**Departamento de Ciencias Fisiologicas, Faculdade de
Ciencias Medicas da Santa Casa de Misericordia, Caixa
Postal 20372, 04023 S. Paulo, Brazil

ABSTRACT

Proteases which inactivate bradykinin were partially purified from the fresh exsanguinated liver of rat, man, dog, guinea-pig, chicken, frog and snake. The enzymes which are present in the soluble fraction of the liver homogenates, were prepared by DEAE-cellulose chromatography, in 0.025M tris-HCl, pH 7.4. The peptidase activity was eluted with 0.09M KCl; and further purification was achieved by gel-filtration in Sephadex G-150. The kininases are present in the same range of activity in all studied preparations, and final specific activities are also comparable. The molecular weight of the enzymes, as determined by gel filtration, are in the range of 70,000-100,000. All preparations were completely inhibited by 10mM PMSF and 1mM Tos-PheCh$_2$Cl; 10uM 2-mercaptoethanol, and 1mM Tos-LysCH$_2$Cl do not affect the enzymatic activity. The major site for the cleavage of bradykinin is the Phe$_5$-Ser$_6$ peptide bond. The serine-peptidase is found in the liver of all vertebrates so far studied.

INTRODUCTION

Kininase is the general name given to enzymes which are able to inactivate bradykinin (Arg-Pro-Pro-Gly-Phe-Ser-Pro-Phe-Arg) and related kinins. Carboxypeptidases, angiotensin-converting enzyme, chymotrypsin and several other enzymes display the ability to cleave peptide bonds in the kinins causing inactivation of its biological properties.[1] Plasma contains at least a carboxypeptidase and an angiotensin-converting enzyme able to cleave kinins.[2] The lung is considered the major site for inactivation of bradykinin, but the passage of blood through the isolated rat liver also causes considerable destruction of kinins.[3] The site of cleavage of bradykinin by the liver was studied by perfusion of the organ "in situ".[4] A serine-peptidase purified from rat liver homogenates could be the enzyme involved in this process.[5] The enzyme was also removed from the liver by perfusion with a detergent.[6] The enzyme from liver homogenates did not cleave high molecular weight substrates, such as kininogens, which contains the bradykinin moiety. The cleavage of other proteins was not detected so far.[5]

No physiological role has been yet assigned to such a neutral peptidase, since no natural substrate has been identified. The aim of this work is to verify the presence of this peptidase in the liver homogenate of different animal species, and to characterize some of the enzyme properties.

METHODS

Bradykinin and related peptides were synthesized by Dr. A. C. M. Paiva, from the Department of Biophysics of Escola Paulista de Medicina, by the solid-phase method. Kininases were prepared by a modification of a described procedure for the rat liver.[5,7] Livers from rat, guinea-pig, and dog were extensively perfused "in situ" with cold 0.14M NaCl. Man, chicken, frog and snake (Bothrops jararaca) livers were chopped into small pieces and they were washed with saline, as soon as possible after death, to remove all visible blood. The organs were homogenized in 0.025M tris-HCl, pH 7.4 with 0.25M sucrose in a final volume of 50ml for each 10g of wet tissue.

The homogenates were centrifuged at 40,000xg for 30 minutes and the supernatants were applied to a DEAE-cellulose (Cellex-D) column (1.5x5.0cm), equilibrated with the same tris- buffer. The kininases were eluted by increasing KCl. The pool of active kininase, corresponding to the serine peptidase, was concentrated by ammonium sulfate precipitation between 50 and 70% saturation. This material was applied to a Sephadex G-150 column (1.5x100cm), in the same tris-buffer.

Kininase activity was followed by the remaining biological activity of bradykinin incubated with the enzyme preparations at different time intervals.[8] The site of cleavage was determined by incubation at 200 ug bradykinin with the enzyme in the tris-buffer, at 37°C and at convenient time intervals. The products were measured in an amino-acid analyzer with a special buffer system.[5] Proteins were estimated by absorbance at 280nm.

RESULTS

Rat, man, dog, guinea-pig, chicken, frog and snake liver kininase was prepared following the same procedure. The separation of the 40,000 x g supernatant of liver homogenates in DEAE-cellulose column followed the same pattern. In Figure 1 the elution profile for human and canine enzymes are shown and these results are essentially the same for other mammals studied; the fractionation of the kininase from chicken and frog also followed the same general profile (Figure 2). Kinin-destroying enzymes are eluted at the beginning of the chromatography, and also when the ionic strength was raised to 0.05M KCl. Part of this activity is due to the angiotensin-coverting enzyme and probably lysosomal cathepsins.

Most of the serine-peptidase is eluted at 0.09M KCl; in some preparations of the guinea-pig enzyme, an activity was obtained at 0.12M KCl, but in the other cases all kininases were removed with 0.09M KCl. Other proteolytic enzymes such as aminopeptidases are eluted at higher salt concentrations. The enzyme concentrated by ammonium sulfate was chromatographed in a Sephadex G-150 column. The elution patterns for the

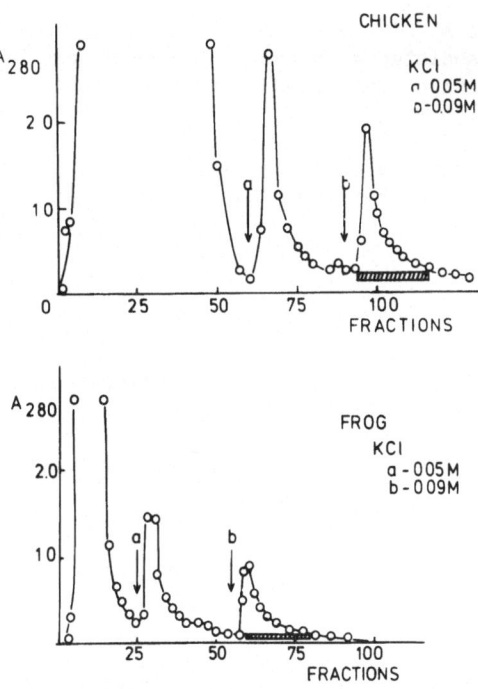

Figure 1.   Chromatography of the homogenates (10g of wet liver) of man and dog in a Cellex-D column (1.5 x 5.5cm), with 0.025M tris-HCl buffer, pH 7.4, and KCl (0.05M and 0.09M, as indicated); flow rate was 80ml/per hour and 6.5 ml - fractions were collected at 4°C.

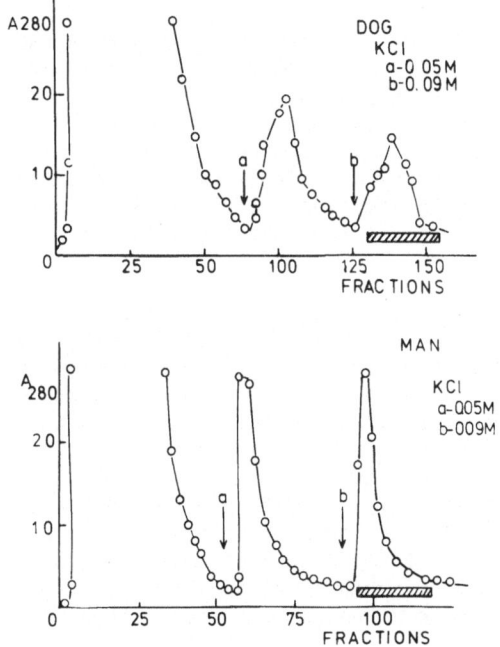

Figure 2.   Chromatography of liver homogenates of chicken and frog in the same sample and running conditions expressed in Figure 1.

enzymes from different species are compared in Figure 3. Kinin inactivating activity is associated only with the second peak of a preparation,
being the activity profile correspondent to the protein as followed by
its UV-absorbance at 280nm.

The molecular weight was estimated from the gel filtration for the
different preparations and they are between 70,000 and 100,000 (Table 1).

Table 1. Molecular weight determined by gel filtration of the serine-
peptidase from different species.

Animal	Molecular Weight
Rat	80,000
Man	100,000
Dog	92,000
Guinea-pig	70,000
Chicken	88,000
Frog	98,000
Snake	82,000

The degree of purification of the kininases from the different
species is difficult to calculate since the stability of the enzymes is
poor, and there is more than one enzyme at the initial phases of the
purification able to inactivate bradykinin. In Table 2 the final yield
is compared, after gel-filtration of the various kininases. The initial
and final specific activities are also shown. In order to avoid differences
due to the stability of the peptidases, the activity was determined as soon
as the pools were made, at the end of the gel-filtration step.

The properties of the enzymes were compared by their susceptibility
to different low molecular inhibitors (Table 3). All preparations were
readily inhibited by PMSF, and only the activity of the chicken enzyme
was not completely destroyed in the used concentration of PMSF, but the
inhibition of captopryl and the site of cleavage of bradykinin indicated
that this preparation is still contaminated by an angiotensin-converting
enzyme. The inhibition of Tos-PheCh$_2$Cl indicated that the enzyme is
related to the specifity of chymotrypsin; Tos-LysCH$_2$Cl were tested as a
control to an unspecific inhibition of chloro-methyl ketones, and did not
cause any change in activity. Lower concentrations of 2-mercaptoethanol
did not cause any activiation of the kininases, but dithiothreitol in the
same concentrations caused inhibition; in this case disulfide bridges
are being reduced, causing an unspecific modification of the enzymes.

The sites of cleavage of the bradykinin molecule were compared, in
order to verify the specifity of the kininase partially purified by this
procedure. The results in Table 4 indicate that in all preparations the
main peptide formed is Arg_1-Phe_5, but free Arg also occurs. The large
amounts of Arg in the incubations of man, rat, dog and chicken enzyme

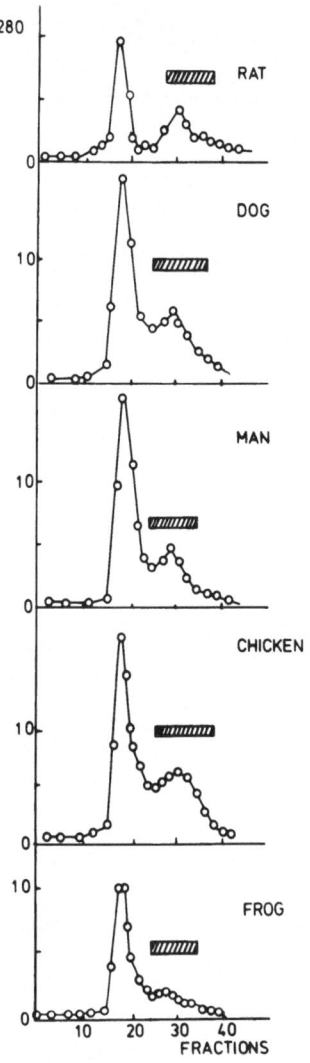

Figure 3. Chromatography of liver kininase in Sephadex G-150 (1.8 x 100cm), developed with 0.025M tris-HCl buffer, pH 7.4, containing 0.01mM 2-mercaptoethanol; 5.5ml-fractions were collected under 7.0ml flow-rate, at 4°C. The applied sample was the concentrated pool from the Cellex-D column; the different animal species are indicated in the figure.

are probably due to contaminations with a carboxypeptidase B-type enzyme. The appearance of Arg_1-Pro_7 in incubation of man and chicken preparations are compatible with contamination with an angiotensin converting enzyme.

DISCUSSION

All animals studied so far contain a serine-peptidase in the soluble fraction of the liver homogenates, which inactivates bradykinin by cleavage of at least one peptide bond. The rat enzyme, which has been studied previously, cleaves only small peptide substrates.[5] The amount of the enzyme in liver homogenates is of the same order, except for the amphibia species.

The specific activity of the kininase in the homogenates from different species is in the same range. The value for the preparation from frog is lower, what could be due to the fact that in this case the liver was not perfused; the same reason could explain the slightly lower value for the preparation from human liver. The variations in final specific activity may be reflecting differences in the activity of the enzyme particular to each species. However it is possible that these

Table 2. Comparative results of the purification of the liver kininase from different species

Animal	Initial Specific Activity	Final Specific Activity	Yield (%)
Rat	1.69	63.0	10.2
Guinea-pig	1.04	65.6	29.2
Dog	1.18	16.1	8.3
Man	0.73	14.5	8.5
Chicken	1.60	17.1	6.6
Frog	0.38	7.6	24.9
Snake	1.52	15.7	8.4

Specific activity is expressed as the hydrolysis of 1.0ug of bradykinin in the conditions of the assay per A280nm as described previously.[5,6]

Table 3. Inhibition of kininases by low molecular weight compounds

Animal	Inhibition (%)			
	PMSF 10mM	TPCK 1.0mM	2-mercaptoethanol 0.1nM	Captopryl 0.01mM
Rat	100	100	4	-
Guinea-pig	97	94	2	18
Dog	98	97	6	47
Man	91	96	0	59
Chicken	86	91	2	51
Frog	94	88	5	23
Snake	98	95	-	25

The enzymes were preincubated with the inhibitor in 0.025M tris-HCl buffer, pH 8.0, 30°C, for 30 minutes, (-) not determined

Table 4. Hydrolysis of bradykinin by liver kininases

Formed peptide (nmol)	Animal				
	Rat	Guinea-pig	Dog	Man	Chicken
Arg_1-Phe_5	47.5	38.6	85.9	31.3	47.9
Ser_6-Arg_9	15.5	28.0	3.6	2.6	5.6
Phe_8-Arg_9	nd	nd	nd	0.05	nd
Arg_1-Pro_7	nd	nd	nd	2.9	3.7
Arg	35.5	4.6	65.0	9.9	67.0

Incubation of bradykinin (170nmols) with 20 to 40ug of the kininases from the gel-filtration pool.
nd = not detected

differences are related to the poor stability of the enzymes after the last step of purification.

The molecular weight is in the range of 70,000-100,000, as determined by gel filtration. These values may be different if the enzymes are glycoproteins, but anyway they are molecules large enough to be distinguished from other neutral serine proteinases found in the liver or in neutrophiles which display a similar specificity towards derivatives of Tyr or Phe.

The major site of cleavage of bradykinin is the Phe_5-Ser_6 for all these peptidases and the complentary peptide Ser_6-Arg_9 was not found in ·stoichiometric amounts. Contaminants like carboxypeptidase N or angiotensin converting enzymes could explain these findings, although previous observations have shown that the rat liver kininase cleaves, besides Phe_5-Ser_6, the Phe_8-Arg_9 bond.[5] This cleavage pattern was also found for a well characterized endopeptidase, chymotrypsin.[8,10] The preparations of human and chicken livers, which were not submitted to perfusions, produced more peptides including a cleavage which can be associated with angiotensin converting enzyme (formation of the peptide Phe-Arg).

The role of these peptidases is probably not associated only to the cleavage and the inactivation of bradykinin; more broadly they may play a role in processing hormone peptides which reach the cytoplasma of the liver cells, or they may be involved in the steps of the intracellular degradation of proteins.

REFERENCES

1. Erdos, E. G., Kininases, Hand. exp. Pharm. 25 (suppl.), 428-487, (1979).

2. G. Oshima, J. Kato, and E. Erdos, Plasma carboxypeptidase N, subunits and characteristics, Arch. Biochem. Biophys., 170:132-138, (1975).

3. D. R. Borges, E. A. Limaos, J. L. Prado, and A. C. M. Camargo, Catabolism of vasoactive peptides by perfused rat liver, Naunyn-Schmiedeberg's Arch. Pharmac., 295:33-40, (1976).

4. D. R. Borges, J. A. Guimaraes, E. A. Limaos, J. L. Prado, and A. C. M. Camargo, Bradykinin inactivation of perfused rat liver. Role of a thiol activated endopeptidase, Naunyn-Schmiedeberg's Arch. Pharmac., 309:197-201, (1979).

5. M. G. N. Mazzacoratti, C. A. M. Sampaio, Rat liver kininase, a serine peptidase, Biochem. Pharmac., 31:799-804, (1982).

6. M. Kouyoumdjian, D. R. Borges, and J. L. Prado, Kinin inactivating endopeptidase from rat liver, Int. J. Biochem., 16:733-739, (1984).

7. C. A. M. Sampaio, M. G. N. Mazzacoratti, and M. U. Sampaio, Characterization of a soluble kininase in the rat liver homogenates, Agents & Actions, 9 (suppl.):430-434, (1982).

8. C. A. M. Sampaio, S. T. Nunez, M. G. N. Mazzacoratti, and J. L. Prado, Inactivation of kinins by chymotrypsin, Biochem. Pharmac., 25:2391-2394, (1975).

9. A. J. Barret, Introduction to the history and classification of tissue proteinase, in: Proteinases in Mammalian Cell and Tissues, A. J. Barret (ed.), Elsevier, pp. 1-52, (1977).

10. D. F. Elliot, G. P. Lewis, and E. W. Horton, The structure of bradykinin, A plasma kinin from ox blood, Biochem. Biophys. Res. Com., 3:87-93, (1960).

VASCULAR, POST PROLINE CLEAVING ENZYME: METABOLISM OF VASOACTIVE PEPTIDES

Hester H. Bausback and Patrick E. Ward

Department of Pharmacology
New York Medical College
Valhalla, New York 10595

SUMMARY

Vasoactive peptides contain a high proportion of proline residues which make them resistant to hydrolysis by many peptidases. However, post proline cleaving enzyme (PPCE; EC 3.4.21.26), a proline specific endopeptidase which specifically hydrolyzes internal peptide bonds on the carboxyl side of proline residues, has been shown to inactivate numerous vasoactive peptides including angiotensins, kinins, substance P, vasopressin and oxytocin. In order to determine whether PPCE could be involved in vascular metabolism of vasoactive peptides, we carried out localization and characterization studies of PPCE-like activity in hog aorta and mesenteric artery. PPCE was assayed fluorometrically at pH 7.0 using the specific PPCE substrate CBZ-Gly-Pro-4-methyl-coumarinylamide. The subcellular distribution of vascular PPCE was essentially the same as that of the cytosolic marker enzyme lactic dehydrogenase (LDH). PPCE was enriched six-fold in the cytosolic fraction (11.4 ± 2.7 units/mg) and, unlike the plasma membrane-bound proline specific exopeptidase dipeptidyl-(amino)peptidase IV (DAP IV; EC 3.4.14.5), little or no activity could be detected in the microsomal or plasma membrane fractions. Similar to PPCE characterized from other sites, vascular PPCE was stabilized and activated by dithiothreitol and EDTA, and inhibited by DFP, p-chloromercuriphenyl sulfonic acid, L-1-tosylamido-2-phenylethylchloromethyl ketone, Cu^{++}, Ca^{++}, and Zn^{++}. Vascular PPCE was unaffected by inhibitors of trypsin and kallikrein (Aprotinin, ABTI), aminopeptidase M (bestatin, amastatin), neutral endopeptidase (phosphoramidon), angiotensin I converting enzyme (captopril) or carboxypeptidase N (MERGETPA). These data demonstrate that PPCE is present in vascular endothelium and/or smooth muscle. Although PPCE may participate in vascular metabolism of vasoactive peptides, its cytosolic localization and endopeptidase specificity suggests that its role is limited to peptide degradation after transport into the cell.

INTRODUCTION

Angiotensin I converting enzyme (ACE, EC 3.4.15.1) is present on the cell surface of vascular endothelium, and its importance to _in vivo_ formation of angiotensin II and degradation of kinins is well established.[1,2] Over the last several years, our laboratory has been involved in determining whether other specific peptidases are also present in the vasculature, and whether such enzymes participate in the metabolism of vasoactive peptides. These studies have identified two peptidases (AmM, DAP IV) on the cell surface of vascular endothelium and/or smooth muscle which can differentially metabolize vasoactive peptides.[3-5]

Aminopeptidase M (AmM, EC 3.4.11.2) hydrolyzes basic and neutral amino acids (but not Glu or Asp) from the N-terminus of peptides, except where the penultimate amino acid is Pro.[6] Consistant with this substrate specificity, vascular AmM can convert kallidin to bradykinin and inactivate des(Asp[1])angiotensin I, angiotensin III, hepta(5-11)substance P and met-enkephalin.[4] AmM does not, however, hydrolyze bradykinin, angiotensin I, angiotensin II, saralasin, vasopressin, oxytocin or any form of substance P containing the Arg-Pro-Lys-Pro sequence.

Vascular dipeptidyl(amino)peptidase IV (DAP IV; EC 3.4.14.5) specifically hydrolyzes X-Pro dipeptides from the N-terminus of polypeptides.[5,7] Substance P, which has sequential Arg-Pro and Lys-Pro dipeptides at its N-terminus, is the only vasoactive peptide which fits DAP IV's specificity. Although bradykinin also has an Arg-Pro N-terminus, it is not hydrolyzed by DAP IV because of the presence of a second Pro in position three.[8]

During the course of these studies, we found that a vascular plasma membrane (VPM)-enriched fraction inactivated angiotensin II and des(Arg[9])-bradykinin (R-Pro-Phe) by hydrolysis of the Pro-Phe bond. Since this metabolism involved hydrolysis of a proline bond, several proline specific enzymes were considered likely candidates. One of these, post proline cleaving enzyme (PPCE; EC 3.4.21.26), is an endopeptidase which specifically hydrolyzes peptides on the carboxyl side of internal proline residues.[9] Purified PPCE has been shown to inactivate a wide variety of vasoactive peptides,[10,11] and its specificity is consistant with the above hydrolysis of angiotensin II and des(Arg[9])bradykinin (Figure 1). Thus, the present study was carried out to determine whether PPCE is present within the vasculature, and whether it could account for vascular degradation of angiotensins and des(Arg)kinins.

METHODS

Vessel Subcellular Fractionation

Aorta and mesenteric arteries were obtained from freshly slaughtered hogs, cleaned in 0.9% (w/v) saline, and subfractionated to low speed pellet (LSP), cytosolic (CYT) and microsomal (MIC) fractions. As shown in Figure

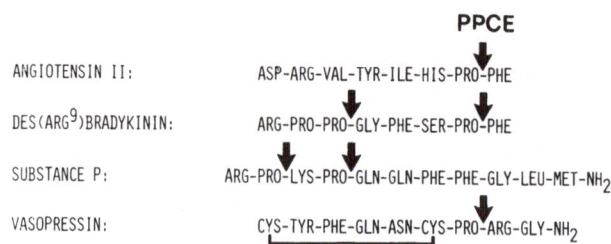

Fig. 1. Hydrolysis of vasoactive peptides by post proline cleaving enzyme (9-11).

2, the microsomal fraction was then separated into four subfractions (V_{1-4}) according to the procedure of Kwan et al.[12] as described previously.[3-5] The layer at the top of the gradient was designated the vascular plasma membrane (VPM)-enriched fraction since, as found previously,[3-5] it was enriched in the plasma membrane marker enzyme 5' nucleotidase (EC 3.1.3.5). Further, ACE, AmM and DAP IV activities were comparably enriched.

Enzyme Assays

Marker enzymes, ACE, AmM and DAP IV were assayed as previously described.[3-5] PPCE was assayed according to the procedure of Yoshimoto et al.[13] using CBZ-Gly-Pro-4-methyl-coumarinylamide (Bachem, Torrance, CA) as substrate. The reaction mixture consisted of 3.45 ml of 0.1 M phosphate buffer (pH 7.0), 50 µl of 0.5 mM substrate in dioxane, 400 µl of 10 mM dithiothreitol and 100 µl of enzyme. The fluorescence of the 7-amino-4-methyl-coumarin product was monitored at 37°C using a Turner 111 Fluorometer with excitation and emission set at 360 and 455 nm respectively. Increases in fluorescence were directly proportional to both time of incubation and amount of enzyme added. Enzyme specific activity is expressed as units/mg protein where one unit equals the change in relative fluorescence per minute. For inhibition studies, inhibitors were pre-incubated for 15-30 minutes before addition of substrate. Protein was determined by the method of Lowry et al.[14] using bovine serum albumen as the standard.

Peptide Metabolism

Qualitative analysis of peptide metabolism was carried out by thin layer chromatography (TLC) on MN 300 cellulose plates.[4] The standard incubation consisted of a 500 µM final concentration of peptide in 40 µl of 100 mM Tris/HCl (pH 7.0) and 10 µl of the VPM. At sequential time

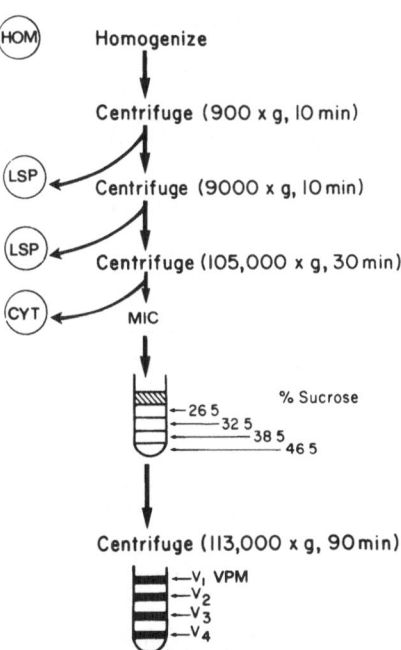

Fig. 2. Isolation of vascular plasma membrane.

intervals, 5 μl aliquots were spotted on the plate and immediately dried. Plates were developed in butanol:acetic acid:water (4:1:5) and the products visualized by staining with 0.4% (w/v) ninhydrin in acetone according to Toennies and Kolb.[15]

RESULTS

Peptide Metabolism

Incubation of the VPM with angiotensin II or des(Arg[9])bradykinin confirmed our previous observation that both peptides were hydrolyzed at the Pro[7]-Phe[8] bond. Hydrolysis was not affected by ACE, AmM or DAP IV inhibitors, but could be completely inhibited by EDTA and o-phenanthroline.

PPCE - Localization and Characterization

As previously found,[3-5] the cytosolic marker enzyme LDH was enriched 3.6-fold in the vascular cytosol fraction. Similarly, PPCE-like activity was concentrated in the same fraction with a specific activity of 11.4 ± 1.7 units/mg (Figure 3). This activity represented a more than six-fold enrichment over homogenate activity (1.9 ± 0.4). Further, whereas membrane-bound DAP IV was localized to the VPM fraction, little or no PPCE-like activity could be detected in the microsomal (MIC) or vascular plasma membrane (VPM)-enriched fractions. These data indicated that if PPCE was responsible for the observed VPM hydrolysis of angiotensin II and des(Arg[9]) bradykinin, such hydrolysis must be an artifact of vessel subfractionation (i.e., trace contamination of the VPM fraction with cytosolic PPCE). Thus,

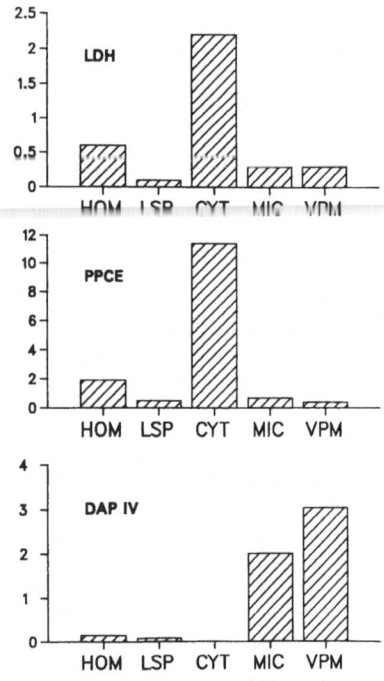

Fig. 3. Distribution of lactic dehydrogenase (LDH), post proline cleaving enzyme (PPCE) and dipeptidyl(amino)-peptidase IV (DAP IV) in subcellular fractions of hog aorta.

in order to confirm that the cytosolic activity was true PPCE, and to determine whether such activity was responsible for VPM angiotensin II and des(Arg[9])bradykinin hydrolysis, a complete inhibition profile of the cytosolic PPCE-like activity was conducted and compared to that obtained with the VPM activity.

As shown in Table 1, vascular cytosolic PPCE was inhibited by the divalent cations Zn^{++}, Ca^{++} and Cu^{++}, whereas Mg^{++}, Co^{++} and Mn^{++} were ineffective. Pre-incubation with EDTA resulted in a slight increase of activity which was completely inhibited by p-chloromercuriphenyl sulfonic acid, L-1-tosylamido-2-phenylethylchloromethyl ketone and DFP. Substance P, a reported substrate for PPCE, was also an effective inhibitor. However, inhibitors of trypsin and kallikrein ($protinin, SBTI), AmM (bestatin, amastatin), neutral endopeptidase (phosphoramidon),[16] ACE (captopril) or carboxypeptidase N (MERGETPA)[17] had no effect. This inhibition profile, essentially the same as that reported for purified PPCE,[9] confirmed that the vascular cytosolic activity being measured was true PPCE. Further, since the hydrolysis of angiotensin II and des(Arg[9])bradykinin was effectively inhibited by chelating agents which had no inhibitory effect on PPCE, these data ruled out the possibility that the vascular plasma membrane metabolism of these peptides was due to contamination by cytosolic PPCE.

Table 1. Inhibition of vascular post proline cleaving enzyme.

COMPOUND	Conc (mM)	% Control
-	-	100
$ZnCl_2$	0.1	33
$CaCl_2$	0.1	35
$CuSO_4$	1.0	9
$MgCl_2$	1.0	102
$CoCl_2$	1.0	80
$MnCl_2$	1.0	95
EDTA	1.0	110
p-Chloromercuriphenyl- sulfonic acid	1.0	6
L-1-Tosylamido-2-phenylethyl- chloromethyl ketone	1.0	3
Substance P	0.01	40
Aprotinin	0.1 TIU	104
SBTI	2000 IU	87
Bestatin	0.1	107
Amastatin	0.1	87
Phosphoramidon	0.1	101
Captopril	1.0	92
MERGETPA	0.1	91

DISCUSSION

The biologic effects of vasoactive peptides are related not only to receptor stimulation, but also to the net effect of peptide metabolism occuring in the micro-environment of the vascular cell surface receptors. However, with few exceptions (i.e., ACE), little progress has been made in identifying specific peptide-peptidase pathways of physiologic significance. This is due to the fact that few studies have been able to identify specific vascular peptidases in a definitive manner, and may also be due to the idea that the "apparent" broad substrate profile of many peptidases precludes specificity. Nevertheless, as pointed out by Hughes,[18] a combination of the correct enzyme substrate specificity/peptide structure and the appropriate anatomical (cellular and subcellular) distribution can constitute a physiologically significant "functional specificity" for metabolism of locally released and/or circulating peptides. For example, despite its accepted role as the rate-limiting enzyme in the conversion of angiotensin I to angiotensin II, and in the inactivation of kinins, it is important to remember that vascular ACE is not substrate specific. Rather, ACE can hydrolyze a variety of dipeptides from low molecular weight peptides. Thus, it is a combination of both the substrate specificity and the vascular endothelial/plasma membrane localization of ACE which collectively accounts for its pivotal role in endogenous angiotensin II formation and kinin inactivation.

ACE, AmM and DAP IV are present as intrinsic proteins on the cell surface (brush border) membrane of renal proximal tubule cells.[19] We have recently reported[3] that all three enzymes are also present on a vascular, plasma membrane-enriched fraction prepared from hog aorta and mesenteric artery. All three enzymes are bound to the membrane in a similar manner, and immunologically indistinguishable forms of each are also present in plasma. Although the endothelial localization of ACE is well established,[1,2] the relative cellular (endothelial, smooth muscle) distribution of AmM and DAP IV remain to be determined. Vascular plasma membrane DAP IV can specifically convert substance P to hepta(5-11)-substance P and AmM can differentially metabolize a number of vasoactive peptides.[4,5] Thus, both enzymes have the correct subcellular localization and substrate specificity to modulate both the form and concentration of vasoactive peptides in the micro-environment of the vascular cell surface receptors. Nevertheless, further studies on the cellular distribution and substrate affinity of these enzymes will be required before their significance to _in vivo_ peptide metabolism can be established.

In view of the above, the physiologic significance of vascular PPCE is less clear. PPCE's specificity for hydrolyzing internal proline bonds gives it the capacity to degrade essentially all vasoactive peptides, and such specificity would seem to preclude selective, differential metabolism. Although further work may establish that PPCE has a significantly higher affinity for specific peptides (and thus favor their inactivation at low _in vivo_ substrate concentrations), such hydrolysis could occur only after uptake of the peptide into the cell. Thus, although such a process cannot be ruled out, it is unlikely that vascular PPCE plays a significant role in _in vivo_ metabolism of vasoactive peptides, at least under normal conditions. Nevertheless, since PPCE has been identified in the circulation,[20] plasma PPCE may play a role in the inactivation of circulating vasoactive peptides.

Although the results of our studies to date have not identified the vascular plasma membrane enzyme responsible for inactivation of angiotensin II and des(Arg)kinins, the present data have established that such metabolism is not artifact related to cytosolic (PPCE) contamination of the plasma membrane fraction. Further, hydrolysis of the Pro^7-Phe^8 bond is consistant with the reports of Regoli and co-workers[21,22] regarding in-activation of these peptides. Identifying, localizing and characterizing this enzyme could be particularly important since its activity may be the major, and like ACE, common pathway for vascular inactivation of angiotensins and kinins (specifically des(Arg)kinins).

ACKNOWLEDGEMENTS

This work was supported by NIADDKD grant #1 R01 AM 28184. We would like to thank the Karl Ehmer Co. for supplying fresh porcine tissues.

REFERENCES

1. R. L. Soffer, Angiotensin I converting enzyme and the regulation of vasoactive peptides, Ann. Rev. Biochem., 45:73-94 (1976).
2. U. S. Ryan, J. W. Ryan, C. Whitaker, and A. Chiu, Localization of angiotensin converting enzyme (kininase II). II. Immunocytochemistry and immunofluorescence, Tissue Cell, 8:125-146 (1976).
3. P. E. Ward, Immunoelectrophoretic analysis of vascular, membrane bound angiotensin I converting enzyme, aminopeptidase M, and dipeptidyl (amino)peptidase IV, Biochem. Pharmacol., 33:3183-3193 (1984).
4. F. E. Palmieri, J. J. Petrelli, and P. E. Ward, Vascular, plasma membrane aminopeptidase M: Metabolism of vasoactive peptides, Biochem. Pharmacol. (In press).
5. F. E. Palmieri and P. E. Ward, Mesentery vascular metabolism of substance P, Biochim. Biophys. Acta, 755:522-525 (1983).
6. A. J. Kenny and A. G. Booth, Microvilli: Their ultrastructure, enzymology and molecular organization, Essays Biochem., 14:1-44 (1978).
7. E. Heymann and R. Mentlein, Liver dipeptidyl aminopeptidase IV hydrolyzes substance P, FEBS Lett., 91:360-364 (1978).
8. T. Kato, T. Nagatsu, K. Fukasawa, M. Harada, I. Nagatsu, and S. Sakakibara, Successive cleavage of N-terminal Arg^1-Pro^2 and Lys^3-Pro^4 from substance P but no release of Arg^1-Pro^2 from bradykinin, by X-Pro dipeptidyl-aminopeptidase, Biochim. Biophys. Acta, 525:417-422 (1978).
9. R. Walter, W. H. Simmons, and T. Yoshimoto, Proline specific endo- and exopeptidases, Mol. Cell. Biochem., 30:111-127 (1980).
10. H. Shlank and R. Walter, Enzymic cleavage of post proline peptide bonds: Degredation of arginine-vasopressin and angiotensin II, Proc. Soc. Exp. Biol. Med., 141:452-455 (1972).
11. L. B. Hersh, Immunological, physical and chemical evidence for the identity of brain and kidney post-proline cleaving enzyme, J. Neurochem., 37:172-178 (1981).
12. C. Y. Kwan, R. Garfield, and E. E. Daniel, An improved procedure for the isolation of plasma membranes from rat mesenteric arteries, J. Mol. Cell. Cardiol., 11:639-659 (1979).
13. T. Yoshimoto, K. Ogita, R. Walter, M. Koida, and D. Tsuru, Post proline cleaving enzyme. Synthesis of a new fluorogenic substrate and distribution of the endopeptidase in rat tissues and body fluids of man, Biochim. Biophys. Acta, 569:184-192 (1979).
14. O. H. Lowry, N. J. Rosebrough, A. L. Farr, and R. J. Randall, Protein measurement with folin phenol reagent, J. Biol. Chem., 193:265-275 (1951).
15. G. Toennies and J. J. Kolb, Techniques and reagents for paper chromatography, Anal. Chem., 23:823-826 (1951).
16. J. Almenoff and M. Orlowski, Membrane bound neutral metalloendopeptidase: Interaction with synthetic substrates, natural peptides and inhibitors, Biochemistry, 22:590-599 (1983).

17. T. H. Plummer and T. J. Ryan, A potent mercapto bi-product analogue inhibitor for human carboxypeptidase N, _Biochim. Biophys. Res. Commun._, 98:448-454 (1981).

18. J. Hughes, Biogenesis, release and inactivation of enkephalins and dynorphins, _Brit. Med. Bull._, 39:17-24 (1983).

19. P. E. Ward and M. A. Sheridan, Immunoelectrophoretic analysis of renal and intestinal brush border converting enzyme, _Biochem. Pharmacol._, 32:265-274 (1983).

20. T. Kato, M. Okada, and T. Nagatsu, Distribution of post proline cleaving enzyme in human brain and the peripheral tissues, _Mol. Cell. Biochem._, 32:117-121 (1980).

21. J. Magnan and D. Regoli, Metabolism of angiotensin II and some analogs in intact strips and in muscle preparations of rabbit aortae, _Can. J. Physiol. Pharmacol._, 56:39-47 (1978).

22. F. Marceau, M. Gendreau, J. Barabe, S. St-Pierre, and D. Regoli, The degredation of bradykinin and of des-Arg[9]-bradykinin in plasma, _Can. J. Physiol. Pharmacol._, 59:131-138 (1981).

SYNTHETIC INHIBITORS OF CARBOXYPEPTIDASE N

George H. Fisher*, James W. Ryan and Alfred Chung

Department of Medicine
University of Miami School of Medicine
Miami, FL 33101

Thomas H. Plummer, Jr.

Center for Laboratories and Research
New York State Department of Health
Albany, NY 12201

SUMMARY

Further to explore the functions of carboxypeptidase N (CPN) in vivo, we undertook two studies to find CPN inhibitors of high potency and relatively long duration of action. In each study we examined for inhibition of hydrolysis of [^{3}H]benzoyl-Ala-Arg using pure bovine serum CPN or human serum. In the first such study we synthesized a series of acyl amino acids and acyl di - and tripeptides containing arginine, lysine or both. All proved to be weak inhibitors (Ki = 10^{-3} to 10^{-4} M). N$^\alpha$-carbamoyl-Arg was the strongest: Ki = 3.5 x 10^{-5} M.

In the second study we prepared S-acyl (thio ester) derivatives of the highly potent CPN inhibitor 2-mercaptomethyl-3-guanidinoethylthiopropionic acid (2-MGP), as certain S-acyl groups markedly increase the duration of captopril, another mercapto-containing compound. Acetyl-, Boc-phenylalanyl-, phenylalanyl-, benzoyl-alanyl-, alanyl-, and Boc-alanyl-2-MGP retained the high potency of 2-MGP in vitro. Although Ala-2-MGP exerted maximum effects in vivo, like those of 2-MGP, the duration of action of Ala-2-MGP was slightly shorter than that of 2-MGP. These results indicate that the mercapto group of 2-MGP can be taken up in some forms of thioester linkage and still retain virtually the full potency of 2-MGP itself. Thus, it appears that a free mercapto function is not essential for the action of 2-MGP.

*Present Address: Department of Chemistry, University of Miami, Coral Gables, FL 33124

INTRODUCTION

Carboxypeptidase N (CPN) is a zinc-containing metalloenzyme with actions similar to those of carboxypeptidase B which cleaves basic amino acids (arginine or lysine) from the carboxyl terminus of peptides. Although CPN is sometimes called "Kininase I," the enzyme has a surprisingly low affinity for bradykinin (Kc/Km = 2 x 10^4 $M^{-1}sec^{-1}$)[1]. Inhibitors of CPN do not potentiate blood pressure effects of bradykinin but markedly potentiate spasmogenic effects of C3a and markedly worsen the course of aggregate anaphylaxis[2,3].

One of the most potent inhibitors of CPN is 2-mercaptomethyl-3-guanidinoethylthiopropionic acid (2-MGP, Ki = 3 x 10^{-9} M)[4]. However, 2-MGP has a short duration of action, presumably because of its ability to form disulfides, symmetrical or mixed. In efforts to obtain longer-acting analogs of 2-MGP, we sought derivatives which would maintain the potency of 2-MGP but be less prone to form inactive disulfides. In order to accomplish this goal, we have synthesized a series of derivatives in which the mercapto function of 2-MGP has been incorporated into a thioester bond as a means of minimizing formation of disulfides.

In further studies to explore the functions of CPN in vivo, we have synthesized a series of acyl analogs of arginine or lysine or acyl di- and tripeptides containing arginine and lysine or both. These compounds and the 2-MGP thioester derivatives were assayed for inhibition of hydrolysis of ^{3}H benzoyl-Ala-Arg by pure bovine serum CPN or human serum as the enzyme source. All of the Arg and Lys analogs proved to be weak inhibitors of CPN (Ki 10^{-3} to 10^{-4} M) while the 2-MGP thioester derivatives were approximately as potent as 2-MGP, with Ki values in the range of 10^{-8} to 10^{-9} M.

EXPERIMENTAL

Syntheses

Unless specified otherwise, acyl-Arg and acyl-Lys derivatives and peptides were synthesized by the solid-phase technique on a Schwarz-Mann automatic peptide synthesizer. Boc-N^g-tosyl-Arg or Boc-N^ϵ-ClBzl-Lys were attached to chloromethylated, 1% cross-linked Merrifield resin by refluxing in ethanol in the presence of triethylamine. The Boc protecting group was removed with 30% TFA/CH_2Cl_2 and the resulting TFA salt was neutralized with 10% Et$_3$N/CH_2Cl_2. A 2- to 3-fold excess of the next Boc-protected amino acid or organic acylating acid was coupled to the free α-amino group of Arg or Lys by the dicyclohexylcarbo-diimide (DCC)-mediated coupling procedure for 2 to 4 hours in CH_2Cl_2. Completeness of coupling was monitored by ninhydrin.

Cleavage of the final product from the resin with simultaneous removal of protecting groups was accomplished with anhydrous, liquid hydrogen fluoride in the presence of 10% anisole. The products were purified by combinations of gel filtration on Sephadex G-10 with 1% acetic acid, partition chromatography on Sephadex G-10 with n-butanol-acetic acid-water (4:1:5), and chromatography on Sephadex LH-20 with n-butanol-water (6:94). The purity of the final products was monitored by thin layer chromatography.

N^α-carbamoyl-Arg was synthesized by the procedure of Chauhan[5] by reaction of potassium cyanate with N^g-nitroarginine in aqueous ethanol at pH 9 (Et$_3$N), followed by removal of the guanidino nitro group by catalytic hydrogenolysis. N^α-(4-t-butylbenzoyl)-Arg was prepared by coupling 4-t-butylbenzoic acid to N^g-nitro-Arg-OBzl ester using DCC-CH_2Cl_2, followed by catalytic hydrogenolysis. Biotinyl-Arg was synthesized by coupling biotin N-hydroxy-succinimide ester to arginine in aqueous dimethylformamide

(DMF) solution with recrystallization of the resulting product from aqueous methanol. N^α-formyl-Arg was prepared by the procedure of Sheehan and Yang[6] by addition of acetic anhydride dropwise to a cold (5°C) solution of arginine in 98% formic acid. Maleoyl-Arg was formed by acylating arginine with maleic anhydride in water with recrystallization of the product from aqueous methanol.

S-Acetyl-2-MGP was isolated as an intermediate product during the synthesis of 2-MGP by the procedure described by Plummer and Ryan[4]. 2-MGP was purified on a column of CM-Sephadex with 0.2M pyridine-formate buffer. Boc-Phe-ONSu active ester was allowed to react with 2-MGP in aqueous tetrahydrofuran (THF) solution to give the Boc-Phe-thioester of 2-MGP as a white solid, mp 185-186°C after recrystallization from methanol-water. The same Boc-Phe-2-MGP thioester was also obtained by coupling Boc-Phe to 2-MGP using carbodiimidazole (CDI) in DMF as the coupling agent. The Boc group was removed by treatment with 30% TFA/CH_2Cl_2 with purification of Phe-2-MGP thioester on a column of Sephadex LH-20 with n-butanol-water (6:94).

Similarly, Boc-Ala-2-MGP thioester was obtained by coupling Boc-Ala to 2-MGP using CDI in DMF solution, and removal of the Boc group with TFA gave Ala-2-MGP thioester. The free α-amino group of Ala-2-MGP was acylated with benzoylchloride in aqueous dioxane to give Bz-Ala-2-MGP which was purified on a column of Sephadex G-15 with 1% HOAc to give a few milligrams of white solid product.

Assay of Inhibition Potencies

[^{3}H] Benzoyl-Ala-Arg (25 Ci/mmol), prepared in this laboratory, was used as substrate in a final concentration of 40 nM), and reactions obeyed first order enzyme kinetics. Typically, human serum was used as the source of carboxypeptidase N in a final concentration of 1:80. Some experiments used pure bovine serum CPN. The assay buffer was 0.05 M Hepes buffer, pH 7.5, containing 0.15 M NaCl and 0.05% sodium azide.

The assay protocol was adapted after that described previously (7): To each of a series of 7-ml liquid scintillation vials was added 50 µl). Each vial then received 50 µl of buffer (for blank and control reaction mixtures) or 50 µl of inhibitor in buffer. Reactions were started by adding 100 µl of human serum, 1:40 dilution in assay buffer. Blank reaction mixtures received 100 µl of buffer instead of serum dilution. Reaction mixtures were incubated at 37°C for 10 min, and reactions were stopped by adding 200 µl of 0.5 M HCl. Each vial received 3 ml of Ventrex LSC #1, a cocktail formulated to extract hippuric acid from acidified aqueous solution. The cocktail also extracts [^{3}H]benzoyl-Ala, the radioactive product formed by CPN, but does not extract unhydrolyzed substrate. Vials were capped, inverted 20 times and submitted for liquid scintillation counting. Substrate was measured by counting ^{3}H of a vial containing 50 µl of buffered substrate and 5 ml of the aqueous compatible LSC Scint A (Packard Instruments). Results were computed using the integrated form of the first order rate equation and using the relationship $v/v_i = 1 + (i/K_i)$ where v_0 is the velocity in the absence of inhibitor and v_i the velocity in the presence of a given inhibitor concentration, i[8,9].

RESULTS

The Arg and Lys analogs and the 2-MGP thioester derivatives were assayed as described in the experimental section for their potencies as CPN inhibitors. All of the acyl-Arg and acyl-Lys analogs were weak inhibitors of CPN (Table 1, Ki's 10^{-3} to 10^{-4} M). N^α-Carbamoyl-Arg, H_2NCNH-$CH(CH_2)_3$-$NHCNH_2$, was the strongest: Ki = 3.5 x 10^{-5} M.

Table 1

CPN INHIBITION POTENCIES OF ACYL ARG AND LYS ANALOGS

Analog	Ki (I_{50}) (M)
N^α-Carbamoyl-Arg	3.5×10^{-5}
Benzoyl-Arg-Arg-Arg	2.4×10^{-4}
Benzoyl-Arg-Arg	1.4×10^{-4}
Benzoyl-Pro-Arg	9.3×10^{-4}
Benzoyl-Phe-Arg	3.2×10^{-4}
Benzoyl-Arg-Lys	1.1×10^{-4}
Benzoyl-Lys-Lys	1.1×10^{-4}
Benzoyl-Lys-Lys-Lys	2.9×10^{-4}
Benzoyl-Lys-Arg-Lys	2.0×10^{-4}
Ala-Arg	3.1×10^{-4}
N^α-Acetyl-Ala-Arg	7.8×10^{-4}
N^α-(4-t-butylbenzoyl)-Arg	1.3×10^{-4}
Acetylsalicylyl-Arg	1.3×10^{-4}
Maleoyl-Arg	2.5×10^{-4}
Cinnamoyl-Arg	3.1×10^{-4}
Biotinyl-Arg	3.6×10^{-4}
D-Penicillamine-Arg	2.1×10^{-4}
N^α-Formyl-Arg	1.9×10^{-3}

Table 2

CPN INHIBITION POTENCIES OF 2-MGP DERIVATIVES

Derivative	Ki (I_{50}) (M)
2-MGP	3.0×10^{-9}
Acetyl-2-MGP	4.9×10^{-9}
Phe-2-MGP	5.0×10^{-9}
Boc-Phe-2-MGP	2.2×10^{-9}
Ala-2-MGP	4.6×10^{-9}
Boc-Ala-2-MGP	3.8×10^{-8}
Bz-Ala-2-MGP	9.8×10^{-8}

Table 2 gives the potencies of the 2-MGP thioester derivatives as CPN inhibitors. All of the acyl derivatives of 2-MGP, e.g. acetyl, alanyl, phenylalanyl, Boc-alanyl, Boc-phenylalanyl, were approximately as potent as 2-MGP with Ki values in the range of 10^{-8} to 10^{-9} M. Thus far only one of the acyl-2-MGP derivatives has been assayed in vivo. Ala-2-MGP and 2-MGP were tested using anesthetized Sprague-Dawley rats. Either drug was given iv, and arterial blood samples were collected at 5 min, 10 min, and 30 min following drug administration. Plasma CPN activity was measured for each sample taken after drug injection and for a control sample. As expected from results of our in vitro assays, Ala-2-MGP exerted maximum effects like those of 2-MGP:

	iv ED_{50}	$t_{\frac{1}{2}}$*
2-MGP	0.22 µmol/kg	32 min
Ala-2-MGP	0.26 µmol/kg	23 min

However, the duration of action of Ala-2-MGP was shorter than that of 2-MGP (*$t_{\frac{1}{2}}$ for 0.3 µmol/kg). Whether other of the acyl derivatives of 2-MGP have longer durations of action remains to be determined.

DISCUSSION

CPN, like angiotensin converting enzyme (ACE), is a zinc containing metalloenzyme (cf 10 with 11), and thus it is assumed that the free mercapto group of 2-MGP binds to the Zn^{++} of CPN much as the free mercapto group of captopril (D-2-methyl-3-mercaptopropionyl-L-proline) binds to the Zn^{++} of ACE[4,11]. However, our results indicate that the mercapto group of 2-MGP can be taken up in some forms of thioester linkage to yield acyl derivatives that retain virtually the full potency of 2-MGP itself. Similar acyl derivatives of captopril retain the affinity of captopril for ACE yet have markedly increased durations of action[13]. Thus, it is far from clear that a free mercapto function is essential for the actions of captopril or 2-MGP.

Presumably, the acyl derivatives of 2-MGP and captopril provide recognition groups for the S_1 and possibly the S_2 binding sites of their respective target enzymes. Thus, it is conceivable that any disadvantage incurred by taking up the mercapto functions in thioester linkages is offset by binding at the S_1 binding sites of the target enzymes. Unlike many other thioester compounds, the acyl derivatives of 2-MGP and captopril are chemically stable and do not act as active esters. However, we cannot rule out the possibility that, e.g., Ala-2-MGP is hydrolyzed by CPN to yield 2-MGP at the enzyme's catalytic site. Alternatively, Ala-2-MGP may be hydrolyzed by an aminopeptidase to release free 2-MGP.

Thus, while it is unclear whether the thioesters themselves can bind the zinc of CPN, it seems eminently reasonable that acylation per se prevents the formation of mixed and symmetrical disulfides, products that are themselves largely unreactive with CPN (and ACE, see 11). Indeed, it is far from clear how much of 2-MGP (and captopril) remains in a form reactive with its target enzyme following iv injection. Although Ala-2-MGP did not increase the duration of action of 2-MGP, it seems clearly possible that other acyl-functions (perhaps not vulnerable to the actions of aminopeptidase enzymes) will be found that have prolonged durations of action.

ACKNOWLEDGEMENTS

This work was supported in part by funds from the U.S. Public Health Service (HL 22986) and from the Council of Tobacco Research.

REFERENCES

1. Ryan, J.W. and Ryan, U.S., Endothelial Surface Enzymes and the Dynamic Processing of Plasma Substrates. Intl. Rev. Exp. Pathol. 26: 1-43 (1984).
2. Huey, R., Bloor, C.M., Kawahara, M.S. and Hugli, T.E., Potentiation of the Anaphylatoxins in vivo Using an Inhibitor of Serum Carboxypeptidase N. I. Lethality and Pathologic Effect on Pulmonary Tissue. Amer. J. Pathol. 112: 48-60 (1983).
3. Ryan, J.W., Berryer, P., Hart, M.A. and Ryan, U.S., Aggregate Anaphylaxis and Carboxypeptidase N. This Meeting. (1984).
4. Plummer, T.H. and Ryan, T.J., A Potent Mercapto Bi-Product Analogue Inhibitor for Human Carboxypeptidase N. Biochem. Biophys. Res. Commun. 98: 448-454 (1981).
5. Chauhan, V.S., Young, G.T. and Bowery, N.G., Structure-Activity Studies in the Bradykinin Series: Synthesis of Analogs Modified in Position. Bioorg. Chem. 8: 333-338 (1979).
6. Sheehan, J.C. and Yang, D.-D.H., Use of N-Formyl Amino Acids in Peptide Synthesis. J. Amer. Chem. Soc. 80: 1154-1158 (1958).

7.   Ryan, J.W., Chung, A. and Ryan, U.S., A Radioassay for Carboxypeptidase N. Adv. Exp. Med. Biol. 156B: 867-874 (1983).

8.   Ryan, J.W., Angiotensin I Converting Enzyme (Kininase II). In: Methods of Enzymatic Analysis, vol. V, Enzymes 3: Peptidases, Proteases and Their Inhibitors, Ed. by Bergmeyer, Verlag Chemie, Weinheim, 20-34 (1984).

9.   Carlin, G., Ryan, J.W. and Saldeen, T., Assays of Components of the Kallikrein-Kinin System Based on First Order Reaction Kinetics. Adv. Exp. Med. Biol. 156B: 797-804 (1983).

10. Soffer, R.L., Angiotensin Converting Enzyme and the Regulation of Vasoactive Peptides. Ann. Rev. Biochem. 45: 73-94 (1976).

11. Plummer, T.H. and Hurwitz, M., Human Plasma Carboxypeptidase N: Isolation and Characterization. J. Biol. Chem. 253: 3907-3912 (1978).

12. Cushman, D.W., Cheung, H.S., Sabo, E.F. and Ondetti, M.A., Design of Potent Competitive Inhibitors of Angiotensin-Converting Enzyme. Carboxyalkanoyl and Mercaptoalkanoyl Amino Acids. Biochemistry 16: 5484-5491 (1977).

13. Ryan, J.W. and Chung, A., A New Class of Inhibitors of Angiotensin Converting Enzyme. Adv. Exp. Med. Biol. 156B: 1133-1139 (1983).

CARBOXYALKYL PEPTIDE INHIBITORS OF KININASE II: CHIRAL SYNTHESIS

Alfred Y.K. Chung and James W. Ryan

Department of Medicine, University of Miami

Miami, FL 33101

SUMMARY

Heretofore, carboxyalkyl peptide inhibitors of kininase II (e.g. N-[1-carboxy-3-phenylpropyl]-Ala-Pro, "enalaprilic acid") have been synthesized by means that yield racemic product. Typically, the secondary amine bond is formed by reacting an amino acid or dipeptide with a 2-keto carboxylic acid ester or imide. The group providing the 2-keto function must be used in excess, and the desired S,S,S isomer must be obtained by resolution procedures. We have developed a procedure whereby enalaprilic acid, RAC-X-64 and related compounds are synthesized stereospecifically and in relatively high yields.

INTRODUCTION

Carboxyalkyl-dipeptides in which the 2-amino group of the dipeptide moiety is alkylated comprise a series of highly potent inhibitors of angiotensin converting enzyme (ACE) and a series of moderately potent inhibitors of "enkephalinase A"[1,2]. The carboxyalkyl-dipeptide inhibitors of ACE not only have high affinities for the target enzyme, they also are capable of entering into slow, tight-binding complexes having apparent Ki values as low as 10^{-11}M (Ryan, J.W. et al, this meeting). Heretofore, however, methods of synthesis of carboxyalkyl-dipeptides have yielded racemized products, and yields have been low. Perhaps the most commonly used method of reductive alkylation has been the procedure in which a 2-keto carboxylic acid is reacted with a dipeptide in the presence of cyanoborohydride. Alternatively, an amino acid can be reacted with an alpha keto-carboxylic acid in amide linkage with a second amino acid, again in the presence of cyanoborohydride or under conditions of hydrogenation[1]. In either case, the moiety bearing the alpha keto function is racemized in the final product. In the case of the carboxyalkyl-dipeptide inhibitors of ACE (e.g. N-[1-carboxy-3-phenylpropyl]-Ala-Pro), the S,S,S form is the desired isomer. Hence, resolution is required after synthesis to obtain the desired isomer. In addition, the known synthetic methods require that the alpha keto-bearing residue be used in excess (5-40 equivalents in respect to the amino-bearing function), and reactions require 1-10 days to approximate completion. Yields are low and scale-up from mg to kg quantities is difficult and expensive.

Recently, Effenberger et al[3] have described a method for the chiral synthesis of carboxyalkyl-amino acids in which an amino acid ester is reacted with the triflate ester (trifluoromethane sulfonate ester) of a 2-hydroxy-carboxylic acid ester. In the present study, we have used a similar approach to prepare carboxyalkyl-dipeptides in their S,S,S isomeric forms.

MATERIALS AND METHODS

D-(-)-lactic acid was from Aldrich Chemical Co., and D-homophenylalanine was from Chemical Dynamics. [^{3}H]Benzoyl-Phe-Gly-Pro, the substrate used for assay of ACE, 25 Ci/mmol, was prepared as described by Chung et al (this meeting).

Thin Layer Chromatography
The thin layer chromatography solvent systems used silica gel plates (Analtech).

Solvent system 1 [$R_f(1)$] = benzene:acetic acid: water, 9:9:1 (by vol).
Solvent system 2 [$R_f(2)$] = 1-butanol:acetic acid:water, 75:13:12.
Solvent system 3 [$R_f(3)$] = 1-butanol:pyridine:acetic acid:water, 15:10:3:12.
Solvent system 4 [$R_f(4)$] = chloroform:methanol:ammonium hydroxide, 12:9:4.
Solvent system 5 [$R_f(5)$] = 1-butanol:ethyl acetate: acetic acid: water, 1:1:1:1.
Solvent system 6 [$R_f(6)$] = ethyl acetate:pyridine:acetic acid:water, 5:5:1:3.
Solvent system 7 [$R_f(7)$] = ethyl acetate:pyridine:acetic acid:water, 200:20:6:11.
Solvent system 8 [$R_f(8)$] = methanol:chloroform, 1:1.

EXPERIMENTAL

D-(+)-Lactic Acid Benzyl Ester   The dry lithium salt of D-(-)-lactic acid, 52 mmol, was mixed with 30 ml of benzyl alcohol. The resulting solution was saturated with hydrogen chloride at 0-5°C for 3.5 h, and then stored at 4°C overnight. Excess hydrogen chloride was removed by rotary evaporation at 35°C. A small amount of ether was added, and the organic phase was washed with water, saturated sodium chloride solution, cold 1 N sodium bicarbonate, and finally with saturated sodium chloride solution. The organic phase was dried over magnesium sulfate and recovered by filtration. D-(+)-lactic acid benzyl ester was recovered by vacuum distillation between 113-123°C at about 1 mm Hg. Yield 4.6 g (49%).

D-(-)-2-Hydroxy-4-Phenylbutanoic Acid   D-Homophenylalanine, 46.3 mmol, ([α]$_D$ = -47° (C = 1; 1 N HCl) was added to 250 ml of water containing 3.86 ml of sulfuric acid. The solution was cooled to 2°C and 69.5 mmole of sodium nitrite was added in small portions over a period of 3 h. The solution was stirred at 2°C for 1 h and then 30 ml of diisopropyl ether was added. Another 14 mmol of sodium nitrite was added, and the solution was stirred at 2°C for 1 h and at room temp overnight. The solution was extracted with ethyl acetate and then with diisopropyl ether. The combined organic phases were washed with water and saturated aqueous sodium chloride solution, dried over magnesium sulfate and then filtered. Solvent was removed from the filtrate in vacuo. The residue was crystallized in diisopropyl ether/light petroleum ether: white crystals, mp 113.5-114.5°C. Elementary analysis for $C_{10}H_{12}O_3$

calc   C 66.65, H 6.71, o 26.64
found   C 66.13, H 6.59

Ethyl-D-(-)-2-Hydroxy-4-Phenyl Butyrate   Thionyl chloride, 35.6 mmol, was
added dropwise at -10°C into 15 ml of dry ethanol. The mixture was stirred
at -10°C for 10 min and then 10 mmol of D-(-)-2-hydroxy-4-phenylbutyric
acid in 4 ml of dry ethanol at -10°C was added dropwise. The resulting
solution was stirred at -10°C for another 10 min, slowly warmed to room
temp and then stirred overnight. Solvent was removed in vacuo, and the
residue was taken up in 50 ml of ether. The organic phase was washed with
cold saturated sodium chloride solution, 1 N sodium bicarbonate, and saturated sodium chloride solution, dried over magnesium sulfate and then
filtered. Solvent was removed from the filtrate under reduced pressure;
yield 2.15 g of yellow oil. NMR (CDCl$_3$): triplet at 1.27δ(3H; CH$_3$ of ethyl
ester); broad band at 2.05 δ (2H; -CH$_2$-); an unsymmetrical triplet at 2.78δ
(2H; -CH$_2$-C$_6$H$_5$); a multiplet at 3.48 δ (1H; -CH(O)); a quartlet at 4.19 δ
(-CH$_2$- of ethyl ester) overlapping with a singlet at 4.36 δ OH; total of
3H); a singlet at 7.2 δ (5H; C$_6$H$_5$-). Optical rotation: [α]$_D^{25}$ = -2.87°
(C = 5, ethanol).

D-1-(1-Carbethoxy)-3-Phenylpropyl Triflate

Trifluoromethanesulfonic anhydride, 9 mmol, in 2 ml of dry dichloromethane was added dropwise over 5 min, with stirring, into a solution of
9.45 mmol of dry pyridine in 27 ml of dichloromethane. Immediately thereafter, 9 mmol of ethyl D-(-)-2-hydroxy-4-phenylbutyrate in 2 ml of dichloromethane was added, all at -22°C. The reaction temperature was raised to
22°C for 10 min. The mixture was filtered, the precipitate was washed with
dichloromethane, and solvent was removed from the combined filtrates by
rotary evaporation at 30°C. The residue was suspended in 5 ml of n-hexane
and poured onto a silica gel plug (1.1 x 6.5 cm). The product was recovered by elution with 25 ml of n-hexane. Evaporation of solvent in vacuo
yielded a light red oil, 1.472 g. Infra-red spectrum (liquid film): carbonyl band at 1760 cm^{-1}.

Nα-Cbo-α-Ethyl-L-Glutamate, Dicyclohexylamine salt   Fifty mmol of Nα-Cbo-
L-glutamic acid was added in portions to a stirred cold solution of 50 mmol
of triethylamine in 30 ml of dry dichloromethane. The resulting mixture
was stirred in an ice bath to obtain a clear solution. Diethyl sulfate,
55 mmol (obtained by vacuum distillation, 72-74°C at about 1 mm Hg) was
added, and the resulting mixture was stirred at room temp for 3 days.
Solvent was removed in vacuo to yield an oily residue. The residue was
taken up in a small volume of ethyl acetate, and washed with dilute cold
sulfuric acid and then with a solution of saturated aqueous sodium chloride.
The organic phase was dried over magnesium sulfate and filtered, and solvent in the filtrate was reduced to a small volume. The dicyclohexylamine
salt was formed by adding 40 mmol of dicyclohexylamine in ethyl acetate.
The mixture was left at room temp overnight, cooled, and the precipitate
obtained was collected by filtration. The precipitate was washed with
ethyl acetate and anhydrous ether, and then dried to yield 9.2 g of white
crystals; mp 154.5 - 156.5°C. The product was recrystallized in water;
yield 6.1 g of white needles; mp 158-159°C.

Nα-Cbo-α-Ethyl-γ-Anilido-L-Glutamate   A suspension of 30 mmol of
Nα-Cbo-α-ethyl-L-glutamate dicyclohexylamine salt in 40 ml of water at
0°C was acidified to pH 2 with a cold, 5% solution of potassium sulfate
and potassium hydrogen sulfate (2:1 by weight). The mixture was extracted
3 times with ethyl acetate, and the combined organic phases were then washed
with cold water and then with saturated sodium chloride sohution and the
solvent removed under reduced pressure to yield 9.5 g of a clear oily residue. To a stirred solution of this oily residue in 15 ml of dichloromethane in a dry ice/ice/ice/acetone bath was added dropwise a solution of
dichloromethane. One min after this addition was completed, 35 mmol of
freshly distilled aniline in 20 ml of dichloromethane was added dropwise.

The reaction mixture was stirred in the dry ice/ice acetone bath for 1 h, then in an ice bath for 2 h and finally at room temp overnight. A precipitate was removed by filtration and was washed with ethyl acetate and ether. The combined organic phases were cooled and then washed with cold dilute hydrochloric acid, saturated sodium chloride solution, 1 N sodium bicarbonate and saturated sodium chloride solution. The organic phase was dried over anhydrous sodium sulfate and filtered, and solvent was removed from the filtrate to yield a gel-like residue. The residue was crystallized from isopropanol and isopropyl ether. The white gel-like crystals obtained were broken up in isopropyl ether, recovered by filtration and washed with isopropyl ether to yield 9.85 g of white powder, mp 96–98°C. Thin layer chromatography: $R_f(1) = 0.74$; $R_f(2) = 0.75$; $R_f(5) = 0.835$; $R_f(7) = 0.87$. Infra-red (CHCl$_3$) spectrum: carbonyl bands from 1660–1750 cm (strong, broad); no absorption between 2300–2500 cm ; NH band of urethane at 3432 cm^{-1} (moderately strong, sharp); aromatic at 1605 cm^{-1}. Optical rotation: $[\alpha]^{25}_D = 13.8°$ (C = 3, methanol).

α-Ethyl-γ-Anilido-L-Glutamate   2.2 g of Nα-Cbo-α-ethyl-γ-anilido-L-glutamate was submitted to hydrogenolysis using 0.75 g of 10% palladium on carbon, 30 ml of tetrahydrofuran and ethyl acetate (1:1 by volume) and hydrogen gas at 25 psi for 2.5 h to give the corresponding deprotected compound. Thin layer chromatography: $R_f(1) = 0.58$; $R_f(2) = 0.45$; $R_f(7) = 0.20$; $R_f(8) = 0.65$.

RESULTS

   Preparation of N-(L-1-Carbethoxy-3-Phenylpropyl)-L-Alanyl-L-Proline
D-1-(1-carbethoxy)-3-phenylpropyl triflate (1.9 mmol) in 6 ml of dry dichloromethane was added at room temp, dropwise over 15 min, to a solution of 3.8 mmol of L-alanyl-L-proline t-butyl ester in 6 ml of dichloromethane. The solution was stirred at room temp for 2.5 h. Solvent was removed in vacuo at 30°C to yield an oily residue. The residue was dissolved in 40 ml of ethyl acetate/ether (2:1 by volume) and was washed with water and saturated sodium chloride solution. The organic phase was dried over magnesium sulfate and filtered. Solvent was removed to yield 0.96 g of a yellow oil. The residue was applied to an LH-20 column (2.5 x 96.5 cm) developed with ethanol. Fractions of 7.45 ml were collected. Fractions 26–28 were pooled, solvent was removed in vacuo to yield 0.297 g of an oily residue. The crude material was deprotected with anhydrous trifluoroacetic acid and solvent was removed in vacuo. The residue was dissolved in 10 ml of water and then recovered by lyophilization. The dried solid dissolved in concentrated ammonium hydroxide was applied to a column (2.2 x 36.5 cm) of Amberlite XAD-2 resin developed with 0.1 M aqueous amonium hydroxide containing 5% acetonitrile. Fractions of 8.55 ml were collected. Fractions 10–13 were pooled, and solvent was removed to yield 124 mg. The Amberlite column was then eluted with 95% ethanol. Fraction 53 contained 36 mg of the desired product. The crude product of fractions 10–13 was further purified by LH-20 chromatography (2.5 x 96.5 cm column) developed with 95% ethanol, 6.0 ml fractions. Fractions 35–37 were pooled.

N-(1-Carbethoxy-3-Carboxanilidopropyl)-L-Alanine
Nα-Cbo-α-ethyl-γ-L-glutamyl anilide, 12.5 mmol, was deprotected by hydrogenolysis using 1 g of 10% palladium on carbon in 40 ml of tetrahydrofuran/ethyl acetate (1:1 by volume) at 20 psi at room temp for 2 h. The catalyst was removed by filtration, and solvent was removed in vacuo to yield a clear oily residue. Crystals formed at room temp overnight.

   D-1-benzyloxycarbonylethyl triflate (6.3 mmol) in 26 ml of dichloromethane was added dropwise over a period of 30 min at room temp to a vigorously stirred solution of the above-prepared deprotected product in 26 ml

of dichloromethane. Thirty min later, a solution (4.1 mmol) of triethylamine in 5 ml of dichloromethane was added dropwise over 5 min. The mixture
was then stirred for 30 min, following which solvent was removed in vacuo
at 25°C. A 50 ml mixture of ethyl acetate/ether (1:1 by volume) was added
to the residue and was washed with water and then saturated sodium chloride
solution. The organic phase was dried over anhydrous sodium sulfate and
filtered, and solvent was removed under reduced pressure to yield 3.65 g
of a yellow oily residue. Hydrogenolysis of this oily residue was carried
out using 1 g of 10% palladium on carbon in 30 ml of ethanol at 20 psi at
room temp for 2.5 h. The catalyst was removed by filtration and was washed
with ethanol. The volume of the combined filtrates was reduced in vacuo
to about 7 ml, and 10 ml of ether were then added. White crystals formed
at room temp and were collected by filtration. The crystals were washed
with ethanol/ether (1:1 by volume) and dried in a vacuum desiccator over
phosphorus pentoxide to yield 0.9 g of product; mp 137-137.5°C. Another
0.365 g was obtained from the mother liquor by LH-20 column chromatography;
column developed with ethanol.

Optical rotation: $[\alpha]_D^{25}$ = 12.6° (C = 1; ethanol)
Elementary analysis for $C_{16}H_{22}N_2O_5$

calc   C = 59.61;   H = 6.88;   N = 8.69
found   C = 58.11;   H = 6.71;   N = 8.41

Thin layer chromatography: $R_f(1)$ = 0.27; $R_f(2)$ = 0.39;
$R_f(5)$ = 0.62; $R_f(7)$ = 0.23
NMR $(CD_3)_2SO$ and (CD_3COCD_3): A triplet at 1.25 δ (CH_3 of ethyl ester)
overlapping with a doublet at 1.29 δ (CH_3 of Ala) (total of 6H); a multiplet overlapping with acetone at 2.05 δ (CH_2 of Glu); a triplet at 2.55 δ
(2H, δ -CH_2 of Glu); two sets of multiplets of 3.31 δ (CH of Glu) and
3.39 δ (CH of Ala) (total of 2H); a quartlet at 4.10 δ (2H, CH_2 of ethyl
ester); a broad singlet at 4.57 δ (2H, NH): a multiplet at 7.04 δ (1H);
and apparent triplet at 7.27 δ (2H) and an apparent doublet at 7.68 δ
(2H) (aromatic); a broad singlet at 9.51 δ (1H, COOH). Infra-red spectrum (KBr): Zwitterion at 1597 cm^{-1} (strong, broad); carbonyl of anilide
at 1670 cm^{-1} (strong, sharp) and carbonyl of ester bond at 1742 cm^{-1}
(strong, sharp).

N-(L-1-Carbethoxy-3-Carboxanilidopropyl)-L- Alanyl-L-Proline (RAC-X-64)

Diphenylphosphoryl azide (2.685 mmol) in 3 ml of dry dimethylformamide
was added slowly to a solution of 2.49 mmol of Nα-(L-1-carbethoxy-3-car-
boxanilidopropyl)-L-alanine and 2.73 mmol of L-proline benzyl ester hydrochloride salt in 7.0 ml of dimethylformamide, with stirring at 0°C. The
mixture was stirred at 0°C for 5 minutes and then 5.15 mmol of triethylamine in 5 ml dimethylformamide was added dropwise over 15 minutes. The
mixture was then stirred at 0°C for 3 h, then slowly warmed to room temp
and stirred overnight. The solution was concentrated to a small volume
in vacuo at 40°C and then diluted with 8 ml of ethyl acetate. The organic
phase was washed successively with half-saturated aqueous solution of
sodium bicarbonate, and then with saturated aqueous sodium chloride solution. The organic phase was dried over anhydrous sodium sulfate and
filtered, and solvent was removed in vacuo to yield 1.55 g of oily residue (solidified on standing at room temp for 1 h). Addition of absolute
ethanol and ethyl acetate caused the formation of salt crystals, which
were removed by filtration. The filtrate was submitted to hydrogenolysis
with 300 mg of 10% palladium on carbon in ethanol at 20 psi at room temp
for 2 h. Catalyst was removed by filtration and solvent was removed from
the filtrate in vacuo. The residue was chromatographed on silica gel
(2.6 x 48 cm column) developed with n-butanol/acetic acid/water (75:13:
12 by volume). Fractions of 6.25 ml were collected. Fractions 68-85
were pooled. Solvent was removed with a rotatory evaporator. The residue

was diluted with water and then recovered by lyophilization resulting in 0.409 gm of white powder. The material was further purified using an LH-20 column (215 x 96.5 cm) developed with ethanol. Fractions of 6.0 ml were collected and fractions 35-38 were pooled. Thin layer chromatography: $R_f(1) = 0.52$; $R_f(2) = 0.38$; $R_f(3) = 0.69$; $R_f(5) = 0.58$; $R_f(6) = 0.745$.

Optical notation: $[\alpha]_D^{25} = 57.25°$ (C = 1; ethanol).

Intravenous ED_{50} of RAC-X-64 before and after saponification

RAC-X-64, or its dicarboxylic acid analog obtained by saponification, was administered i.v. to an anesthetized Sprague-Dawley rat in increasing doses (n=3). Starting at 25 min before the first drug dose, the rat was injected i.v. with angiotensin I, 120 ng/kg, and the same dose of angiotensin I was injected every 10 min thereafter for 220 min. 5 min after the second injection of angiotensin I, prodrug or drug was injected in a dose of 30 nmol/kg. Ten min later, another 30 nmol/kg was injected and was followed 20 min after the first dose by injection of 60 nmol/kg and 30 min after the first dose by injection of 120 nmol/kg. Thus, cumulative drug or prodrug dosing was 30, 60, 120 and 240 nmol/kg. Drug effects were measured in terms of mean arterial blood pressure responses to challenge with i.v. angiotensin I and were expressed as % of the control response. The ACE inhibitory effects were long-lasting (t 1/2 > 150 min). ED_{50} values were computed from linear regression equations for % control response v. log inhibitor dose. The following Table also shows effects of Captopril.

Compound	ED_{50}	t 1/2*
RAC-X-64	96 nmol/kg	> 210 min
RAC-X-64	9.5	165
Captopril	105	16

*time required for half-recovery from maximum drug effects.

Inhibitor Potencies In Vitro
N-[1(S)-carbethoxy-3-phenylpropyl]-L-Ala-L-Pro (MK 421) and N-[1(S)-carbethoxy-3-carboxanilidopropyl]-L-Ala-L-Pro (RAC-X-64) were treated for effects on human serum ACE activity. Also shown are results obtained after saponification (1 mg of compound in 100 µl of M KOH in ethanol at 37°C for 30 min) of the corresponding prodrug. I_{50} values (concentration of inhibitor required to reduce ACE activity by half) are shown below:

Compound	I_{50}
N-[1-carbethoxy-3-phenylpropyl]-Ala-Pro*	125.0 nM
N-[1-carboxy-3-phenylpropyl]-Ala-Pro	0.83
N-[1-carbethoxy-3-carboxanilidopropyl]-Ala-Pro	34.1
N-[1-carboxy-3-carboxanilidopropyl]-Ala-Pro	0.45

*MK 421; **RAC-X-64.

DISCUSSION

Formation of the secondary amine bond of carboxyalkyl-dipeptides by reacting an alpha-amino function with the triflate ester of an alpha-hydroxy function provides a major advance over previous methods of reductive alkylation. The reaction is relatively rapid and is efficient under mild conditions. When the chiral center provided by the alpha-hydroxy-bearing function is in the R-form, the center is inverted to the S-form in the final product. Conversely, the S-form of the alpha-hydroxy-bearing function yields an R-form in the final product. Of the known highly potent carboxyalkyl-dipeptide inhibitors of ACE, each has no fewer than 3 centers of asymmetry, and, as discussed above, methods of reductive alkylation used heretofore have guaranteed racemization (of unpredictable degree) at one of the 3 chiral centers: For example, the (R,S,),S,S isomer is obtained when 2-keto-4-phenylbutanoate is reacted with S-Ala-S-Pro, and the S,(R,S), S isomer is obtained when (S)-homophenylalanine is reacted with pyruvoyl-S-proline (cf Patchett et al, 1980). Thus, the synthetic procedures described in this paper not only improve yields at reduced elapsed times, the new procedures eliminate the need for resolution steps to obtain the desired S,S,S-isomer. In addition, the starting materials and intermediates required by our synthetic approaches are either available commercially or are readily prepared. Reaction conditions are not limiting in terms of scale of synthesis, hence conversion from mg scale to kg scale poses no unfamiliar problems. Typically, large scale synthesis favors purification by crystallization. Whether such will be true for carboxyalkyl-dipeptides remains to be seen.

ACKNOWLEDGEMENTS

This work was supported by a grant from the Council of Tobacco Research.

REFERENCES

1. Patchett, A.A. and 26 co-authors. A new class of angiotensin converting enzyme inhibitors. Nature, 288:280-283 (1980).
2. Mumford, R.A., Zimmerman, M., Broeke, J., Taub, D., Joshua, H., Rothrock, J.W., Hirshfield, J.M., Springer, J.P. and Patchett, A.A., Inhibition of porcine kidney "enkephalinase" by substituted-n-carboxymethyl dipeptides. Biochem. Biophy. Res. Commun., 109:1303-1309 (1982).
3. Effenberger, F., Burkhard, U. and Willfahrt, J., Angew. Chem., 95:50 (1983).
4. Ryan, J.W., Angiotensin I converting enzyme (kininase II) peptidyl-dipeptide hydrolase EC 3.4.15.1. In Methods of Enzymatic Analysis, (ed. H.U. Bergmeyer), Verlag Chemie GmbH, Weinheim, Germany, Vol. 5, pp. 20-34 (1984).

SLOW TIGHT BINDING INHIBITORS OF ANGIOTENSIN CONVERTING ENZYME

James W. Ryan, Alfred Y. K. Chung, Pierre Berryer
Marjoire A. Murray and James P.A. Ryan

Department of Medicine, University of Miami, Miami, FL 33101

SUMMARY

We have found that apparent Ki values of some, but not all, carboxyalkyl-dipeptide inhibitors of angiotensin converting enzyme decrease as a function of incubation time. The most potent of the ACE inhibitors tested so far is RAC-X-65 (N-[1(S)-carboxy-3-carboxanilidiopropyl]-L-Ala-L-Pro). When RAC-X-65 is not preincubated with human serum ACE (2.4×10^{-11} M), the apparent Ki value is 4.4×10^{-10} M. Preincubation of RAC-X-65 with ACE for 15 min before addition of substrate yields an apparent Ki of 4.1×10^{-11} M. a 90 min preincubation of the inhibitor with ACE yields an apparent Ki of 1.2×10^{-11} M, i.e., the reaction of the inhibitor with enzyme is virtually stoichiometric. The enzyme:inhibitor complex is poorly separated by molecular sieve chromatography or by dilution. That such tightly bound complexes are formed _in vivo_ is suggested by the following results: The intravenous ED_{50} (anesthetized rats) of RAC-X-65 is 9.43 nmol/kg, and the time for half recovery (t ½) of responsiveness to i.v. angiotensin I, 120 ng/kg, following a cumulative dose of 240 nmol/kg of the inhibitor is 165 min. For comparison, the i.v. ED_{50} of captopril is 105 nmol/kg, and its t ½ following a cumulative dose of 240 nmol/kg is 16 min. Implied is the possibility that slow tight binding inhibitors of ACE may be used in a 1 pill per day regimen for the treatment of hypertension.

INTRODUCTION

While screening a series of carboxyalkyl-dipeptide inhibitors of angiotensin converting enzyme (ACE), we noted that apparent Ki values of some such inhibitors decrease as a function of time of incubation of inhibitor with enzyme. Thus, when MK 422 (N-[1(S)-carboxy-3-phenylpropyl]-L-Ala-L-Pro) is not preincubated with enzyme (2.4×10^{-11} M) before adding substrate, its apparent Ki value is 8.1×10^{-10} M. However, if MK 422 is preincubated with enzyme for 15 min before starting the reaction by adding substrate, the apparent Ki falls to 1.7×10^{-10} M. Even more striking results are obtained with RAC-X-65 (N-[1(S)-carboxy-3-carboxanilidopropyl]-L-Ala-L-Pro). The apparent Ki falls from 4.4×10^{-10} M (no preincubation) to 1.2×10^{-11} M when the inhibitor is preincubated with enzyme for 90 min. The text that follows describes an analysis of slow tight binding of RAC-X-65 with ACE.

MATERIALS AND METHODS

RAC-X-65 and MK 422 were synthesized as described by Chung et al (this meeting). In vitro assays of inhibitor potencies used pooled human serum (Seralc). The undiluted serum contained ACE at a concentration of 6.72 x 10^{-9} M. Assays were performed using [^{3}H]benzoyl-Phe-Gly-Pro as substrate as described by Chung et al (this meeting; see also 1). The buffer used throughout was 0.05 M Hepes, pH 8.0, containing 0.1 M NaCl, 0.6 M Na_2SO_4 and chlorhexidine gluconate, 0.01% by vol. In vivo assays of inhibitor potencies were performed using Sprague-Dawley rats anesthetized with pento-barbital, 50 mg/kg i.p. Each rat was treated with heaprin, 500 u/kg, and cannulas were placed in the superior vena cava and the right femoral artery. Arterial blood pressure and mean arterial blood pressure were recorded continuously. The blood pressure response to i.v. angiotensin I, 120 ng/kg, was measured, and the rats were challenged every 10 min thereafter for up to 300 min with the same i.v. dose of angiotensin I. Drugs were given in the cumulative dose schedule indicated in Fig. 2.

RESULTS

MK 422 and RAC-X-65 were prepared from their respective l-carbethoxy forms (MK 421 and RAC-X-64) by saponification in 1 M KOH in ethanol at 37°C for 30 min. Structures of MK 422 and RAC-X-65 are shown in Fig. 1. Each monoethyl ester analog was synthesized chirally (see Chung et al, this meeting) to yield the desired S, S, S isomer.

Effects of Time of Incubation on Degree of Inhibition

Table 1 shows that the potency of inhibition of ACE by RAC-X-65 increased as a function of time of incubation. In the absence of inhibitor, fractional substrate utilization, $\ln[S/(S-P)]$ ([^{3}H]benzoyl-Phe-Gly-Pro used as substrate), increased linearly with time (control V/Km = 0.0091 min^{-1} for [E]=2.4 x 10^{-11} M, r = 0.9996 for n = 12). However, apparent (V/Km) fell progressively as incubation time increased when RAC-X-65, 1.087 x 10^{-10} M, was incubated with ACE, 2.4 x 10^{-11} M. Values of apparent (V/Km) shown in Table 1 are cumulative for the time periods indicated, thus it appeared that after 30 min of incubation, apparent (V/Km) was about 46% of control. However, the appearance is deceptive in that inhibition is progressive with time, e.g. the apparent (V/Km) for the last 3 min of incubation with substrate was 0.00097 min^{-1} (about 10.7% of the control) and asymptotically approached zero.

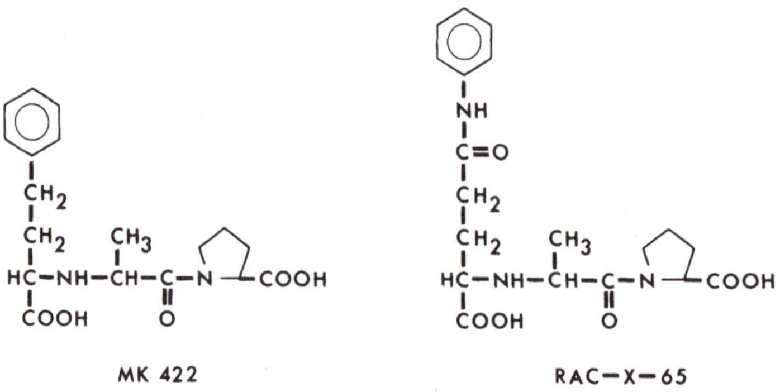

Fig. 1. Structures of MK 422 and RAC-X-65.

Table 1. Effects of Incubation Time on Degree of Inhibition

Incubation Time (min)	ln[S/(S-P)]	Apparent (V/Km)(min^{-1} x 10^{-3})
3	0.02053	6.843
6	0.04144	6.907
9	0.04973	5.526
12	0.06169	5.141
15	0.08320	5.547
18	0.09100	5.056
21	0.10430	4.967
24	0.11167	4.653
27	0.12299	4.555
30	0.12590	4.197

RAC-X-65 (or buffer) and buffered human serum were mixed as quickly as possible (approximately 15 sec) with buffered substrate, [3H]benzoyl-Phe-Gly-Pro, and the reaction mixture was incubated at 37°C. Samples (200 μl) were collected at the indicated time intervals and were worked up to measure fractional substrate utilization (ln[S/(S-P)]) and to comptue rates of fractional substrate utilization [apparent (V/Km)] as described elsewhere (Chung et al, this meeting). Final concentrations of reactants in the reaction mixture: ACE, 2.4 x 10^{-11} M; substrate 4 x 10^{-8} M; RAC-X-65, 0 (results not shown) or 1.087 x 10^{-10} M.

Effects of Dilution of Enzyme:Inhibitor Mixtures on REcovery of Enzyme Activity

As implied by results in Table 1, after binding of inhibitor with enzyme, there follows the formation of a tightly bound enzyme:inhibitor complex. It seemed possible that RAC-X-65 might act initially as a reversible inhibitor and then as an irreversible inhibitor. REsults shown in TAble 2 indicate that dilution of the enzyme:inhibitor complex formed during a 10 min preincubation of relatively large concentrations of ACE and RAC-X-65 sufficed to restore enzyme activity. As indicated in the Table, the time required after dilution for enzyme activity to become manifest was apparently an inverse function of concentration of inhibitor. Thus, when [E] was 2.4 x 10^{-11} M and [I] was 4.22 x 10^{-12} M, apparent (V/Km) increased from 0.00424 min^{-1} to 0.00702 min^{-1} within 9 min. When [I] was 2.09 x 10^{-11} M, apparent (V/Km) rose progressively over a period of at least 60 min but still did not approximate that of the control reaction mixture (V/Km = 0.0091 min^{-1}).

Apparent Ki Values Vary as a Function of Incubation Time

To assess effects of time of incubation on apparent Ki values, we preincubated varying concentrations of RAC-X-65 or MK 422 with a constant concentration of human serum ACE and then added one volume (100 μl) of buffered substrate [3H]benzoyl-Phe-Gly-Pro (4 x 10^{-8} M) to each reaction vial for an additional 10 min incubation, all at 37°C. Results are shown in Table 3. ACE was in a final concentration of 2.8 x 10^{-11} M. Apparent Ki values were obtained graphically by plotting $[I]/[1-(v_i/v_c)]$ versus v_c/v_i for $[I]/[1-(v_i/v_c)]=Ki(V_c/V_i) + [E]$, where [I] is total inhibitor concentration, [E] is enzyme concentration, v_c is velocity of the control reaction and v_i is velocity of the reaction in the presence of inhibitor.

Table 2. Effects of Dilution of the Enzyme:Inhibitor Complex on Recovery of Enzyme Activity

Incubation Time (min	Apparent (V/Km) $(min^{-1} \times 10^3)$ for inhibitor concentrations [I]		
	[I]		
	0	4.22×10^{-12} M	2.09×10^{-11} M
3	8.440	4.237	0.0
6	9.183	5.567	1.250
9	9.062	7.020	2.074
12	10.373	6.578	1.937
15	9.275	7.237	2.097
18	9.197	6.583	2.520
21	9.324	6.902	2.625
24	9.505	6.779	2.859
27	9.153	6.893	3.266
30	9.459	6.937	3.557
40	9.112	7.632	3.799
60	9.268	7.220	4.454

RAC-X-65, at 0.0, 2.11 nM or 0.422 nM was preincubated with human serum ACE, 2.42×10^{-9} M in the assay buffer at 37°C for 10 min. Reaction mixtures were then diluted 1:101 in buffered substrate, [3H]benzoyl-Phe-Gly-Pro, 4×10^{-8} M. At the time intervals indicated above, 200 µl samples were worked up to measure fractional substrate utilization (apparent (V/Km)). Inhibitor concentrations indicated in the Table are final concentrations after dilution in buffered substrate. The final concentration of ACE was 2.4×10^{-11} M.

Estimates of Apparent Ki are Functions of Enzyme Concentration

The close approach to stoichiometric binding of RAC-X-65 to ACE shown in Table 3 suggested that apparent Ki varies as a function of enzyme concentration. Table 4 shows that this is true whether or not inhibitor and enzyme are preincubated together before addition of substrate.

Table 3. Apparent Ki Declines as Time of Preincubation of Inhibitor With ACE is Increased

Preincubation Time (min)	Apparent Ki (pM)	
	RAC-X-65	MK 422
0	437.3	838
15	41.4	174
30	25.3	114
60	17.0	97
90	14.2	89

Table 4. Effects of Enzyme Concentration on Apparent Ki

Without preincubation

[E]	Apparent Ki (pM)	[I]/[E]
2.46×10^{-11} M	190.6	7.75
1.72×10^{-10} M	544.6	3.17

With a 10 min preincubation

[E]	Apparent Ki (pM)	[I]/[E]
2.46×10^{-11} M	90.0	3.66
1.72×10^{-10} M	148.4	0.86

Interestingly, the molar ratio of inhibitor (for [I] = Ki) to enzyme ([I]/[E]) is lower for the higher concentration of enzyme, possibly because of higher concentrations of reactants in the second step of binding of inhibitor to enzyme that precedes isomerization of the enzyme inhibitor complex.

Thus, under the conditions of our experiments, the binding of RAC-X-65 by ACE after 90 min of preincubation is virtually stoichiometric. Also evident, however, is that true Ki cannot be measured by the methods employed here, hence our use of the term apparent Ki. Note that MK 422 also acts as a slow tight binding inhibitor.

As noted elsewhere,[1] for competitive inhibitors of moderate potency, one can measure Ki values directly under conditions of first order enzyme kinetics. The Michaelis-Menten equation can be simplified and inverted to yield an equation of a straight line, apparent (Km/V) = [I](Km/VKi) + (Km/V), such that a plot of apparent (Km/V) versus [I] gives a straight line having true Km/V as its y-intercept and -Ki as its x-intercept. The Ki of captopril is readily assessed by this procedure (Ki = 1×10^{-9} M). If several concentrations of RAC-X-65 are incubated with ACE and substrate for shrot intervals (e.g. 3 - 5 min), the results plotted as noted above approximate a straight line (apparent Ki = 4.4×10^{-10} M). However, a 10 min preincubation of RAC-X-65 with ACE before addition of substrate yields a curve concave upward. As [I] is decreased, apparent (Km/V) approaches true Km/V asymptotically, and there is no x-intercept.

Are Slow Tight Binding Enzyme:Inhibitor Complexes Formed in Vivo?

As suggested by their relative apparent Ki values (measured without preincubation of inhibitor with enzyme), RAC-X-65 is somewhat more than twice as potent as captopril. Under the same conditions, MK 422 has an apparent Ki approximately 20% lower than that of captopril. However, and as noted above, the apparent Ki of RAC-X-65 preincubated with ACE can fall to values on the order of 1×10^{-11} M. Thus, it seemed possible that RAC-X-65 could be as much as 100 times as potent as captopril in _vivo_ if it enters into a tightly bound complex sith ACE.

To examine for the latter possibility, we performed intravenous ED_{50} studies using anesthetized rats as described in Materials and Methods. We compared effects of cumulative doses of RAC-X-65, RAC-X-64 (the l-carbethoxy analog of RAC-X-65), and captopril and effects of a single, relatively large dose of captopril. Results are shown in Fig. 2. The cumulative dose i.v. ED_{50} of RAC-X-65 was 9.3 nmol/kg, and time for half-recovery (t $\frac{1}{2}$) of responsiveness to angiotensin I, 120 ng/kg, was 165 min. Captopril given in cumulative doses had an ED_{50} of 109 nmol/kg and a t $\frac{1}{2}$ of 16 min (data not shown). Thus, RAC-X-65 is at least 10-times more potent than captopril in vivo. These results are consistent with the concept that RAC-X-65 and ACE enter into a tightly bound complex in vivo. Given that captopril administered in three doses per day is a highly effective antihypertensive agent, it seems likely that RAC-X-65 should be no less effective when administered once per day. The onset of action of the prodrug RAC-X-64 is relatively slow, and its i.v. ED_{50} is 98 nmol/kg. However, given in the same cumulative doses as used for RAC-X-65, the $\frac{1}{2}$ for the monoethyl ester was greater than 215 min.

DISCUSSION

The phenomenon of slow tight binding of some inhibitors to their target enzymes is now widely recognized (cf 2, 3). The slow tight binding of methotrexate to dihydrofolate reductase and that of pepstatin to pepsin are perhaps among the better characterized. In terms of kinetics, a minimum of two steps must be postulated: 1) binding of inhibitor to enzyme, and 2) progression of the initial enzyme:inhibitor complex into a more stable, poorly dissociable conformer. Within the limits of our analysis, it appears that the binding of RAC-X-65 (and that of MK 422) to ACE is understandable in terms of the relatively slow formation of a tightly bound enzyme:inhibitor complex.

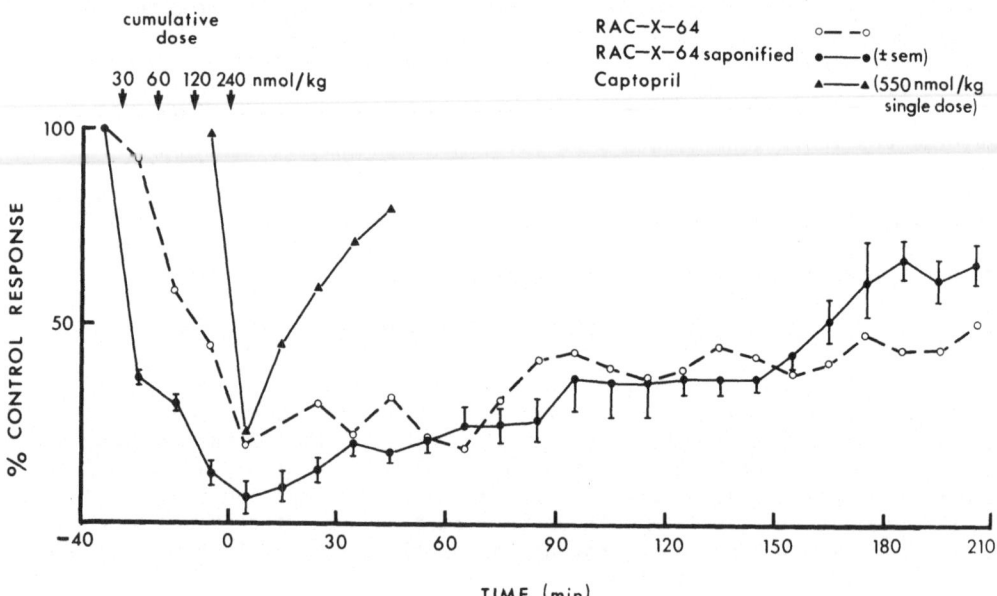

Fig. 2. Intravenous ED_{50} studies. See text for details. RAC-X-65 was prepared by saponification of RAC-X-64. Effects were measured in terms of inhibition of blood pressure response to i.v. angiotensin I, 120 ng/kg.

424

A priori, it is reasonable to believe that formation of such tightly bound complexes is dependent in part on pH, ions, ionic strength, temperature and possibly other factors readily manipulated in in vitro experiments. Relationships of incubation conditions used in in vitro experiments to those that obtain in vivo are generally unclear. Thus results of such in vitro experiments may or may not give insights into the likelihood of the formation of tightly bound enzyme:inhibitor complexes in vivo. The question of whether tightly bound complexes of inhibitor and ACE can be formed in vivo is made more complicated by the knowledge that a major portion of ACE is in solid phase, disposed on surfaces of cells continuously washed by plasma containing the inhibitor.[4] Thus, it is not inconceivable that hemodynamic factors would favor dissociation of the initial enzyme:inhibitor complex and thus prevent or minimize the secondary formation of the tightly bound complex. However, such evidence as is available at present supports the concept that at least part of intravenously administered RAC-X-65 is taken up into tightly bound complexes with ACE: The cumulative i.v. ED_{50} of RAC-X-65 is less than 1/10th of that of captopril (Ki 1×10^{-9} M), and the time for half recovery of responsiveness of the test animal to i.v. angiotensin I is at least 10-times greater for RAC-X-65 than for captopril. As indicated above, the rapidity with which tightly bound complexes are formed in vitro is in part a function of concentrations of reactants. Hence, the relatively large concentrations of RAC-X-65 achieved in plasma within the first 15 sec of injection, reacting with the relatively large concentrations of ACE disposed on blood vessel surfaces (e.g. see 5), may promote formation of tightly bound complexes within seconds or fractions of a second rather than in minutes. Under the latter conditions, hemodynamic factors may have few if any effects on the formation of tightly bound inhibitor:ACE complexes. It is conceivable, however, that hemodynamic factors, if they influence enzyme:inhibitor complexes at all, may accelerate dissociation of the tightly bound complexes as plasma concentrations of inhibitor decline to levels far below enzyme concentrations.

ACKNOWLEDGEMENTS

This work was supported in part by grants from the U.S. Public Health Service (HL 22896) and from the Council of Tobacco Research, 814D.

REFERENCES

1. J. W. Ryan, Angiotensin I converting enzyme (kininase II) peptidyl-dipeptide hydrolase EC 3.4.15.1, in: "Methods of Enzymatic Analysis," H. U. Bergmeyer, ed., Verlag Chemie GmbH, Weinheim, Germany, Vol. 5 (1984).
2. J. W. Williams, J. F. Morrison, and R. G. Dugleby, Methotrexate a high-affinity pseudosubstrate of dihydrofolate reductase, Biochemistry, 18:2567-2573 (1979).
3. D. H. Rich and E. T. O. Sun, Mechanism of inhibition of pepsin by pepstatin, Biochem. Pharmacol., 29:2205-2212 (1980).
4. J. W. Ryan and U. S. Ryan, Pulmonary endothelial cells, Fed. Proc., 36:2683-2691 (1977).
5. J. W. Ryan and U. S. Ryan, Endothelial surface enzymes and the dynamic processing of plasma substrates, Int. Rev. Pathol., 26:1-43 (1984).

RADIOLABELLED SUBSTRATES FOR ANGIOTENSIN CONVERTING ENZYME

Alfred Y.K. Chung, James W. Ryan, James P.A. Ryan
and Una S. Ryan

Department of Medicine, University of Miami
Miami, FL 33101

SUMMARY

Six [^{3}H]benzoyl-tripeptides were prepared and tested as substrates for angiotensin converting enzyme. Each was prepared first as its [4-iodo]-benzoyl-analog, and an atom of ^{3}H per molecule was introduced by catalytic dehalogenation in ^{3}H$_2$-gas. Kinetic parameters were measured at 37°C using as buffer 0.05 M Hepes, pH 8.0, containing 0.1 M NaCl and 0.6 M Na$_2$SO$_4$. When the substrates were used at concentrations far below their respective Km values, fractional rates of substrate utilization per unit time for constant enzyme concentration were direct functions of respective second order rate constants (Kc/Km). Although absolute values of Kc/Km differed for human enzyme as opposed to rabbit enzyme, relative values of Kc/Km were virtually identical. Similarly, relative rates of substrate utilization during passage through lungs of anesthetized rats were similar to relative values of Kc/Km measured in vitro. Thus, there is now a range of ACE substrates usable, in vitro and in vivo, under conditions of first order enzyme kinetics, conditions under which values of V/Km and Ki can be measured directly.

INTRODUCTION

Angiotensin converting enzyme (ACE) is known to be reactive with a wide range of acyl-tripeptides[1-3]. No fewer that eight such compounds are in use for the assay of ACE for both research and clinical purposes. However, no single ACE substrate now known suffices for every assay purpose. Further, there are certain assay needs not adequately met by any of the known ACE substrates. For example, those substrates adequate for measuring the abundant ACE of human serum are too unreactive for measuring the small amounts of ACE that occur in association with vascular endothelial cells in culture. Similarly, those substrates useful for monitoring ACE activities of cell cultures, e.g. benzoyl-Phe-Ala-Pro, tend to be far too reactive for measuring pulmonary ACE concentrations in vivo[4,5]. The two substrates in commonest use for measuring serum ACE, hippuryl-Gly-Gly and hippuryl-His-Leu, are not sufficiently reactive for measuring pulmonary ACE in vivo.

In the present study, we set out to design and prepare substrates less reactive with ACE than benzoyl-Phe-Ala-Pro but more reactive than hippuryl-Gly-Gly and hippuryl-His-Leu. Further, to overcome the disadvantages of

chromophoric and fluorophoric assays in terms of use under conditions of
first order enzyme kinetics and in terms of uses in in vivo assays, we designed each of the new substrates to bear one atom of ^{3}H per molecule of
substrate[4,6,7]. For each substrate, ^{3}H was introduced into the acyl-moiety
such that the radioactive product formed would have precisely the same
specific radioactivity as that of the substrate. Because each substrate
was obtained at high specific radioactivity (~25 Ci/mmol), each could be
used at concentrations far below Km. Advantages of the use of substrate
at S<<Km have been described[8,9], and many of these advantages are apparent
from results shown below.

MATERIALS AND METHODS

[3H]Hippuryl-Gly-Gly, [3H]hippuryl-His-Leu, [3H]benzoyl-Phe-His-Leu,
and [3H]benzoyl-Phe-Ala-Pro, each at approx 25 Ci/mmol, were either synthesized here or were obtained from Ventrex Laboratories, Inc. Portland,
Maine. The two new substrates were prepared as follows:
[4-iodo]Benzoyl-Phe-Gly-Pro Z-Glycine, 20 mmol in dimethylformamide at
-5°C, was reacted with 20 mmol of dicyclohexylcarbodiimide in dichloromethane and then 21 mmol of proline-t-butyl ester in dichloromethane was
added to the reaction mixture. The reaction proceeded at 0°C for 1 h and
at room temp for 4 h. After work-up, the crude product was hydrogenated
(1g of 10% Pd on C, 25 psi for 3 h). Gly-Pro-t-butyl ester was converted
to its HCl salt and was crystallized in methanol/tetrahydrofuran/benzene/
ether: 1.65 g white crystals, mp 161.5-162°C. HCl.Gly-Pro-t-butyl ester,
1 mmol, was reacted with 1 mmol of [4-iodo]benzoyl-phenylalanine-2,4,5-
trichlorophenol ester in a mixture of dimethylformamide, and 6 ml of tetrahydrofuran containing 1 mmol of N-methyl morpholine at room temp for
24 h. Work-up yielded white crystals, 0.485 g, mp 184-185°C. Recrystallization in methanol/ethyl acetate: 0.47 g of white crystals, mp 185-185.5°C;
amino acid analysis: Phe 1.00, Gly 0.99, Pro 1.025. The t-butyl ester
was removed with anhydrous trifluoroacetic acid (1 h, room temp).
[4-iodo]Benzoyl-Ala-Gly-Pro [4-iodo]Benzoyl chloride, 6.84 mmol in dioxane and 6.84 mmol of Na_2CO_3 in water were added dropwise to 6.84 mmol of
Ala-Gly in a mixture of water and dioxane, all at 0°C. The reaction proceeded at 0°C for 30 min and at room temp overnight. Solvent was removed
in vacuo, and the residue was dissolved in a small vol of water. After
extraction with ether, the aqueous phase was cooled to 0°C and adjusted
to pH 2 with HCl. A white precipitate formed and was collected by fil
tration. The product was crystallized in methanol/isopropyl ether: 1.44 g
white crystals, dp 182-183°C. The product, 2 mmol, proline-t-butyl ester,
2 mmol, and 2 mmol of hydroxybenzotriazole were dissolved in dimethylformamide at -5°C. Dicyclohexylcarbodiimide, 2 mmol in dichloromethane,
was added. The reaction proceeded at -5°C for 1 h and at 4°C for 48 h.
Crude product obtained by work-up was dissolved in trifluoroacetic acid/
ether (1:1 by vol) and left at room temp for 1 h. Residue obtained by
rotary evaporation was chromatographed on silica gel developed with butan-
1-ol/acetic acid/water (75:13:12 by vol). The final product, 29 mg of
white powder, had the following amino acid analysis: Ala 1.07, Gly 1.00,
Pro 0.98.

Tritiation procedures Each of [4-iodo]benzoyl-Phe-Gly-Pro and
[4-iodo]benzoyl-Ala-Gly-Pro was treated as follows: 10 mg of compound was
dissolved in 2 ml of water/dimethylformamide (1:1 by vol) and was reacted
with 10 Ci of $^3H_2$ gas in the presence of 10 mg of 10% Pd on $CaCO_3$ for 4 h
at room temp. Catalyst was removed by filtration, and labile ^{3}H was removed by repeated lyophilization.

Enzyme sources A pool of human serum was provided by Seralc. Pure
rabbit lung ACE was the kind gift of Dr. Richard Soffer, Cornell University Medical College.

Abbreviations

Benzoyl-Phe-Ala-Pro	BPAP
Benzoyl-Phe-Gly-Pro	BPGP
Benzoyl-Ala-Gly-Pro	BAGP
Benzoyl-Phe-His-Leu	BPHL
Hippuryl-His-Leu	HHL
Hippuryl-Gly-Gly	HGG

Methods of assay   Each substrate was used, except as noted below, in concentrations far below its K_m. The assay buffer was 0.05 M Hepes, pH 8.0, containing 0.1 M NaCl, 0.6M Na_2SO_4 and chlorhexidine gluconate, 0.01% by vol. All reactions were conducted in 7 ml liquid scintillation vials. Typically, each vial received 100 μl of buffered enzyme (or buffer for blanks) and reactions were started by adding 100 μl of buffered substrate (0.1 μCi). Incubations were at 37°C. Reaction mixtures containing BPAP, BPGP, BAGP, or BPHL as substrate were incubated for 10 min. Reaction mixtures containing HHL or HGG as substrate were incubated for 30 to 60 min. Reactions were stopped by adding 1,000 μl of 0.1 M HCl (for BPAP, BPGP, or BAGP) or 200 μl of 0.5 M HCL (for BPHL, HHL or HGG). Each vial then received 1,000 μl of toluene containing Omnifluor, 0.4 g% (for BPAP and BPGP), or 3,000 μl of Ventrex LSC #1 (for BAGP, BPHL, HHL or HGG). Vials were capped, inverted 20-times and submitted for liquid scintillation counting. Substrate was quantified by liquid scintillation counting of vials containing 100 μl of buffered substrate and 5 ml of RIAfluor or Scint A. Results were computed using the integrated form of the first order rate equation. In experiments in which inhibitors or carrier or alternative substrates were used, each reaction vial received 50 μl of buffered ^{3}H-labelled substrate and 50 μl of buffered inhibitor or substrate. Reactions were started by adding 100 μl of buffered enzyme. Incubations and work up of reaction mixtures were as described above.

RESULTS

Linearity and precision   As shown in Table 1, the reaction of BPGP with pure rabbit lung ACE is linear over a wide range of enzyme concentrations. When V/Km is plotted versus enzyme concentration ([E]), one obtains a straight line of slope Kc/Km (2.51×10^5 M^{-1} for Table 1). The reactions of pure ACE with all other substrates studied were also linear, and results were obtainable at high precision (overall coefficient of variation of less than 4%). Table 2 shows results obtained when BPGP was reacted with human serum at relatively high dilution (1:80 - 1:640). Again reactions are essentially linear.

Effects of natural inhibitors   However, when high fractional concentrations of serum are used (dilutions of 1:5 - 1:40), reaction rates are not a linear function of serum concentration. As noted elsewhere[9,10], serum and other body fluids contain low molecular mass inhibitors of ACE, and the effects of these natural inhibitors become more pronounced as serum concentration is increased. However, one can capitalize on the inhibitor effects: Under conditions of first order enzyme kinetics, the Michaelis-Menten equation can be simplified, rearranged and inverted to give an equation of a straight line[9].

app (Km/V) = (Km/[VKi])i + (Km/V)

Thus, by plotting apparent (app) (Km/V) versus fractional serum concentration as inhibitor concentration, one obtains a straight line having true Km/V as the y-intercept and fractional concentration of serum required for 50% inhibition as the -x-intercept. Still, as a practical matter, it is better to assay serum ACE by using serum at relatively high dilution 1:80-1:160) such that effects of natural inhibitors are negligible.

Table 1

REACTION OF RABBIT LUNG ACE WITH BPCP

[E]** (pM)	V/Km $(min^{-1} \times 10^2)$	V/Km for [E] = 1 nM
3.125	0.763 $\pm$ 0.036*	2.442 $\pm$ 0.115
6.5	1.560 $\pm$ 0.086	2.496 $\pm$ 0.138
12.5	3.188 $\pm$ 0.155	2.550 $\pm$ 0.124
25	6.320 $\pm$ 0.303	2.528 $\pm$ 0.121
50	12.566 $\pm$ 0.488	2.513 $\pm$ 0.098

* $\bar{x} \pm$ 1 S.D., n = 20

** [E] represents enzyme concentration.

Table 2

REACTION OF HUMAN SERUM WITH BPGP

fractional concentration of serum	apparent (V/Km) $(min^{-1} \times 10^{-2})$	apparent (V/Km) for undiluted serum
1.5625E - 03	0.494 $\pm$ 0.033*	3.162 $\pm$ 0.211
3.125 E - 03	0.988 $\pm$ 0.048	3.162 $\pm$ 0.154
6.25 E - 03	1.944 $\pm$ 0.081	3.190 $\pm$ 0.130
1.25 E - 02	3.736 $\pm$ 0.095	2.989 $\pm$ 0.076

* $\bar{x} \pm$ S.D., n = 20

better to assay serum ACE by using serum at relatively high dilution 1:80-1:160) such that effects of natural inhibitors are neglibile.

Specificity   Each of the six substrates reacted with ACE with high selectivity. Effects of captopril or BPP$_{9a}$ on serum-catalyzed hydrolysis of substrates were much like those on pure rabbit lung ACE (Table 3). There was, however, an interesting exception: BPP$_{9a}$ was approx 6-times more potent in inhibiting human ACE as opposed to rabbit ACE.

Kinetics   Using pure ACE, one can readily measure Kc, Km and Kc/Km, values shown in (Table 4). Kc/Km is the second order rate constant and is a direct function of (1/t)ln[S/(S - P)]. Thus, relative values of Kc/Km can be measured even when [E] is not known.

Table 5 shows values of Kc/Km for human serum ACE based on our best estimate of the actual concentration of ACE in the serum sample used. Tables 4 and 5 show relative values of Kc/Km for pure rabbit lung ACE and for human serum ACE, values in remarkable agreement even though actual values of Kc/Km for one enzyme source as compared with the other differed by approx 6-fold.

<u>Kinetics in vivo</u>   Table 6 shows relative rates of hydrolysis of five of the substrates during a single passage through the pulmonary vascular beds of anesthetized rats. Amax/Km is a term recommended by Dr. John Catravas to represent the product of microvascular volume times V/Km or app (V/Km). As a practical matter Amax/Km is obtained by multiplying plasma flow (F) times ln[S/(S - P)]. Relative slopes of lines produced by plotting Amax/Km versus plasma flow are essentially the same as relative values of Kc/Km as measured <u>in vitro</u>. Thus, extent of hydrolysis of a given substrate during passage through the pulmonary vascular bed is apparently a function of Kc/Km.

DISCUSSION

In terms of our goals, it should be noted that each of BPGP, BAGP and BPHL is of a reactivity greater than those of HGG and HHL and clearly less than that of BPAP. Of the three new substrates, BPHL and BAGP have the degrees of reactivity most favorable for assay of ACE activity <u>in vivo</u> (respective degrees of hydrolysis during a single pass through rat lungs: 45 and 55%). BPGP is probably too reactive.

Of the two substrates most favorable for assay of ACE <u>in vivo</u>, BAGP seems the better candidate. BPHL is prone, during the tritiation procedure, to take up 2 atoms of ^{3}H: one in exchange with the iodo-group and another on the imidazole ring of histidine. As is obvious, generation of two ra-dioactive products ([^{3}H]benzoyl-Phe plus [^{3}H]His-Leu) makes computation of enzyme activity very much more difficult. In addition, BPHL appears to

Table 3

EFFECTS OF INHIBITORS ON ACE
Apparent Ki (nM)

Substrate	BPP (9a)		Captopril	
	R-ACE*	H-ACE*	R-ACE	H-ACE
BPAP	5.1	0.6	1.0	0.6
BPGP	7.2	1.2	1.0	0.7
BAGP	6.0	1.2	0.9	0.6
BPHL	6.9	0.5	1.5	0.7
HHL	5.6	0.2	0.2	0.1
HGG	4.0	0.2	0.7	0.1

*R-ACE represents pure rabbit lung ACE, and H-ACE represents ACE of human serum.

Table 4

KINETIC PARAMETERS: PURE RABBIT LUNG ACE

Substrate	Km (μM)	Kc/Km (M^{-1}min^{-1})	Ratio* Kc/Km
BPAP	0.5	2.87E+09	39.9
BPGP	10.7	2.51E+09	34.9
BAGP	27.6	1.42E+09	19.7
BPHL	13.5	9.60E+08	13.3
HHL	82.5	1.17E+08	1.63
HGG	4000.0	7.20E+07	1.0

*Relative Kc/Km with Kc/Km of HGG taken as 1.0

Table 5

KINETIC PARAMETERS: ACE OF HUMAN SERUM

Substrate	Km (μM)	Kc/Km ($M^{-1}min^{-1}$)	Ratio* Kc/Km
BPAP	0.82	5.24E+08	40.2
BPGP	13.7	4.72E+08	32.5
BAGP	42.6	2.87E+08	21.6
BPHL	11.3	1.48E+08	11.5
HHL	176	1.88E+07	1.56
HGG	3920	1.30E+07	1.0

*Relative Kc/Km with Kc/Km of HGG taken as 1.0.

undergo radiolysis to a far greater extent than does BAGP. In experience so far, no radiolysis of BAGP has been detected over a period of 3 years.

Although we did not make a systematic study of structure-activity relationships, our results (relative values of Kc/Km) make certain such relationships evident. Gly as a P_1' residue is clearly less favorable than Ala (compare BPAP and BPGP). Similarly, Phe as a P_1 residue is markedly superior to Ala or Gly (compare BPGP with BAGP and BPHL with HHL). As is well known, Pro is markedly preferred over Leu or Gly as a P_2' residue. A somewhat surprising result is that the high Kc/Km of BPAP is obtained in spite of an extremely low Kc. In contrast, the high Kc/Km of BPGP is obtained along with a high Kc. Presumably, Gly-Pro is a very much better leaving group than is Ala-Pro. Nonetheless, a point to be emphasized is that, under conditions of first order enzyme kinetics, degree of reactivity of substrate with enzyme is determined entirely by Kc/Km and not by Kc[8,10,11].

Acknowledgements

This work was supported in part by grants from the U.S. Public Health Service (HL 22896 and HL 21568) and the Council of Tobacco Research 814D.

Table 6

RELATIVE VALUES OF Kc/Km IN VIVO

Substrate	Slope of Amax/Km v. F	Ratios** of slopes
BPAP	2.3464	47.21
BAGP	0.9901	19.92
BPHL	0.6753	13.59
HHL	0.0796	1.60
HGG	0.0497	1.00

* Amax/Km is the product of plasma (F) times the natural log of fractional substrate utilization (ln[S/(S-P]) where S is the initial concentration of substrate and P is the concentration of product formed during a single passage of substrate through the lungs of an anesthetized rat. Thus, Amax/Km is equivalent to the product of capillary plasma volume times V/Km.

** Note that the ratios of slopes (slope for HGG taken as 1.0) are very similar to relative values of Kc/Km measured in vitro (see Tables 4 and 5).

REFERENCES

1. Cushman, D.W. and Cheung, H.S., Spectrophotometric assay and properties of the angiotensin-converting enzyme of rabbit lung. Biochem. Pharmac. 20: 1637-1648 (1971).
2. Ryan, J.W., Chung, A., Martin, L.C. and Ryan, U.S., New substrates for the radioassay of angiotensin converting enzyme of endothelial cells in culture. Tissue and Cell 10: 555-562 (1978).
3. Bunning, P., Holmquist, B. and Riordan, J.F., Substrate specificity and kinetic characteristics of angiotensin converting enzyme. Biochemistry 22: 103-110 (1983).
4. Ryan, J.W., Assay of peptidase and protease enzymes in vivo. Biochem. Pharmacol. 32: 2127-2137 (1983).
5. Catravas, J.D. and Gillis, C.N., Metabolism of [^{3}H]benzoyl-phe-ala-pro by pulmonary angiotensin converting enzyme in vivo: Effects of bradykinin, SQ 14225 or acute hypoxia. J. Pharmacol. Exp. Ther. 217: 263-270 (1981).
6. Ryan, J.W., Chung, A., Ammons, C. and Carlton, M.L., A simple radio-assay for angiotensin converting enzyme. Biochem J.167: 501-504, (1977).
7. Chung, A., Ryan, J.W., Peña, G. and Oza, N.B., A simple radioassay for human urinary kallikrein. Adv. Exp. Med. Biol. 120A: 115-125 (1979).
8. Carlin, G., Ryan, J.W. and Saldeen, T., Assays of components of the kallikrein-kinin system based on first order reaction kinetics. Adv. Exp. Med. Biol. 156B: 797-804 (1983).
9. Ryan, J.W., Angiotensin I converting enzyme (kininase II) peptidyl-dipeptide hydrolase EC 3.4.15.1. In Methods of Enzymatic Analysis, ed. H.U. Bergmeyer, Verlag Chemie GmbH, Weinheim, Germany Vol. 5 pp. 20-34 (1984).
10. Ryan, J.W., Martin, L.C., Chung, A. and Peña, G., Mammalian inhibitors of angiotensin converting enzyme (kininase II). Adv. Exp. Med. Biol. 120B: 599-606 (1979).
11. Cornish-Bowden, A., Introduction to enzyme kinetics. In Fundamentals of Enzyme Kinetics, ed. A. Cornish-Bowden, Butterworth, London, pp. 16-38 (1979).

AGGREGATE ANAPHYLAXIS AND CARBOXYPEPTIDASE N

James W. Ryan, Pierre Berryer, Mary Ann Hart and Una S. Ryan

Department of Medicine, University of Miami, Miami, FL 33101

SUMMARY

Bradykinin (BK) is widely believed to play a role in the pathogenesis of anaphylaxis. To help clarify any such roles, we examined for effects of inhibitors of kininase II (angiotensin converting enzyme, ACE) and "kininase I" (carboxypeptidase N, CPN), on the early course of egg albumin-induced aggregate anaphylaxis in anesthetized guinea pigs. In this model, pulmonary and systemic arterial blood pressure (BP) rise (unless pulmonary fibrillation occurs), lung wgt increases by ~ 60% and pulmonary microvessels are occluded by cell-rich thrombi, all within 5 min of i.v. antigen. The 30 min mortality rate is ~ 2%. ACE inhibitors (BPP$_{9a}$, Captopril and MK 422; doses up to 140 µmol/kg) do not make anaphylaxis more nor less severe in terms discernible by changes in BP, lung wgt, EKG or intravascular coagulation. In marked contrast, an inhibitor of CPN (2-mercaptomethyl-3-guanidinoethylthiopropionic acid, 2-MGP; 8-16 µmol/kg) increases the 30 min mortality rate to 94% and lung wgt to 180% of control. The animals die in ventricular fibrillation. Given the enormous BK potentiating effects of BPP$_{9a}$, Captopril and MK 422, it seems likely that little if any BK is formed in the early min of anaphylaxis. 2-MGP does not potentiate BP effects of BK but markedly potentiates effects of C3a anaphylatoxin. Thus, our data support the views that 1) BK is neither a primary nor secondary mediator of aggregate anaphylaxis, and 2) the adverse effects of 2-MGP are best explained in terms of preservation of anaphylatoxins and not in terms of preservation of kinins.

INTRODUCTION

Because of its ability to lower blood pressure, increase vascular permeability, increase insufflation pressure and induce a transient leucocytosis,[1-3] bradykinin has been postulated to act as a humoral mediator of anaphylaxis (for review see 4). In addition, immunologic challenge of basophils is known to cause release of a kallikrein-like enzyme.[5]

Further to examine for possible roles of the kallikrein-kinin system in anaphylaxis, we have studied effects of inhibitors of two kininase enzymes (kininase I and kininase II) on the early course of egg albumin-induced aggregage anaphylaxis in guinea pigs. Our rationale was as follows: Inhibitors of kininase II (angiotensin converting enzyme) are known to potentiate blood pressure effects of intravenously administered bradykinin by up to

1,000-fold (e.g. see 6). These inhibitors also potentiate blood pressure effects of kallidin-10 and glandular kallikrein. Thus if bradykinin and/or kallidin-10 is formed in the early min of aggregate anaphylaxis, the effects of the kinin(s) should be greatly exaggerated. If, then, the kinin is a primary mediator, severity of anaphylaxis should be enhanced. Conversely, if the kinin is a secondary mediator, severity of anaphylaxis might be lessened.

Whether kininase I is in fact a functionally significant kininase is in doubt (cf 7,8). Nonetheless, an excellent inhibitor (2-mercaptomethyl-3-guanidinoethylthiopropionic acid, 2-MGP; Ki 2 x 10^{-9} M) is available and was used in the present studies. The inhibitor, 2-MGP, does not potentiate blood pressure effects of intravenously administered bradykinin but very strongly potentiates effects of at least one of the anaphylatoxins, C3a.[9] Thus, while our primary interest was in the effects, if any, of kinins on the course of anaphylaxis, we were also interested in seeing effects of a CPN inhibitor in a disorder characterized in part by fulminant complement activation.

MATERIALS AND METHODS

Ft. Deitrick-hartley guinea pigs were used throughout. Approx 2/3rd's were immunized and the remainder were not. Half of those immunized were subsequently challenged with antigen and the other half were sham-challenged with saline. All of the non-immunized gunea pigs were challenged with antigen.

Immunization

Each of the guinea pigs selected for immunization received three i.p. injections of egg albumin, 1 mg in complete Freund's adjuvant. The first injection was given on day zero, the second on day 2 and the third on day 5. Three to four weeks after the first injection, the guinea pigs were used for induction of anaphylaxis.

Induction of Anaphylaxis

Each guinea pig was anesthetized with i.p. pentobarbital, 30 mg/kg. A tracheostomy was performed, and the naimal was ventilated mechanically. Heparin, 500 units/kg, was given i.v., and cannulas were inserted into the right external jugular vein and the right femoral artery. Systemic arterial blood pressure, mean arterial blood pressure and insufflation pressure were measured continuously. Lead II of the EKG was recorded. At time zero, 2 mg of egg albumin in 0.1 ml of saline was injected i.v. Observations were made for 30 min or until any earlier time of spontaneous death. Those that did not die spontaneously were killed with an overdose of pentobarbital. Lungs were removed en bloc, rinsed in saline and weighed. One group of guinea pigs received an infusion of captopril, 30 mg/kg, 1.5 mg/kg/min for 20 min. Ten min after beginning the infusion, antigen was injected. Others received bolus injections of other kininase II inhibitors (BPP$_{9a}$ or MK 422), 2.5 mg/kg. Another group received an infusion of the carboxypeptidase N inhibitor, 2-MGP, 0.8 or 1.6 µmol/kg/min for 10 min. Five min after start of the infusion, antigen was injected.

Specificity of Inhibitors

In all experiments in which enzyme inhibitors were used, blood samples (0.3 ml) were collected before, during and after infusion of inhibitor. Plasmas of these samples were assayed for kininase Ii, CPN, DAP IV and aminopeptidase A activities, using as substrates, respectively,

[^{3}H]hippuryl-Gly-Gly but did not inhibit hydrolysis of the substrates for CPN, DAP IV nor aminopeptidase A. The CPN inhibitor, 2-MGP, inhibited hydrolysis of [^{3}H]benzoyl-Ala-Arg and, on occasion, slightly inhibited hydrolysis (25-30% inhibition) of the kininase II substrate. 2-MGP did not inhibit aminopeptidase A nor dAP IV.

RESULTS

Control Studies

The immunization and antigen challenge procedures that we used produce a moderate anaphylactic reaction. Figure 1 shows typical changes in blood pressure and insufflation pressure.   EKG changes include an almost immediate atrial tachycardia that occasionally progresses to A-V block. Approx 2-3% of the experimental animals progress to ventricular fibrillation, which is usually fatal. The 30 min mortality rate is about 2%.

Effects of Kininase II Inhibitors

Over the course of these studies, we used kininase II inhibitors of three different chemical classes: captopril, BPP$_{9a}$ and MK 422, each in doses capable of inhibiting intrinsic serum kininase II by >99% (see 10 for method of assay). Effects of a large dose of captopril (30 mg/kg) on the course of aggregate anaphylaxis are shown in Figure 2. Two points are notable: 1. Inhibition of kininase II does not make anaphylaxis better nor worse (see Tables below). 2. Blood pressures of pentobarbital-anesthetized guinea pigs appear to be dependent in large degree on the renin-angiotensin system (see BP trace before injection of antigen).

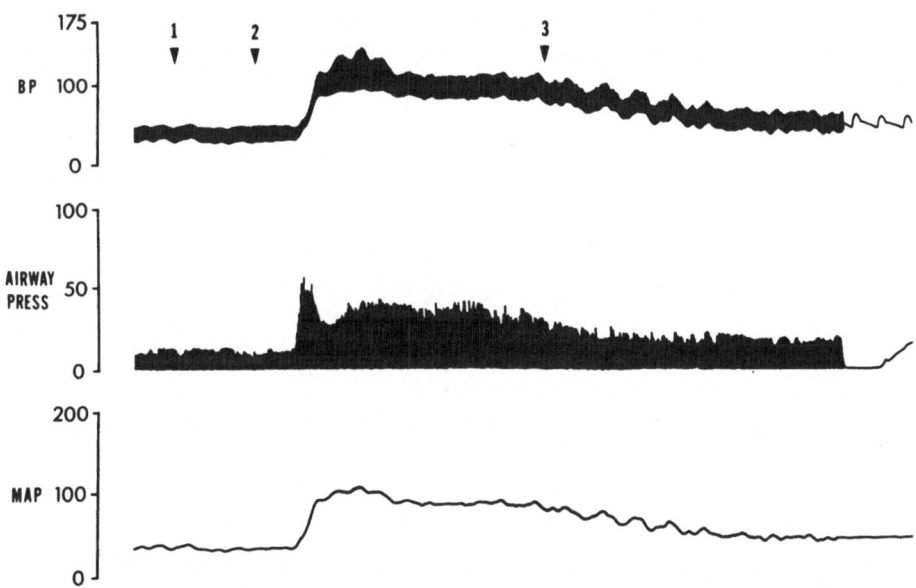

Fig. 1.   Figure 1 shows typical changes of blood pressure and airway pressure in our model of aggregate anaphylaxis. Symbols: 1, start of saline infusion, 0.103 ml per min; 3, termination of infusion; 2, injection of antigen. Chart speeds: 2.5 mm per min and 25 mm per sec.

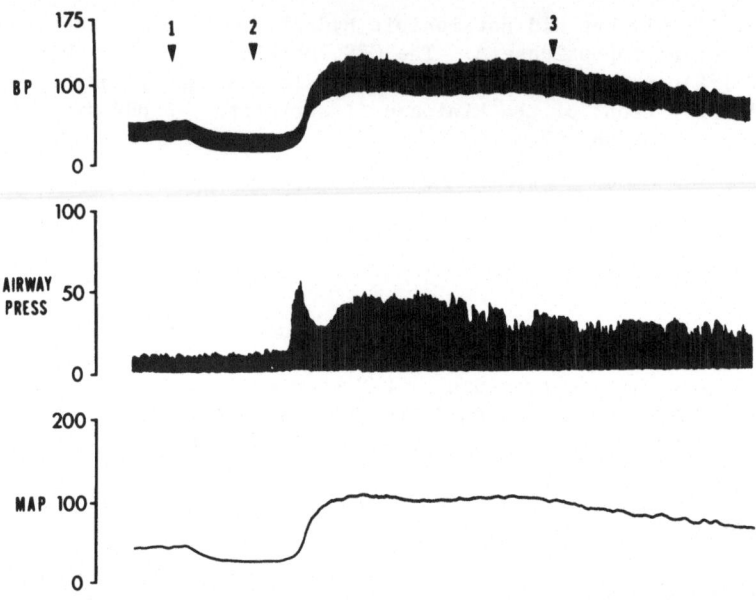

Fig. 2. Figure 2 shows results obtained when anaphylaxis was induced in
guinea pig receiving an infusion of captopril (8 µmol/kg/min),
a kininase II inhibitor. Symbols: 1, start of captopril infusion;
3, termination of infusion; 2, injection of antigen. Chart speed:
2.5 mm per min. Note effects of captopril on baseline blood pressure (BP).

Effects of 2-MGP

The name "kininase I" may represent more than one enzyme. Nonetheless,
the enzyme generally referred to as "kininase I" is carboxypeptidase N,
an enzyme known in other circles as "anaphylatoxin inhibitor" (cf 9,11).
Carboxypeptidase N (CPN) is capable of degrading each of C4a, C3a and C5a
in vitro and probably degrades at least C3a in vivo.[9] When the CPN inhi-

Table 1. Effects of an Inhibitor of Carboxypeptidase N on Lung Weight as
Percent of Body Weight

Group	Antigenic Challenge	Inhibitor Treatment	Lung wgt / Body wgt %
I non-sensitized	+	+	0.62 ± 0.05 (S.D.)
II sensitized	0	+	0.57 ± 0.08
III sensitized	0	0	0.63 ± 0.05
IV non-sensitized	+	0	0.59 ± 0.06
V sensitized	+	0	0.87 ± 0.12
VI sensitized	+	+	0.99 ± 0.09

Student's t-test

n for Groups I, II, III, IV, V and VI: 6, 8, 6, 6, 14 and 12.
Group I versus II, III, or IV: p > 0.1
Group I, II, III, or IV versus V: p < 0.0005
Group I, II, III, or IV versus VI: p < 0.0005
Group V versus VI: p < 0.01

438

Table 2. Effects of a Carboxypeptidase N Inhibitor on Insufflation Pressure

Group	Antigenic Challenge	Inhibitor Treatment	Insufflation Pressure (mm Hg)
A non-sensitized	+	+	25.67 ± 1.5 (S.D.)
B sensitized	0	+	25.57 ± 1.62
C sensitized	+	0	113.60 ± 36.28
D sensitized	+	+	143.17 ± 14.68

Student's t-test

n for Groups A, B, C and D: 9, 7, 5 and 12.
Group A versus B: $p > 0.1$
Group A or B versus C: $p < 0.0005$
Group A or B versus D: $p < 0.0005$
Group C versus D: $p < 0.05$

bitor, 2-MGP[12] is infusd at a rate of 0.8 μmol/kg/min for 10 min, intrinsic CPN of guinea pig serum is completely inhibited throughout the last 8 min of the infusion and about 20 min thereafter.[7] Figure 3 shows effects of antigenic challenge at 5 min after starting the 2-MGP infusion. Severity of anaphylaxis is markedly increased, and the 30 min mortality rate is 94% (approx 47-fold increase over control).

Morphologic Findings

Electron micrographs of lungs collected 30 min after antigenic challenge reveal widespread deposition of cell-rich microthrombi (and/or cell-rich microemboli). Although the lungs of anaphylactic guinea pigs pretreated with a kininase I inhibitor (2-MGP) are markedly heavier than those of anaphylactic guinea pigs either not treated or treated with a kininase II

Table 3. Effects of Captopril on Lung Weight as Percent of Body Weight

Group	Antigenic Challenge	Captopril* Treatment	Lung wgt / Body wgt %
I non-sensitized	+	+	0.60 ± 0.06 (S.D.)
II sensitized	0	+	0.56 ± 0.08
III sensitized	0	0	0.63 ± 0.05
IV non-sensitized	+	0	0.59 ± 0.06
V sensitized	+	0	0.87 ± 0.12
VI sensitized	+	+	0.82 ± 0.14

Student's t-test (x ± 1 S.D.)

n for Groups I, II, III, IV, V and VI: 6, 8, 6, 6, 14 and 12.
Group I versus II, III, or IV: $p > 0.1$
Group I, II, III, or IV versus V: $p < 0.0000$
Group I, II, III, or IV versus VI: $p < 0.0005$
Group V versus VI: $p < 0.1$

*Captopril infusion 14 μmol/kg/min x 10 min.

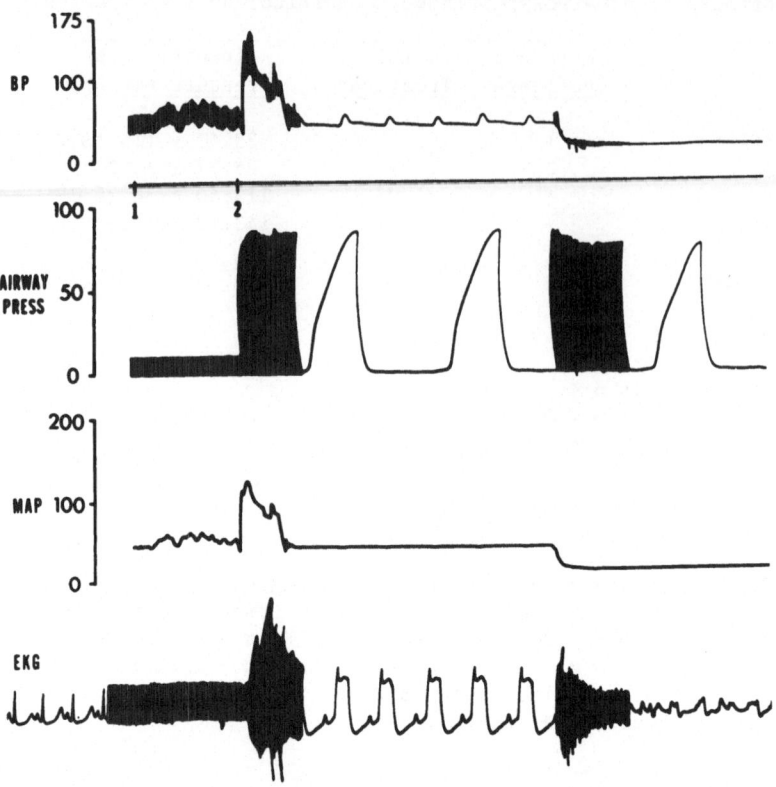

Fig. 3.   Figure 3 shows results obtained when anaphylaxis was induced in
          a guinea pig receiving an infusion of 2-MGP, a carboxypeptidase
          N inhibitor. Symbols: 1, start of infusion; 2, injection of
          antigen. Chart speed: 2.5 mm per min and 25 mm per sec.

inhibitor, the morphologic picture differs little: Cell-rich thrombi are
widespread and extravasation of erythrocytes is more prominent (see Tables
for lung wgts and insufflation pressures).

Lung Weights and Airway Pressures

     The most striking effects of CPN inhibition are on insufflation pres-
sures, EKG (see Figure 3), lung wgts and mortality. Not only is insufflation
pressure markedly increased, the increase is strikingly prolonged. All
anaphylactic animals pretreated with 2-MGP developed severe A-V block and
well-over 90% developed ventricular fibrillation. Of a group of 8 non-
sensitized guinea pigs infused with 2-MGP and challenged with i.v. egg
albumin, none showed changes in blood pressure, airway pressure nor cardiac
rhythms and none died. Thus, adverse effects of 2-MGP are clearly dependent
on events set in motion by union of antibody and antigen. As shown in the
Tables, lungs of anaphylactic guinea pigs treated with 2-MGP were significantly heavier than those of anaphylactic guinea pigs either not treated
or treated with captopril. Curiously, increases in lung wgts occurred almost
immediately following antigenic challenge. For those anaphylactic guinea
pigs pretreated with 2-MGP, lungs collected 2, 3 and 5 min after challenge
with antigen (i.e., lungs from guinea pigs that died shortly after challenge)
were as heavy as those collected at 10, 20 and 30 min following challenge.
Also shown in the Tables are effects of 2-MGP on insufflation pressure.
Clearly, pulmonary compliance fell precipitously and (see Figure 3) never

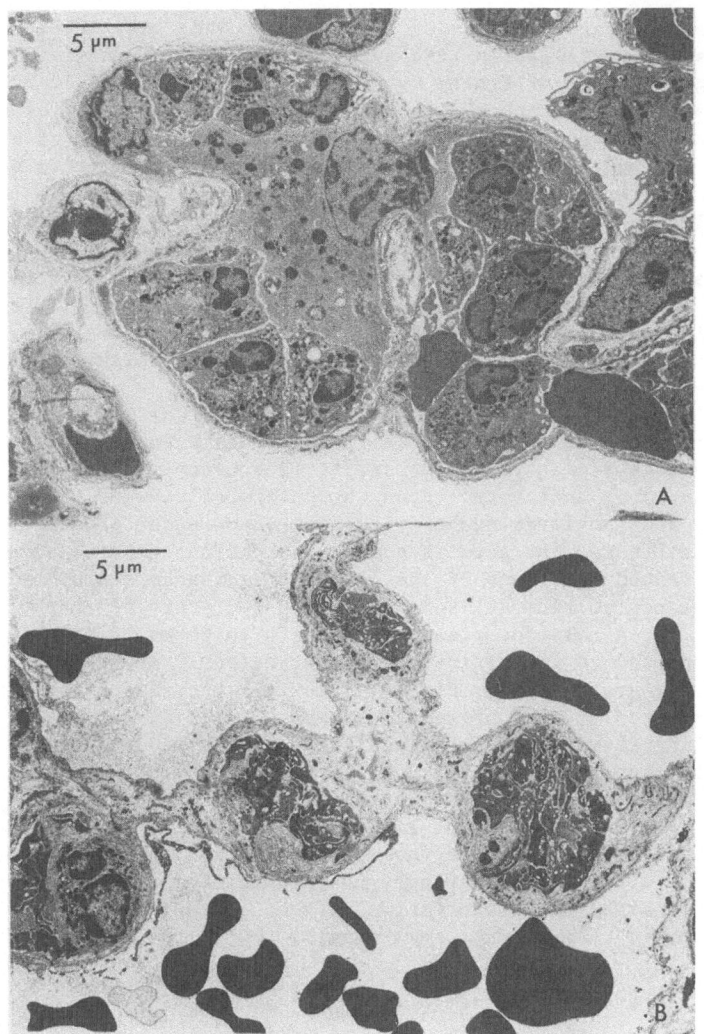

Fig. 4. Electron micrographs of guinea pig lungs collected and fixed 10
min after induction of anaphylaxis. Fig. 4A: Lungs of a guinea
pig not infused with 2-MGP. Fig. 4B: Lungs of a guinea pig infused with 2-MGP. As indicated by results shown in Tables 1 and
2, lungs of guinea pigs treated with 2-MGP were consistently
heavier than those of guinea pigs not treated with the CPN inhibitor. Similarly; 2-MGP pretreatment markedly enhanced the decrease
in compliance of aggregate anaphylaxis. As indicated by Fig.
4B, alveolar hemorrhage was also more prominent among anaphylactic
guinea pigs treated with 2-MGP. Cell-rich thrombi occurred extensively in both groups.

recovered to baseline during the observation period.

DISCUSSION

Initially, we believed that it would be a simple matter to demonstrate
the presumed roles of kinins in aggregate anaphylaxis. Indeed, prior
studies by Brocklehurst and Lahiri[13] and Jonasson and Becker[3] suggested

that antigenic challenge of lungs of sensitized guinea pigs _in vitro_ causes a large release of a kallikrein-like enzyme. Further, given similarities of pharmacologic effects of kinins to hemodynamic changes widely believed to occur in anaphylactic "shock", we postulated that inhibition of kininase II, a maneuver known to markedly potentiate effects of kinins (cf 6,14,15), would convert aggregate anaphylaxis from a serious disease into a disaster. Our hypothesis was wrong. In our experience, what has heretofore been called anaphylactic "shock" in this model of aggregate anaphylaxis is not owing to profound and sustained peripheral vasocilation, it is owing to profound and sustained peripheral vasodilation, it is owing to ventricular fibrillation. Indeed systemic arterial blood pressure invariably rises unless fibrillation occurs. Further, in tissues such as the lungs, the microvascular beds are largely occluded and are highly unlikely sites for pooling of blood.

Because kininase II inhibitors (all bradykinin potentiating agents) do not make aggregate anaphylaxis worse, it is extremely unlikely that kinins act as humoral mediators. From the points of view of the pharmaceutical industry and the large number of patients now under treatment with kininase II inhibitors, the news is good. The patients may be at no special risk for exaggerated reactions of the class of aggregate anaphylaxis. Although kinins _per se_ seem unlikely to act as mediators of anaphylaxis, we cannot rule out a role for plasma kallikrein in terms of its hemostatic functions as opposed to its kinin-generating actions. As is evident in the electron micrographs above, disseminated intravascular coagulation is a major characteristic of aggregate anaphylaxis in guinea pigs. Clearly the most striking results were obtained using sensitized guinea pigs infused with a CPN inhibitor, 2-MGP. apparently, the activity of CPN is of major importance in defense of the host against aggregate anaphylaxis and very possibly other forms of complement-linked injury. While our data do not directly implicate one or more of the anaphylatoxins, our data taken with those of Huey et al.[9] suggest strongly that inhibition of CPN markedly exaggerates (presumably by potentiation) effects of anaphylatoxins released early in the course of aggregate anaphylaxis.

ACKNOWLEDGEMENTS

This work was supported in part by grants from the U.S. Public Health Service (HL 22896, HL 22087 and HL 21568) and the Council of Tobacco Research, 814D.

REFERENCES

1. W. T. Beraldo, Formation of bradykinin in anaphylactic and peptone shock, _Am. J. Physiol._, 163:283-289 (1950).
2. H. O. J. Collier, The action and antagonism of kinins on bronchioles, _Ann. N. Y. Acad. Sci._, 104:290-298 (1963).
3. O. Jonasson and E. L. Becker, Release of kallikrein from guinea pig lung during anaphylaxis, _J. Exp. Med._, 123:509-522 (1966).
4. P. J. Piper, Anaphylaxis and the release of active substances in the lungs, _Pharmac. Ther. B._, 3:75-98 (1977).
5. H. H. Newball, R. W. Berninger, R. C. Talamo, and L. M. Lichtenstein, Anaphylactic release of a basophil kallikrein-like activity. I. Purification and characterization, _J. Clin. Invest._, 64:457-465 (1979).
6. J. Roblero, P. Hernandez, J. W. Ryan, and P. Berryer, A simple bioassay for rat glandular kallikrein, _Adv. Exp. Med. Biol._, 156A:437-443 (1983).

7. J. W. Ryan, A. Chung, and U. S. Ryan, A radioassay for carboxypeptidase N, Adv. Exp. Med. Biol., 156B:867-874 (1983).

8. J. W. Ryan and U. S. Ryan, Endothelial surface enzymes and the dynamic processing of plasma substrates, Intern. Rev. Exp. Pathol., 26:1-43 (1984).

9. R. Huey, C. M. Bloor, M. S. Kawahara, and T. E. Hugli, Potentiation of the anaphylatoxins in vivo using an inhibitor of serum carboxypeptidase N (SCPN). I. Lethality and pathologic effects of pulmonary tissue, Amer. J. Pathol., 112:48-60 (1983).

10. J. W. Ryan, Angiotensin I converting enzyme (kininase II) peptidyl-dipeptide hydrolase EC 3.4.15.1, in: "Methods of Enzymatic Analysis," H. U. Bergmeyer, ed., Verlag Chemie GmbH, Weinheim, Germany, Vol. 5 (1984).

11. V. A. Bokisch and H. J. Müller-Eberhard, Anaphylatoxin inactivator of human plasma: Its isolation and characterization as a carboxypeptidase, J. Clin. Invest., 49:2427-2436 (1970).

12. T. H. Plummer and T. J. Ryan, A potent mercapto bi-product analog inhibitor for human carboxypeptidase N, Biochem. Biophys. Res. Comm., 98:448-454 (1981).

13. W. E. Brocklehurst and S. C. Lahiri, The production of bradykinin in anaphylaxis, J. Physiol., 160:15-16 (1962).

14. S. H. Ferreira, A bradykinin-potentiating factor (BPF) present in the venom of Bothrops jararaca, Br. J. Pharmac. Chemother., 24:163-169 (1965).

15. Y. S. Bakhle, Converting enzyme in vitro measurement and properties, in: "Handbook Exp. Pharmac.," I. H. Page and F. M. Bumpus, eds., Springer-Verlag, New York, Vol. 37 (1974).

MICHAELIS-MENTEN KINETICS OF PULMONARY ENDOTHELIAL
ANGIOTENSIN CONVERTING ENZYME IN THE CONSCIOUS RABBIT

John D. Catravas

Department of Pharmacology and Toxicology
Medical College of Georgia
Augusta, GA   30912

SUMMARY

Estimations of Michaelis-Menten constants Km and Amax (product of Vmax and pulmonary microvascular plasma volume) of pulmonary, endothelial-bound angiotensin converting enzyme (ACE) for the synthetic substrate ^{3}H-Benzoyl-Phe-Ala-Pro (BPAP) were performed in rabbits, in vivo, utilizing indicator dilution techniques. The animals were conscious and equipped with permanent right atrial and left carotid catheters. For each determination of Km and Amax, two consecutive bolus injections of BPAP were given into the right atrial catheter, the first containing 0.1 and the second 1622 nmol of substrate, producing first order and mixed order substrate concentrations, respectively, in the pulmonary circulation. Arterial blood was withdrawn at 0.7 sec intervals for 15 sec after each injection and from the family of substrate concentrations thus created (usually 14-20) and resulting range of substrate utilization (10-90%), Km and Amax values were calculated utilizing the Lineweaver-Burk, Eadie-Scatchard, Woolf-Augustinsson-Hofstee or Hanes-Woolf transformations of the integrated Henri-Michaelis-Menten equation. All four methods produced similar values of Km (10-12 µM), Amax (6-7 µmol/min) and Amax/Km (600-720 ml/min); however, linear regression analysis of data from the Hanes-Woolf transformation resulted in a higher correlation coefficient (0.96 vs 0.86-0.88 for the other three methods). Values for the kinetic constants reported here were similar to those previously reported in anesthetized rabbits utilizing the Woolf-Augustinsson-Hofstee transformation, but higher than those reported for purified rabbit lung ACE, in vitro.

INTRODUCTION

Recent reports from our laboratory (1) as well as from Gillis' (2) and Pitt's (3) have introduced methods for estimating Michaelis-Menten kinetics of pulmonary endothelial-bound angiotensin converting enzyme for a synthetic tripeptide (benzoyl-phenylalanyl-alanyl-proline; BPAP) in vivo. Although it is too early to assess the impact of these new methodologies, it is hoped that they may provide a variety of information including a) new knowledge on the function of enzymes in their natural milieu, b) improved means of assaying clinically useful enzyme inhibitors, in vivo, in experimental animals and in man, and c) new diagnostic procedures for the early detection of lung microvascular injury.

All of the aforementioned reports have been based on the Woolf-Augustinsson-Hofstee transformation of the integrated Henri-Michaelis-Menten equation, originally proposed by Linehan and Dawson (4) for studying the uptake of prostaglandin E by the dog lung lobe, in vitro. The present study examines additional methods of analyzing such data and compares the values of in vivo determined Michaelis-Menten kinetic constants between conscious and anesthetized rabbits.

METHODS

Male New Zealand albino rabbits weighing approximately 3.5 kg were anesthetized with a mixture of ketamine (50 mg/kg) and xylaxine (5 mg/kg) im; catheters were introduced into the right jugular vein and left carotid artery and exteriorized at the back of the neck; each animal was fitted with a protective jacket and allowed to recover for 20-24 hours. At the time of the experiment, the rabbit was placed in a restraining holder and indicator dilution-type determinations of single pass trans-pulmonary metabolism of ^{3}H-BPAP were performed. Each animal received two consecutive bolus injections of the substrate, the first containing only the radioactive tracer (2 μCi, 10 μCi/nmol) and the second containing ^{3}H-BPAP and 1622 nmol of BPAP, in order to achieve first and mixed order substrate concentrations, respectively, in the pulmonary circulation. Detailed description of the technique and equipment is presented in reference (1). Each pair of determinations produced 14-20 substrate concentrations ranging from approximately 0.2 nM to 50 μM. At each concentration substrate utilization was estimated as $([S_o] - [S])/[S_o]$ and ranged from 0.9 (at low $[S_o]$) to 0.1 (at high $[S_o]$), with $[S_o]$ and $[S]$ reflecting the initial and final substrate concentrations in the effluent arterial blood, estimated in nmol/ml as $[S_o] = [BPAP] + [BP]$ (benzoyl-phe, product of BPAP metabolism by ACE) and $[S] = [BPAP]$. Because these types of experiments do not measure initial reaction velocities (i.e. $([S_o] - [S])/[S_o]$ is greater than 0.05), data analysis is performed utilizing the integrated Henri-Michaelis-Menten equation (5) which is based on substrate utilization rather than initial velocities. As it is described in (1), the Henri-Michaelis-Menten equation

$$v = \frac{-d[S]}{dt} = \frac{Vmax \cdot [S]}{Km + [S]} \tag{1}$$

can be integrated and rearranged to the form:

$$[S_o] - [S] = -Km \cdot \ln([S_o]/[S]) + Vmax \cdot t_c \tag{2}$$

where t_c is the microvascular mean transit time of the substrate, i.e. incubation time. As with equation (1), Vmax in equation (2) is defined as:

$$Vmax = [E] \cdot K_{cat} \tag{3}$$

or

$$Vmax = \frac{E}{n \cdot Q_c} \cdot K_{cat} \tag{4}$$

where [E] is the concentration of enzyme in mol/l, E is the enzyme mass in mol, Q_c is the pulmonary microvascular plasma volume and $n \cdot Q_c$ (where $0 < n < 1$) is the volume of distribution or reaction volume for E. If E distributes in the total microvascular plasma volume, then $n = 1$. For the remainder of the discussion, it will be assumed that $n = 1$. If we then define

$$Amax = E \cdot K_{cat} \qquad (5)$$

with units $mol \cdot min^{-1}$, and substitute $\dot{Q}$ (pulmonary plasma flow) for Q_c/t_c, then equation 2 becomes

$$[S_o] - [S] = -Km \cdot \ln([S_o]/[S]) + Amax/\dot{Q} \qquad (6)$$

The advantage of equation (6) is that the term t_c, which cannot as yet be estimated from our experiments, is eliminated, and the equation is of the form $y = ax + b$. Values for Km and Amax can thus be determined by fitting the values of $[S_o]$ and $[S]$ obtained from each pair of indicator-dilution type determinations, to equation 6 using linear regression. Equation (6) is actually the Woolf-Augustinsson-Hofstee (W-A-H) transformation of the integrated Henri-Michaelis-Menten equation, the linear form of this transformation being:

$$v = Km \cdot \frac{v}{[S]} + Vmax \qquad (7)$$

Three other commonly used linear transformations of the Henri-Michaelis-Menten equation have been used to analyze the data. They are:

Lineweaver-Burk (L-B) transformation.

$$\frac{1}{[S_o] - [S]} = \frac{\dot{Q} \cdot Km}{Amax} \cdot \frac{\ln([S_o]/[S])}{[S_o] - [S]} + \frac{\dot{Q}}{Amax} \qquad (8)$$

Eadie-Scatchard (E-S) transformation.

$$\ln([S_o]/[S]) = -\frac{1}{Km} ([S_o] - [S]) + \frac{Amax}{\dot{Q} \cdot Km} \qquad (9)$$

Hanes-Woolf (H-W) transformation.

$$\frac{1}{\ln([S_o]/[S])} = \frac{\dot{Q}}{Amax} \frac{[S_o] - [S]}{\ln([S_o]/[S])} + \frac{\dot{Q} \cdot Km}{Amax} \qquad (10)$$

The coefficients in each of equations 6, 8, 9 and 10 and the equations used to calculate Km and Amax are shown in Table 1.

RESULTS AND DISCUSSION

There were no differences in the values of Km, Amax or Amax/Km calculated in conscious rabbits with any of the four transformations of the Henri-Michaelis-Menten equation, as shown in Table 2. However, the Hanes-Woolf method resulted in a correlation coefficient (0.96 ± 0.01) which was significantly higher than the other three ($p < 0.05$).

An advantage of the Hanes-Woolf transformation probably lies in that

Table 1. Coefficients of the Equation (y = ax + b) Used to Calculate Km and Amax Values of ACE for BPAP In Vivo

	L-B	E-S	W-A-H	H-W
a	$\dot{Q} \cdot$ Km/Amax	-1/Km	-Km	$\dot{Q}$/Amax
b	$\dot{Q}$/Amax	Amax/($\dot{Q}$ Km)	Amax/$\dot{Q}$	$\dot{Q} \cdot$ Km/Amax
Km	a/b	-1/a	-a	b/a
Amax	$\dot{Q}$/b	$-\dot{Q} \cdot$ b/a	$\dot{Q} \cdot$ b	$\dot{Q}$/a

Table 2. Kinetic Constants of Pulmonary Endothelial ACE for BPAP in Conscious Rabbits (Means ±1 S.E., n = 6)

	TRANSFORMATION			
	L-B	E-S	W-A-H	H-W
Km (μM)	11.9±1.1	12.2±1.1	9.5±1.2	10.6±1.1
Amax (μmol/min)	7.4±1.0	7.7±0.7	6.4±0.7	6.8±0.7
Amax/Km (ml/min)	614±46	654±63	715±76	658±54
Correlation coefficient	0.86±0.04	-0.88±0.03	-0.88±0.03	0.96±0.01

it minimizes the error in $\ln([S_o]/[S])$ factor occurring from high substrate utilizations during the trace injection, by including it in both the dependent and the independent variables. For example, a difference between 85% and 90% substrate utilization (i.e. a 5.9% error) will produce a difference in $\ln([S_o]/[S])$ between 1.897 and 2.303 (i.e. a 21.4% error). Another advantage may occur from the utilization of the inverse of $\ln([S_o]/[S])$ which further minimizes the error. A Hanes-Woolf plot from an experiment in a conscious rabbit is shown in Figure 1.

A problem occurred frequently when analyzing data with the L-B transformation. Utilizing all data from the experiment, the L-B transformation often produced regression coefficients which were not significantly different from zero. The reason appears to be the high variance in values of the dependent variable with data from the first injection containing trace substrate concentrations (<0.1 nmol). Even small errors in $[S_o]$ - $[S]$ from the first injection will produce disproportionally large errors when inversed as is the case with the independent variable of the L-B transformation. To avoid this problem kinetic constant calculations with the L-B method utilize data from the second injection only.

The Km values of lung endothelial ACE for BPAP in conscious rabbits are very similar to those previously reported in anesthetized rabbits in two separate studies (1,2) suggesting no significant effects of allobarbital and urethane (anesthetics used in both instances) on the enzyme-substrate interaction, in vivo. Furthermore, similar Km values were reported by Pitt and Lister (3) in neonatal and adult conscious sheep (Table 3). Interestingly, all these values measured in vivo are two to three times higher than the Km of partially purified rabbit lung ACE or purified human serum ACE for BPAP (6,7). These consistent differences

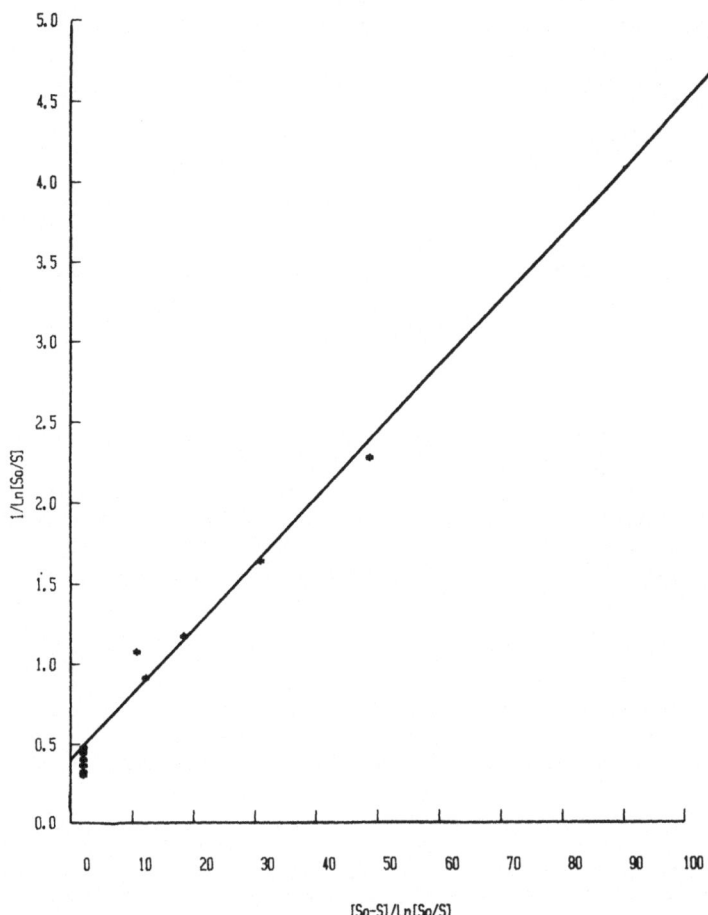

Fig. 1. Hanes-Woolf plot (equation (10)) of data from a pair of indicator dilution type determinations of single pass transpulmonary
metabolism of ^{3}H-BPAP in a conscious rabbit. Plot includes
14 data points, 7 from the first bolus injection (trace) and 7
from the second (1622 nmol BPAP) injection. Km = 10.0 μM,
Amax = 6.4 μmol/min, Amax/K$_m$ = 640, correlation coefficient:
0.99, Km is calculated as the ratio of the y-intercept to the
slope. Amax is calculated as the ratio of pulmonary plasma flow
to the slope.

Table 3. Kinetic constants of pulmonary endothelial ACE for BPAP

Species	Km (µM)	Amax (µmol/min/kg)	Amax/Km (ml/min/kg)	Reference
Rabbit anesthetized	11±1	2.1±0.2	198	1
Rabbit conscious	10±1	2.0±0.2	203	*
Rabbit anesthetized	9±1	1.1±0.2	117	2
Sheep conscious-- adult	15±3	4.1±0.6	276	3
Sheep conscious-- newborn	15±3	2.8±0.4	187	3

*Present data. All values were obtained from the Woolf-Augustinsson-Hofstee transformation; however, values from references 2 and 3 utilized the non-linear model to correct for possible heterogeneity in substrate transit times.

could be readily accounted for by the presence of circulating inhibitors for lung ACE. Recently, Ryan (8) described a procedure for estimating relative levels of endogenous ACE inhibitors and their effect on serum ACE. He estimated that under normal conditions human serum ACE is inhibited by more than 95%. Although similar calculations have not been performed with rabbit serum, it would be reasonable to expect a significant but perhaps lower level of inhibitors: ACE activity in rabbit serum is about four times greater than that in human serum (9,10). We have preliminary evidence that in rabbit lungs perfused in situ with an albumin-rich, blood free medium, Km values of lung endothelial ACE for BPAP are comparable to those observed with the purified enzyme, in vitro. Interpretation of these data, however, is complicated by the differences in the pressure flow relationship between the in vivo and in situ preparations.

Even when expressed as "per kg of body weight," Amax values of lung ACE for BPAP vary somewhat among different studies and, perhaps, among species (Table 3). As it is shown in equation (5), Amax is directly proportional to the enzyme mass E. Assuming identical Kcat (as for example with conscious vs anesthetized rabbits where the anesthetic has no effect on the enzyme), Amax will change with E, i.e. with endothelial surface area. Endothelial surface area undergoes continuous changes as a result of capillary recruitment and derecruitment and, in a not fully recruited bed, it can be influenced by changes in pulmonary blood flow and pressures. Perhaps differences in the fraction of the microvascular bed recruited with the experimental preparations used among the various laboratories contribute to this variability in Amax.

ACKNOWLEDGEMENTS

These studies were supported in part by the U.S. Public Health Service (HL 31422) and by the Georgia Affiliate of the American Lung Association. The expert technical assistance of Ms. Julia Andrieni and the meticulous preparation of the manuscript by Ms. Marianne Reneau are gratefully acknowledged.

REFERENCES

1. J. D. Catravas and R. E. White, Kinetics of angiotensin converting enzyme and 5´-nucleotidase, in vivo, J. Appl. Physiol. 57:1173-1181 (1984).
2. R. E. Howell, R. Moalli, and C. N. Gillis, Analysis of rabbit pulmonary angiotensin converting enzyme kinetics, in vivo, J. Pharmacol. Exp. Ther. 228:154-160 (1984).
3. B. R. Pitt and G. Lister, Kinetics of pulmonary angiotensin converting enzyme activity in conscious developing lambs, J. Appl. Physiol. 57:1158-1166 (1984).
4. J. H. Linehan and C. A. Dawson, A kinetic model of prostaglandin metabolism in the lung, J. Appl. Physiol. 47:411-424 (1979).
5. I. H. Segal, "Enzyme Kinetics," Wiley, New York (1975).
6. J. W. Ryan, L. C. Martin, A. Chung, and G. Pena, Mammalian inhibitors of angiotensin converting enzyme (Kininase II), Adv. Exp. Med. Biol. 120B:599-606 (1979).
7. J. W. Ryan, Assay of peptidase and protease enzymes, in vivo, Biochem. Pharmacol. 32:2127-2137 (1983).
8. J. W. Ryan, Angiotensin I converting enzyme (Kininase II) peptidyl-dipeptide hydrolase EC 3.4.15.1, in: "Methods of Enzymatic Analysis, Vol. 5," H. O. Bergmeyer, ed., Verlag Chemie GmbH, Weinheim, Germany (1984).
9. J. S. Lazo, J. D. Catravas, and C. N. Gillis, Reduction in rabbit serum and pulmonary angiotensin converting enzyme activity after subacute bleomycin treatment, Biochem. Pharmacol. 18:2577-2584 (1981).
10. J. J. Lanzillo and B. L. Fanburg, Development of competitive enzyme immunoassays for human serum angiotensin-1-converting enzyme: A comparison of four assay configurations, Anal. Biochem. 126:156-164 (1982).

IN VIVO DETERMINATIONS OF Ki VALUES FOR

ANGIOTENSIN CONVERTING ENZYME INHIBITORS

John D. Catravas and Betty L. Anthony

Department of Pharmacology and Toxicology
Medical College of Georgia
Augusta, GA   30912-3368

SUMMARY

We present two methods for calculating Ki values of angiotensin converting enzyme (ACE) inhibitors, such as captopril, in anesthetized or conscious rabbits. Both methods are based on indicator-dilution type determinations of single pass transpulmonary metabolism of the ACE substrate benzoyl-phe-ala-pro (BPAP). The first method involves two determinations of Michaelis-Menten constants Km and Amax (product of Vmax and lung capillary plasma volume) of endothelial-bound ACE for BPAP. Thirty seconds before the second determination of kinetic constants, the inhibitor is administered iv (e.g. captopril, 12 nmol/kg). Comparisons of the apparent Km and Amax values, obtained after the inhibitor to the control values obtained from the first determination, provide Ki values. With the second method, the ratio Amax/Km is obtained, under first-order reaction conditions, before and 30 sec after administration of inhibitor. These apparent and control ratios are used to calculate Ki values. In both methods, plasma levels of the inhibitor at the time of the determination of apparent kinetic constants are estimated by injecting radio-labelled inhibitor (e.g. ^{3}H-captopril), analyzing radioactivity in arterial samples and correcting for plasma protein binding. These methods are potentially applicable to the clinical evaluation of new ACE inhibitors, in vivo, under normal or pathologic conditions.

INTRODUCTION

We have reported earlier in this volume, and before (1), on a method for the determination of Michaelis-Menten constants of endothelium-bound angiotensin converting enzyme (ACE) for the synthetic substrate benzoyl-phe-ala-pro (BPAP) in conscious and anesthetized rabbits, in vivo. One potentially useful application of this methodology is the evaluation of ACE inhibitors, in vivo, based on measurements of control and apparent Km values of ACE for BPAP in the absence and presence of the inhibitor, respectively. ACE inhibitors prevent the formation of angiotensin II from angiotensin I and the breakdown of bradykinin. They represent a new class of antihypertensive agents. At present two ACE inhibitors, captopril and enalapril are approved for clinical use and several others are in various stages of development. Testing of these drugs in vivo has largely relied on monitoring their ability to reduce or prevent the rise in systemic blood pressure induced by various stimuli, a response dependent not only on enzyme-drug interaction, but also on tissue distribution and uptake, mechanisms of metabolism and excretion and drug binding to circulating macromolecules. It would thus follow that a method of directly monitoring the drug-induced enzyme inhibition, in vivo, would be of value to drug development. It would further allow observations on possible disturbances in drug enzyme interaction in the presence of clinically relevant pathologies.

METHODS

The experiments were performed on ten New Zealans white male rabbits weighing approximately 3.5 kg. They were anesthetized with a mixture of urethane (200 mg/ml) and allobarbital (50 mg/ml), artificially ventilated and equipped with carotid arterial and right atrial catheters. In six animals, four determinations of single plass transpulmonary conversion of the synthetic ACE substrate ^{3}H-BPAP (10 µCi/nmol) were performed utilizing indicator dilution techniques, previously described in detail (1,2). Substrate mass injected during the first and third determinations was 0.1 nmol (i.e. 2 µCi of tracer/determination, only), whereas 1600-1800 nmol BPAP were included with the tracer in determinations two and four. Exactly thirty seconds prior to the third determination, each animal received 12 nmol captopril/kg body weight, i.v. Data were analyzed as follows.

Mixed-Order Method

Utilizing the Eadie-Scatchard transformation (equation (1)) of the integrated Henri-Michaelis-Menten equation (3), first we calculated Km and Amax constants of ACE for BPAP with data from determinations 1 and 2 and then apparent Km and Amax values from determinations 3 and 4 (after captopril administration). A more detailed description of this procedure is published elsewhere in this volume (2). Briefly, data were fitted by linear regression to the equation:

$$\ln([S_o]/[S]) = -\frac{1}{Km}([S_o] - [S]) + \frac{Amax}{\dot{Q} \cdot Km} \tag{1}$$

where $[S_o]$ is the initial substrate concentration (i.e., total ^{3}H concentration in each arterial blood sample), $[S]$ is the final substrate concentration (i.e., ^{3}H-BPAP concentration remaining in each arterial blood sample), $\dot{Q}$ is pulmonary plasma flow, and

$$Amax = Vmax \cdot n \cdot Q_c = E \cdot K_{cat} \tag{2}$$

where Q_c is capillary plasma volume (liters), n is the fraction of Q_c in which E distributes, assumed = 1 and E is enzyme mass (mol).

Km or apparent Km (Km´) were calculated as the negative of the inverse of the slope of the regression line. Ki values for captopril were determined from the following relationships (3); assuming captopril behaved as:

Competitive inhibitor.

$$Km´ = Km(1 + \frac{[I]}{K_i}) \tag{3}$$

$$Amax' = f \cdot Amax \tag{4}$$

where f reflects the fraction of E accessible to substrate in the presence of the inhibitor. For a reversible inhibitor, f = 1; for an irreversible inhibitor, 0 < f < 1.

<u>Mixed inhibitor.</u>

$$Km' = \frac{Km(1 + \dfrac{[I]}{Ki})}{1 + \dfrac{[I]}{\alpha \cdot Ki}} \tag{5}$$

$$Amax' = \frac{Amax}{1 + \dfrac{[I]}{\alpha \cdot Ki}} \tag{6}$$

where $\alpha > 1$.

<u>First-Order Method</u>

Under first order conditions, $[S] \ll Km$, $Km \sim Km + [S]$ and the Henri-Michaelis-Menten equation can be written as:

$$V = \frac{-d[S]}{dt} = \frac{Vmax}{Km} \cdot [S] \tag{7}$$

When integrated from $t = 0$ to t_c (mean capillary transit time) and from $[S_o]$ to $[S]$ (at time t_c), equation (7) becomes

$$\ln \frac{[So]}{[S]} = \frac{Vmax}{Km} \cdot t_c \tag{8}$$

Substituting $Amax/Q_c$ for Vmax and $\dot{Q}$ for Q_c/t_c, equation (8) becomes

$$\dot{Q} \cdot \ln \frac{[So]}{[S]} = \frac{Amax}{Km} \tag{9}$$

or, since the fraction of substrate metabolized (M) is $(S_o - S)/S_o$, equation (9) can be expressed as:

$$\dot{Q} \cdot \ln \frac{1}{1 - M} = \frac{Amax}{Km} \tag{10}$$

Considering the Km of ACE for BPAP <u>in vitro</u> (5 µM, ref. 5) or <u>in vivo</u> (15 µM, ref. 1,2), the substrate concentrations achieved with the injection of 0.1 nmol BPAP in determinations 1 and 3 of this study allow us to assume that the substrate-enzyme interaction in these experiments proceeds at first order conditions. Under these circumstances, the apparent (Amax/Km) ratio is reduced in the presence of an inhibitor to:

$$\left(\frac{Amax}{Km}\right)^{'} = \frac{Amax}{Km} \cdot \frac{f}{1 + ([I]/Ki)} \tag{11}$$

This relationship holds true for competitive, non-competitive or mixed type inhibition (3), as it can be seen from equations (3), (4), (5) and (6). The value of f is 1 for a mixed type or reversible competitive inhibitor. When captopril was assumed to act as an irreversible inhibitor f was computed as Amax'/Amax from individual Amax and Amax' values obtained with the mixed order method (equation (1)). In these experiments, the ratios Amax/Km and (Amax/Km)', before and after captopril, respectively, were computed as the integral over the entire transpulmonary passage using equation (9).

With both methods [I] is the concentration of free captopril in plasma at the time of the determination (i.e., thirty seconds after administration). To calculate [I], a separate group of 4 rabbits were similarly anesthetized, catheterized and ventilated. At time = 0, 1.2 µCi ^{3}H-captopril/kg body weight (12 nmol/kg; 0.1 µCi/nmol) was injected together with 0.2 mg Evans Blue dye (T-1824) into the right jugular catheter. At t = 30 sec and 60 sec arterial blood (3 ml) was withdrawn into heparinized syringes. After centrifugation, radioactivity (tritium) was determined in 0.5 plasma aliquots and in 0.5 ml eluents of Amicon disposable microconcentrators (>99% rejection of compounds with molecular weight >67,000). The latter sample provided estimates of the free (non-protein-bound) captopril levels in plasma. Dye concentrations were estimated spectrophotometrically (605 nm) in 1 ml plasma. Tissue uptake of captopril at 30 and 60 sec ws estimated as

$$U_t = \frac{FC_D - FC_C}{FC_D} \tag{12}$$

where FC_D and FC_C are the fractional concentrations of the dye and captopril in plasma, respectively. As it is shown in Table 1, there was considerable tissue uptake but minimal binding of ^{3}H-captopril under these experimental conditions. Concentration of free captopril in plasma was calculated as the ratio of ^{3}H-dpm in one ml of the Amicon microconcentrator eluent to the specific activity of ^{3}H-captopril injected (0.1 µCi/nmol or 220,000 dpm/nmol).

All calculations were performed with the aid of a DEC Rainbow computer.

RESULTS AND DISCUSSION

Apparent Km values of ACE for BPAP increased almost three-fold 30 sec after administration of captopril (Table 2), an expected observation indicative of a competitive inhibitor. Concentrations of captopril in plasma at the time of estimation of apparent kinetics ranged from 32.3 nM (30 sec after captopril: beginning of third determination of BPAP transpulmonary metabolism) to 29.7 nM (60 sec after captopril: end of fourth determination of BPAP transpulmonary metabolism). Since these two values were close, their average (31 nM) was used at [I] in Ki calculations, with equations (3), (5) and (6), while [I] = 32.3 nM with equation (11).

Concomitant with the increase in apparent Km (Km'), apparent Amax (Amax') decreased significantly from Amax = 12 µmol/min to Amax = 6 µmol/min after captopril. Since Amax = E · Kcat, a decrease in apparent

Table 1. Plasma Dilution, Tissue Uptake and Plasma Protein Binding of ^{3}H-captopril (C) 30 Sec and 60 Sec after IV Injection (12 nmol/kg) into Anesthetized Rabbits (n = 4).

	30 sec	60 sec
C-Plasma protein binding	2%	2%
C-Total plasma fraction (FC_C)	0.001266	0.001166
Dye-Total plasma fraction (FC_D)	0.022220	0.022210
C-Tissue uptake	94.3%	94.8%
C-Free plasma concentration	32.3 nM	29.7 nM

Table 2. Control and Apparent Michaelis-Menten Constants of BPAP for Pulmonary Endothelial ACE, in Anesthetized Rabbits, In Vivo (n = 6; Means ±1 S.E.).

Mixed Order Method

Km	16.9 ± 4.4 µM
Km´	43.2 ± 7.8 µM
Amax	12.0 ± 2.4 µmol/min
Amax´	6.0 ± 1.7 µmol/min
[I]	31.0 nM

First Order Method

Amax/Km	763 ± 100 ml/min
(Amax/Km)´	128 ± 37 ml/min
[I]	32.3 nM

Amax together with a rise in apparent Km after administration of an inhibitor suggests a) mixed-type inhibition, b) competitive-type inhibition with an irreversible inhibitor tightly binding to a fraction of the enzyme and thus effectively reducing E, or c) competitive-type inhibition where the available enzyme has decreased by a factor (f) after the inhibitor administration, due to reduction in lumenal microvascular surface area.

Possibility (c) is the least likely in this study. We have indirect evidence that microvascular surface area may not have changed significantly. Table 3 shows no differences in mean systemic blood pressure, BPAP volume of distribution (roughly equivalent to cardiac and pulmonary plasma volume), BPAP mean transit time through the lung or pulmonary blood flow, before and after captopril administration. Furthermore, in three of the six rabbits single transpulmonary metabolism of 5´-AMP by endothelial bound 5´-nucleotidase was estimated together with BPAP conversion by ACE. No significant changes in Amax/Km ratio of 5´-AMP for nucleotidase were observed after captopril (data not shown) further

Table 3. Hemodynamic Parameters Measured during the Determination of Ki Values of Captopril for ACE in Anesthetized Rabbits (n = 6, Mean ±1 S.E.)

	Control	Post-Captopril
Systemic Blood Pressure (mmHg)	112 ± 6	102 ± 6
BPAP volume of distribution (ml)	60 ± 6	49 ± 3
BPAP mean transit time (sec)	5.0 ± 0.2	5.0 ± 0.2
Pulmonary blood flow (ml/min)	488 ± 72	413 ± 40

reducing the probability for a significant decrease in surface area (de-recruitment) to have occurred.

With data from the present experiments, it is not possible to distinguish between mixed type and competitive irreversible inhibitions. If a mixed type inhibition is assumed, Ki can be computed with the first order method using equation (11) (Ki = 6.3 nM), or with the mixed order method, from solving equations (5) and (6) (Ki = 7.5 nM), as shown in Table 4. Similarly, if a competitive, irreversible inhibition is assumed, Ki values can be estimated using the mixed order method from equation (3) (Ki = 23 nM) or with the first order method using equation (11). In the latter case f is computed as the ratio of Amax to Amax from equation (4) (Ki = 17 nM) as shown in Table 4.

Whether irreversible or mixed-type inhibition is assumed, the first order and the mixed order methods produced similar results (Table 4); however, there is a three-fold difference in the Ki values between the calculations for the two types of inhibition.

Early reports on the mechanism of inhibition of purified ACE by captopril indicated a simple competitive-type inhibition (5,6). However, these reports utilized the Lineweaver-Burk graphic approach in which the points away from the ordinate (1/v) are more heavily weighted in the fitting of the line, and errors in determination of Vmax are magnified because reciprocals are plotted (3). More recently, captopril was reported to act as a mixed-type inhibitor towards rat lung ACE, in vitro (7). Although labelled "mixed-type," the inhibition could well be of the irreversible type, since the characterization was based solely on the

Table 4. Calculations of Ki Values of Captopril for Pulmonary Endothelial ACE In Vivo (n = 6; Mean ±1 S.E.)

	α	f	Ki
Mixed Type Inhibition			
First Order – eq. 11	–	1	6.3 ± 1.3 nM
Mixed Order – eq. 5,6	2.05	–	7.5 ± 1.2 nM
Irreversible Inhibition			
First Order	–	0.47 ± 0.09	17.1 ± 4.1 nM
Mixed Order – eq. 3	–	–	23.4 ± 4.4 nM

concomitant increase in apparent Km and decrease in apparent Amax. Indeed, thiol containing compounds, such as captopril, can form strong bonds with Zn^{++}, present in ACE, which may be responsible for the long duration of action of the drug. In a recent study it was demonstrated that lung ACE in conscious rabbits was significantly inhibited even three days after captopril (2 mg/kg, iv) administration (8). Our Ki values calculated assuming mixed-type inhibition are very close to those previously reported (4,5,6). This observation, although suggestive, could well be coincidental and cannot be used as an argument towards determining the mechanism of inhibition. Since it is conceivable that captopril may interact differently with purified ACE vs ACE in vivo, we are currently attempting to elucidate the mode of inhibition in vivo utilizing the techniques presented here at varying [I] and [E].

ACKNOWLEDGEMENTS

We are pleased to acknowledge the expert technical assistance of Nancy Quinn and Julia Andrieni. We thank Marianne Reneau for her meticulous preparation of the manuscript. Supported in part by the U.S. Public Health Service (HL 31422) and the Georgia affiliates of the American Heart Association.

REFERENCES

1. J. D. Catravas and R. E. White, Kinetics of angiotensin converting enzyme and 5´-nucleotidase, in vivo, J. Appl. Physiol. 57:1173-1181 (1984).
2. J. D. Catravas, Michaelis-Menten kinetics of pulmonary angiotensin converting enzyme in the conscious rabbit, in: "Kinin IV" (1986).
3. I. H. Segel, "Enzyme Kinetics," Wiley, New York (1975).
4. J. W. Ryan, Assay of peptidase and protease enzymes, in vivo, Biochem. Pharmacol. 32:2127-2137 (1983).
5. D. W. Cushman, H. S. Cheng, E. F. Sabo, and M. A. Ondetti, Design of new antihypertensive drugs: Potent and specific inhibitors of angiotensin converting enzyme, Prog. Cardiovasc. Dis. 21:176-182 (1978).
6. D. W. Cushman, H. W. Cheng, E. F. Sabo, and M. A. Ondetti, Design of potent competitive inhibitors of angiotensin converting enzyme. Carboxyalkanoyl and marcapto alkanoyl amino acids, Biochem. 16:5484-5491 (1977).
7. F. A. O. Mendelsohn, J. Csicsmann, and J. S. Hutchinson, Complex competitive and non-competitive inhibition of rat lung angiotensin-converting enzyme by inhibitors containing thiol groups: Captopril and SA 446, Clin. Sci. 61:277s-280s (1981).
8. X. Chen, B. R. Pitt, R. Moalli, and C. N. Gillis, Correlation between lung and plasma angiotensin converting enzyme and the hypotensive effect of captopril in conscious rabbits, J. Pharmacol. Exp. Ther. 229:649-653 (1984).

RAT TESTICULAR ANGIOTENSIN I CONVERTING ENZYME: PURIFICATION AND COMPARISON

WITH RAT PULMONARY ENZYME

Takamasa Yamaguchi, Masaharu Hiratsuka, Masahiko Ikekita,
Kazuyuki Kizuki and Hiroshi Moriya

Department of Biochemistry, Science University of Tokyo
Shinjuku-ku, Tokyo 162, Japan

SUMMARY

Enzymological properties of rat testicular angiotensin I converting
enzyme (RT-ACE) were compared with those of rat pulmonary angiotensin I
converting enzyme (RP-ACE). The molecule of RT-ACE was different from that
of RP-ACE with respect to the molecular weight, i.e., the molecular weight
of RT-ACE was estimated to be 104 kilo-dalton (kd) and that of RP-ACE (150
kd) on SDS-polyacrylamide gel electrophoresis. On the other hand, the enzy-
mochemical properties of RT-ACE were very similar to those of RP-ACE, with
regard to activation by NaCl, optimum pH, Km value for N*-hippuryl-His-
Leu-OH hydrolysis and sensitivities to various inhibitors. Therefore, it
was speculated that the portions contributing to the appearance of catalytic
activity would be similar between RT-ACE and RP-ACE.

INTRODUCTION

In some mammals, i.e., dog, cat, guinea pig and rat, it has been reported that a large amount of angiotensin I converting enzyme (EC 3.4.15.1,
kininase II, abbreviated as ACE) present in testes.[1,2] Especially, in rat,
the content of ACE in testes was reported to be much more than those in
lungs and kidneys.[1] And it has been demonstrated that the amounts of ACE
in rat testes increase with the sexual maturation of the rat and high concentration of ACE is maintained after puberty.[2] Considering of these matters,
the ACE would have somewhat important role in male reproductive system.
However, there has been no evidence to demonstrate that the ACE participates
in the physiological function of testes. Furthermore, rat testicular ACE
has not been studied in detail on the enzymological properties as the isolated enzyme. Thus, we attempted to purify the ACE from rat testes in order
to clarify the enzymo-chemical and structural properties as the first stage
of the studies to elucidate the physiological significance of the ACE in
male reproductive system. For this purpose, it would be useful to compare
the properties of RT-ACE directly to those of the ACE from popular source
such as lung, whose properties had been well understood. However, in rat,
the enzymo-chemical properties of the purified pulmonary ACE have not been
studied in detail. So that, we also attempted to purify ACE from rat lungs
in the present investigation. In some respects, the properties of RT-ACE
were studied comparing with those of the purified rat pulmonary ACE (RP-
ACE).

MATERIALLS AND METHODS

N*-hippuryl-His-Leu-OH (HHL), H-His-Leu-OH, angiotensihns I and II, bradykinin, Leu[5]-enkephaline and Met[5]-enkephaline were purchased from Peptide Institute Inc. (Osaka, Japan). Captopril was a kind gift from Sankyo Co. Ltd. (Tokyo, Japan). Other chemicals were of guaranteed reagent grade.

When HHL was used as substrate of ACe, the amounts of enzymatically liberated hippuric acid were measured according to the method of Cushman and Cheung.[3] One unit (U) was defined the amounts of the enzyme that can hydrolyze one μmol of HHL per min at 37°C in 0.1 M borate-bicarbonate buffer, pH 8.3, containing 5 mM HHL and 0.8 M NaCl.

When angiotensin I was used as substrate, the amounts of enzymatically liberated H-His-Leu-OH were determined by the fluorescence method of Conroy and Lai.[4]

RESULTS

Purification of RT-ACE and RP-ACE

RT-ACE   Results of the purification of RT-ACE were summarized in Table 1. All of the procedures described below were carried out at 4°C.

Step 1   Frozen tstes (400 g) of Wistar rats were thawed and homogenized with Polytron (Kinematica, Switzerland) in 3 vol. of 5 mM Tris-HCl buffer, pH 8.0. Homogenate was filtered through nylon mesh and the filtrate was centrifuged. Sodium deoxycholate (DOC) was added to the supernatant to make the final concentration 0.25% (W/V). Then, the suspension was stirred for 3 hr to solubilize ACE from testicular membrane. After centrifugation, the supernatant was dialyzed twice against 10 vol. of 5 mM Tris-HCl buffer, pH 8.0, for 9 hr each. Dialysate (DOC extract) was used as the starting material for the purification of RT-ACE. About 2,600 U of the enzyme was obtained.

Step 2   DOC extract was dialyzed against 20 mM sodium acetate buffer, pH 4.6, for 3 hr (acid treatment). White precipitate which generated during

Table 1. Purification of Rat Testicular Angiotensin I Converting Enzyme (From 400 g Tissues)

Purification step	Activity (U)	Recovery (%)	Protein (A_{280})	U/A_{280}	P.F.
1) Deoxycholate extraction	2602	100	59466	0.044	1
2) Acid treatment (pH 4.6)	2343	90	4373	0.54	12.3
3) Ammonium sulfate fractionation (45 - 75%)	2093	80.4	1744	1.20	27.3
4) First DEAE-Sepharose CL-6B chromatography	1831	70.4	317	5.78	131.4
5) Second DEAE-Sepharose CL-6B chromatography	663.7	25.5	13.2	50.28	1143
6) Sephadex G-200 gel filtration	153.3	5.9	1.7	90.18	2050

this dialysis was removed by centrifugation. The supernatant was immediately adjusted to pH 8.0 with one tenth vol. of 0.5 M Tris-HCl buffer, pH 8.0. Most of ACE were recovered in this solution at 90% yield and 1the enzyme was purified 12.6 fold from DOC extract.

Step 3   Ammonium sulfate fracitonation of the solution was carried out. The precipitated materials between 45-75% ammonium sulfate saturation were collected by centrifugation. And the pellet was resolved in 5 mM Tris-HCl buffer, pH 8.0. Most of ACE were recovered in this solution and the enzyme was purified 27.3 fold from DOC extract.

Steps 4 and 5   The sample from step 3 was dialyzed twice against 20 vol. of 50 mM Tris-HCl buffer, pH 8.0, for 12 hr each. And the dialysate was applied to a DEAE-Sepharose CL-6B column equilibrated with the same buffer. After the column was washed with the same buffer, adsorbed materials were eluted with linear gradient of 0-0.2 M NaCl in 50 mM Tris-HCl buffer, pH 8.0. Sample from this chromatography was thoroughly dialyzed against 0.1 M borate-NaOH buffer, pH 8.5. And the dialysate was applied to a DEAE-Sepharose CL-6B column equilibrated with the same buffer. And adsorbed materials were eluted with linear gradient of 0.1-1 M borate-naOH buffer, pH 8.5. By these ion exchange chromatographies, ACE was purified 1,143 fold from DOC extract.

Step 6   The sample from step 5 was concentrated and applied to a Sephadex G-200 column. Gel filtration was carried out using 25 mM Tris-HCl buffer, pH 8.0, containing 0.1 M NaCl as running buffer.

By these purification procedures, RT-ACE was purified 2,050 fold from DOC extract and final preparation whose specific activity was 90.18 U/A_{280} was obtained at the yield of 5.9%.

RP-ACE   Purification of ACE from lungs of Wistar rats was performed according to the purification method for RT-ACE. However, RP-ACE could not be completely purified only by the purification procedures that were employed in RT-ACE. Therefore, hydrophobic chromatography on a Phenyl-Sepharose CL-4B column was supplemented after acid treatment (step 2) was done. Finally, ACE was purified 1,100 fold from DOC extract of rat lungs (210 g) and final preparation whose specific activity ws 59.55 U/A_{280} was obtained at the yield of 7.7% (data were not shown).

SDS-Polyacrylamide Gel Electrophoresis

Fig. 1 shows electrophorograms of SDS-polyacrylamide gel electrophoresis of RT-ACE and RP-ACE on 5% gels. Final preparations of both RT-ACE (A) and RP-ACE (B) appeared as a single protein band. RT-ACE was migrated faster than RP-ACE. This shows that the molecule of RT-ACE was smaller than that of RP-ACE. The estimated molecular weights of RT-ACE and RP-ACE were 104 ± 3 kilo dalton (kd) (n=5) and 150 ± 6 kd (n=7), respectively.

Fig. 1-C shows the electrophorogram of RT-ACE that was developed with PAS reagent. A single stained band was observed at the position related to 104 kd (indicated with arrow). This shows that the molecule of RT-ACE would have sugar moiety.

Comparisons of Enzymo-Chemical Properties Between RT-ACE and RP-ACE

Actions of RT-ACE and RP-ACE on angiotensins I and II, bradykinin, Leu[5]-enkephaline and Met[5]-enkephaline. Actions of RT-ACE and RP-ACE on angiotensins I and II, bradykinin, Leu[5]-enkephaline and Met[5]-enkephaline were analyzed by thin layer chromatographies using silica gel 60 plates (Merck, Japan).

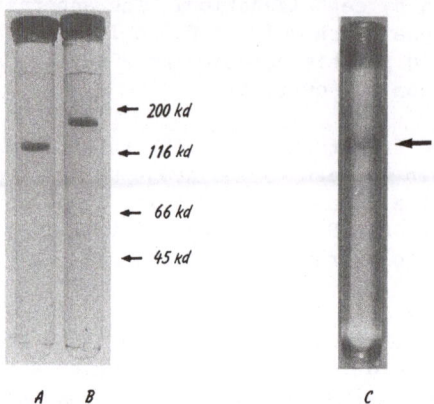

Fig. 1.　SDS-Polyacrylamide gel electrophoresis of RT-ACE and RP-ACE.
Samples; A: RT-ACE (0.05 A_{280}), B: RP-ACE (0.06 A_{280}), C: RT-ACE
(0.15 A_{280}).　SDS-polyacrylamide gel electrophoresis was performed
according to the method of Weber and Osborn[5] using 5% gels.　After
electrophoresis, gels A and B were stained with Coomassie Brilliant
Blue R-250 and gel C was stained with PAS reagent.　High molecular
weight protein standards were the product of Bio-Rad (California,
USA).

　　　Both RT-ACe and RP-ACE hydrolyzed angiotensin I into two peptide fragments.　Rf values of these fragments coincided with those of authentic angiotensin II and H-His-Leu-OH, respectively.　In both ACEs, further degradation
of angiotensin II was not observed.　On the other hand, bradykinin, Leu[5]-
enkephaline and Met[5]-enkephaline were all hydrolyzed into two peptide fragments by the incubation with RT-ACE or RP-ACE (products from each substrate
were 1not identified).　These angiotensin I converting, bradykininase and
enkephalinase activities of both ACEs were all inhibited by the addition
of 1 µM captopril.

　　　Effects of NaCl on the HHL hydrolyzing activities of RT-ACE and RP-
ACE　　As shown in Fig. 2, HHL hydrolyzing activities of RT-ACE and RP-ACE
were both strongly activated by the addition of NaCl.　In both ACEs, maximum
activities were obtained at 0.8 M NaCl.　At 0.4 M NaCl, the activities of
both ACEs were reduced to 80% of their full activities that were observed
in the presence of 0.8 M NaCl.　At 0.2 M NaCl, the activities of RT-ACE
and RP-ACE were reduced to 43 and 50% of their full activities, respectively.
And　when NaCl was almost omitted, the residual activities of RT-ACE and
RP-ACE were only 3 and 5% of their full activities, respectively.　Thus,
the reduction of NaCl concentration diminished the HHL hydrolyzing activities of both ACEs to similar extent.

　　　Optimum pHs　　RT-ACe had most potent HHL hydrolyzing activity at the
pHs between 8.1-8.3 when assays were carried out in 0.1 M Tris-H_2SO_4 buffers
of various pHs in the presence of 0.8 M NaCl.　On the other hand, the highest
HHL hydrolyzing activity of RP-ACE was observed at pH 8.3 when the activity
of RP-ACE was measured in the same buffers.

　　　Meanwhile, the highest angiotensin I converting activity of RT-ACE
was observed at pH 6.8-7.0.　And that of RP-ACE was observed at 7.0 (analyses
were performed using 50 mM MES-NaOH buffers at pH range from 5.8 to 7.0
and 0.1 M Tris-H_2SO_4 buffers at pH range from 7.5 to 7.9).

　　　Km values for HHL hydrolysis of RT-ACE and RP-ACE　　From Lineweaver-
Burk plots, Km values for HHL hydrolysis of RT-ACE and RP-ACE were estimated

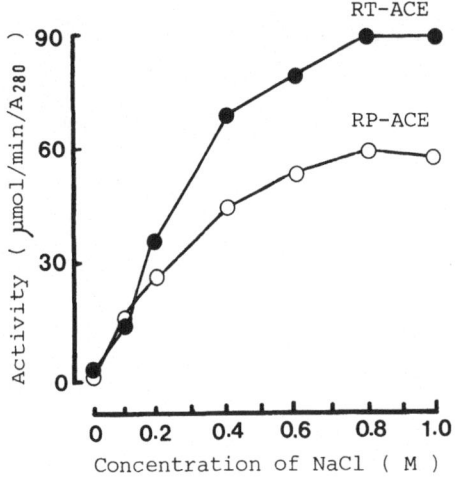

Fig. 2.   Effects of NaCl on the HHL hydrolyzing activities of RT-ACE and
RP-ACE.   The final preparations of both ACEs were thoroughly dialyzed against 5 mM borate-NaOH buffer, pH 8.3, to remove chloride
ion.   HHL hydrolyzing activity of eac ACE was determined in 0.1
M borate-bicarbonate buffers, pH 8.3, containing various concentrations of NaCl.

to be same (2.5 mM).

Effects of various compounds on the HHL hydrolyzing activities of RT-
ACE and RP-ACE   Effects of various compounds on the HHL hydrolyzing activities of RT-ACE and RP-ACE were summarized in Table II.

The activity of RT-ACE was partially or completely inhibited by the
addition of such chelating agents as EDTA and o-phenanthroline or the addition of such suylfhydryl compounds as L-cysteine and reduced glutathione.
From these results, RT-ACE was considered to be classified in a group of
metallo-peptidases.   HHL hydrolyzing activity of RT-ACE was inhibited by
captopril, a specific inhibitor of ACE, at lower concentrations (10^{-8}-10^{-6} M)
in contrast with the case of the other inhibitors described in Table II.
The influence of captopril concentrations on the inhibition of RT-ACe was
very similar to the case of RP-ACe.

DISCUSSION

We purified two molecular types of ACEs from rat organs, one from testes
(RT-ACE) and the other from lungs (RP-ACE).   RT-ACE was distinguishable
from RP-ACE by its smaller molecular weight than that of RP-ACE.   In the
present investigation, further analyses were not done on the structural
differences between RT-ACE and RP-ACE.   Therefore, it has been unclear which
portions of the molecules are different from each other between both ACEs.

Difference of molecular weights between testicular and pulmonary ACEs
also had been reported in other mammal.   El-Dorry et. al., demonstrated
that the purified rabbit testicular ACE had smaller molecular weight
(100,000) than rabbit pulmonary ACE (140,000).[6]   It is intriguing to speculate that the presence of low molecular weight ACE in testis might be in
common in various mammals.

On the other hand, it was anticipated that RT-ACe would have

Table 2. Effects of Various Compounds on the HHL Hydrolyzing Activities of RT-ACE and RP-ACE

| Compound | Final Conc. (M) | Residual Activity (%) | |
		RT-ACE	RP-ACE
EDTA	10^{-4}	17	**
	10^{-3}	ND*	ND*
o-phenanthroline	10^{-4}	50	**
	10^{-3}	ND*	**
L-cysteine	10^{-4}	51	49
	10^{-3}	ND*	23
Reduced glutathione	10^{-4}	80	80
	10^{-3}	ND*	20
Captopril	10^{-8}	51	65
	10^{-7}	6	7
	10^{-6}	ND*	ND*

ND*; not detected, **; not tested. HHL hydrolyzing activity of each puri-fied ACE (3.3 mU) was determined in the presence of each compound in the assay medium during incubation period at the concentration described ib this table.

distinctive enzymo-chemical properties from RP-ACE since the molecule of RT-ACe was different from RP-ACE. However, the enzymo-chemical properties of RT-ACE were found to be very similar to those of RP-ACE with regard to activation by NaCl, optimum pH, Km value for hydrolysis and sensitivities to various inhibitors. These results show that the sites contributing to the appearances of enzyme activities might resemble between both ACEs inspite of the difference in their molecular sizes. From this point of view, also in vivo, RT-ACE would be able to have similar catalytic function to RP-ACE.

Recently, some investigators demonstrated the presence of renin and angiotensin I in Leydig cells of rat testis by immunochemical, enzymo-chemi-cal and immuno-histochemical techniques.[7,8] Therefore, renin-angiotensin system would actually exist in rat testis. However, since detailed localiza-tion of RT-ACE in rat testis has not been investigated, it is still unclear whether angiotensin I which was generated by the action of the testicular renin can be a substrate of RT-ACE in vivo. Meanwhile, bradykinin and en-kephalines were hydrolyzed by the action of RT-ACE. So that, RT-ACE is also considered to participate to the inactivation of these bio-active pep-tides in testis. But on these peptides, any clear evidences for the distri-bution of themselves, their precursors (such as kininogen) and generating enzyme (such as kallikrein) in rat testis have not been demonstrated.

Accordingly, substrate(s) of RT-ACE is(are) not necessarily clarified at present stage. ACEs from various mammalian sources are known to be flexi-ble peptidases, i.e., the ACEs act on various oligopeptides and release dipeptides or tripeptides from carboxy termini of peptides in vitro.[9-11] Although substrate specificity of RT-ACE was not studied in the present investigation, judging from that RT-ACE had similar enzymo-chemical proper-ties to RP-ACE, RT-ACE is also thought to have flexibility toward various peptides. Therefore, it seems undesirable to restrict the consideration of physiologicall significance of RT-ACE only to the metabolism of angio-tensin I, kinins and enkephalines. It also should be anticipated that RT-ACE might contribute to the metabolisms of the other known or unknown biologically important peptides.

REFERENCES

1. D. W. Cushman and H. S. Cheung, Concentrations of angiotensin-converting enzyme in tissues of the rat, Biochem. Biophys. Acta, 250:261-265 (1971).
2. D. W. Cushman and H. S. Cheung, Studies in vitro of angiotensin-converting enzyme of lung and other tissues, in: "Hypertension," J. Genest and E. Koiw, eds., Springer-Verlag (1972).
3. D. W. Cushman and H. S. Cheung, Spectrophotometric assay and properties of angiotensin-converting enzyme of rabbit lung, Biochem. Pharmacol., 20:1637-1748 (1971).
4. J. M. Conroy and C. Y. Lai, A rapid and sensitive fluorescence assay for angiotensin-converting enzyme, Anal. Biochem., 87:556-561 (1978).
5. K. Weber and M. Osborn, The reliability of molecular weight determinations by dodecyl sulfate-polyacrylamide gel electrophoresis, J. Biol. Chem., 244:4406-4412 (1969).
6. H. A. El-Dorry, H. G. Bull, K. Iwata, N. A. Thornberry, E. H. Cordes, and R. L. Soffer, Molecular and catalytic properties of rabbit testicular dipeptidyl carboxypeptidase, J. Biol. Chem., 257:14128-14133 (1982).
7. M. Parmentier, T. Inagami, R. Pochet, and J. C. Desclin, Pituitary-dependent renin-like immunoreactivity in the rat testis, Endocrinology, 112:1318-1323 (1983).
8. K. N. Pandy, K. S. Misano, and T. Inagami, Evidence for intracellular formation of angiotensins; coexistence of renin and angiotensin-converting enzyme in Leydig cells of rat testes, Biochem. Biophys. Res. Commun., 122:1337-1343 (1984).
9. E. G. Erdös, Kininases, in: "Hand. Exp. Pharm., Vol. XXV, Supple.," E. G. Erdös, ed., Springer-Verlag (1979).
10. J. Inokuchi and A. Nagamatsu, Tripeptidyl carboxypeptidase activity of kininase II (angiotensin-convrting enzyme), Biochem. Biophys. Acta, 662:300-307 (1981).
11. H. Yokosawa, S. Endo, Y. Ogura, and S. Ishii, A new feature of angiotensin-converting enzyme in the brain: Hydrolysis of substance P, Biochem. Biophys. Res. Commun., 116:735-742 (1983).

KININASE II OF HUMAN SEMINAL FLUID: KINETICS AND INHIBITION

Marc van Sande, Hugo Neels, Simon Scharpé
and Barton Holmquist*

Faculty of Medicine, University of Antwerp, Universiteitsplein
1, B-2610 Wilrijk, Belgium

*Center for Biochemical and Biophysical Sciences and Medicine
Harvard Medical School, 250 Longwood Avenue, Boston
MA

SUMMARY

The activity of kininase II in crude human sperm was measured continuously by measuring the hydrolysis of a blocked tripeptide 3-(2-furylacryloyl)-L- phenylalanyl-glycl-glycine (1 mmol/l). Mean seminal plasma activity was 335±61 U/g protein; the K_m was 0.7 mmol/l; pH optimum was 8.8 in a 50 mmol/l HEPES buffer and the chloride optimum was 300 mmol/l. This male genital tract enzyme is inhibited by several kininase II inhibitors. Captopril (SQ 14225) showed IC_{50} = 1.6 x 10^{-8} mol/l, with a competitive pattern (K_1 = 7.3 x 10^{-9}). 3-(Mercaptomethyl)-oxo-piperidineacetic acid showed the same kind of inhibition with an IC_{50} = 1.8 x 10^{-6} mol/l (K_1 = 6.8 x 10^{-7} mol/l). Enalapril diacid was the most potent inhibitor and had an IC_{50} of 4.1 x 10^{-9} mol/l and showed a mixed competitive and non-competitive inhibition (K_1 = 10^{-9} mol/K_1' = 9.5 x 10^{-10} mol/l). These in vitro inhibition data suggest that, in vivo, such drugs may effect the function of kininase II in the male reproductive system. The observed 50% inhibition constants are comparable to those observed in lung enzyme suggesting similar kinetic properties.

INTRODUCTION

Although kininase II activity[1] is generally considered to be highest in the lung on a per g protein basis, high kininase II activity is also observed in human prostate, prostatic fluid and seminal fluid. However, since seminal fluid contains no detectable angiotensin II,[2] and the uterus is one of the most sensitive organs to bradykinin stimulation,[2] it would appear that the role of human seminal fluid kininase II is to degradade bradykinin. Kininase II's function in the seminal fluid is also implied by experiments[3,4] demonstrating that sperm motility is influenced both by bradykinin and by kininase II inhibitors. As these effects have been studied solely by examination of sperm motility, the aim of this study is to obtain kinetic data about seminal kininase II activity and its inhibition.

MATERIAL AND METHODS

Human seminal fluid was obtained from sperm donors. It was frozen within 12 h at -25°C. After pooling, the suspension was homogenized with a Teflon pestled Elvejhem glass homogenizer, in the presence of 0.5% (vol/vol) Nonidet P 40 (LKB, Bromma, Sweden)[5] and centrifuged at 2000 x g for 60 min (4°C). The resulting supernatant was emulsified with Lipoclean (1,1,2 trichloro-1,2,2 trifluoroethane) (Behringwerke A.G., Marburg, F.R.G.) to remove remaining lipids and centrifuged at 3000 x g (10 min). The supernatant enzyme preparation was stored at -25°C until use.

Substrate   3-(2-furylacryloyl)-L-phenylananyl-glycyl-glycine) was synthesized by one of us (B.H.). All other reagents used were from E. Merck (Darmstadt, F.R.G.). Substrate solutions were made at 8 different concentrations ranging from 2 mmol/l to 0.25 mmol/l (HEPES buffer, 50 mmol/l, pH 8.8 at 25°C, containing 0.3 mol/l NaCl). A substrate concentration of one 1 mmol/l was used for determination of the pH optimum, the optimum salt concentration and IC_{50}'s.

Inhibitors   Captopril (SQ 14225)[6] was a generous gift of Squibb, Belgium. 3-(Mercaptomethyl)-2-oxo-1-piperi-dineacetic acid[7] was a kind gift from the Warner Lambert Foundation (Parke-Davis, Ann Arbor, Michigan, U.S.A.) and enalapril ethylester (MK 421) and enalapril diacid (MK 422)[8] were a gift from the Merck Institute (Rahway, New Jersey, U.S.A.). Bovine serum albumin 1 g/l, was added to stock inhibitor solutions to prevent adsorption to glass or plastic. At this concentration no effect in activity by the albumin was observed, although serum albumin is known to inhibit kininase II.[9]

Procedures

Kinetic experiments   Reactions were initiated by adding 30 µl of enzyme or enzyme-inhibitor mixture (prepared by preincubating 40 µl of enzyme with 20 µl of inhibitor for 15 min) to 500 µl of substrate.

Continuous spectrophotometric readings   A model 8450A spectrophotometer (Hewlett-Packard, Palo Alto, CA 94304) was used throughout. Since the furylacryloyltripeptide is itself a chromophore[10] different wavelengths were chosen to follow hydrolysis such the absorbance was less than 2 at each substrate concentration while maintaining a 1 cm pathlength for convenience. Thus for the lowest substrate concentration, 2.5×10^{-4} mol/l, a wavelength of 334 nm was used, producing an initial absorbance A_o of 1.55 with $\Delta A = 0.49$. The second wavelength, 345 nm, was used for the concentration range of 0.5 to 1.5×10^{-3} mol/l ($A_o = 0.60 - 1.8$, $\Delta A = 0.25 - 0.78$). At each substrate concentration, hydrolysis was allowed to go to completion with 5 samples to obtain accurate ΔA values in order to convert ΔA/min to moles/min.

The direct linear plot introduced by Eisenthal and Cornish-Bowden[11] was used for kinectic analysis.

This method is used throughout this study because it provides clear and accurate information about the quality of the observations, identifies aberant measurements while providing unbiased estimates of the kinetic constants.[12]

Kinetic analysis and calculations of inhibition constants   The enzyme velocities (dA/dt) were calculated either with the spectrophotometer or manually. K_i and K_i' were calculated for each set of experiments from K_m/V_{max} and $1/V_{max}$ against I.[13] IC_{50}'s were calculated from a Hill plot.[14]

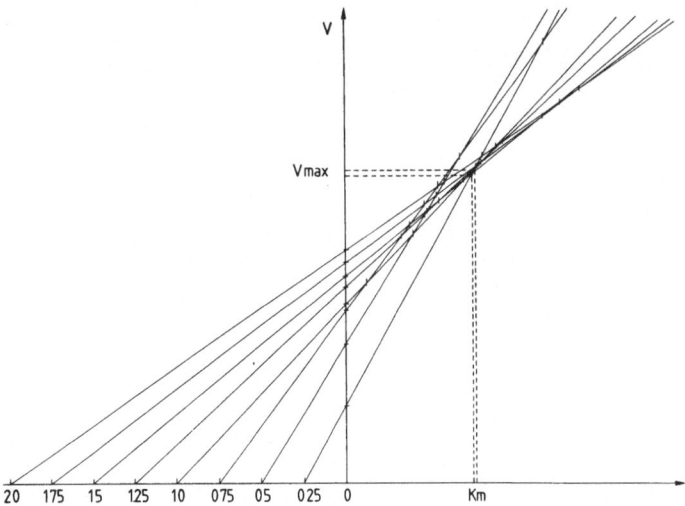

Figure 1.   Direct linear plot of V_{max} against K_m. Each line represents
one observation, and is drawn with intercepts – s on the
abcissa and V on the ordinate. The points of intersection form
a non parametric distribution from which the best estimate,
V_{max} and K_m, are taken as medians.

RESULTS AND DISCUSSION

Human seminal fluid   The mean kininase II activity in normal seminal
plasma using 1 mmol FAPGG was 335 61 U/g protein (n=5). The ratio of this
activity vs the serum activity (n=100, 90 U/1)[15] is 250 in accord with the
data of Cushman and Cheung.[16] The pH optimum (Figure 2) is 8.8 for HEPES
and HEPPS and is practically independent of the buffers used (Tris,
Tricine, glycineamide). The pH optimum is slightly higher than that of
serum.[17] The use of different substrates may account for this phenomenon,
although an isoenzymatic difference cannot be excluded. Kininase II is
characteristically activated by chloride ion and that dependence was established for the seminal plasma enzyme used here (Figure 3). The shape
of the curve and the optimum (300 mmol/1) are similar to those found for
FAPPG with enzyme of rabbit lung and human serum.[18,19]

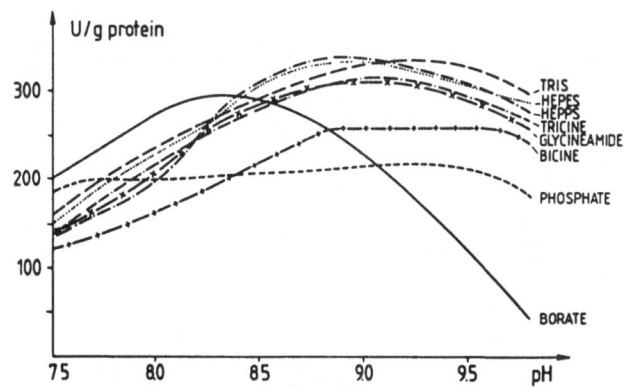

Figure 2.   pH effect on FAPGG hydrolysis by human seminal fluid kininase II.

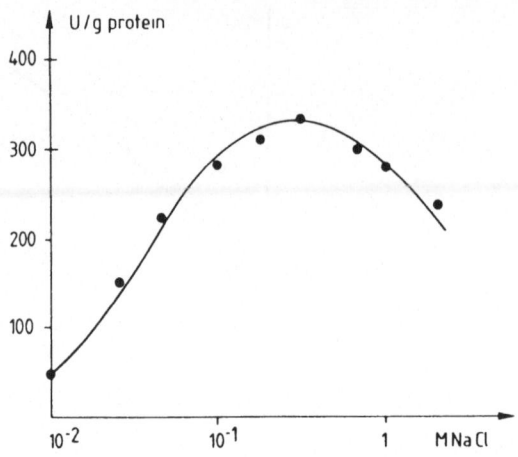

Figure 3.   Chloride ion effect on FAPGG (1 mmol/1) hydrolysis by human
seminal fluid kininase II.

Kinetic studies   The direct linear plot for FAPGG hydrolysis (Figure 1)
over the concentration range of 0.25 to 2 x 10^{-3} mM reveals a K_m of 7 x
10^{-4} mol/1 with a V_{max} of 335 µmol/min/g protein for the pool used in the
kinetic procedures (see Procedures). This K_m value is consistent with
that of kininase II from human serum[19] and rabbit lung,[10] indicating that
differences such as found in electrophoretic behaviour (unpublished results) can only be attributed to side chains, and not to the active site.

Table 1.   Kinetic properties of four kininase II inhibitors.

Inhibitor	Inhibitor concentration(a)	Apparent K_m (a)	Apparent V_{max}(b)	Inhibition constants (a)
1. Dipeptide Analogs				
Captopril (SQ 14225)	0	6.8×10^{-4}	563	$K_i = 7.3 \times 10^{-9}$
	8×10^{-10}	6.7×10^{-4}	560	
	1×10^{-9}	7.1×10^{-4}	567	
	2×10^{-9}	8.5×10^{-4}	567	
	5×10^{-9}	12.2×10^{-4}	570	
	1×10^{-8}	13.5×10^{-4}	570	
3-(Mercapto-methyl)- 2-oxo-1-piperidine acetic acid	0	7.0×10^{-4}	567	$K_i = 6.8 \times 10^{-7}$
	4.0×10^{-7}	9.2×10^{-4}	570	
	6.3×10^{-7}	12.1×10^{-4}	573	
	1.0×10^{-6}	12.2×10^{-4}	567	
	1.6×10^{-6}	16.6×10^{-4}	543	
2. Tripeptide Analogs				
Enalapril ethyl ester (MK 421)	0	6.8×10^{-4}	570	$K_i = 4.2 \times 10^{-6}$
	5.6×10^{-7}	7.6×10^{-4}	497	
	1.0×10^{-6}	8.5×10^{-4}	467	$K_i' = 6.4 \times 10^{-6}$
	3.2×10^{-6}	9.2×10^{-4}	387	
	5.6×10^{-6}	10.4×10^{-4}	327	
Enalapril diacid (MK 422)	0	1.56×10^{-3}	572	$K_i = 10^{-9}$
	3.9×10^{-10}	1.63×10^{-3}	390	
	7.9×10^{-10}	1.60×10^{-3}	325	$K_i' = 9.5 \times 10^{-10}$
	10^{-9}	1.65×10^{-3}	273	
	1.5×10^{-9}	1.70×10^{-3}	273	

(a) : mol/L   ;   (b) : µmol/min/g protein

472

Table 2. IC_{50} of the four inhibitor studies with regard to other data available in the literature.

IC_{50} (mol/l)	Tissue used
1. Dipeptide Analogs - Mercapto-acyl Amino Acids	
Captopril	
23×10^{-9}	rabbit lung (6)
4.5×10^{-9}	human lung (23)
12×10^{-9}	guinea-pig serum (7)
$2.9-34 \times 10^{-9}$ (mean 20)	hog plasma (8)
16×10^{-9}	human seminal plasma*
3-(Mercaptomethyl)-2-oxo-1-piperidineacetic acid	
1.0×10^{-6}	guinea-pig serum (7)
1.8×10^{-6}	human seminal plasma*
2. Tripeptide Analog-Carboxyalkyl Dipeptide	
Enalapril ethylester	
1.2×10^{-6}	hog plasma (8)
5.6×10^{-6}	human seminal plasma*
Enalapril diacid	
4.1×10^{-9}	human seminal plasma*

* present study

Inhibition Enalapril diacid was the most potent inhibitor tested (IC_{50} = 4.1×10^{-9} mol/l; $K_i = 10^{-9}$ mol/l; $K_i' = 9.5 \times 10^{-10}$ mol/l (Tables 1 and 2). In contrast, Enalapril ethylester proved to be less potent (IC_{50} = 5.6×10^{-6} mol/l), but it also produced a mixed competitive, non-competitive inhibition pattern ($K_i = 4.2 \times 10^{-6}$; $K_i' = 6.4 \times 10^{-6}$). Captopril gives IC_{50} = 1.6×10^{-8} mol/l; $K_i = 7.3 \times 10^{-9}$ and it acted as a purely competitive inhibitor.

3-(Mercaptomethyl)-2-oxo-1-piperidineacetic acid had an IC_{50} of 1.8×10^{-6} and was purely competitive ($K_i = 6.8 \times 10^{-7}$). In our experimental setting, however, this compound lost its inhibiting properties rather quickly, probably due to oxidation of the mercaptan.

This study, as well as most of the published in vitro work on these inhibitors, is based on inhibition models using N-terminal blocked tri-peptide substrates. Assays using Hip-His-Leu the most frequently employed substrate are prone to large errors due to very low enzymatic activities originating from substrate inhibition. These difficulties, which arise especially at low substrate and high inhibitor concentrations, are probably the reason why so few kinetic data are known about these important inhibitors. More recent methods, such as the one used here, or the one using an intramolecularly quenched substrate[17] have proven more appropriate for kinetic studies, not in the least because they allow continuous measurements. Although the enzyme preparation used was obtained from another species organ than that used in the original inhibitor studies, our results are very similar for both the dipeptide and tripeptide inhibitor analogs (Table 2). Captopril has been reported to act as a competitive inhibitor of rabbit lung kininase II with a K_i almost identical with that found in the current experiments.[20]

Kinetic studies of 3-(mercaptomethyl)-2-oxo-1-piperidineacetic acid have not been published. The IC_{50} here reported agrees closely with the IC_{50} for kininase II from guinea-pig serum. The competitive nature of the inhibition is not surprising, because the molecule is mainly rearranged, albeit less potent, version of captopril. The IC_{50} and the kinetic inhibition constants, obtained for the tripeptide analog, Enalapril ethylester and its diacid form are in close accorance with those originally reported for hog plasma enzyme by Patchett et al.[8] While diacid form is a carboxyalkyldipeptide devoid of thiol groups, it nonetheless effectively inhibits the seminal fluid enzyme.

It is of interest to note that the activity of Enalapril ethylester, which in this study has mixed competitive and non-competitive inhibition, last longer than that of competitive captopril.[21] Kininase II activity in the male genital tract is remarkably high. Its function and its natural substrate(s) in human seminal plasma being still unknown, the relation of the in vitro inhibition to possible in vivo effects of these inhibitors remains to be elucidated. Because the captopril concentration in plasma is 10^3 times greater than that used in these inhibition studies, an influence on sperm motility has to be considered. In a recent study,[22] 18% of male infertility was treated with a proteinase inhibitor, and in another study,[4] it was shown that sperm motility could be enhanced by adding captopril. Hence, this effect of captopril or other potent kininase II inhibitors needs thorough examination.

ACKNOWLEDGEMENTS

We are highly indebted to Mr. E. Cuypers and Mr. R. Verkerk for their skillful technical assistance.

REFERENCES

1. M. A. Hollinger, Serum angiotensin-converting enzyme. Status report on its diagnostic significance in pulmonary disease, Chest, 83: 589-590, (1983).

2. D. Depierre, J. P. Bargetzi, and M. Roth, Dipeptidyl carboxypeptidase from human seminal sperm, Biochim. Biophys. Acta, 523:469-476, (1978).

3. S. Kaneko, & C. Moriwaki, Studies on dipeptidyl carboxypeptidase in the male reproductive organs; its biological and pathological status, J. Pharm. Dyn., 4:175-183, (1981).

4. S. Kaneko, & C. Moriwaki, Effects of kinins and dipeptidyl carboxypeptidase on the motility of highly washed human sperm, J. Pharm. Dyn., 4:443-450, (1981).

5. M. Horiuchi, K. I. Fukumura, T. Terashima, & T. Iso, Method for determination of angiotensin-converting enzyme activity in blood and tissue by high performance liquid chromatography, J. Chromatogr., 233:123-130, (1982).

6. M. A. Ondetti, B. Rubin, & D. W. Cushman, Design of specific inhibitors of angiotensin-converting enzyme: new class of orally active antihypertensive agents, Science, 166:441-444, (1977).

7. S. Klutcho, M. L. Hoefle, R. D. Smith, et al., Synthhsis and angiotensin-converting enzyme inhibitory activity of 3-(mercaptomethyl)-2-oxo-1-pyrrolidineacetic acids and 3-(mercaptomethyl)-2-oxo-1-piperidineacetic acids, J. Med. Chem., 24:104-109, (1980).

8. A. A. Patchett, E. Harris, E. W. Tristram, et al., A new class of angiotensin-converting enzyme inhibitors, Nature, 288:280-283, (1980).

9. R. J. Klauser, C. J. G. Robinson, D. V. Marinkovic, & E. G. Erdös, Inhibition of human peptidyl dipeptidase (angiotensin-I converting enzyme: kininase II) by human serum albumin and its fragments, Hypertension, 1:281-286, (1979).

10. B. Holmquist, P. Bünning, & J. F. Riordan, A continuous spectrophotometric assay for angiotensin converting enzyme, Anal. Biochem., 95:540-548, (1979).

11. R. Eisenthal, & A. Cornish-Bowden, The direct linear plot. A new graphical procedure for estimating enzyme kinetic parameters, Biochem. J., 139:715-720, (1974).

12. G. L. Atkins, & I. A. Nimmo, Current trends in the estimation of Michaelis-Menten parameters, Anal. Biochem., 104:1-9, (1980).

13. A. Cornish-Bowden, Principles of enzyme kinetics. Inhibitors and activators, Butterworths, London, p. 52, (1976).

14. R. B. Loftfield, & E. A. Eigner, Molecular order of participation of inhibitors (or activators) in biological systems, Science, 164:305-308, (1969).

15. H. M. Neels, S. L. Scharpé, M. E. van Sande, & G. A. Fonteyne, Single-reagent micro centrifugal assay for antiotensin converting enzyme, Clin. Chem., 30:163-164, (1984).

16. D. W. Cushman, & H. S. Cheung, Concentrations of angiotensin converting enzyme in tissues of the rat, Biochim. Biophys. Acta, 250:261-265, (1971).

17. H. M. Neels, S. L. Scharpé, G. A. Fonteyne, et al., Fluorometric assay for angiotensin converting enzyme in human serum by centrifugal analysis, Clin. Chim. Acta, 141:281-286, (1984).

18. H. M. Neels, S. L. Scharpé, M. E. Van Sande, et al., Improved micromethod for assay of serum angiotensin converting enzyme, Clin. Chem., 28:1352-1355, (1982).

19. S. Ronca-Testoni, Direct spectrophotometric assay for angiotensin converting enzyme in serum, Clin. Chem., 29:1093-1096, (1983).

20. D. W. Cushman, H. S. Cheung, E. F. Sabo, & M. A. Ondetti, Design of potent competitive inhibitors of angiotensin converting enzyme. Carboxyalkanoyl and mercaptoalkanoyl aminoacids, Biochem., 16:5484-5491, (1977).

21. H. Gravas, J. Biollaz, B. Waeber, et al., Effects of the oral angiotensin converting enzyme inhibitor MK-421 in human hypertension, Clin. Sci., 6:281s-283s, (1981).

22. H. Sato, Components of kallikrein kinin system and treatment of male infertility, Keio J. Med., 29:19-38, (1980).

23. C. Gronhagen-Riska, & F. Fyhrquist, Purification of human lung angiotensin converting snzyme, Scand. J. Clin. Lab. Invest., 40:711-719, (1980).

INVESTIGATIONS ON THE FUNCTIONAL ROLE OF ANGIOTENSIN CONVERTING ENZYME

(ACE) IN HUMAN SEMINAL PLASMA

Franz Krassnigg, Harald Niederhauser, Rainer Placzek,
Julian Frick* and Wolf-Bernhard Schill

Department of Dermatology, Andrology Unit, Ludwig-Maximilians
University of Munich, D-8000 Munich 2, German Federal Republic
and *Urological Department, General Hospital, A-5020 Salzburg
Austria

SUMMARY

The investigations were carried out with partially purified angiotensin
converting enzyme (E.C.3.4.15.1) from human seminal plasma and from human
blood plasma. The Km-constants for angiotensin converting enzyme (ACE)
from both sources, estimated by the use of synthetic substrates, were in
the same order. The catalytic properties of the enzymes were characterized
by a series of known peptidase inhibitors. The male antifertility drug
gossypol (1,1',6,6',7,7'-hexahydroxy-3,3'-dimethyl-5,5'-bis-isopropyl-(2,2'-
naphthalene)-8,8'-dicarboxaldehyde) was identified as a potent ACE-inhibitor.
The inhibitory constants of several kinins and other biologically active
peptides were determined. Any regulatory influence of the peptides investigated on the ACE-activity in vivo is not probably. The inhibitor of Zn-
containing metalloproteases 2-(N-hydroxycarboxamido)-4-methylpentanoyl-
L-alanylglycine amide) (Zinkov[TM]) selectively inhibited ACE from blood
plasma, whereas ACE from seminal plasma was not influenced. In seminal
plasma the majority of the enzyme is associated with macromolecular structures, identified as membrane vesicles. These vesicles contain also other
enzymatic activities usually detectable in seminal plasma. In the male
genital tract ACE is synthesized in the prostate, epididymis and testis.
As our data indicate ACE seems not to be involved in the regulation of
sperm motility.

INTRODUCTION

Synthesis and inactivation of vasoactive peptides is controlled in
vivo to a large extent by four different enzymes: kallikrein, renin, angio-
tensinases and ACE. Originally ACE was discovered in the blood of animals.
Studies in this field increased, when the biologically important conversion
of blood-borne angiotensin I to angiotensin II by ACE, located on the luminal
surface of small blod vessels in the lung and other tissues, was detected.[1]
Quantitative measurements of ACE-activities in various tissues are normally
carried out by spectrophotometric assays.[2]

In man the highest ACE-activities are detectable in the lung and in
tissues and secretory products of the male reproductive organs.

In testis and epididymis of the rat ACE-levels were also investigated under different experimental conditions.[3] In the brain, retina and adrenal cortex the primary vascular localization of ACE was shown by immunofluorescent techniques. High ACE-levels could also be demonstrated in cultured vascular endothelial cells. These cells are able to release up to 40 times of their initial ACE-activity thus supporting the view that the vascular endothelium is the main source for ACE in blood. The diagnostically valuable estimation of ACE-activities in blood in certain diseases is due to an increase of the enzyme activity in macrophages, as it is shown in leprosy, in epitheloid granuloma cells tyupical for sarcoidosis and in Gaucher cells in Gaucher's disease. The functional role of ACE in seminal plasma, where the enzyme is present in significantly higher amounts than in all other body fluids and tissues, is still elusive, although there are reports indicating an involvement of components of the kallikrein-kinin system in the regulation of sperm motility.[4]

MATERIALS AND METHODS

Semen samples were obtained from healthy donors and from patients with fertility disorders seeking advice at our outpatient clinic. Fresh ejaculates were allowed to liquify for 60 min at 22°C. Sperm count and viability (percentage of motile spermatozoa) were determined. After centrifugation at 600 x g for 30 min the seminal plasma was pooled and stored at -24°C. Blood plasma was received from patients of the Dermatological Department.

ACE-Activity Determination

The release of hippuric acid from the substrate hippuryl-L-His-L-Leu was measured for 30 min at pH 8.3 and 37°C, as described by Cushman.[5] Additionally, n-butanol was added for the suppression of unspecific proteolytic activities. All peptidase inhibitors and the applied biologically active peptides were dissolved in substrate puffer. For the dissolution of gossypol acetic acid, a solvent system consisting of 0.8% (v/v) N,N'-dimethylformamide in substrate puffer was used.

Isolation of ACE from Seminal Plasma and From Blood Plasma

Pooled human seminal plasma and blood plasma were dialyzed and submitted to DEAE-sephacel ion exchange chromatography. Elution was performed by a step-wise gradient of NaCl ranging from 0-0.3 M/l in Tris-HCl puffer pH 7.32.[6] The eluted ACE-activities were concentrated and submitted to gel chromatography with Sepharose 6B as gel matrix.

Sedimentation of ACE-Activity by Ultracentrifugation

Pooled, native seminal plasma was centrifuged at 106000 x g for 6 hours. The pellet was resuspended in Tris-HCl puffer, pH 7.32.[6] For the final purification of the sediment gel chromatography (Sepharose 6B) was used. Equilibration and elution of the column was performed with Tris-HCI puffer, pH 7.32.[6]

Determination of Sperm Motility

The motility of washed human spermatozoa was measured in Tyrode solution, pH 7.30. Sperm count was adjusted to 60-70 x 10^6 x ml^{-1}.

Protein concentratons were estimated by the method of Lowry with bovine serum albumine as a standard.

Preparation of Tissue Extracts

Samples of prostatic, epididymis, testis and skeletal muscle tissue, received from the Urological Department, General Hospital Salzburg, were homogenized at 0-4°C and extracted with isotonic Tris-HCl puffer, pH 7.32.[6] The specific ACE-activities were determined in the supernatants after centrifugation (600 x g, 30 min).

RESULTS

ACE-Determination

All ACE-activity data presented here have been identified as specific by control experiments with the specific ACE-inhibitor captopril.

Properties of ACE Isolated from Seminal Plasma and From Blood Plasma

ACE from blood plasma and from seminal plasma showed in the assay pH optima of about 8.3 and Km's in the range of 10^{-6} M. The Vmax of both enzymes were 3.7 and 4.0 x 10^{-6} M x min^{-1} (Table 1).

Distribution of the ACE-Activity in Seminal Plasma

Gel chromatography of human seminal plasma (Sephrose 6B) demonstrated the association of the ACE-activity with macromolecular structures, identified in the electron microscope as membrane vesicles with diameters of 100 nm or less (Figure 1). The same was found for ACE from blood plasma, where also a partially association of ACE with large particles is demonstrable (Figure 2).

Distribution of the ACE-Activity in Tissues of the Male Genital Tract

Determination of the ACE-activity in extracts of tissues from the male genital tract, prepared under identical conditions, revealed significant activity differences. The highest ACE-levels were present in extracts from prostatic tissue, but epididymis and testis contained also significant activities, in comparison to the levels present in skeletal muscle (Figure 3).

Table 1. Properties of Angiotensin Converting Enzyme Isolated from Blood Plasma and from Seminal Plasma

	ACE(seminal plasma)	ACE(blood plasma)
Km(10^{-6}M x 1^{-1})	2.45 ± 0.28	2.90 ± 0.40
Vmax(10^{-6}M x min^{-1})	3.7 ± 0.2	4.0 ± 0.2
pH optimum	8.2 - 8.5	8.3
temperature optimum (° C)	32 - 37	37 - 38

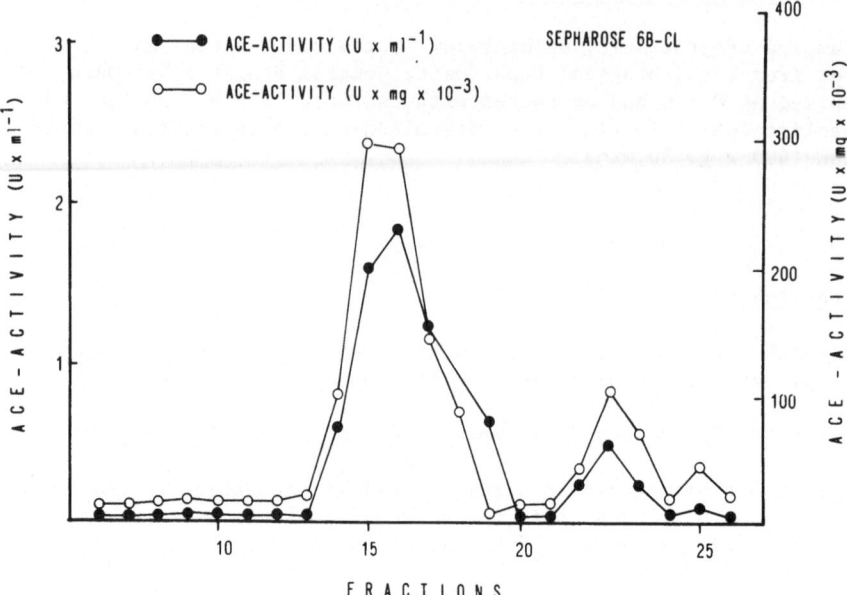

Fig. 1.   Gel chromatography of human seminal plasma.   Distribution of ACE-
activity.   Elution was performed with Tris-HCl puffer.[6]

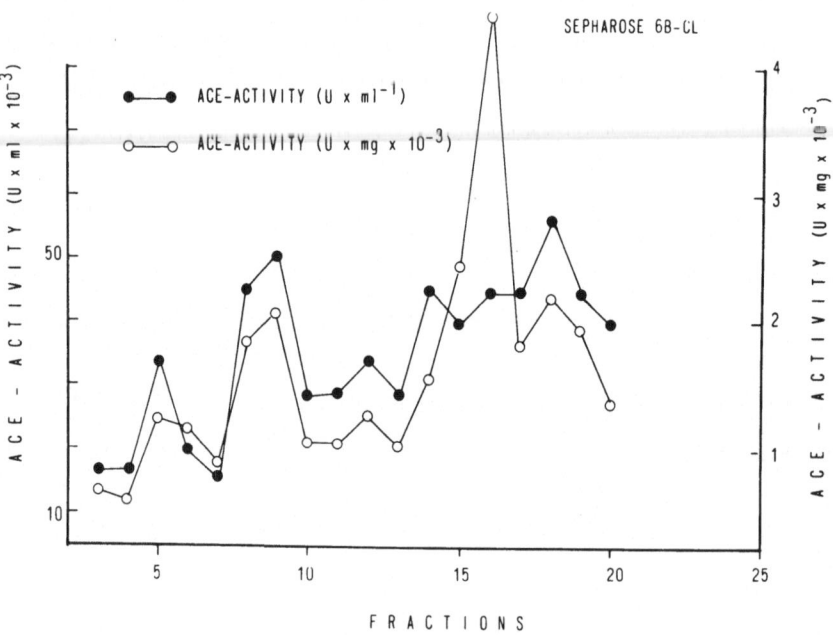

Fig. 2.   Gel chromatography of blood plasma.   Distribution of ACE-activity.
Elution was performed with Tris-HCl puffer.[6]

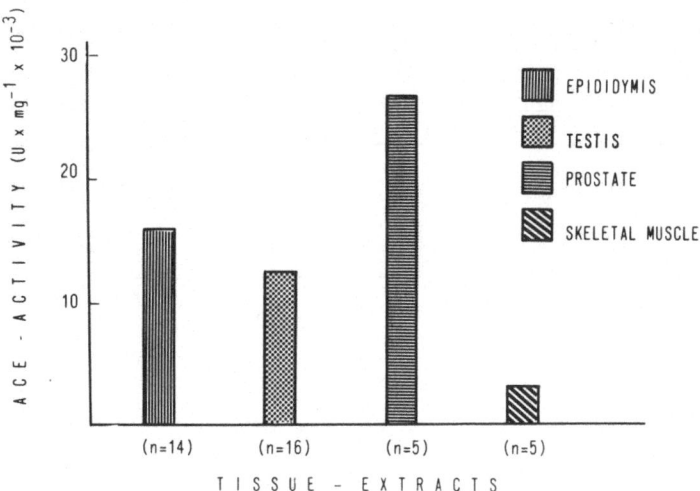

Fig. 3. Distribution of ACE-activity in extracts from tissues of the male
         genital tract.

Preparation of ACE From Seminal Plasma and From Blood Plasma

     The partially purified ACE showed specific activities of 125 U x
mg^{-1} for ACE from seminal plasma and of 83 U x mg^{-1} for the enzyme from
blood plasma. The purification led to a nearly hundredfold enrichment of
the specific activities.

Inhibition of ACE-Activity

     A number of peptidase inhibitors were able to inhibit the enzymes from
both sources with inhibitory constants in the range of 10^{-3} to 10^{-9} M x
1^{-1}. However Zinkov^{TM}, well characterized as inhibitor of Zn-containing
metalloproteases, inhibited only ACE from blood plasma (Table 2).

Influence of Kinins and Other Biologically Active Peptides on the ACE-Activity

     Kinins and other active peptides were assayed for their influence on
the ACE-activity. The estimated inhibitory constants for ACE from both
sources were low in every case (Table 3).

Determination of the Regulatory Influence of ACE on the Motility of Spermatozoa

     The effects of the ACE-inhibitors gossypol acetic acid and captopril
(3-SH-2-methylpropionyl-L-proline) on the motility of human spermatozoa
were determined. Only gossypol acetic acid completely inhibited the sperm
motility in an irreversible manner at concentrations of 10^{-4} M x 1^{-1} (Figure
4). Captopril has no inhibitory influence on sperm motility in vitro.
At concentrations of more than 10^{-3} M x 1^{-1} a motility enhancement was measured (Figure 5).

DISCUSSION

     Many studies about the action of kinins in blood and other body fluids
e.g. seminal plasma are limited by the fact that these peptides undergo

Table 2. Inhibition of ACE-Activity by Peptidase Inhibitors

	50% inhibition (M x 1^{-1})	
	ACE(plasma)	ACE(seminal plasma)
Captopril	2.9×10^{-9}	5.0×10^{-9}
Gossypol acetic acid	8.8×10^{-5}	7.0×10^{-5}
Pyr-Gly-Leu-Pro-Pro Arg-Pro-Lys-Ile-Pro-Pro	1.3×10^{-4}	8.3×10^{-3}
Pepstatin	no inhibition	no inhibition
Neurotensin	5.8×10^{-1}	6.6×10^{-1}
Zinkov^{TM}	5.2×10^{-5}	no inhibition
D-Phe-Ala-L-Phe-Ala-L-Arg-chloromethyl-ketone	1.0×10^{-1}	1.4

Table 3. Influence of Biologically Active Peptides and Kinins on the ACE-Activity

	50% inhibition (M x 1^{-1})	
	ACE(plasma)	ACE(seminal plasma)
Met-kallidin	3.7×10^{-2}	5.0×10^{-2}
Kallidin	1.2×10^{-1}	1.0×10^{-1}
Bradykinin	2.3×10^{-3}	6.0×10^{-1}
Angiotensin I	no inhibition	no inhibition
Angiotensin II	1.1	no inhibition
Angiotensin III	2.8×10^{-1}	5.1×10^{-1}
Met-enkephalin	2.8	6.3×10^{-1}

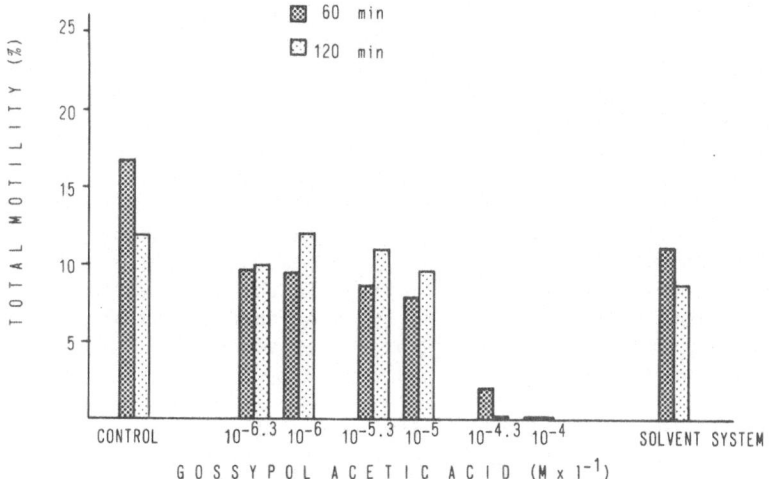

Fig. 4. Inhibition of sperm motility by gossypol acetic acid. Sperm count was $65 \times 10^6 \times ml^{-1}$.

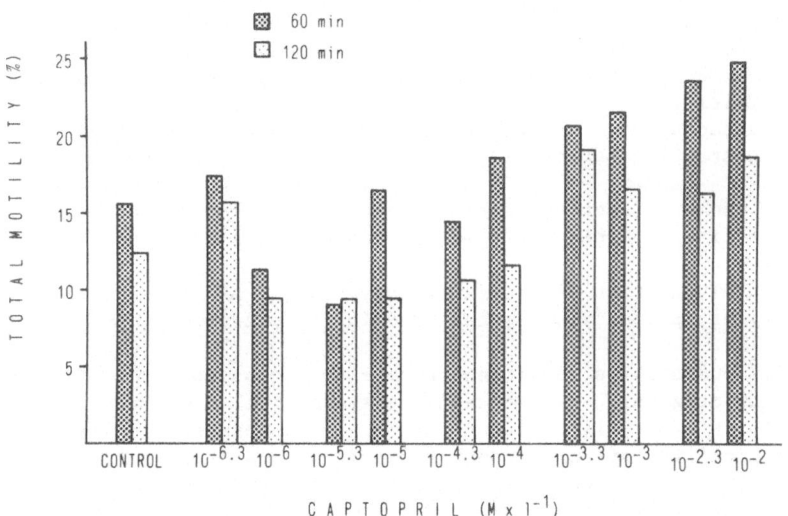

Fig. 5. Influence of captopril on the motility of human spermatozoa. Sperm count was adjusted to $65 \times 10^6 \times ml^{-1}$.

a rapid turnover. The inactivation depends to a large extent on the action of unspecific kininases and probably more important in vivo on the action of ACE. So far no differences in the catalytic properties of ACE from seminal plasma and other body fluids and tissues have been reported. By the use of a series of inhibitors we could demonstrate that many of the substances investigated revealed only small differences in their inhibitory properties on ACE derived from seminal plasma and from blood. The exception was Zinkov[TM], already characterized as an inhibitor of the Zn-containing metalloprotease thermolysin, of a bacterial elastase and of the membrane-bound enkephalinase from mouse striatum, which inhibited selectively ACE from blood plasma, whereas the activity of ACE from seminal plasma was not influenced. The easiest explanation for this finding is the assumption that induced steric differences in the binding sites of ACE exist, which enable only the attachment of more or less hydrophobic compounds. The coordination of the central zinc atom of ACE could be in addition of great importance for the binding of inhibitors. This seems to be the case for the specific ACE-inhibitor captopril, an aliphatic thiol derivative which appears to be an efficient monodentate ligand for the central zinc atom of the enzyme. After binding of the inhibitor the attachment of substrate molecules is completely impossible.

As we have shown, the ACE-activity in seminal plasma is associated with macromolecular structures, which were identified in the electron microscope as membrane vesicles. In blood plasma we could also demonstrate at least in part an association of the ACE-activity to macromolecular structures. These vesicles contain in addition the whole ATPase-activity of the seminal plasma together with activities of L-leucineaminopeptidase and acid phosphatase. The functional role of the vesicles in the fertilization process is unknown.

The different distribution of ACE in the male genital tract of mammals was already reported.[3] This study has shown that in man the highest ACE-levels are detectable in the prostate, but epididymis and testis also contain elevated values in comparison to the activities present in the skeletal muscle. These data are in good accordance with the results of ACE-determinations in split ejaculates, where the first fraction always contains the highest activities. Our findings are further supported by the fact that ACE-levels detectable in seminal plasma after vasectomy are significantly reduced demonstrating the partial origin of ACE from epididymis and testis.

Kinins and other active peptides seem to have no regulatory influence on the ACE-activity of blood plasma and seminal plasma, as our data show.

For the elucidation of the functional role of ACE in seminal plasma the motility of spermatozoa was measured in the presence of ACE-inhibitors.

At this occasion we could demonstrate that gossypol, the only male antifertility drug which has reached the stage of clinical trial so far,[8] is a potent inhibitor of ACE from both sources. Gossypol is also able to inhibit the motility of human spermatozoa.[9] On the other hand we could demonstrate that the specific ACE-inhibitor captopril has no inhibitory influence on the motility of human spermatozoa at low concentrations, whereas at higher concentrations an improvement of the sperm motility was observed.

These results support the view that ACE is not directly involved in the regulation of sperm motility.

In summary, our studies brought evidence for heterogenities in the catalytic properties of ACE. The data are first indications for the existence of tissue-specific angiotensin converting enzymes.

ACKNOWLEDGEMENT

This study was supported by the DFG, SFB 0207, LP-20.

REFERENCES

1. M. A. Ondretti and D. W. Cushman, Enzymes of the renin-angiotensin system and their inhibitors, Ann. Rev. Biochem., 51:283-308 (1982).
2. D. W. Cushman and H. S. Cheung, Concentrations of angiotensin converting enzyme in tissues of the rat, Biochem. Biophys. Acta, 250:261-265 (1971).
3. G. Hohlbrugger, H. Schweisfurth, and H. Dahlheim, Angiotensin converting enzyme in rat testis, epididymis and vas deferens under different conditions, J. Reprod. Fertil., 65:97-103 (1982).
4. W.-B. Schill and G. L. haberland, Kinin-induced enhancement of sperm motility, Hoppe-Seyler's Z. Physiol. Chem., 355:229-231 (1974).
5. D. W. Cushman and H. S. Cheung, Spectrophotometric assay and properties of the angiotensin converting enzyme in rabbit lung, Biochem. Pharmacol., 20:1637-1648 (1971).
6. B. Stegmayr and G. Ronquist, Promotive effect on human sperm progressive motility by prostasomes, Urol. Res., 10:253-257 (1982).
7. A. Makler, A new multiple exposure photography method for objective sperm motility determination, Fertil. Steril., 30:192-199 (1978).
8. G. Z. Liu, Clinical study of gossypol as a male contraceptive, Reproduction, 5:189-193 (1981).
9. N. R. Kalla and M. Vasudev, Studies on the male antifertility agent gossypol acetic acid. I. In vitro studies on the effect of gossypol acetic acid in human spermatozoa, IRCS Med. Sci. Biochem., 8:375-379 (1980).

BIOLOGICAL REGULATION OF TESTICULAR ANGIOTENSIN I-CONVERTING ENZYME

Paul A. Velletri and Walter Lovenberg

Section of Biochemical Pharmacology
National Heart, Lung and Blood Institute
Bethesda, Maryland 20205

SUMMARY

Angiotensin I-converting enzyme (ACE) from rat testes and lung was purified to homogeneity and partially characterized with respect to physicochemical parameters. Additionally, the biological regulation of testicular ACE by gonadotropins and androgens was investigated and the cell type with which ACE is associated in testes was identified. Rat testicular ACE is a lower molecular weight, isozymic version of the lung enzyme. Partial proteolysis of each isozyme produces different peptide maps, suggesting unique primary structures for each protein. The sensitivity of each isozyme to Co^{2+}, chelators and thermal denaturation is different, a finding that further supports the hypothesis that structural differences exist between the two isozymes. The pituitary gland is essential for the development during puberty and maintenance during adulthood of testicular ACE. In hypophysectomized mature rats, gonadotropins or androgen can maintain ACE activity to near sham-operated levels. ACE activity in testes appears to be associated almost entirely with various stages of germinal cell development. The function(s) of testicular ACE awaits definition. The mechanism of androgen-maintenance of testicular ACE is unclear. Whether androgen specifically induces gene expression of testicular ACE or simply allows for ACE activity to develop in parallel with spermatogenesis is an unresolved question.

INTRODUCTION

Angiotensin I-converting enzyme (kininase II; E.C. 3.4.15.1; ACE) is a metal-containing dipeptidyl carboxypeptidase that is ubiquitously distributed in mammals. Its role in the conversion of blood-borne angiotensin I to angiotensin II in the pulmonary circulation has been well documented,[1] and it now appears as though ACE can recognize a number of biologically active peptides, or their precursors, as substrates. The pulmonary source of ACE has been the most extensively characterized due to its well established physiological role in peptide processing.

However, in 1971, Cushman and Cheung undertook a regional tissue distribution study of ACE activity in the rat,[2] and found that testes possessed a converting enzyme of a specific activity comparable to or in excess of that found in rat lung. They further noted that the testicular enzyme developed during puberty and that hypophysectomy arrested the pubertal development of testicular ACE.

Recently, a comparison of purified rabbit pulmonary and testicular ACE indicated that the testicular enzyme had a markedly lower molecular weight and a different amino- and carboxyl-terminal peptide sequence than the pulmonary enzyme.[3] Furthermore, the rabbit testicular enzyme displayed certain physicochemical and immunological differences when compared to the pulmonary enzyme. Michaelis-Menten estimations of kinetic parameters indicated that the rabbit pulmonary and testicular isozymes shared similar catalytic properties. However, the above-cited structural and immunological differences between pulmonary and testicular ACE appeared to be due to tissue-specific expression of mRNA.

It is unclear what the biological consequences, if any, of the presence of ACE isozymes in different tissues might be. Furthermore, the endocrinological control of testicular ACE and the cell type with which gonadel ACE is associated have not been explored. It is possible that the structural variations in the isozymes may affect their thermodynamic stability and therefore their rate of degradation or turnover in vivo. The relationship between thermodynamic stability and in vivo turnover is predicted by the conformer equilibria hypothesis, which suggests that for many proteins the rate of unfolding (thermal stability) is the rate-limiting step in proteolysis (see Ref. 4). Differences in the turnover of each isozyme in a specific tissue is an intriguing hypothesis in light of the potential for tissue-specific hormonal control of testicular, but not pulmonary, ACE.

The studies reported in this paper were conducted in an attempt to assess the functional significance of the different structures of pulmonary and testicular ACE and to determine the hormones responsible for the pubertal development and maintenance during adulthood of testicular ACE. Additionally, the cell type with which testicular ACE is associated was explored. The thermal denaturation of pulmonary and testicular ACE was studied in the presence and absence of chelators to assess the role of divalent cations in maintaining structural integrity of each isozyme, and these studies were related to the endocrinological control of testicular ACE.

METHODS

Methodologies for the quantitation of ACE activity, the purification of ACE from rat lung and testes, the generation of proteolytic peptide maps, the kinetic analysis of inhibitory effects of reagents on ACE and comparisons of the thermal stabilities of purified ACE isozymes have been described in detail by Velletri et al.[4] Descriptions of hypophysectomy and hormone-replacement protocols, separation of testicular cell types by centrifugal elutriation and captopril binding to intact germinal cells can be found in Velletri et al.[5] The results presented in the five tables of this paper represent preliminary data first reported at the International Kinin Congress 1984 in Savannah, GA, USA, and subsequently described in considerably greater detail in Refs. 7 and 8.

RESULTS AND DISCUSSION

1. Physicochemical Properties

The data summarized in Table 1 clearly indicate that rat pulmonary
and testicular ACE are isozymes of each other. Pulmonary ACE is 55,000
daltons larger than testicular ACE and, upon proteolytic digestion,
generates a different peptide map than the testicular enzyme. Halide
activation of each isozyme appears to be identical, although the response
of purified ACE from each tissue to Co^{2+} is different: at pH 8, Co^{2+} has
virtually no effect on pulmonary ACE, but is a strong inhibitor of testicular ACE. Although the response of purified pulmonary or testicular ACE to
site-directed inhibitors or sulfhydryl compounds was identical, pulmonary
ACE was one order of magnitude more sensitive to chelators than the
testicular enzyme. The above data indicate that reagents (i.e., Co^{2+} and
chelators) that may interact with the divalent metal ion present in the
holoenzyme have different effects on each isozyme of ACE. Such findings
suggest, but by no means prove, distinct interactions of the divalent
cation with its respective ACE isozymic apoenzyme. Although it is well
known that Zn^{2+} is an essential component of pulmonary ACE,[1] the nature
of the divalent cation in the testicular isozyme remains to be elucidated,
and it is therefore possible that the different actions of Co^{2+} and
chelators on each isozyme may reside in the type of cation present in each
isozyme.

The thermodynamic stabilities of purified pulmonary and testicular
ACE were markedly different (Table 1). Residual ACE activity was
measured following incubation of ACE at 55°C for varying periods of time.
Pulmonary ACE was three times more stable to denaturation and loss of
activity at 55°C than its testicular counterpart. Thermal denaturation
of each isozyme was markedly potentiated by the presence of chelators such
as EDTA. In fact, the differences in the thermal stabilities of each
enzyme were attenuated by carrying out the thermal denaturation studies
in the presence of chelators. These data suggest that the divalent
cation associated with each ACE isozyme may play an integral role not only
in the catalytic activity of each enzyme but in the maintenance of its
tertiary structure. Because the tertiary structure of a protein may re-
late to its thermodynamic stability and susceptibility to proteolysis (as
predicted by the conformer equilibria hypothesis described in Ref. 4),
the fact that native pulmonary ACE is more resistant to heat denaturation
than its testicular counterpart might signify that different rates of
proteolysis of each isozyme occur in vivo. As the specific activities
of crude pulmonary and testicular ACE in rat are comparable, one might
predict a more rapid turnover of testicular ACE in vivo if its susceptibility to proteolytic digestion is greater than that of pulmonary
ACE. A more rapid turnover of the testicular enzyme is consistent with
the potential endocrinological control of testicular ACE.

2. Hypophysectomy and Hormone Replacement

To explore the regulation of testicular ACE by hormones, hypophysectomy studies were conducted on pre-pubescent and mature rats. As
shown in Table II, hypophysectomy of pre-pubescent rats prevented the
development of testicular ACE activity. Values of testicular ACE
activity were only 5% of levels detected in sham-operated animals.
Levels of pulmonary ACE were unaffected by hypophysectomy and, unlike
testicular ACE activity, pulmonary ACE activity was present from birth
(data not shown). Although protein synthesis decreased in the testes
of hypophysectomized rats (as measured by the protein to wet weight
ratio), the drop in ACE activity was in marked excess to that drop. To

Table I. Summary of Physicochemical Properties of Rat Pulmonary and
Testicular ACE

Property	Pulmonary ACE	Testicular ACE
Molecular Weight[1]	175,000	120,000
Staphylococcus V8 Proteolytic Peptide Maps[2]	6 major peptide fragments	7 major peptide fragments
Effect of Cl^-	Activation ($EC_{50} \simeq 0.15$ M)	Activation ($EC_{50} \simeq 0.15$ M)
Effect of Co^{2+}	Negligible at ph 8.0	Inhibitory at ph 8.0
Inhibition by Chelators		
1. EDTA	$IC_{50} \simeq 10^{-5}$ M	$IC_{50} \simeq 10^{-4}$ M
2. 1,10-phenanthroline	$IC_{50} \simeq 5 \times 10^{-5}$ M	$IC_{50} \simeq 5 \times 10^{-4}$ M
Inhibition by Site-Directed Inhibitors		
1. Captopril	$IC_{50} \simeq 10^{-9}$ M	$IC_{50} \simeq 10^{-9}$ M
2. Teprotide	$IC_{50} \simeq 5 \times 10^{-8}$ M	$IC_{50} \simeq 5 \times 10^{-8}$ M
Thermal Denaturation at 55°C		
1. Control	$t1/_2 \simeq 6$ min	$t1/_2 \simeq 2$ min
2. + 100 μM EDTA	$t1/_2 \simeq 1.5$ min	$t1/_2 \simeq 1$ min

These data are summarized from experiments that have been described in
detail in Velletri et al.[4]

[1] Molecular weight determined by SDS-PAGE (7.5% polyacrylamide).

[2] Peptide fragments generated from pulmonary ACE did not possess molecular
weights comparable to those peptide fragments generated from
testicular ACE.

our knowledge, this report is the first that confirms the original observation of Cushman and Cheung[2] that the pituitary gland is necessary
for the pubertal development of testicular ACE.

Furthermore, hypophysectomy of mature rats that have been allowed to
develop testicular ACE activity results in an almost total loss of gonadal
enzyme activity within three weeks (Table III). The drop in enzyme
activity was far greater than the drop in testicular wet weight following surgery. Hence, the studies reported above clearly suggest that the
pituitary gland is required for both the pubertal development and maintenance during adulthood of testicular ACE activity.

Table II. Pubertal Development of Testicular ACE Requires Presence of
Pituitary Gland

Tissue	Tissue Wet Weight	Protein/Wet Weight	ACE Activity
	grams	mg. protein/g. wet wt.	mUnits/mg. protein
Lung			
Sham-Operated	3.06 ± 0.102	125 ± 3.51	26.6 ± 1.19
Hypophysectomized	1.47 ± 0.11 (*)	109 ± 7.16	32.7 ± 2.67
Testis			
Sham-Operated	3.12 ± 0.086	95.4 ± 1.58	11.3 ± 2.08
Hypophysectomized	0.084 ± 0.005 (*)	83.1 ± 1.71	0.59 ± 0.183 (*)

All values represent means ± one standard error of 10 sham-operated or 9
hypophysectomized rats. Animals were hypophysectomized at 3 weeks of age
and allowed to undergo puberty and mature to 10 weeks of age. These data
are based on experiments presented for publication in greater detail in
Velletri et al.[5]

(*) p<0.001 compared to sham-operated value.

Table III. Maintenance of Testicular ACE in Adulthood Requires Presence
of Pituitary Gland

Treatment	Testicular Wet Weight	Protein/Wet Weight	ACE Activity
	g. wet wt.	mg. protein/g. wet wt.	mUnits/mg. protein
Sham-Operated	3.64 ± 0.10	112 ± 1.9	5.63 ± 0.63
Hypophysectomized	1.09 ± 0.062 (*)	116 ± 3.3	0.66 ± 0.072 (*)

All values represent mean ± one standard error of 5 sham-operated and 7
hypophysectomized rats. Animals were hypophysectomized at 10 weeks of
age and the study concluded 13 days following surgery. Further details
can be obtained from data presented for publication in Velletri et al.[5]

* p<0.001 compared to sham-operated value.

Three protocols of hormone replacement therapy were employed in an attempt to assess which hormones regulate ACE activity in testes: (1) follicle stimulating hormone/luteinizing hormone (FSH/LH) at 7.5 units/rat x day; (2) human chorionic gonadotropin (hCG) at 10 units/rat x day; and (3) testosterone (Test) at 3 mg/rat x day. Eight to 10 days of hormone replacement therapy with any one of the above regimens failed to elevate testicular ACE activity in mature rats that were hypophysectomized when pre-pubescent and therefore had never developed enzyme activity, or in mature rats that were hypophysectomized following development of enzyme activity but were allowed to lose all testicular ACE prior to the initiation of hormone replacement therapy. Hence, it was difficult to re-initiate ACE synthesis if the enzyme had never developed or if it were allowed to disappear completely (data not shown).

However, if the same hormone replacement protocol were initiated on the first day following hypophysectomy of mature rats possessing ACE activity and maintained for 21 days, all three hormone regimens were capable of maintaining over 80% of control testicular ACE activity seen in sham-operated rats (Table IV). Untreated, hypophysectomized rats lost virtually all testicular ACE activity within 21 days. The fact that maintenance of testicular ACE activity following hypophysectomy was sensitive to all three hormone regimens strongly suggested that enzyme activity was associated primarily with germinal cells. Such a conclusion was warranted by the fact that germinal cells are sensitive to gonadotropins (due to indirect actions) and androgen (due to direct actions). However, to conclude that testicular ACE was in fact associated primarily with germinal cells, more direct evidence was required.

Table IV. Maintenance of Testicular ACE in Hypophysectomized Adult Rats by Various Hormone Regimens

Treatment	Testicular Wet Weight	Protein/Wet Weight	ACE Activity
	grams	mg. protein/g. wet wt.	mUnits/mg. protein
Sham-Operated	3.10 ± 0.085	112 ± 1.7	5.38 ± 0.19
Hypophysectomy	0.94 ± 0.062	124 ± 5.1	0.82 ± 0.23
+ FSH/LH	2.95 ± 0.048	117 ± 1.1	4.34 ± 0.13
+ hCG	2.86 ± 0.078	118 ± 1.6	4.78 ± 0.19
+ Testosterone	2.68 ± 0.090	120 ± 2.8	4.46 ± 0.27

All values represent mean ± one standard error of 10 rats, except for the testosterone-treated group, which consisted of 9 rats. Animals were hypophysectomized at 10 weeks of age and hormone therapy was initiated on the first day following surgery and continued for 21 days. Further details can be obtained from data presented for publication in Velletri et al.[5]

3. Cellular Localization of Testicular ACE

As shown in Table V, following centrifugal elutriation of dispersed testicular cells, ACE activity was associated primarily with the germinal cells of rat testes. Leydig and Sertoli cells possessed virtually no detectable ACE activity. The above observations held true whether values were expressed as total ACE activity or specific ACE activity. Crude germinal cells also bound the site-directed inhibitor, [3H]captopril, specifically, which indicated that the carboxypeptidase activity associated with germinal cells was in fact ACE.

Table V. Elutriation of Dispersed Testicular Cells and Determination of Associated ACE Activity and Captopril Binding

Fraction	Total ACE Activity	Specific ACE Activity	Specific Captopril Binding
	Units	mUnits/mg. protein	$fmol/2 \times 10^6$ cells
Starting Material	65.6	18.7	–
Crude Germinal Cells	9.69	22.2	664
Leydig Cells	0.0457	0.457	–
Sertoli Cells	0.0197	0.206	–

Values represent averages of duplicate determinations from a representative experiment. Cells were prepared for centrifugal elutriation as described by Velletri et al.[5] and more extensive treatment of data can be found in that paper.

The experiments summarized in this paper clearly indicate that in the rat, testicular ACE is a lower molecular weight version of the pulmonary enzyme. Testicular ACE appears to be less thermodynamically stable than its pulmonary counterpart and might therefore be more susceptible to proteolysis. In vivo degradation might therefore be faster for the testicular enzyme. Because specific ACE activity in testis is comparable to that found in lung, the testicular enzyme might be subject to a greater rate of turnover. The testicular enzyme requires the presence of an intact pituitary gland for its development and maintenance. Testosterone appears to act directly in maintaining testicular ACE activity, whereas the effects of gonadotropins may be indirect by stimulating steroidogenesis in Leydig cells and/or nutrient factor production by Sertoli cells. Both centrifugal elutriation studies and captopril binding studies indicate that the majority of testicular ACE activity is present in germinal cells, although the precise stages of gametogenesis with which activity is associated has not been identified. What remains to be determined is the function of testicular ACE and whether the actions of androgen are to induce gene expression for ACE or simply to allow for spermatogenesis to occur and with it a non-specific parallel increase in ACE.

ACKNOWLEDGEMENTS

The authors wish to thank D. Aquilano, M. Billingsley, E. Bruckwick, C. Cutler, M. L. Dufau and C. M. Tsai-Morris, who were all involved with various aspects of this work, and whose contributions are to be more clearly discerned in Refs. 4 and 5.

REFERENCES

1. Soffer, R. L., Angiotensin-converting enzyme, in: Biochemical Regulation of Blood Pressure, ed., R. L. Soffer, John Wiley and Sons, pp. 123-164, (1981).
2. Cushman, D. W. and Cheung, H. S., Concentration of angiotensin-converting enzyme in tissues of the rat, Biochim. Biophys. Acta 250:261-265, (1971).
3. Soffer, R. L. and El-Dorry, H. A., Angiotensin-converting enzyme: immunologic, structural and developmental aspects, Fed Proc. 42:2735-2739, (1983).
4. Velletri, P. A., Billingsley, M. L. and Lovenberg, W., Thermal denaturation of rat pulmonary and testicular angiotensin converting enzyme isozymes: effects of chelators and $CoCl_2$, Biochim. Biophys. Acta, submitted.
5. Velletri, P. A., Aquilano, D. Bruckwick, E., Tsai-Morris, C. H., Dufau, M. L. and Lovenberg, W., Endocrinological control and cellular localization of rat testicular angiotensin converting enzyme (E.C. 3.4.15.1), Endocrinology, submitted.

ROLE OF KININASE II (ACE; E.C.3.4.15.1) IN THE REGULATION OF RENIN

SECRETION

V. Eisen, M.R. Munday and J.D.H. Slater

Middlesex Hospital Medical School

London, W1, UK

The activities of most proteolytic enzymes in plasma are checked by inhibitors of great versatility and capacity. In contrast, the activity of plasma renin is mainly regulated by the rate of its release from the cells of its origin. Renin is synthesized by a dozen or more cell species, yet only certain cells of the juxtaglomerular (jg) apparatus and chorionic cells secrete the active enzyme into extracellular fluids. All other renin-producing cells are also the site of angiotensin I and II (AI and AII) formation, and it is the latter which is secreted[1]. Inactive renin, also described as prorenin, is secreted by non-renal sources as well[2]. Its contribution to changes in concentrations of active renin is not certain.

Our aim was to study in vivo the short loop negative feedback (SLNF) which is the principal local regulator of jg secretion. It is called short because it is postulated that renin - as soon as it is secreted - leads to AI and then AII formation. This AII potently suppresses jg renin secretion. There is good evidence that AII achieves this inhibition by combining with AII receptors, thus depolarizing the jg cell membrane. This increases, through a transduction mechanism, the calcium influx into jg cells. The raised cytosol calcium then - in what may be a unique pattern in stimulus-secretion coupling - depresses renin secretion[3,4].

Conflicting views have been expressed as to the type of channel through which AII influences calcium flux. Churchill[5] postulates that AII acts on channels which are distinct from the voltage-operated channels affected by verapamil-type blockers. Fray et al[4] found that these blockers effectively counteracted AII and concluded that the same channels were affected.

To complete the loop from renin to AII, angiotensin I converting enzyme (ACE; kininase II) is essential. ACE thus assumes the role of a peptidase which controls the secretion of another peptide. Certain aspects of the SLNF, relevant to the role of ACE, are not yet fully understood. Jg cells contain high concentrations not only of renin, but also of its substrate and of ACE[6]. The short loop may therefore be even shorter in that the crucial AII may originate and act in the cells themselves. This may be important because jg cells appear to secrete much more renin into the surrounding interstitium than into the afferent arteriole; the bulk of renin enters the vascular space only at the level of the peritubular capillaries. Furthermore, jg cells not only secrete renin, but also take it up - a process which may inhibit renin secretion[4,7]. Such feedback inhibition by renin itself could of course supplement the depressant action of AII which may not be sufficient, as estimates of overall AI conversion in the kidney range from negligible to about 20%[6].

We have studied some of these points by observing acute effects on the SLNF of the ACE inhibitor captopril and the calcium channel blocker verapamil, infused singly or together into the ear vein of conscious rabbits. The limitations imposed by the use of non-anesthetized animals were accepted to avoid the potent effects of anesthetics on renin secretion.

METHODS

Conscious rabbits lightly tranquillized with diazepam (0.2 mgKg^{-1} i.m.) were placed unrestrained into open cardboard boxes with access to lettuce and water. Thin plastic cannulae were inserted into the ear vein and artery for infusion of drugs, sampling of blood and monitoring of the blood pressure. Plasma renin activity (PRA; rate of AI formation by the endogenous plasma renin and angiotensinogen) was measured by a miniature version of a described assay[8]. AI formation was linear over 2 hours with PRA values of 1 - 70 pmole.hr^{-1}.ml^{-1}. The mean intra-assay coefficient of variation (CV) was 6.6 and 5.2% for PRA measurements of 4 and 28.5 pmole.hr^{-1}.ml^{-1}, respectively (both n = 5). Plasma renin concentration (PRC) was measured as PRA, but in presence of sheep angiotensinogen (1.4 nmole per ml of rabbit plasma). Total renin concentration (TRC) was measured as PRC, but after activation of the inactive renin in plasma by trypsin (1 mg. ml^{-1}; 30 min at room temperature). AI formation was linear over 2 hours in PRC and TRC assays ranging from 7 to 150 pmole.hr^{-1}.ml^{-1}. The CV of PRC was 7.3% and of TRC 5.8% (n = 24). Inactive plasma renin concentration (IPRC) was calculated as TRC - PRC. ACE was measured as rate of hydrolysis of Hip-His-Leu[9].

To minimize the blood volume required, some assays were not carried out in all samples. The volume of fluid infused in the course of one experiment, exceeded the volume of blood collected by 30 per cent; the haematocrit fell by 5-10 per cent.

RESULTS

Captopril (50 µgmin^{-1}.ml^{-1}) promptly inhibited serum ACE. Extremely high bolus doses of AI (up to 10 µg.kg^{-1}) had absolutely no effect on the blood pressure. We therefore assumed that conversion of endogenous AI was also effectively inhibited. The increase in PRA and PRC was accompanied by a moderate fall in blood pressure (Fig 1a). The low concentrations of IPRC did not change significantly. The hyperreninaemia produced by ACE inhibition is mainly due to the absence of AII. We therefore tested whether the response to infused angiotensin amide (AIIa) would reveal signs of up-regulation of AII receptors. Indeed, AIIa depressed PRA and PRC effectively. When AIIa was discontinued, PRA and PRC rose again, but did not attain the levels seen at the beginning of the captopril infusion.

Blockade of calcium channels (Fig 1b) usually produced a smaller rise in PRA and PRC, although the fall in blood pressure was as great or greater. PRA raised by verapamil, leads to AI and then AII formation without interference. High circulating AII levels must therefore be assumed, which in turn may down-regulate AII receptors on the jg cells and elsewhere. Indeed, higher doses of AIIa had to be infused to depress PRA and PRC. When AIIa was discontinued, PRA and PRC attained or even exceeded the PRA and PRC levels seen before the AIIa infusion.

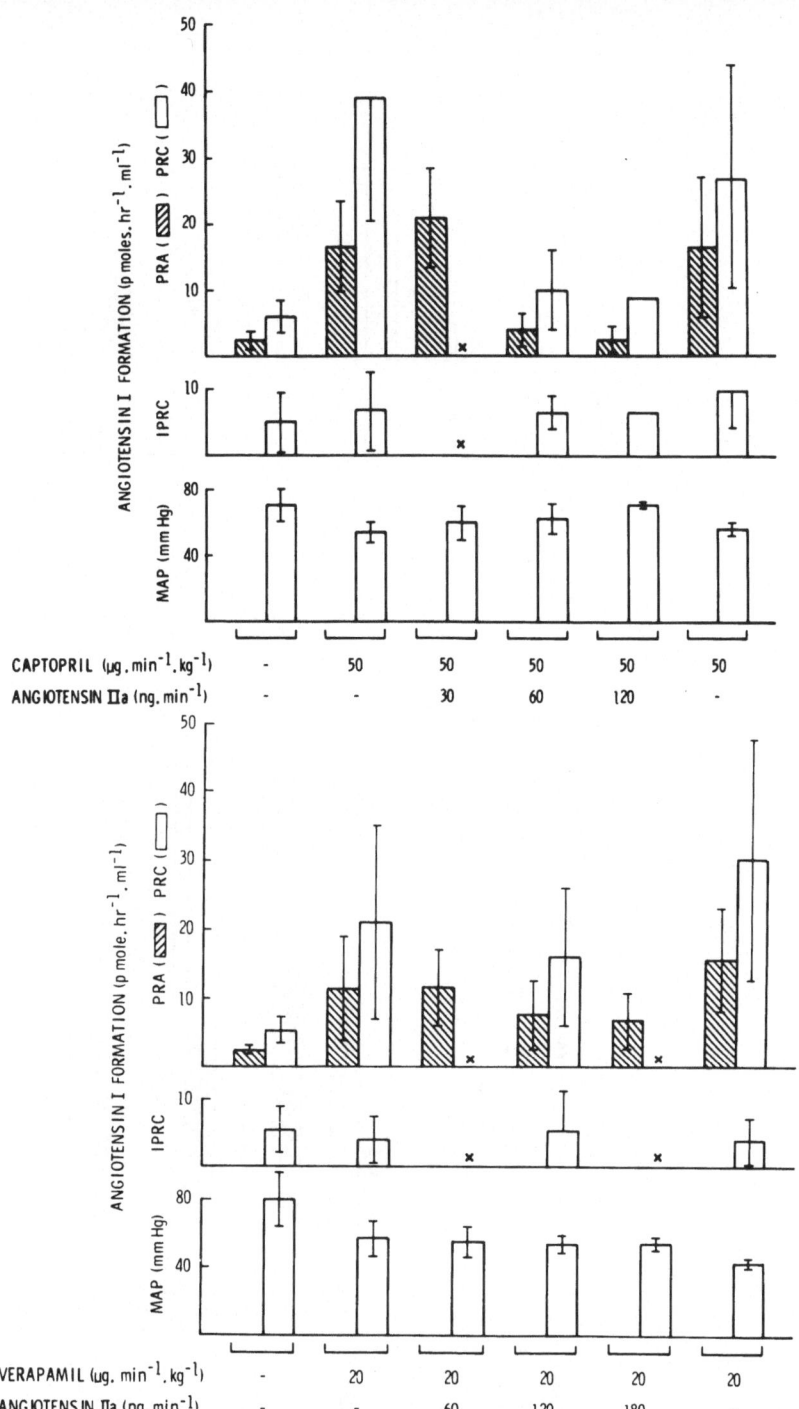

Fig. 1a/b Effects of captopril, verapamil and angiotensin II amide on PRA, IPRC and mean atrerial pressure (MAP). Drugs were infused iv in saline at the rates specified, each horizontal bracket indicating a 50 min infusion peroid. Intervals between these periods were less than 2 min. Assays were carried out on blood samples collected at 40 and 50 min. of a period and the average value used to calculate the m + s.d.; s.d. was omitted when number of samples was less than 4. MAP was calculated from the binned measurements at 42.5,45 and 47.5 min. x = not measured;n = 6.

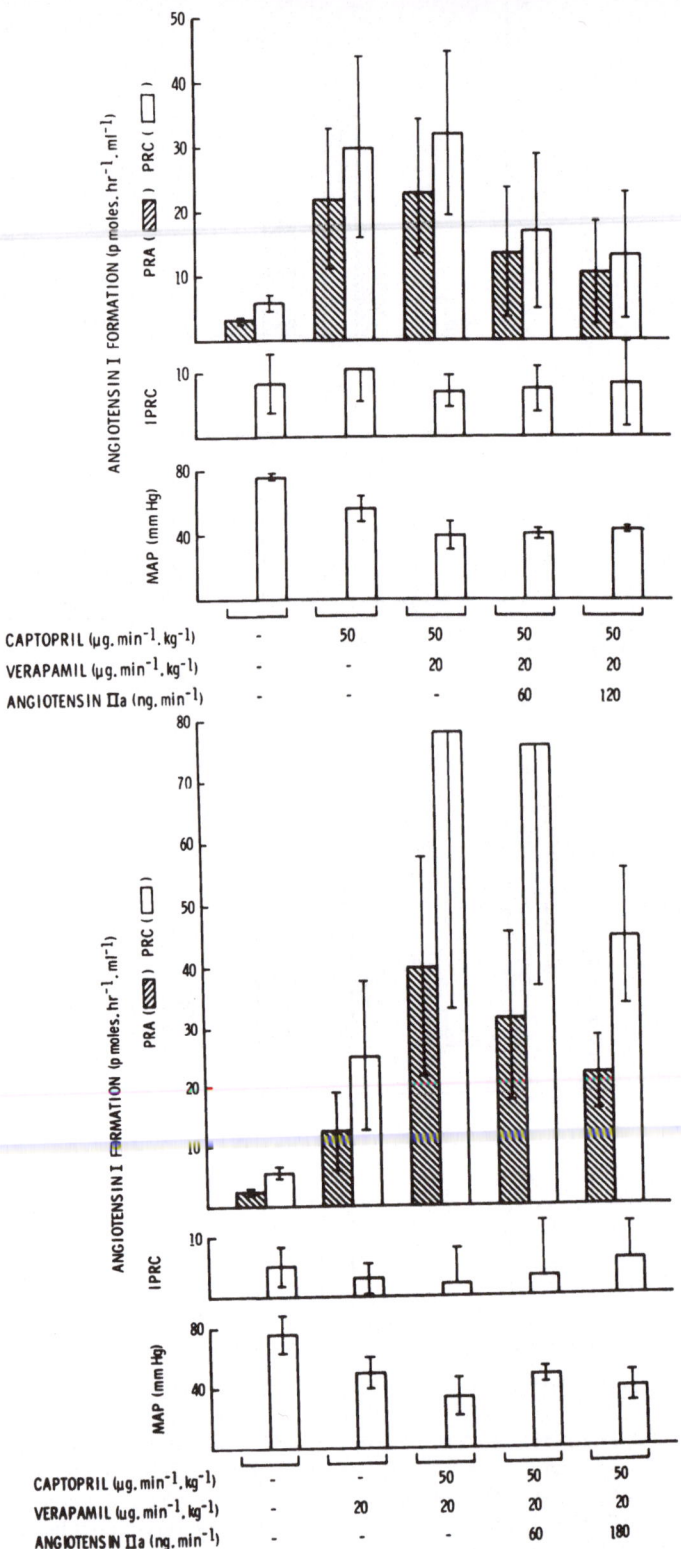

Fig. 2. Effects of captopril with subsequent addition of verapmil (a), and of verapmil with subsequent addition of captopril(b). Data presented as in Fig. 1. n = 6. Note that effect of combined drugs was much graeter when verapamil, rather than captopril was given first.

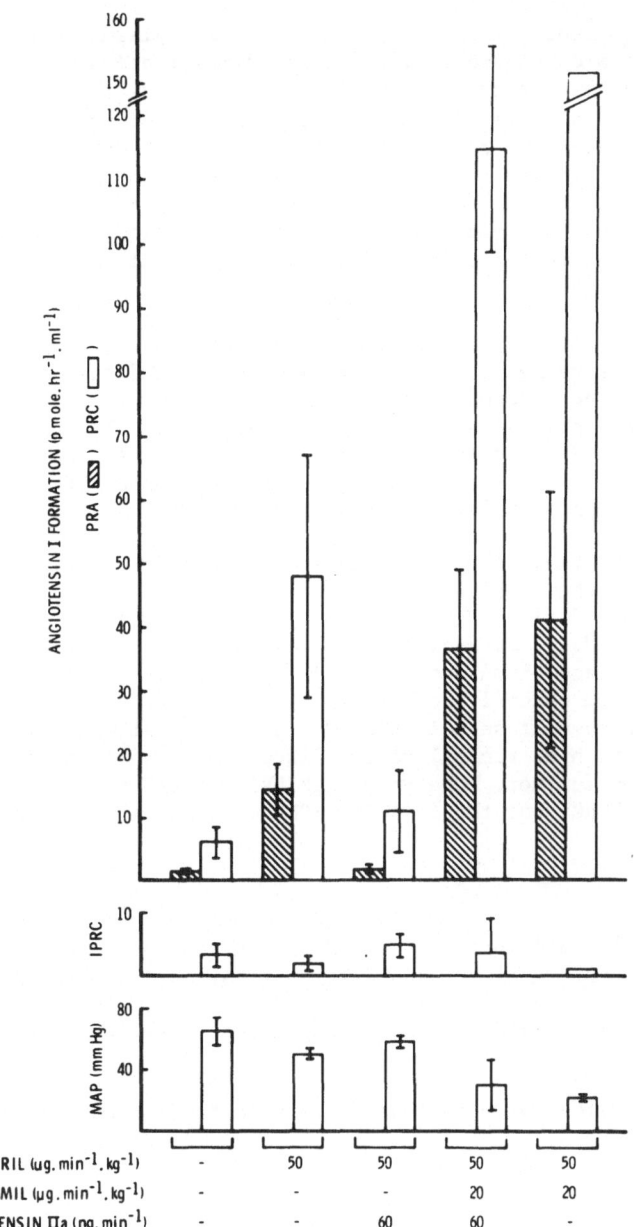

Fig. 3. Modification of experiment in Fig. 2a Data presented as in Fig. 1. Exposure to AII amide greatly enhanced subsequent jg response to captopril + verapmil.

The difference between the actions of captopril and verapamil emerged more clearly when the means ± s.d. of the percentage changes induced by the infusions in individual rabbits were considered. Captopril increased in individual rabbits PRA by 918 ± 350% (m ± s.d.) above control values; mean arterial pressure (MAP) fell by 24 ± 8%; the mean ratio PRA change/MAP change was 38.2. Verapamil raised PRA by 456 ± 252% and reduced MAP by 27%, giving a mean ratio of 16.9.

Since both captopril and verapamil increase plasma renin, but have opposite effects on plasma AII, combined administration was used to examine _in vivo_ whether even short-lasting changes in circulating AII influenced the secretory responsiveness of jg cells. When captopril was infused first and verapamil added later (Fig. 2a), AII formation was inhibited from the beginning. The combination captopril + verapamil therefore acted after and during a phase of low or absent circulating AII, and probable up-regulation of AII receptors; this view was supported by the finding that addition of verapamil did not increase PRA and PRC (p > 0.2), although it lowered blood pressure.

When the initial hyperreninaemia was produced by verapamil (Fig. 2b) it resulted - as we believe - in high AII levels and down-regulation of AII receptors. If the endogenous AII formation was now inhibited by captopril, PRA and PRC rose dramatically (p < 0.01), exceeding PRA and PRC produced by the two drugs in Fig. 2a (p < 0.05 and p < 0.01). Thus, when a phase of high circulating AII was terminated by ACE inhibition, greatly exaggerated responses to absence or lack of AII were seen.

To test the view that preceding short exposure of AII enhanced _in vivo_ the response to the combination captopril + verapamil, the experiment shown in Fig. 2a was modified (Fig. 3). Endogenous AII was abolished by captopril as in Fig. 2a. Next, sufficient AIIa was infused to restore pre-captopril values of renin and blood pressure and - we assume - down-regulate AII receptors. Calcium channel blockade was now instituted. In clear contrast to the non-enhancement seen in Fig. 2a, the combination captopril + verapamil now induced very high renin levels. Discontinuation of AIIa appeared to raise them even further. The very high PRA and PRC were associated with low levels of IPRC, but the falls in IPRC were not significant (p > 0.1).

DISCUSSION

The prompt impairment of the SLNF by infused captopril or verapamil, and the prompt effect of infused AIIa, suggest that agents arriving in the renal artery have ready access to the critical sites in the jg apparatus. However, the part played by AII formed inside jg cells requires further study.

The very different relationship between the percentage changes in PRA and in MAP produced by captopril and by verapamil provide _in vivo_ evidence that jg renin secretion is more potently influenced by local AII levels than by arterial pressure.

The responses of jg cells appeared to be rapidly modulated by changes in surrounding AII concentrations. The findings suggested that the up- and down-regulation of AII receptors of jg cells can be more rapid _in vivo_ than has hitherto been demonstrated[10]. The cellular mechanisms of this AII action require further study. The enhanced secretory responses occurred at a time when plasma AII ($t_{\frac{1}{2}}$ = 1-4 minutes) would have returned to low values after an AIIa infusion had been stopped and/or captopril started. This implies that jg responsiveness was changed after the influence of AII on calcium fluxes had ceased. It is also unlikely that changes in intracellular calcium levels were the responsible factor, because jg responses were increased after either verapamil or exogenous AIIa, in spite of the opposite effects of these drugs on free calcium in the cytosol. In any event, if the observed changes in jg responsiveness are indeed due to modulation of AII receptors, these are likely to be located - like most receptors for peptides - on the cell surface, and their modulation may not require transduction by altered calcium fluxes or other mechanisms.

As apparent from a comparison of figures 2a and 3, down-regulation of AII receptors enhances jg responses to blockade of voltage-dependent-calcium channels, as well as reducing the effectiveness of AII. Such down-regulation may therefore lead to a more general increase in jg reactivity, a phenomenon reminiscent of the rebound hyperexcitability underlying withdrawal syndromes in some drug addictions. However, as verapamil is a use-dependent blocker and far more effective on open channels, its greater effectiveness after AII (Fig. 3) could partly be due to its facilitated access into channels opened by AII. Both interpretations imply that at least some jg calcium channels respond both to AII and to blockers, as postulated by Fray[4]. Actions on a common channel may also account for the observation that AIIa was more effective against captopril than against verapamil (cf figures 1a and 1b). A model of a calcium channel which is linked both to a voltage gate and a receptor gate, has been proposed by Glossmann et al[11].

Extreme rises in active plasma renin occurred without accompanying increases in inactive renin, or definite evidence of its enhanced activation. This appears to support the view[12] that active and inactive renin are released under separate controls. However, our findings would also be compatible with a common control, provided that changes in the rate of release of inactive renin were co-ordinated with a precisely parallel change in the rate of its activation.

REFERENCES

1. Inagami, T., Pandey, K., Naruse, K. and Nakamaru, M., Abst. S73 in 4th Int. Congress Endocrinol., Excerpta Med. Amsterdam, p. 87 (1984).
2. Sealey, J.E., Atlas, S.A. and Laragh, J.H., Fed. Proc. 42: 2681 (1983).
3. Vandongen, R. and Peart, W., Br. J. Pharmacol. 50: 125 (1974).
4. Fray, J.C.S., Circ. Res. 47: 485 (1980).
5. Churchill, P.C., J. Physiol., 304: 449 (1980).
6. Navar, L.G. and Rosivall, L., Kidney Internat. 25: 857 (1984).
7. Meignan, M. Menard, J. Bonvalet, J.P. and de Rouffignac, C., Eur. J. Clin. Invest. 10: 407 (1980).
8. Menard, J. and Catt, C.J., Endocrinology 90: 422 (1972).
9. Friedland, J. and Silverstein, E., Am. J. Clin. Pathol. 66: 416 (1976).
10. Leboff, M.S., Dluhy, R.G., Hollenberg, N.K., Moore, T.J., Koletsky, R.J. and Williams, G.H., J. Clin. Invest. 70: 335 (1982).
11. Glossman, H., Ferry, D.R., Lubbecke, F., Mewes, R. and Hofmann, F., TIPS 3: 431 (1982).
12. Ginesi, L.M., Munday, K.A. and Noble, A.R., J. Physiol. 344: 453 (1983).

THE EFFECT OF ALPHANAPTHYLTHIOUREA (ANTU)-INDUCED ACUTE INJURY ON LUNG

BINDING OF ANTIBODY TO ANGIOTENSIN CONVERTING ENZYME (ACE)

James R. McCormick, Michael Moore, Robert Chrzanowski, and William Cieplinski

Departments of Medicine, VA Medical Centers, Newington, CT
and Augusta, GA and Medical College of Georgia, Augusta, GA
and University of Connecticut Health Center, Farmington, VT

SUMMARY

The effects of ANTU-induced acute pulmonary capillary injury on lung
and serum ACE functional activity and the specific accumulation of radio-
labelled anti-ACE in lung were explored. Rats were injected either with
ANTU or the solvent and sacrificed at various intervals up to one week
after injection. All ANTU-injected animals developed pulmonary edema and
bilateral pleural effusions which resolved by the one week time point. At
no time was there any significant change in serum ACE levels. The
specific activity of total lung ACE however rose from $11.0 \pm .95$ (mean$\pm$SEM)
to 18.4 ± 1.1 by two hours after ANTU; by 24 hours, however, solubilized lung
ACE had fallen significantly to $6.9 \pm .79$ (p<.01). Total lung ACE had returned to control values by one week. In parallel groups of animals the
accumulation of ^{125}I-labelled anti-ACE (AA) or normal sheep immunoglobulin
(NSG) was compared in control and ANTU-treated rats. The ratio of the
radioactivity in the lungs of AA - injected animals to that in NSG -
injected animals fell significantly after ANTU administration ($5.0 \pm .88$ to
$1.2 \pm .28$ at 2 hours) suggesting that immunoreactive ACE had fallen despite
an increase in ACE functional activity. The decreased binding of AA at
the early time points perhaps reflects internalization of endothelial cell
ACE in response to injury and an inability of the antibody to interact with
the enzyme. The reduction in binding at 24 hours ($1.38 \pm .47$) correlates
with a reduction in total lung ACE. ANTI-ACE may be a useful reagent for
quantitating endothelial cell damage following lung injury.

INTRODUCTION

Angiotensin converting enzyme (ACE) is a peptidyl dipeptidase which
activates angiotensin I to the potent vasopressor angiotensin II and inactivates bradykinin.[1] As such, it plays an important role in the
regulation of systemic blood pressure and probably local vascular tone.
It is principally synthesized by vascular endothelial cells and localized
upon the luminal surface membrane which facilitates its access to substrates within the circulating blood.[2] Serum ACE appears to be derived
from the endothelial cell[3] but a variety of other cell types and tissues
synthesize the enzyme and the range of its substrates and thus possibly
its functions may be broader than originally believed.[4-6]

Apparently all endothelial cells produce ACE; thus, its detection serves as a convenient, if not completely specific, marker for this cell type. The lung is rich in converting enzyme, most of which is associated with the capillary endothelium.[7] Acute or chronic lung injury is associated with changes in serum or lung ACE in experimental animals and man and it has been suggested that changes in the serum enzyme reflect pulmonary vascular injury.[8-11] Hollinger et al. demonstrated a rapid increase in serum ACE following thiourea-induced pulmonary edema in rats at a time when total lung ACE apparently declined[8] and suggested that release of ACE by injured vascular endothelial cells was the source. The increase was transient, however, returning toward control values by 2-3 hours after injury, rendering this measurement an unreliable marker of persistent endothelial damage.

Other investigators have documented altered metabolic function of the lung vascular bed following acute injury induced by high inspired oxygen concentrations. Dobuler et al. demonstrated reduced catalytic activity of lung ACE in vivo in rabbits infused with a synthetic substrate following hyperoxia. The metabolic change occurred before significant morphologic alterations were observed; their technique may therefore prove to be a sensitive indicator of early endothelial cell damage.[12] In an effort to develop a lung endothelial cell marker that can be used in conjunction with assays of metabolic function, we have produced an antibody to rat lung converting enzyme and compared changes in its specific accumulation in lung with the effect of acute pulmonary injury on serum and total lung ACE catalytic activity.

MATERIALS AND METHODS

Production of Lung Injury

Specific pathogen-free male, hooded, Long-Evans rats (268±15 grams) were used in these studies. Alphanapthylthiourea (ANTU) was purchased from the Aldridge Chemical Company and dissolved in one part propylene glycol and three parts distilled water for a final concentration of 5mg/ml. After ketamine anesthesia, the animals were injected intraperitoneally with 3.5 mg/kg of ANTU or solvent and sacrificed at 2, 4, and 24 hours and 1 week. At the time of sacrifice, blood was collected and the serum separated and assayed for ACE activity. The chest cavity was opened and any pleural fluid present was quantitated and assayed for ACE and total protein. The lungs were perfused in situ with sterile saline, removed, trimmed and homogenized individually in a polytron (Brinkman Instruments) in 15 ml of 20mM potassium phosphate buffer containing .125% deoxycholate. They were then agitated at 4°C for 1 hour, sedimented at 15,000 x G and the supernatant was assayed with ACE activity.

Parallel groups of animals were sacrificed for histologic studies. In these animals, the lungs were not perfused with saline but were inflated via the trachea with 10% cold buffered formalin and processed for light microscopy.

ACE Purification and Production of Specific Antibodies

Converting enzyme from rat lungs was purified as previously described using detergent solubilization and ion exchange, hydroxylapatite and gel filtration chromatography.[13] The resulting preparation had a 1400-fold increase in specific activity over the original rat lung homogenate and showed a single band on 8% polyacrylamide SDS gel.

Sheep were injected at monthly intervals with 100–200 µg of purified converting enzyme in Freund's adjuvant and serum was tested periodically for antibody to ACE by immunodiffusion. Once a significant titer had been obtained, serum was heat-inactivated at 56°C for 30 minutes to denature complement and native ACE activity; the IgG fraction was prepared by ammonium sulphate fractionation and ion-exchange chromatography. Pre-immune serum was collected and processed in a similar fashion to yield normal sheep IgG (NSG).

Assay of ACE Enzymatic Activity

ACE activity was determined by its ability to cleave a standard (Hip-his-leu) substrate at 37°C using the spectrophotometric assay of Cushman and Cheung[14] as modified by Lieberman.[15] The activity was expressed in units (U), defined as the number of micromoles of substrate cleaved per minute per milliliter. Specific activity was defined as U/mg protein assayed. Total protein was determined by the method of Lowry et al.[16]

Lung Accumulation of Radiolabelled Immunoglobulins

Normal sheep immunoglobulin or specific polyclonal anti-ACE was radio-labelled with ^{125}I for in vivo studies using a modified chloramine-T technique.[17]

The radiolabelled immunoglobulins (0.5µci/0.6mg protein) were administered to ANTU or solvent-injected rats 30 minutes before sacrifice. At sacrifice, anesthetized animals were exsanguinated by sectioning the abdominal aorta and the lungs were perfused in situ with saline at 20 cm water pressure until the perfusate was clear. Because ANTU treatment results in the non-specific exudation of plasma proteins into the pulmonary interstitium, we homogenized each pair of lungs individually and washed the pellets to remove as much unbound labelled immunoglobulin as possible. Radioactivity in the pellet of both trimmed lungs per gram of wet weight was divided by that in 1 ml of blood from the same animal. This ratio reflects the amount of immunoglobulin retained in the lung and appears to correlate with binding to the bascular bed.[13]

Immunohistology

Rat lungs were inflated with a 1:1 mixture of OCT embedding medium and normal saline and frozen at −70° overnight. Cryostat sections of lung were cut to six micron thickness, placed on gelatin-coated slides, air dried at room temperature and fixed in 95% ethanol. The tissue sections were then incubated with polyclonal anti-ACE or normal sheep immunoglobulin for 60 minutes at 37°C in a humidified chamber. The slides were then rinsed twice with phosphate-buffered saline and incubated for 30 minutes at 37°C with FITC-conjugated rabbit-anti-sheep IgG (Miles Laboratories). After completing the incubation with the second antibody, the slides were rinsed thoroughly with PBS and a coverslip was applied using glycerol: veronal buffered saline (pH8.6) as mounting media. Photomicrographs of the tissue specimens were taken immediately using an AO Series 10 Microstar with a vertical immunofluoresence unit.

RESULTS

Histology

All ANTU-injected animals developed acute, interstitial pulmonary
edema and bilateral pleural effusions which largely resolved by 24
hours (Figure 1, a-d; Table 1). The edema fluid was largely restricted
to bronchial and perivascular lymphatics and was associated with a mild
interstitial and alveolar inflammatory response. The ACE activity and
protein content of the pleural fluid suggested that it originated by
exudation from serum (Table 1).

Table 1. ACE levels in pleural fluid

	Volume (ml)	mU/ml	Units
Control	0	0	0
2°	5.4±1.9*	71.6±4.0	.37±.14
4°	7.8±2.0	72.3±14.5	.51±.14
24°	2.6±2.3	42.1±25.4	.15±.13

* = Mean ± SEM
mU/ml = milli units per ml pleural fluid

There was no significant change in serum ACE at any time point
(Table 2). However, solubilized lung ACE increased significantly at 2
and 4 hours after ANTU but fell below the original value by 24 hours.
By one week, there were no differences in total lung ACE between the
control and ANTU-treated animals (Table 2).

Lung Accumulation of Radiolabelled Immunoglobulins in Control or ANTU-
Treated Rats

As shown in Table 3, control animals accumulated significantly more
of the radiolabelled anti-ACE (AA) than normal sheep immunoglobulin in their
lung pellets. All ANTU-treated rats developed high-permeability pulmonary
edema which was associated with the accumulation of water and plasma proteins in lung. For this reason, there was an absolute increase in the
amount of injected radioactivity in the lungs of these animals at the
very early time points. Therefore, we constructed a ratio comparing the
lung radioactivity in AA injected animals to those injected with NSG.
As shown in Table 3, five times more radioactivity was accumulated in the
lungs of AA injected normal animals. After ANTU treatment, however, the
ratio fell to approximately 1:1 but recovered to pre-ANTU levels by one
week (Table 3). We believe this decline in the ratio of AA to NSG
accumulation after ANTU treatment represents a decrease in the specific
binding of AA in the ANTU-treated lungs.

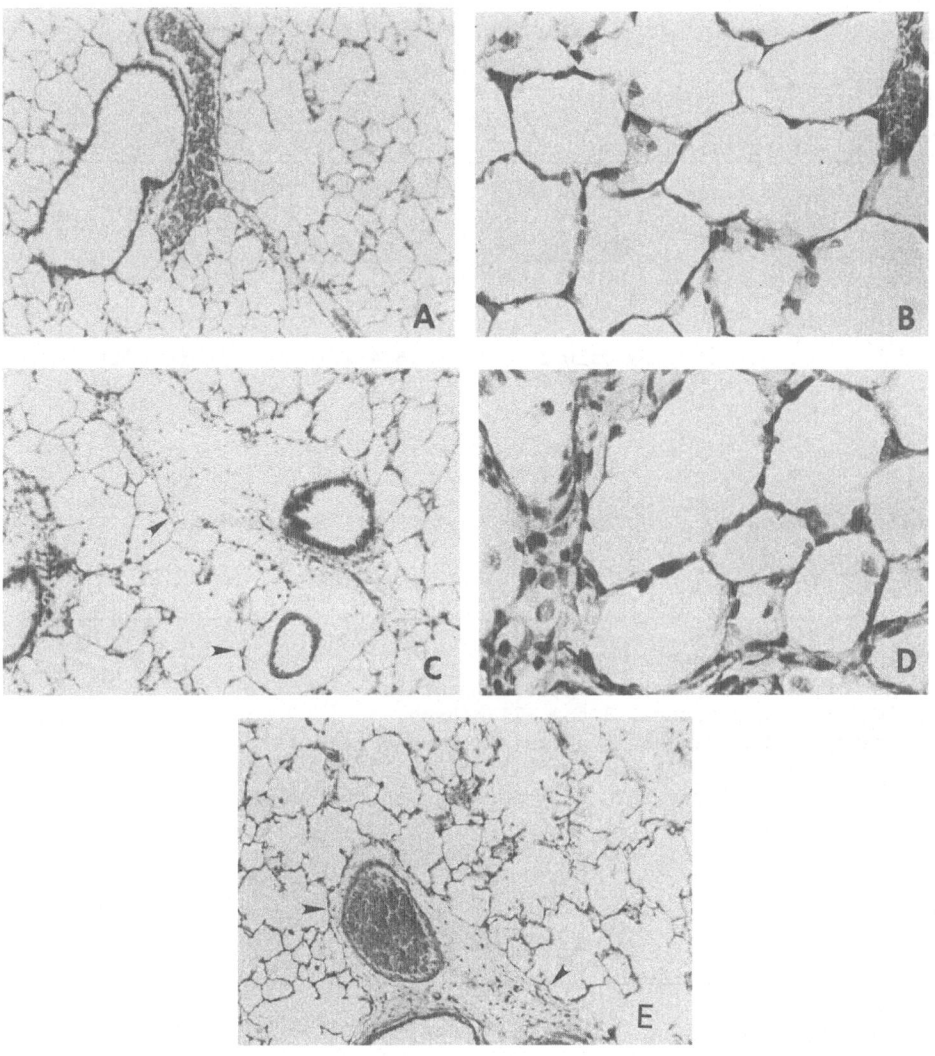

Figure 1. A. The lung of a control animal sacrificed 4 hours after solvent injection demonstrating normal alveolar architecture
(H&E, 100%). B. A higher power of a control animal's lung.
Note the normal venule in the right hand corner (450%).
C. The lung of an ANTU-injected animal at 4 hours. Marked
peribronchial and perivascular lymphatic congestion with edema
fluid is present (arrowheads) (H&E, 100%). D. ANTU-4 hours.
Interstitial edema is present (450%). E. ANTU-24 hours. Far
less interstitial and perivascular edema is seen. There is a
mild influx of inflammatory cells into the alveolar spaces.
(H&E, 100%).

Immunohistology

Control animals demonstrated the typical curvilinear immunofluorescence
associated with binding of AA to the pulmonary vasculature.[18] Four hours
after ANTU, there was little demonstrable difference in this binding but
by 24 hours, the intensity of the immunofluorescence was markedly diminished

Table 2.

	SERUM ACE* (mU/ml)	SOLUBILIZED LUNG ACE (mU/mg)	
Control	77.7±10.6	11.0±.95**	
ANTU 2°	79.3±10.2	18.4±1.1	p<.001†
4°	76.2± 9.6	16.2±2.3	p<.05
24°	76.8±16.4	6.9±.70	p<.01
Control (1 Week)	82.2± 7.0	9.8±.71	
ANTU (1 Week)	78.5± 5.9	8.0±.61	N.S.

mU/ml = milliunits per ml serum
mU/mg = milliunits per mg lung total protein
N = 10 for 1 week groups, 7 for all others
* No significant changes in serum ACE were observed
** Mean ± SEM
† Total lung ACE after ANTU compared with controls using the Student's unpaired t test

Table 3.

	LUNG RADIOACTIVITY*		
	AA	NSG	AA/NSG
Control	.15±.03(8)†	.03±.01(8)	5.00±.88
ANTU 2°	.23±.05(9)	.19±.03(9)	1.21±.28
4°	.19±.01(8)	.16±.03(8)	1.18±.24
24°	.11±.01(8)	.08±.02(8)	1.38±.47
Control (1 Week)	.15±.03(7)	.03±.01(7)	5.00±.68
ANTU (1 Week)	.16±.04(7)	.03±.01(7)	5.32±.57

AA = Anti-ACE; NSG = Normal sheep immunoglobulin
* = Mean ± SEM
() = Number of animals in each group

and the pattern had changed to a more granular appearance (Figure 2:a-c). One week later ANTU-treated animals exhibited no significant difference in the binding of AA when compared with control animals.

DISCUSSION

Acute and chronic lung injury has been shown to have significant effects on the metabolic function of the pulmonary microvasculature in experimental animals and man.[19] These effects may be observed in the absence of obvious structural damage to the capillary endothelial cell. In addition interference with one metabolic function may occur prior to or in the absence of a change in another.[19] For example, in paraquat-induced lung injury in rats, a significant reduction in the uptake of serotonin was observed by three days after the administration of the toxin.[20] At this time there was minimal evidence of injury to the endothelial cell morphologically and no effect on the conversion of angiotensin I to angiotensin II in the isolated, perfused lung model employed in these studies.

In an effort to complement these observations, we studied the effect of ANTU on total lung and serum ACE activities and compared these values to the specific accumulation of radiolabelled AA in lung and the binding of anti-ACE to lung by immunofluorescence. ANTU produces specific injury, primarily to the pulmonary capillary endothelial cell, which begins at one hour after injection, peaks at 24 hours and completely resolves over the ensuing few days.[21] Our studies demonstrate that the initial response to ANTU-induced pulmonary edema involves an increase in total lung ACE followed by a gradual decline to sub-control levels by 24 hours (Table 2). These results are at variance with those reported by Hollinger et al.[8] who, using thiourea, observed a fall in total lung ACE during the early hours after injection of the toxin. These investigators apparently did not detergent-solubilize their lung preparations, a procedure necessary for optimum extraction of the converting enzyme from rat lung.[13]

The reason for the observed increase in converting enzyme in lung is not clear. It may represent a metabolic response of the endothelial cell to ANTU injury. Cunningham and Hurley[21] have observed modest endothelial cell swelling and subendothelial blebbing from 3 to 6 hours after ANTU administration to rats. These lesions progress such that by 24 hours much of the endothelium is thickened and there are greatly increased numbers of cellular organelles. There is one notable exception however; pinocytotic vescicles are greatly reduced within these cells. Since the converting enzyme is localized to the luminal surface membrane of the endothelial cell and pinocytotic vesicles, the ultrastructural change may explain the reduction in total lung ACE seen at 24 hours.

Our immunofluorescence studies are compatible with these findings. During the early hours after ANTU administration, there is no significant change in the binding of antibody to frozen sections of lung. At these times, there is, in fact, an increase in total lung ACE. By 24 hours, however, a reduction in total lung ACE is accompanied by obviously reduced binding of AA to the frozen sections (Figure 2).

In contrast, the studies using the radiolabelled immunoglobulins correlate better with histopathologic and electron microscopic evidence of endothelial damage at the early time points. ANTU clearly reduces the specific accumulation of AA in the lung suggesting that there is a reduced amount of surface-bound ACE available for interaction with the antibody. This effect was observed whether total lung ACE was increased

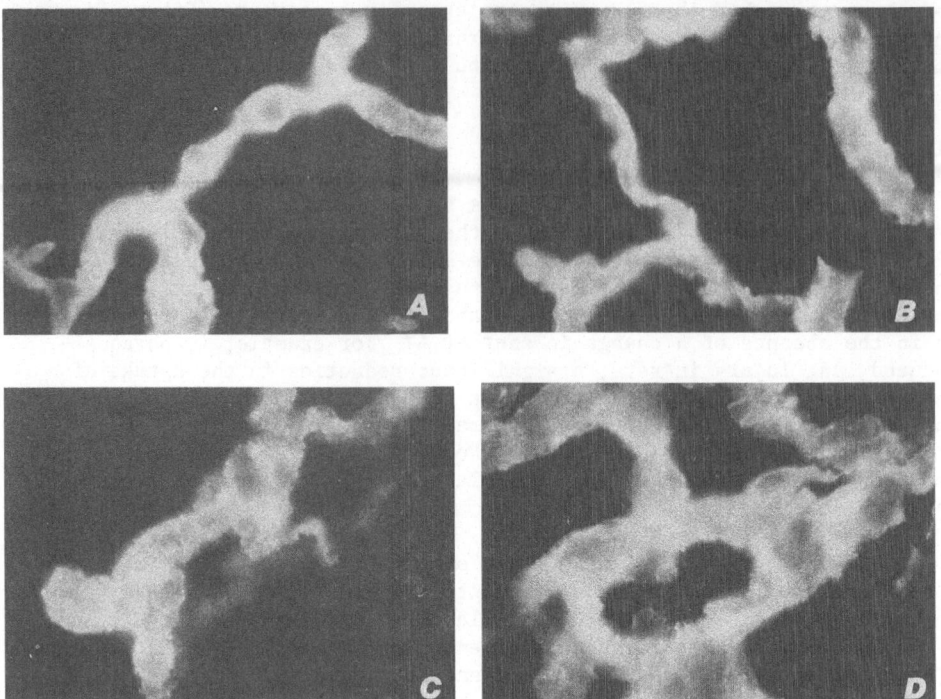

Figure 2. A, B. Frozen sections of normal lung demonstrating curvilinear fluorescence consistent with the binding of polyclonal anti-ACE to capillary endothelial cells (1000X). C, D. At 24 hours after ANTU, the binding of anti-ACE is obviously reduced and demonstrates a more granular staining pattern (1000X). No significant fluorescence was observed when normal sheep globulin was incubated with the lung sections.

or reduced (Table 2). While the mechanism for this response is unknown, it might be postulated that a loss of surface area mediated by endothelial cell swelling and internalization of plasma membrane occurs early in response to ANTU. In support of this hypothesis, Stalcup et al.[22] have recently shown that endothelial cells in tissue culture rapidly reduce surface ACE activity in response to hypoxia, an effect which is reversed within minutes of resuming normoxic conditions. During the early phases of pulmonary edema, alveolar hypoxis almost certainly occurs. Thus, ANTU may directly and indirectly, by way of producing hypoxis, affect the availability of surface-bound ACE for binding to AA.

These studies suggest that changes in the accumulation of radio-labelled AA may be useful for detecting subtle effects of a variety of injurious agents on the pulmonary microvasculature in the intact lung. This technique appears to complement quantitative metabolic studies. For example, Block and Schoen[23] demonstrated a significant reduction in sero-tonin removal by rat lungs exposed to ANTU at times when we observed a reduction in the specific binding of AA. Further studies using models of progressive lung injury are clearly indicated.

Supported by grants from the Veterans Administration Research Service.

ACKNOWLEDGEMENTS

The authors are indebted to Jeanine Leeka and Carolyn Patterson for their excellent secretarial assistance.

REFERENCES

1. R. L. Soffer, Angiotensin-converting enzyme and the regulation of vasoactive peptides, Ann. Rev. Biochem., 45:73-94, (1976).
2. J. W. Ryan, U. S. Ryan, D. R. Schultz, et al., Subcellular localization of pulmonary angiotensin-converting enzyme (Kininase II), Biochem. J., 146:497-499, (1975).
3. A. R. Johnson and E. G. Erdos, Metabolism of vasoactive peptides by human endothelial cells in culture. Angiotensin I converting enzyme (Kininase II) and angiotensinase, J. Clin. Invest., 59: 684-695, (1977).
4. R. Taugner, E. Hockenthal, E. Rix, et al., Immunochemistry of the renin-angiotensin system: Renin, angiotensinogen, angiotensin I, angiotensin II, and converting enzyme on the kidneys of mice, rats, and tree shrews, Kidney Int., 22:S-33-S-43, (1982).
5. D. Ganton, M. Printz, M. I. Phillips, and B. A. Scholkins, The renin angiotensin system in the brain: A model for the synthesis of peptides in the brain, Springer-Verlag, New York, (1982).
6. R. W. Barton and J. R. McCormick, Identification of angiotensin converting enzyme on rat thymocytes, Fed. Proc., 41:738, (1982).
7. P. R. Caldwell, B. C. Seegal, K. C. Hsu, et al., Angiotensin-converting enzyme: Vascular endothelial localization, Science, 191: 1050-1051, (1976).
8. M. A. Hollinger, S. N. Giri, S. Patwell, et al., Effect of acute lung injury on angiotensin-converting enzyme in serum, lung lavage, and effusate, Am. Rev. Respir. Dis., 121:373-376, (1980).
9. T. Nakiwa, R. Matsuoka, T. Hiroshi, et al., Responses of serum and lung angiotensin-converting enzyme activities in the early phase of pulmonary damage induced by oleic acid in dogs, Am. Rev. Resp. Dis., 126:1080-1086, (1982).
10. P. K. Rohatgi, Serum angiotensin-converting enzyme in pulmonary disease, Lung, 160:287-301, (1982).
11. C. W. Bedrossian, J. Woo, W. C. Miller, and D. C. Cannon, Decreased angiotensin-converting enzyme in the adult respiratory distress syndrome, Am. J. Clin. Pathol., 70:244-247, (1978).
12. K. J. Dobuler, J. D. Catravas, and C. N. Gillis, Early detection of oxygen-induced lung injury in conscious rabbits, Am. Rev. Respir. Dis., 126:534-539, (1982).
13. J. R. McCormick, R. S. Thrall, A. Kerlin, and P. A. Ward, In vitro and in vivo effects of antibody to rat angiotensin converting enzyme, Clin. Immunol. Immunopathol., 15:444-455, (1980).
14. D. W. Cushman and H. S. Chung, Spectrophotometric assay and properties of the angiotensin-converting enzyme of rabbit lung, Biochem. Pharmacol., 20:1637-1648, (1971).
15. J. Lieberman and T. H. Rea, Serum angiotensin-converting enzyme in leprosy and coccidioidomycosis, Ann.Int. Med., 87:422-426, (1977).
16. O. H. Lowry, J. J. Rosebrough, A. L. Fau, and R. J. Randall, Protein measurement with the Folin phenol reagent, J. Biol. Chem., 193: 265-276, (1951).

17. P. J. McConahey and F. J. Dixon, A method of trace iodination of proteins for immunologic studies, _Int. Arch. Allergy Appl. Immunol._, 29:185-189, (1966).
18. P. R. Caldwell, H. J. Wigger, L. T. Fernandez, et al., Lung injury induced by antibody fragments to angiotensin-converting enzyme, _Am. J. Pathol._,105:54-63, (1981).
19. C. N. Gillis and J. D. Catravas, Altered removal of vasoactive substances in the injured lung: Detection of lung microvascular injury, _Ann. N.Y. Acad. Sci._, 384:458-474, (1982).
20. R. A. Roth, K. B. Wallace, R. H. Alper, and M. D. Bailie, Effect of paraquat treatment of rats on disposition of 5-hydroxytryptamine and angiotensin by perfused lung, _Biochem. Pharmacol._, 28:2349-2355, (1979).
21. A. L. Cunningham and J. V. Hurley, Alpha-naphthyl-thiourea-induced pulmonary edema in the rat: A topographical and electron-microscope study, _J. Path._, 106:25-35, (1972).
22. S. A. Stalcup, J. S. Lipset, J. M. Woan, P. Leuenberger, and R. B. Mellins, Inhibition of angiotensin converting enzyme activity in cultured endothelial cells by hypoxia, _J. Clin. Invest._, 63: 966-967, (1979).
23. E. R. Block and F. J. Schoen, Effect of alpha-napthylthiourea on uptake of 5-hydroxytryptamine from the pulmonary circulation, _Am. Rev. Resp. Dis._, 123:69-73, (1981).

ISOLATION AND SEQUENCING OF AN ACTIVE-SITE PEPTIDE FROM ANGIOTENSIN I-CONVERTING ENZYME

Robert B. Harris

University of Colorado
Department of Chemistry
Boulder, CO 80309

SUMMARY

A glutamic acid residue at the active-site of bovine lung antiotensin I-converting enzyme was esterified with p-[N,N-bis-(chloroethyl)amino]phenylbutyryl-L-[U-^{14}C]-Proline(chlorambucyl-L-[U-^{14}C]-L-Proline), an affinity label for this enzyme.[2] The radiolabeled enzyme was digested with BrCN and only 1 of the 30 cleavage peptides resolved by reverse-phase HPLC contained the bound radiolabel. This active-site peptide ($M_r \sim 16,000$) was digested with trypsin, and the labeled peptide (T-2) was further degraded with thermolysin. The enzyme digest peptides were also resolved by reverse-phase HPLC. Only 1 of the 5 peptides obtained after thermolysin digestion (Th-1, M_r 1290) contained the bound radiolabel. Th-1 (12 residues) was subjected to manual Edman degradation and the following partial sequence was determined: H$_2$N-Phe-Thr-Glu-Leu-Ala-Asp-Ser-Glu. The radiolabel was released at cycle 3 and the amount recovered was equivalent to the amount of PTH-Glu detected on HPLC. Thus, glutamic acid is esterified with chlorambucyl-L-[U-^{14}C]-Proline which confirms our earlier findings. The sequence that we determined is homologous in five residues with the corresponding sequences of carboxypeptidase A and B, two other mammalian zinc-proteases. There is little sequence homology with thermolysin, a bacterial zinc-protease that also contains an essential active-site glutamic acid residue.

INTRODUCTION

The alkylating agents, p-[N,N-bis(chloroethyl)amino]phenylbutyric acid (chlorambucil), and the chlorambucil derivative of L-Proline, (chlorambucyl-L-Proline) rapidly and irreversibly inactivate angiotensin I-converting enzyme (peptidyl dipeptide carboxyhydrolase, E.C. 3.4.15.1) purified from bovine lung parenchyma tissue.[1] Both compounds behave as affinity labels and chlorambucyl-L-[U-^{14}C]-Proline reacts 1:1 with the enzyme, to produce radiolabeled enzyme. The radioactivity is released by hydroxide ion or hydroxylamine[1] and we have shown that this inhibitor esterifies a Glu residue at the active-site of the enzyme.[2]

We have now sequenced a radiolabeled peptide that contains the active-site glutamic acid. Radiolabeled converting enzyme was prepared by reacting homogeneous enzyme with chlorambucyl-L-[U-^{14}C]-Proline. Radiolaeled enzyme was degraded with cyanogen bromide, trypsin and thermolysin to yield a single radiolabeled dodecapeptide that was partially sequenced by manual Edman degradation. Glutamic acid was confirmed as the site of attachment of the inhibitor. The octapeptide sequence, Phe-Thr-Glu-Leu-Ala-Asp-Ser-Glu, is homologous in five residues with the corresponding sequences of carboxypeptidase A and B. There is little homology with thermolysin, a bacterial zinc protease that also contains an essential Glu residue.

METHODS

Converting Enzyme

Bovine lung converting enzyme was prepared by affinity chromatography.[2,3] We routinely obtain about 3 mgs of enzyme from 500 g of fresh-frozen bovine lung tissue.

The enzyme preparations that we used for these experiments were homogeneous and had specific activities ranging from 11.5-12 units/mg protein.[3] The concentration of converting enzyme was determined using the molar extinction coefficient, $\varepsilon_{278} = 2.1 \times 10^5 M^{-1} \cdot cm^{-1}$.[3]

Amino Acid Analysis

Amino acid analyses were performed on a dual column JEOL JLC-5AH analyzer according to Spackman et al.[4] Peptides were hydrolyzed with 6N HCl (Pierce) in evacuated, sealed glass tubes for 20h at 110°C.

High Performance Liquid Chromatography

HPLC was used to separate the cyanogen bromide and enzyme cleavage peptides and to identify PTH-amino acids after each cycle of the Edman procedure.

All separations were performed on C_{18}-reverse phase columns; the cyanogen bromide and enzyme cleavage peptides were resolved with a linear gradient of 0.1% trifluoroacetic acid to 0.1% trifluoroacetic acid - 50% acetonitrile[3] and were detected at 220 nm (Model 450 Variable Wavelength Detector, Waters Assoc.). The flow rate was 1.2 ml/min (4 mm x 30 cm column, 10 μm packing, A3I Inc.). In order to maximize the resolution of individual cleavage peptides, the entire digest mixture was chromatographed in portions. The fractions containing the peptides of interest from each run were pooled together and lyophilized for further study.

PTH-amino acid derivatives were detected at 254 nm and were resolved using program curve #7 (Model 660 Solvent Programmer, Waters Assoc. Inc.) with a gradient of 90% solvent A (10% acetonitrile - 90% 0.2 N sodium acetate, pH 5.5) to 90% solvent B (90% acetonitrile - 10% 0.2 N sodium acetate, pH 5.5). The flow rate was 1.2 ml/min for 25 min using a 4.6 mm x 25 cm column (5 μm Ultrasphere ODS packing, Altex). PTH-amino acid standards were purchased from Pierce or Sigma and PTH-norleucine (Pierce) was the internal standard. Peak areas were integrated with an on-line Spectra-Physics desktop integrator which also controlled the movement of the fraction collector so that each U.V. absorbing peak was collected in a single test tube.

Radioactivity Measurements

Radioactivity measurements were made with a Beckman model LS-250 scintillation spectrometer using 10 ml of Biofluor (New England Nuclear) as the scintillation solvent.

Gel Permeation Chromatography

The apparent molecular weights of some of the cleavage peptides were determined by gel permeation chromatography on Sephadex G-50 or Sephadex G-25 (Pharmacia). The chromatography columns (1.5 x 60 cm) were equilibrated in 0.1% acetic acid and were calibrated with appropriate molecular weight standards. The cleavage peptides and molecular weight markers were detected at 280 or 206 nm (Model 2138 Uvicord S Monitor, LKB Instruments, Inc.). The elution volume (V_e) of each sample and of the various standards were determined and the gel partition coefficient, K_{av}, was calculated from the formula, $K_{av} = (Ve-Vo)/(Vt-Vo)$. A calibration curve for each column was prepared by plotting log M_r versus K_{av}.

Synthesis of Chlorambucyl-L-[U-14C]Proline

This active-site directed irreversible inhibitor of the converting enzyme was synthesized with a specific radioactivity of 43,000 cpm/μmol as we described previously.[1]

Inhibition of the Converting Enzyme and Uptake of Radioactivity

Bovine lung converting enzyme (25-50 nmol, 3.6 - 7.3 mgs) was dissolved in 0.8 ml 50 mM 1,4-piperazinediethanesulfonic acid buffer, pH 7.5 and inhibited with chlorambucyl-L-[U-14C]-Proline (500 μM) as we described.[1] After 1h, the inhibited enzyme was separated from unbound inhibitor and buffer salts by chromatography on Sephadex G-25 equilibrated in water.[2] The void volume fractions containing the inhibited enzyme were lyophilized.

Cleavage with Cyanogen Bromide

The lyophilized preparation was dissolved in 1 ml of 70% formic acid containing 3.5 M guanidine hydrochloride. Cyanogen bromide (250 mgs, 2.3 mmol) was added and the solution left overnight at room temperature. The solution was then lyophilized at least 3x and the peptides were dissolved in 0.1% trifluoroacetic acid for HPLC.

The cyanogen bromide cleavage peptides were separated by HPLC and the radioactive peptide containing bound chlorambucyl-L-[U-14C]-Proline was identified.[2] This peptide elutes at 85-88% of the linear solvent gradient with a retention time of about 25 min. The fraction containing the radioactive peptide was lyophilized and dissolved in 0.3 ml of 0.2M N-ethylmorpholine acetate, pH 8.1, for digestion with trypsin.

Cleavage with Trypsin

The peptide (25-42 nmol) was digested at 37°C for 4h with 4-7 μg trypsin (weight ratio 1:100) (Sigma, Type XI, dephenyl carbamyl chloride treated-trypsin). The tryptic peptides were separated by HPLC and the radioactive peptide was lyophilized and dissolved in 0.3 ml of 0.2M N-ethylmorpholine acetate for digestion with thermolysin.

Cleavage with Thermolysin

The peptide (21-36 nmol) was digested for 4h at 55°C with 9-16 μg Thermophilic-bacterial protease, (weight ratio 1:20) (Thermolysin, Sigma, Type X-protease). A stock solution of thermolysin was first prepared in 0.5% ammonium bicarbonate, pH 8.0. The thermolytic peptides were separated by HPLC and dried in a stream of nitrogen at 40°C.

Edman Degradation[5]

The radiolabeled peptide (9-15 nmol) was dissolved in 0.3 ml of di-methylallylamine buffer: 5 ml pyridine - 3.3 ml distilled water - 0.4 ml dimethylallylamine (Pierce), adjusted to pH 9.0 with 10% trifluoroacetic acid. Phenyl isothiocyanate (20 µl) was added, the solution was flushed with nitrogen, stoppered, and kept at 50°C for 30 min. The solution was extracted 3 times with 1.2 ml benzene and the aqueous phase was dried in a stream of nitrogen.

Cleavage was done in 100 µl trifluoroacetic acid (40°C, 15 min.) and ethylene chloride was used to precipitate the shortened peptide and to extract the thiazolinone derivative. The ethylene chloride extracts were combined and dried in a stream of nitrogen.

Conversion was carriedout in 0.2 ml 1N HCl (80°C, 10 min.) and the PTH-amino acid was extracted with 3 x 1 ml portions of ethyl acetate. The combined ethyl acetate extracts were dried under nitrogen and dissolve in 0.2 ml of HPLC grade methanol. The aqueous phase was frozen and also sub-jected to HPLC to identify water soluble PTH amino acids.

RESULTS

There are 36 Met residues per mol of bovine lung converting enzyme[3] and we routinely resolve at least 30 of the 37 predicted cyanogen bromide cleavage peptides on HPLC.[2] All of the radioactivity is found in one of the cyanogen bromide cleavage peptides derived from radiolabeled enzyme. This peptide contains the active-site Glu residue that is esterified by chlorambucyl-L-[U-^{14}C]-Proline.[2] The molecular weight of this peptide is about 16,000 (Table 1) determined either by gel permeation chromatography or calculated from its amino acid composition. There are 2 Lys and no Arg equivalents indicating only 2 potential trypsin cleavage sites.

The radioactive cyanogen bromide peptide was digested with trypsin and 3 tryptic peptides (T-1, T-2, and T-3) were resolved on HPLC (Fig. 1). Only T-2 carried the radiolabel and based on the measurement of radioacti-vity, 21-36 nmol (903-1550 cpm) of T-2 was recovered.

The molecular weight of T-2 is about 9,000 (Table 1) and its amino acid analysis shows that T-2 contains no Lys but does contain 1 residue per mol of homoserine lactone. Therefore, T-2 is the C-terminal peptide derived from the cyanogen bromide cleavage peptide. Because many of the residues are neutral or hydrophobic, thermolysin was used to further degrade T-2.

Five peptides were obtained after digestion with thermolysin (Th 1-5) which were resolved on HPLC (Fig. 2). Only Th-1 (M_r 1290) (Table 1) was radioactive. Usually, we recovered 85% of Th-1 (18-31 nmol; 774-1320 total cpm). Th-4 appeared as a single peak on HPLC, but gel permeation chromato-graphy (Sephadex G-25 or Bio-Gel P-4) revealed that Th-4 was actually 2 peptides, Th-4a (M_r 1250) and Th-4b (M_r 1150). The sum total of the resi-dues of the thermolytic peptides is in good agreement with the analysis of T-2 (Table 3) indicating that we probably did not miss any small cleavage peptides.

In 5 separate experiments, Th-1 was subjected to manual Edman degrada-tion to determine its sequence. In 4 experiments, results were obtained through 8 cycles (Table 2). Based on its amino acid composition, Th-1 con-tains 12 residues (Table 2), and its sequence through 8 Edman degradation cycles is:

516

Table 1. Molecular Weights of the Radiolabeled Cyanogen Bromide Cleavage
Peptide and Its Trypsin and Thermolysin Degradation Peptides

Peptide	Molecular Weight	
	Gel Permeation[a]	Amino Acid Analysis[b]
BrCN[c]	15850	16584.1
Trypsin Peptides[d]		
T-1	5300	5282.1
T-2[c]	8600	8278.6
T-3	2200	2663.0
Thermolysin Peptides[e]		
Th-1[c]	1230	1291.6
Th-2	1250	1218.9
Th-3	1000	1048.7
Th-4a	1320	2809.2[f]
Th-4b	1150	–
Th-5	1820	1739.9

[a] Determined by chromatography on a calibrated column (1.5 x 60 cm) of
Sephadex G-50, G-25 or BioGel P-4 equilibrated in 0.1% acetic acid.
[b] Calculated from the nearest integer residues per mol.
[c] Peptides that carry the radiolabel.
[d] Trypsin peptides derived from the BrCN peptide.
[e] Thermolytic peptides derived from T-2.
[f] Calculated from the combined analysis of Th-4a and Th-4b.

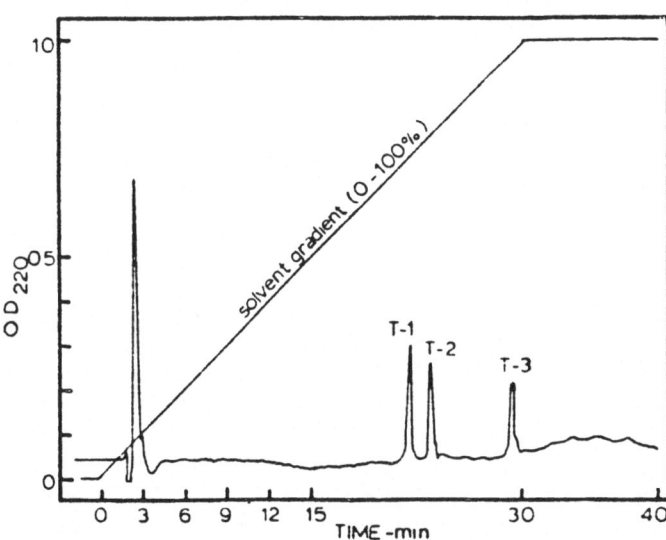

Fig. 1. HPLC separation oj the trypsin degradation peptides derived from
the radiolabeled cyanogen bromide cleavage peptide. All of the
recovered radioactivity (903-1550 cpm) was in peptide T-2. The
fractions containing each peptide were pooled separately and
lyophilized for further studies. The injection peak occurs at
about 3 min.

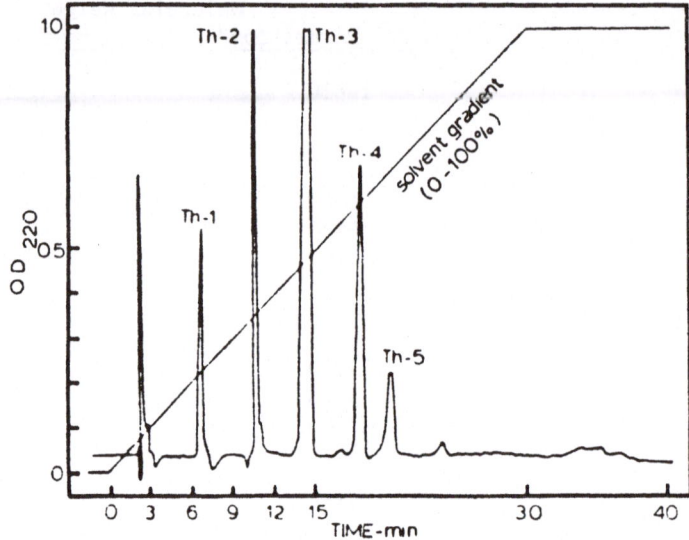

Fig. 2. HPLC separation of the thermolysin degradation peptides derived
from T-2. All of the recovered radioactivity (774-1320 cpm) was
in Th-1. The injection peak occurs at about 3 min.

Table 2. Amino Acid Composition of the Thermolysin Digest Peptides
Derived from T-2[a]

	Th-1[b]	Th-2	Th-3	Th-4a,b[d]	Th-5
			Residues per mol		
Trp[c]	N.D.[e] (0)	N.D. (0)	N.D. (0)	0.9 (1)	N.D. (0)
Asp	0.9 (1)	2.1 (2)	0.9 (1)	N.D. (0)	3.8 (4)
Thr	1.2 (1)	0.3 (0)	0.3 (0)	N.D. (0)	0.4 (0)
Ser	2.2 (2)	0.4 (0)	0.4 (0)	N.D. (0)	0.9 (1)
Glu	1.7 (2)	0.9 (1)	0.8 (1)	1.8 (2)	1.1 (1)
Pro	N.D. (0)	3.2 (3)	1.8 (2)	7.9 (8)	N.D. (0)
Gly	N.D. (0)	3.3 (3)	2.1 (2)	1.8 (2)	5.8 (6)
Ala	0.8 (1)	0.3 (0)	N.D. (0)	N.D. (0)	0.9 (1)
Val	2.1 (2)	4.1 (4)	5.1 (5)	8.2 (8)	N.D. (0)
Ile	0.2 (0)	N.D. (0)	N.D. (0)	0.3 (0)	0.8 (1)
Leu	2.2 (2)	N.D. (0)	N.D. (0)	5.5 (6)	1.7 (2)
Tyr	0.3 (0)	N.D. (0)	N.D. (0)	0.3 (0)	1.0 (1)
Phe	0.9 (1)	N.D. (0)	N.D. (0)	N.D. (0)	1.0 (1)

[a]Results of 20h hydrolyses of 3 nmol Th-1, 13 nmol Th-2, 11 nmol Th-3, 12
nmol Th-4a,b and 12 nmol Th-5 (6N HCl, 110°C). The values for Ser and
Thr are not corrected for decomposition. Figures in parentheses are
nearest integer residues/mol.
[b]Th-1 carries the radiolabel.
[c]Low value due to loss on acid hydrolysis.
[d]A single amino acid analysis was done on peptides Th-4a and Th-4b.
[e]N.D. = Not detected.

Table 3. Sequence Analysis of the Radiolabeled Thermolytic Peptide Derived From Angiotensin Converting Enzyme[a]

PTH-Amino Acid	cycle[b] (nmol detected)							
	1	2	3	4	5	6	7	8
Asp						_4.6_		
Thr		_5.4_	0.9	0.3				
Ser				0.7			_1.7_	0.9
Glu	0.8	0.4	_8.0_	0.6				_1.5_
Leu			0.8	_6.2_	0.9		0.6	
Ala	1.7	0.8	0.4		_3.4_			
Val						0.9		
Phe	_8.5_	0.5	1.1					
Gly	0.9							

[a] 9 nmol of the thermolytic peptide, Th-1, were subjected to manual Edman degradation as described in Methods. The major residue released at each cycle is denoted by underlining. The affinity label was released at cycle 3. As expected, in any one cycle, we often observed the residues from the preceding and succeeding cycles.

H_2 N-Phe-Thr-Glu-Leu-Ala-Asp-Ser-Glu...

Because of the low yields of PTH-Ser and PTH-Glu compared with the amounts of other amino acids that were detected in cycles 7 and 8, there is some uncertainty in the assignment of these last two residues.

At cycle 3, the ester bond between glutamic acid and chlorambucyl-L-[U-^{14}C]-Proline is hydrolyzed during the conversion step of the Edman procedure (1N HCl, 80°C). The bis-hydroxy derivative of chlorambucyl-pro is then extracted into ethyl acetate along with PTH-Glu. The amount of radiolabel that was released was equivalent to the amount of PTH-Glu detected on HPLC. These observations confirmed our earlier findings that Glu is the site of esterification with chlorambucyl-L-[U-^{14}C]-Proline.

DISCUSSION

Obtaining the radiolabeled active-site dodecapeptide of converting enzyme depended on the fortunate circumstances that the ester linkage is stable to the various cleavage procedures. HPLC proved to be very useful in obtaining the labeled peptides in good yield and in good purity. This too was fortunate because a large catalytic polypeptide presents special difficulties in terms of the number of cleavage peptides that are formed and the large amount of material that is needed for study. The fact that we resolve far more than half of the expected cyanogen bromide peptides, 30 out of 37, confirms that the converting enzyme does not contain repeat units either as separate polypeptides or as a single chain.

Chlorambucil and chlorambucyl-L-proline are the only examples of affinity labels for the angiotensin I converting enzyme. In a previous paper[2], we showed that a Glu residue at the active-site is esterified with chlorambucyl-L-proline and in this respect, the converting enzyme is similar to carboxypeptidase A, carboxypeptidase B, or thermolysin in which a catalytic role for Glu is supported by their x-ray structures. The catalytic Glu residues of these other zinc proteases can also be esterified with appropriate affinity labels for these enzymes[6,7].

The sequence that surrounds the catalytic Glu residue of converting enzyme is presented in Figure 3 for comparison with the corresponding amino acid sequences of carboxypeptidase A,[8] carboxypeptidase B,[6] and thermolysin.[9] With the mammalian zinc proteases, there is sequence homology at 5 of the first 8 Thh-1 residues. Only 2 of 8 residues are homologous with thermolysin, a bacterial zinc protease. When the sequences are matched for maximum alignment, it is evident that converting enzyme shows a single amino acid deletion (Phe) on the amino side of the catalytic Glu residue.

Upon binding substrate, thermolysin undergoes a conformational change which brings the catalytic Glu residue and the active-site zinc ion into a non-polar environment.[7] The non-polar environment enhances the ability of the Glu residue to act as a general base.

The sequence, Glu-Leu, is common to each of the zinc proteases (Fig. 3) and in the mammalian protease sequences, one or two Phe residues precede the catalytic Glu. These hydrophobic amino acids may contribute to the non-polar environment of these enzymes during catalysis or if the Leu or other hydrophobic residues are also brought into a non-polar environment along with the Glu residue, it would make the conformational change less favorable.

Converting enzyme is a carboxyl-dipeptidase and does not share substrate specificity with the other zinc proteases. However, the location of a glutamic acid residue at the active-site and the marked homology with the carboxypeptidases near this residue suggests an evolutionary relationship between these enzymes and a similarity in catalytic mechanisms.

```
THERMOLYSIN:          A H  E* L  T H A V T D T Y
CARBOXYPEPTIDASE A:   F T F  E* L R D  T G R T G F
CARBOXYPEPTIDASE B:     T F  E* L R D  K G R T G F
CONVERTING ENZYME:    F T    E* L A D  S E S, V, V, L
```

Fig. 3. Primary sequence neighboring the catalytic Glu residue of bovine lung converting enzyme compared with the analogous sequences of bovine pancreatic carboxypeptidase A and B and bacterial thermolysin. The Glu residue esterified with the appropriate affinity label is indicated by (*). 8 of 12 residues of Th-1 were sequenced; the remaining 4 deduced from its amino acid composition are indicated in brackets. Alignments are marked in boxes.

ACKNOWLEDGEMENTS

This work was supported by a grant (HL22242) from the U.S.P.H.S. National Institutes of Health. These results are excerpted from a full length manuscript, accepted for publication in the Journal of Biological Chemistry.

REFERENCES

1. R. B. Harris and I. B. Wilson, J. Biol. Chem., 257:811-815 (1982).
2. R. B. Harris and I. B. Wilson, J. Biol. Chem., 258:1357-1362 (1983).
3. R. B. Harris and I. B. Wilson, Intl. J. Pep. Prot. Res., 20:167-176 (1983).
4. D. H. Spackman, W. H. Stein, and S. Moore, Anal. Biochem., 30:1190-1206 (1958).
5. P. Edman and A. Henschen, in: "Protein Sequence Determination," S. B. Needleman, ed., Springer-Verlag, New York (1975).
6. M. T. Kimmel and T. H. Plummer, Jr., J. Biol. Chem., 247:7864-7869 (11972), Nature, New Biol., 238:35-37 (1972).
7. D. Rasnick and J. C. Powers, Biochemistry, 17:4363-4369 (1978).
8. R. A. Bradshaw, L. H. Ericsson, K. A. Walsh, and H. Neurath, Proc. Natl. Acad. Sci. USA, 63:1389-1393 (1969).
9. K. Titani, M. A. Hermodson, L. H. Ericsson, K. A. Walsh, and H. Neurath, Nature, New Biol., 238:35-37 (1972).

VALUE OF DETERMINATION OF KININASE II IN BRONCHOALVEOLAR LAVAGE FLUID

Hans Schweisfurth,[1,2] Michael Schmidt, Roland Leppert,
Edgar Brugger and Lucius Maiwald

Marienhospital Gelsenkirchen (Academic Hospital of the University of Essen)[1] and Department of Internal Medicine, University of Würzburg, Federal Republic of Germany. Supported by the Deutsche Forschungsgemeinschaft, Schw. 309/2-1.[2]

SUMMARY

Kininase II (KII), identical with angiotensin-I-converting enzyme (E.C. 3.4.15.1) was characterized biochemically and assayed fluorimetrically in bronchoalveolar lavage fluid and serum of 153 patients with several pulmonary disorders. The albumin concentrations of serum and bronchoalveolar lavage fluid (BLF) have also been measured. The pH optimum of KII derived from BLF (LKII) was 8.0. The Michaelis Menten constant was 38.5 μmol/l using benzyloxycarbonyl-phenylalanyl-histidyl-leucine as synthetic substrate. LKII could be inhibited between 80 and 100% by EDTA, phenanthroline, dimercapto-1-propane-sulfonic adic (DMPS), hydroxyquinoline and captopril. The LKII activity (mU/ml BLF) showed no differences in all lung diseases, but the specific LKII (mU/mg albumin) was significantly elevated in sarcoidosis compared to pneumonia ($p < 0.05$), fibrosis ($p < 0.05$), chronic obstructive bronchitis ($p < 0.005$) and lung cancer ($p < 0.01$), but not in tuberculosis. This study shows that LKII is measurable in native, unconcentrated BLF and the results indicate that LKII could be useful for diagnosis of pulmonary disorders.

INTRODUCTION

Kininase II (KII) is identical with angiotensin-I-converting enzyme (E.C. 3.4.15.1). It is a peptidyldipeptidase which is mainly located in the caveolas of the membranes of the endothelial cells within the pulmonary vasculature.[1] The physiological role of KII is seen in the formation of angiotensin II from angiotensin I by splitting off the dipeptide histidyl-L-leucine and in the degradation of bradykinin[2,3] to an inactive heptapeptide.

KII has become of interest for diagnosis of pulmonary disorders since elevated enzyme activities had been found in serum of patients with sarcoidosis of the lung.[4]

As in other non-pulmonary disorders, increased KII activities also have been observed[5,6,7] the elevation of this enzyme is not to be regarded as pathognomonic for sarcoidosis. Recently KII could also be detected in other body fluids such as urine,[8] pleural effusion,[9] cerebrospinal fluid[10] and seminal plasma.[11]

Since the development of the fiber optic bronchoscopy, bronchoalveolar fluid can be obtained from the alveolar space of the lung.

Several components of this bronchoalveolar lavage fluid (BLF) have already been assayed, but the KII activity has also been estimated after an 50-70 fold enrichment of this enzyme only in some studies.[12,13] The aime of this study was to characterize the biochemical behavior of KII in BLF (LKII). Furthermore, the levels of LKII were to be compared to the KII activities found in serum (SKII) of the patients with pulmonary disorders.

METHODS

The bronchoalveolar lavages were performed by means of a fiber optic bronchoscope of which the tip was wedged into a subsegmental bronchus of the middle lobe or lingula of the lung. In lung cnacer or pneumonia, this procedure has always been practiced in the healthy part of the lung segment. Aliquots of 20 ml of a hypotonic saline solution (80 ml distilled water in 1 l NaCl 0.9%) at 37° C were infused and the fluid was immediately collected through a siphon under light negative pressure (-5 to -10 cm H_2O). This process of lavage was repeated 15 times. The BLF was centrifuged at 400 g for 10 min and stored at -37° C until measurement.

The KII activities in serum and in the non-concentrated, native BLF were measured fluorimetrically as reported elsewhere.[14]

One unit (U) of LKII or SKII is defined as the amount of enzyme required to release 1 μmol histidyl-L-leucine per min at 37° C under standard assay conditions in 1 ml body fluid (i.e. U/ml = μmol/ml/min). If the KII activity is related to one mg albumin, this is regarded as specific enzyme activity.

A total of 153 patients of both sexes has been examined, 44 suffering from sarcoidosis, 10 from tuberculosis, 16 from pneumonia, 15 from fibrosis, 24 from chronic obstructive bronchitis and 44 from lung cancer. The diagnoses were assessed on the basis of clinical features, X-ray, sputum examinations, lung function tests and biopsies obtained by fiberoptic bronchoscopy.

Additionally albumin was determined in serum and BLF by means of colorimetry with bromcresol green at 405 nm wavelength.

RESULTS

The pH optimum of LKII was found to be 8.0 using borax phosphate buffer (Fig. 1). The Michaelis Menten constant was 38.5 μmol/l with benzyloxy-carbonyl-phenylalanyl-histidyl-leucine as synthetic substrate (Fig. 2).

Inhibitors of LKII were also tested. LKII could be blocked by EDTA, 1, 10-phenanthroline, 2, 3-dimercapto-1-propane-sulfonic acid (DMPS), captopril and 8-hydroxyquinoline (Table 1).

In the various pulmonary disorders, the LKII activities (mU/ml BLF) showed no significant differences compared to sarcoidosis. However, if we calculated the specific LKII (mU/mg albumin), the enzyme levels were significantly elevated in sarcoidosis (with the exception of tuberculosis) (Table 2).

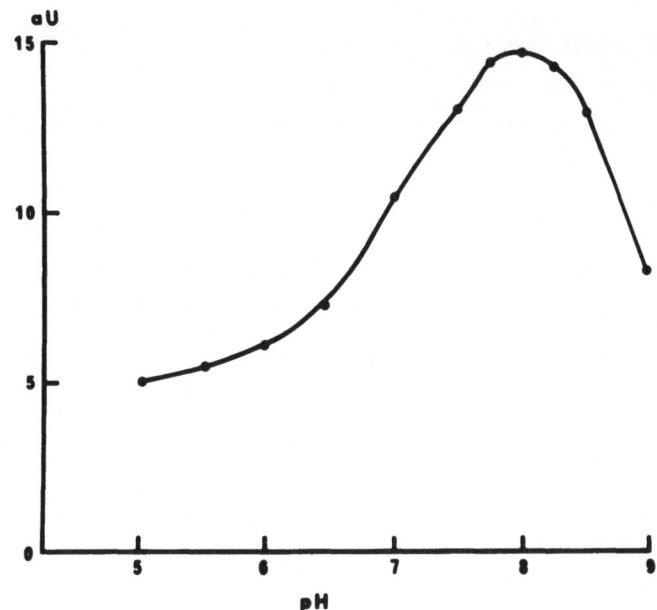

Fig. 1. PH-dependence of KII derived from bronchoalveolar lavage fluid, using borax phosphate buffer (0.05 mol/l borax and 0.1 mol/l KH_2PO_4). aU: Fluorescence intensity in arbitrary units (500 nm wavelength).

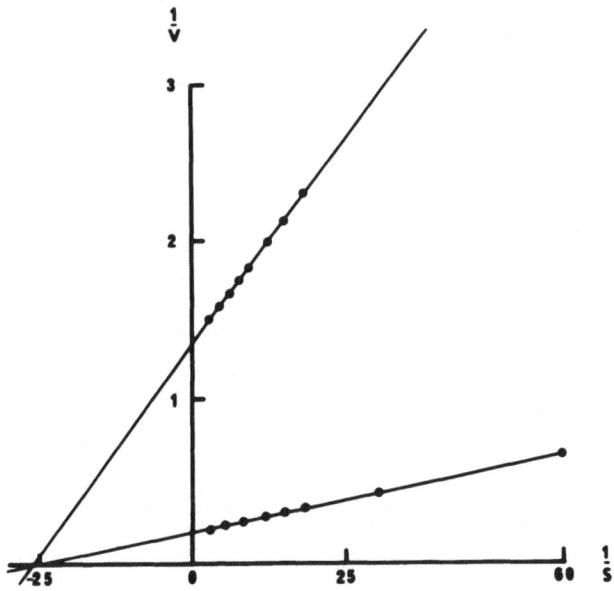

Fig. 2. Determination of the Michaelis Menten constant of LKII by the Lineweaver Burk plot with benzyloxycarbonyl-phenylalanyl-histidyl-leucine as synthetic substrate and borax phosphate buffer, pH 8.0.

Table 1. Inhibition of LKII In Vitro, Using Benzyloxycarbonyl-Phenylalanyl-Histidyl-Leucine as Substrate

	Maximal Inhibition (%)	Concentration (mmol/l)
EDTA	80	0.01
Phenanthroline	90	0.5
DMPS	83	0.01
8-Hydroxyquinoline	100	1.0
Captopril	100	1.0

DISCUSSION

In previous investigations, LKII activities were only measured after
40-70 fold enrichment of the BLF,[12,13] but contradictory results have been
obtained.[15]

With this fluorimetric assay, which based on the method already described,[16] no enrichment of KII was necessary so that we could determine
the KII in native BLF.

The biochemical behavior of the LKII is similar to the KII found in
serum which has the same pH optimum and the K_m was in the range as
reported.[16] This low K_m value indicates that KII has an high affinity the
artificial substrate used. The inhibitory patterns of SKII were also similar to the LKII.

LKII related to 1 ml BLF volume showed no significant differences between the various lung diseases so that the determination of the LKII activities does not seem to be very helpful for diagnosis of lung diseases.
However, if the LKII is related to the albumin concentration of the BLF,

Table 2. Correlation of KII in Serum (SKII) and in BLF (LKII) Between
Sarcoidosis and Different Lung Diseases

	SKII (mU/ml)	LKII (mU/ml)	Specified LKII (mU/mg)
	p <	p <	p <
Tuberculosis	0.05	NS	NS
Pneumonia	0.001	NS	0.05
Fibrosis	0.001	NS	0.05
Chronic obstructive bronchitis	0.001	NS	0.005
Lung cancer	0.001	NS	0.01

in consequence this specific LKII activity (mU/mg albumin) is significantly elevated in the different pulmonary disorders with the exception of tuberculosis.

The distribution of albumin in the BLF was not uniform. The highest albumin concentrations were found in BLF of lung cancer, whereas the lowest albumin concentrations were observed in serum. The ratio between albumin in serum compared to BLF was about 200, the ratio for KII was 80. This is surprising because the molecular weight of albumin is only 65,000 as compared to that of KII which has been reported as 140,000.[17] If only a transudation from the vascular to the alveolar space occurs, the ratios would be expected to be nearly equal. However, our investigations show that the KII with the higher molecular weight would more easily penetrate the membranes. This seems unlikely. Therefore it is presumed that the KII transport is actively facilitated or the KII is secreted by the alveolar cells. In some investigations, no KII could be detected[15] so that it seems to be very possible that the KII could be transported selectively from the endothelial cells into the alveolar space. The pathophysiological role of the KII in the alveolar space is not yet fully understood but it is suggested that the KII acts on natural substrates such as angiotensin I and bradykinin. The generated angiotensin II could also influence the alveolar cells and the degradation of bradykinin should prevent a change in the permeability of the alveolar cells.

Our results show that KII in BLF is similar to the serum KII but the role in the BLF needs to be clarified.

ACKNOWLEDGEMENT

The authors thank Mrs. Wechner for her technical assistance.

REFERENCES

1. J. W. Ryan, U. S. Ryan, D. R. Schultz, C. Whitaker, A. Chung, and F. E. Dorer, Subcellular localization of pulmonary angiotensin converting enzyme (kininase II), Biochem. J., 146:497-499 (1975).
2. K. K. F. Ng and J. R. Vane, Conversion of angiotensin I to angiotensin II, Nature, 216:762-766 (1967).
3. H. Y. T. Yang, E. G. Erdös, and Y. Levin, A dipeptidyl carboxypeptidase that converts angiotensin I and inactivates bradykinin, Biochim. Biophys. Acta, 214:374-376 (1970).
4. J. Lieberman, Elevation of serum angiotensin-converting-enzyme (ACE) level in sarcoidosis, Am. J. Med., 59:365-372 (1975).
5. H. Schweisfurth and H. Wernze, Changes of serum angiotensin I converting enzyme in patients with viral hepatitis and liver cirrhosis, Acta Hepato-Gastroent., 26:207:210 (1979).
6. H. Schweisfurth, Das angiotensin-I-converting enzyme, Dtsch. Med. Wschr. 47:1815-1818 (1982).
7. J. Lieberman and A. Sastre, Serum angiotensin-converting enzyme: Elevations in diabetes mellitus, Ann. Int. Med., 93:825-826 (1980).
8. B. Baggio, S. Favaro, S. Cantaro, L. Bertazzo, A. Frunzio, and A. Borsatti, Increased urine angiotensin I converting enzyme activity in patients with upper urinary tract infection, Clin. Chim. Acta, 109:211-218 (1981).
9. F. K. Romer and H. Geday, Activity of angiotensin-converting enzyme in pleural fluid and serum in non-sarcoid, non-tuberculous pleural effusion, Eur. J. Respir. Dis., 63:102-106 (1982).

10. Schweisfurth, H and S. Schiöberg-Schiegnitz, Assay and biochemical characterization of angiotensin-I-converting enzyme in cerebrospinal fluid, _Enzyme_, 32:12-19 (1984).
11. D. Roth and M. Roth, Purification of angiotensin-converting enzyme from human seminal plasma, _Experientia_, 30:686 (1974).
12. M. Perrin-Fayolle, Y. Pacheco, R. Harf, B. Montagnon, and N. Biot, Angiotensin converting enzyme in bronchoalveolar lavage fluid in pulmonary sarcoidosis, _Thorax_, 34:790-792 (1981).
13. J. J. Lanzillo and B. L. Fanburg, Angiotensin-converting enzyme in bronchoalveolar lining fluid, _Lancet I_:1199-1200 (1979).
14. H. Schweisfurth, M. Schmidt, R. Leppert, E. Brugger, and L. Maiwald, A fluorimetric method for determination of human angiotensin-I-converting enzyme (kininase II) in native, unconcentrated bronchoalveolar lavage fluid, To be published.
15. R. G. Gupta, R. Catchatourian, L. Sicilian, and J. P. Szidon, Angiotensin converting enzyme (ACE) in broncho-alveolar lavage (BAL) in sarcoidosis, _Am. Rev. Resp. Dis._, 119:69 (1979).
16. Y. Piquilloud, A. Reinharz, and M. Roth, Studies on the angiotensin converting enzyme with different substrates, _Biochim. Biophys. Acta_, 206:136-142 (1970).
17. J. J. Lanzillo and B. L. Fanburg, Angiotensin I converting enzyme from human plasma, _Biochem._, 16:5491-5495 (1977).

EVIDENCE FOR A POTENT ANGIOTENSIN I DEGRADING ENZYME DIFFERENT FROM ANGIO-

TENSIN I CONVERTING ENZYME IN RAT VASCULAR TISSUES

Julian Rosenthal,° Johanna Pschorr,* Ingrid C. M. Jacob,*
Nicola von Lutterotti,* Beate Pfeifle,° and Herbert Dahlheim,*

*Department of Physiology, University of Munich, and °Ulm
University Medical Center, Federal Republic of Germany

SUMMARY

There are indications for the existence of an intrinsic renin angiotensin system in vascular walls, which is assumed to participate in blood
pressure regulation and in pathogenesis of arterial hypertension. It was
evaluated if and to what extent the decapeptide angiotensin (A) I, one of
the natural substrates of A I converting enzyme (ACE), is degraded by other
peptidases than ACE in rat vascular tissues. A I and A II degradation was
studied in arterial and venous vascular wall extracts. The activities ranged
between 0.068 ± 0.025 U and 0.044 ± 0.025 U. The enzymes involved were
biochemically characterized by determination of isoelectric points (pI),
pH optima, molecular weights and by investigation of their inhibition behavior in vitro. One potent A I degrading enzyme (AIDE) was identified with
pI between 3.6 and 3.9, and pH optimum at 7.75. In vitro studies revealed
that AIDE activity was not blocked by the specific ACE inhibitors MK 421
or MK 422 (both 11 nMol/ml). The molecular weight of AIDE ranged between
440,000 and 457,000. The results indicate that AIDE is not identical to
ACE (pI 4.2-5.0; pH optimum 8.3). AIDE was also observed in aortic smooth
muscle cells cultured in vitro. AIDE decreased following bilateral nephrectomy or administration of aldosterone combined with sodium chloride loading,
whereas it was elevated in spontaneously hypertensive rats (Okamoto strain).
Since AIDE metabolizes A I, one of the substrates of ACE, it may indirectly
affect A II formation and bradykinin inactivation as well.

INTRODUCTION

The existence of an intrinsic renin angiotensin system (RAS) in arterial
walls has repeatedly been suggested.[1] Nowadays, there is indeed increasing
evidence for the participation of such a hormonal system in regulation of
arterial blood pressure, and also in the pathogenesis of essential and other
forms of hypertension. Recently performed studies with angiotensin I converting enzyme (ACE) inhibitors support this assumption.[2] These blockers
lower blood pressure also in hypertensive patients with normal or even low
plasma renin activities. In a preceding study, enzymatic components of
the RAS in rat vascular tissues were identified and biochemically characterized.[3] In the course of these investigations, a second angiotensin I degrading enzyme (AIDE) beside ACE with an obviously higher angiotensin (A)

I degradation rate than ACE was observed. In the same study, relatively
high amounts of A I and A II immunoreactivities were found in arterial walls.
It was assumed that AIDE was involved in control of local A II formation
and possibly of bradykinin degradation.

The present investigation was undertaken to biochemically characterize
AIDE and to compare its levels in arterial and venous tissues. Beside that,
the effect of varying (patho)physiologic conditions on AIDE activity was
investigated. AIDE activity was also determined in spontaneously hypertensive (SH-) rats of the Okamoto strain and in aortic smooth muscle cells
of the rat cultured in vitro.

METHODS

Sprague-Dawley rats of either sex as well as male SH-rats of the Okamoto
strain and their controls, all weighing between 200 and 250 g,, were anaesthetized with Inactin (Byk-Gulden, Konstanz, FRG; 110 mg/kg b.w. i.p.).
Through a median incision, the thoracic aorta was exposed, removed, and
immediately freed from adjacent fat and blood by repeated rinsing with cold
saline. The V. cava was prepared in the same manner. The tissue was then
frozen in liquid nitrogen for about 15 sec, cut into 0.5 mm pieces, transferred to cold saline (1 ml/0.1 g wet tissue), and homogenized by means
of the Potter-Elvehjem technique (6 times 30 sec with 30 sec intervals)
followed by ultrasonic disintegration (9 times 1 sec with 1 sec intervals;
amplitude: 6 μ). The homogenate was centrifuged (2 min, 8050 x g, Eppendorf
centrifuge 3200, or 1 h, 100,000 x g, Beckman Ultracentrifuge), and the
supernatant used. All procedures were carried out below 4°C.

To 1.0 ml 0.15 M phosphate buffer of the desired pH, 0.075 ml A I (or
A II) (10 ng/ml saline) and 0.1 ml of the supernatant of the tissue extracts
(or saline for the blanks) were added. The mixture was incubated at 37°C.
Samples of 0.05 ml were drawn at several intervals and transferred into
0.5 ml 0.15 M phosphate buffer, pH 7.4, containing bovine gamma-globulin
(Serva, Heidelberg, FRG; final concentration 0.09%). Then, all samples
were measured by radioimmunoassay as described previously.[3,4] The respective
angiotensin levels measured were plotted semilogarithmically against incubation time, and the period of time ($T \frac{1}{2}$) required for a 50% consumption of
the initial substrate was determined. For each sample, $1/T \frac{1}{2}$ (= U) was
taken as a measure for the activity of angiotensin degrading enzymes.[5]

ACE activity was measured either with the method of Piquilloud et
al[4,6] or with a modification of the method of Cushman and Cheung.[3,7] For
determination of IC_{50}-values (measure for the degree of inhibition) ACE
was incubated with the substrate Z-Phe-His-Leu and varying concentrations
of ACE inhibitors. Inhibition of AIDE was investigated with MK 421 (ethyl
ester maleate salt of N-[S]-1-(ethoxy-carbonyl)-3-phenyl-propyl-Ala-L-Pro)
and its diacid form, i.e. MK 422 (both from Merck, Sharpe and Dohme; 11
nM/ml) and with trasylol (Bayer, Leverkusen, FRG; 1333 U/ml).

The isolation and growth of aortic smooth muscle cells in vitro has
been described in detail previously.[8] Suspensions with 60-80 . 10⁵ cells/ml
saline were ultrasonically disintegrated 3 x 2 sec with 1 sec intervals.

To determine isoelectric points (pI), a LKB 8100-1 column, LKB Ampholine
and glycerol gradients were used. Following determination of pH, the eluted
fractions were dialyzed against distilled water, lyophilized, and redissolved
in 0.9% saline.[3]

Estimation of molecular weights was performed by Sephadex gel filtration, using gels G-100 and G-200, 0.9% saline as solvent, and Pharmacia

calibration kits containing ribonuclease A, chymotrypsinogen A, ovalbumin, bovine serum albumin, aldolase, catalase, and ferritin.

Aldosterone was administered for two weeks (CIBA-Geigy, Wehr, FRG; 25 mg/kg b.w. s.c.), combined with 0.9% saline as drinking fluid. Bilateral nephrectomy was performed 20 h prior to the experiments under Nembutal anaesthesia (ABbott/Ceva, Neuilly-sur-Seine, France; 0.84 mg/kg b.w.).

RESULTS

An enzyme kinetic measurement of A I degradation in arterial tissue extract is illustrated in Fig. 1 (upper panel). Within less than 30 min, almost 90% of the initial substrate is consumed. When 0.9% saline is added instead of homogenate extract (blank), reductions of substrate concentrations lower than 10% are observed.

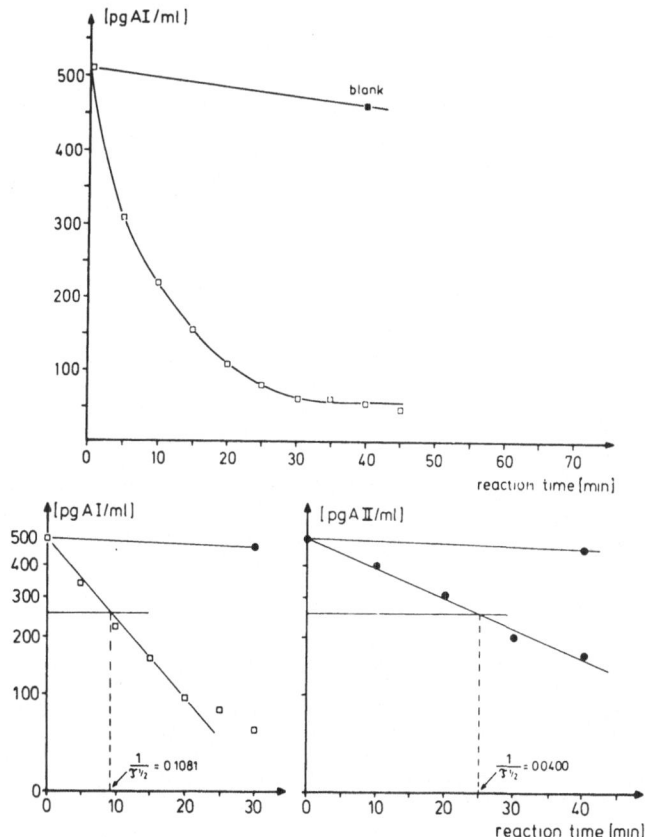

Fig. 1. (Upper panel) Enzyme kinetic determination of A I degradation by rat aortic homogenate extracts. Incubation conditions: 0.15 M phosphate buffer pH 7.75; sample volume: 0.1 ml (0.1 g wet tissue/ ml). Initial substrate concentration of the reaction mixture: approx. 8.7 ng/ml. Incubation temperature: 37°C. For the blank, saline was used instead of homogenate. (Lower panel) A I and A II degradation by rat aortic homogenate extracts (semilogarithmic plot). Incubation conditions for AIDE as above. A II degrading activity was measured at pH 7.4.

In Fig. 1 (lower panels), A I and II degradation for aortic homogenate extracts (0.1 g wet tissue/ml saline) of normal Sprague-Dawley rats are plotted semilogarithmically and demonstrate linearity in both cases. At the optimal pH of the enzymes, the man values are 0.068 ± 0.025 U (n = 13) for A I degradation in arteries and 0.064 ± 0.036 U (n = 6) in veins. For A II degradation, the corresponding values are 0.069 ± 0.017 U (n = 8) for arterial and 0.044 ± 0.025 U (n = 5) for venous tissue. At pH 8.3, the pH optimum for ACE, A I degrading activity was 0.040 ± 0.011 U (n = 9) in the arteries.

The results of isoelectric focusing and pH experiments on arterial A I and II degrading enzymes and ACE are compared in Fig. 2. The second peak measured for A I degrading activity (pI between 4.2 and 4.7) is in the same range as that found for aortic ACE (4.2-5.0). The effect of pH on A I degradation in presence and absence of the specific ACE inhibitors MK 421 or MK 422 revealed a measurable inhibition only between pH 8.0 and 8.8, which is in the range of the ACE pH optimum, whereas at the pH optimum of AIDE (pH 7.0-7.8) no blocking effect was observed (Fig. 3). From these values, a 2- to 3-fold AIDE activity as compared to that of ACE was estimated when using identical initial concentrations of their common substrate A I. Molecular weight values, determined for AIDE, ranged from 440,000 to 457,000, and were different from those of A II degrading enzyme (232,000-315,000).

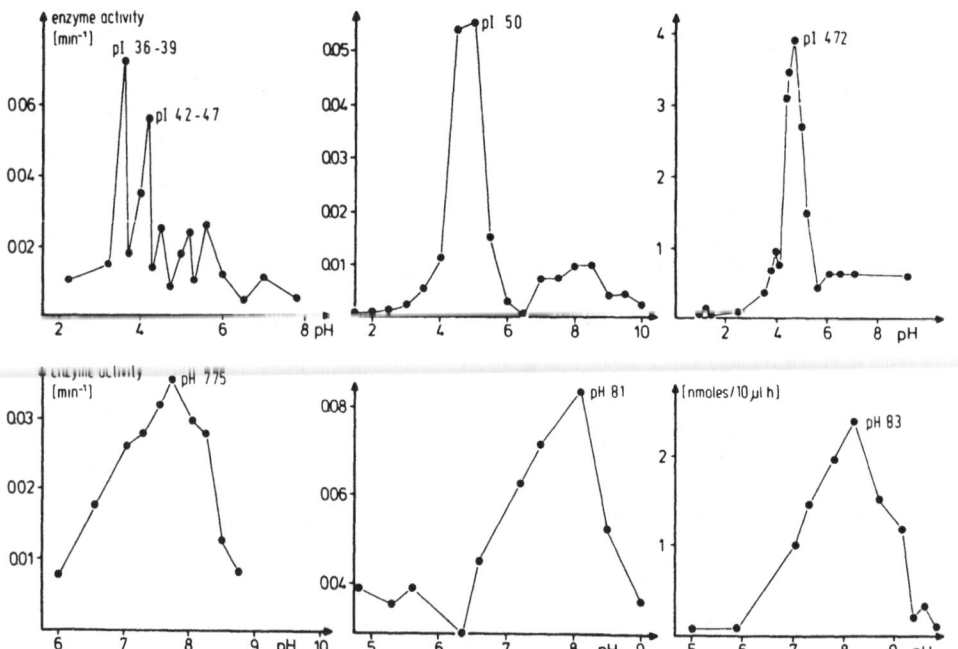

Fig. 2. (Upper panel) Determination of isoelectric points in aortic tissue. pH gradient: 3.5-10. Left: AIDE; starting material: 119 mg wet tissue. Center: A II degrading enzyme; starting material: 806 mg wet tissue. Right: ACE; starting material: 605 mg wet tissue. (Lower panel) Effect of pH. Incubation conditions: A I and A II degradation in 0.15 M phosphate buffer of the desired pH. Other conditions as in Fig. 1; ACE in 0.05 M borax phosphate buffer of the desired pH containing 1% NaCl (Piquilloud-method);[6] incubation time: 60 min; incubation temperature: 37°C.

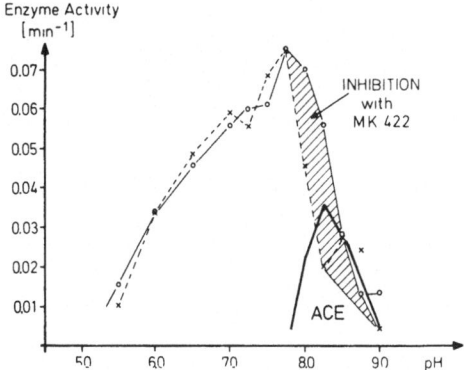

Fig. 3. Effect of pH on AIDE activity of rat aortic homogenate extracts
with and without ACE inhibitor MK 422. Incubation concentration
of the inhibitor: 11 nM/ml incubation mixture. Incubation in 0.15
M phosphate buffer of the desired pH. Other conditions as in Fig.
1.

The IC_{50}-value for ACE fropm arterial walls (in vitro studies) with
the inhibitor MK 422 was 0.0018 nM/ml (Fig. 4). Trasylol (1333 U/ml) did
not affect the activity of AIDE.

The isoelectric focusing behavior of AIDE from aortic smooth muscle
cells revealed two pI values at 5.0 and 6.6 (Fig. 5, left); the effects
of pH (Fig. 5, right) gave further evidence for the presence of two A I
degrading enzymes with pH optima at 6.0 and 8.0, the latter one being identical with the pH optimum of ACE.

Following bilateral nephrectomy, ACE activity was increased in aortic
(32.7 ± 0.9 vs 27.3 ± 1.3 nM/g. min, p < 0.001, 3 rats) as well as in venous
tissue (26.0 ± 0.8 vs 13.6 ± 0.8 nM/g. min, p < 0.001, 6 rats); AIDE was
reduced only in the aorta (0.093 ± 0.006 U vs 0.126 ± 0.013 U, p < 0.005,
3 rats). In aldosterone-treated animals, an increase of ACE activity was
found only in aortic tissue (56.7 ± 2.6 vs 46.3 ± 1.3 nM/g. min, p < 0.001,
4 rats) whereas a decrease occurred in veins (28.3 ± 0.8 vs 31.6 ± 1.2 nM/g.
min, p < 0.005,, 4 rats). AIDE activity decreased in venous tissue (0.114
± 0.003 U vs 0.138 ± 0.005 U, p < 0.005, 4 rats). In SH-rats, there was

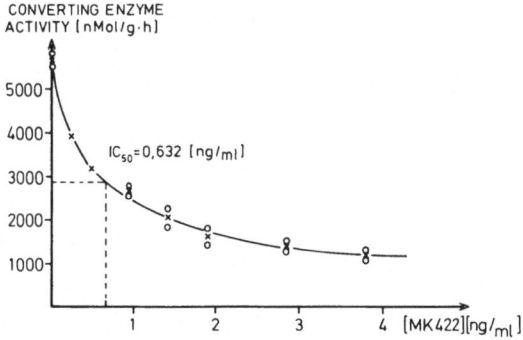

Fig. 4. Determination of IC_{50}-value for ACE activity in aortic tissue.
Measurements were performed with the method of Piquilloud et al.[6]
at pH 8.0. Other conditions as in Fig. 2.

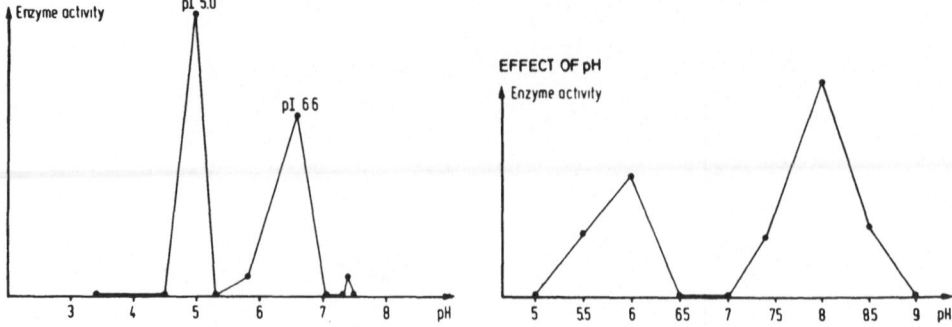

Fig. 5. (Left) Determination of isoelectric points of AIDE activity in
         isolated smooth muscle cells of rat aorta cultivated in vitro.
         pH gradient: 3.5-10. Starting material: 60-80 . 10^5 cells/ml,
         17.5 ml. (Right) Effect of pH. Incubation in 0.15 M phosphate
         buffer of the desired pH. Samples were drawn after 0, 20 and 40
         minutes. Other conditions as in Fig. 1.

an increase of AIDE activity in arterial tissue (0.098 ± 0.002 U vs 0.059
± 0.005 U, p < 0.005, 3 rats) and a significant decrease in venous tissue
(0.027 ± 0.004 U vs 0.040 ± 0.002 U, p < 0.003, 6 rats); ACE activity also
increased in the aorta (80.0 ± 1.8 vs 21.1 ± 0.6 nM/g. min, p < 0.001, 3
rats).

DISCUSSION

     In this report, information on the vascular renin angiotensin system
was extended by emphasizing the existence and action of an enzyme presumably
important for the local A II formation, and possibly for bradykinin inactivation. The analytic approach by enzyme kinetic measurements, employing low
substrate concentrations, was useful in quantifying AIDE activities. The
utilization of substrate saturation would necessitate high dilution of the
samples for radioimmunological measurements, which may lead to inaccurate
values. BEside that, the angiotensin substrate concentrations employed
in these experiments are closer to the physiologic levels of A I in vascular
walls.[3] The optimal homogeniuzation conditions for vascular tissues have
been systematically determined prior to the experiments.

     Under these conditions, and when measuring the enzymatic activities
at their respective pH optima, AIDE activity was 2-3 times higher than that
of ACE. Therefore, AIDE may not be neglected when studying vascular angiotensin formation. This is supported by the fact that the pH optimum of
AIDE is nearer to the physiologic pH of 7.4 than that of ACE. Since it
is known tha tpeptidases degrade various substrates, it has to be considered
that AIDE may consume other peptides than A I. However, in arterial and
venous tissues, A I is mainly degraded by AIDE.

     An AIDE is also present in venous tissue; its specific activity does
not diffeer significantly from that of aortic tissue. At this point we
have no further data on the biochemical characteristics of the venous enzyme.
Since there are indications for the existence of venous renin and ACE
biochemically different from the aortic enzymes, the tentative conclusion
was drawn that the RAS in venous tissue behaves physiologically different
from its arterial counterpart.[3]

AIDE activity was not inhibited by MK 421 or MK 422, two specific A
I converting enzyme inhibitors, in a concentration which blocks ACE at least
to 95%. No inhibition was observed with trasylol either. The latter inhibitor was used, since earlier investigations demonstrated the existence of
an A I degrading enzyme in microdissected glomeruli of rat kidney, which
was obviously suppressed by trasylol at this concentration.[9] Therefore,
AIDE from aortic tissue appears to be different from that observed in renal
cortex.

Experiments in 20 hours bilaterally nephrectomized rats exhibited a
decrease of arterial AIDE activity. The accompanying metabolic acidosis
is likely to enhance this effect in vivo, since the pH in blood is shifted
further away from the pH optimum of AIDE (7.75). However, under these conditions ACe activity increased in both aortic and venous tissues. This disso-
ciative behavior also indicates that AIDE and ACE are not identical.

In SH-rats (Okamoto strain), AIDE activity was significantly elevated
in aortic tissue when compared with normotensive controls of the same strain
or with normal Sprague-Dawley rats. However, this increase was markedly
lower than that of ACE in arterial walls. This experiment was performed
in SH-rats with a mean systolic blood pressure of 190 ± 7.63 mm Hg.
Increased activities of A I and A II-forming enzymes in vascular tissues
of SH-rats have been reported previously,[1,3] indicating a general
stimulation of the enzymatic components of the vascular RAS in this model
of hypertension.

Finally, administration of aldosterone combined with 0.9% saline as
drinking fluid induced a decrease of AIDE, and simultaneously a significant
increase of ACE. In this case, AIDE enhances the physiologic activity
of ACE with regard to A II formation or bradykinin inactivation.

Though it appears that AIDE is important for control of A II steady
state in vascular walls, there may be other, still unknown enzymatic components of the RAS involved in vascular A II formation. This is underlined
by the results obtained for aortic smooth muscle cells, which contain enzymatic components of the RAS different from those present in total vascular
tissue. Since intracellular enzymes of the RAS were also found by Muirhead
and Inagami in juxtaglomerular cells[10] and by Re et al.[11] in canine aortic
smooth muscle cells we expect intracellular, possibly metabolic actions
of the RAS. To what extent the intracellular system is related to that
present in total arterial walls is to be determined by future studies.

Some major questions remain for future investigations. They are mainly
concerned with the physiologic or pathophysiologic role of AIDE and the
nature of its reaction products. In addition, it has to be clarified if
there exist enzymatic effectors influencing this enzyme or other biologically active peptides metabolized by AIDE. In any case, because of its high
specific activity and the presence of relatively high concentrations of
its substrate A I in vascular walls,[3] AIDE is likely to be involved in
local A II and possibly also in bradykinin metabolisms.

ACKNOWLEDGEMENTS

This work was supported by the Deutsche Forschungsgemeinschaft. We
thank Gerhard Wittmann for his technical assistance.

REFERENCES

1. H. Dahlheim, I. C. M. Jacob, J. Pschorr, and J. Rosenthal, The renin angiotensin system in the extrarenal vascular walls: An approach to studies in humans, in: "Hormones in Normal and Abnormal Human Tissues," Vol. 3, K. Fotherby and S. B. Pal, eds., Walter de Gruyter & Co., Berlin, New York (1983).

2. Z. P. Horowitz, Pharmacology and mechanism of action of inhibitors of the renin angiotensin system, in: "Drug Development and Evaluation, Vol 4: Pharmacology and Use of Angiotensin I Converting Enzyme Inhibitors," F. Gross and R. K. Liedtke, eds., Fischer-Verlag, Stuttgart, New York (1980).

3. J. Rosenthal, B. Pfeifle, M. L. Michailov, J. Pschorr, I. C. M. Jacob, and H. Dahlheim, Investigations on components of the renin angiotensin system in rat vascular tissue, Hypertension, 6:383-390 (1984).

4. W. Burghardt, H. Schweisfurth,, and H. Dahlheim, Juxtaglomerular angiotensin II formation, Kidney Int., 22(Suppl. 12):S49-S54 (1982).

5. H. Dahlheim, K. Petschauer, and K. Thurau, Anreicherung und charakterisierung der erythrocytenangiotensinase, Pflügers Arch, 305:105-117 (1969).

6. Y. Piquilloud, A. Reinharz, and M. Roth, Studies on the angiotensin converting enzyme with different substrates, Biochim Biophys Acta, 206:136-142 (1970).

7. D. W. Cushman and H. S. Cheung, Spectrophotometric assay and properties of the angiotensin-converting enzyme of rabbit lung, Biochem Pharmacol, 20:1637-1648 (1971).

8. B. Pfeifle, H. H. Ditschuneit, and H. Distschuneit, Insulin as a cellular growth regulator of rat arterial smooth muscle cells in vitro, Horm. Metab. Res., 12:381-385 (1980).

9. H. Dahlheim and E. Schmidmeier, Determination and characterization of angiotensinase activity of microdissected juxtaglomerular apparatuses (JGA) of the rat kidney, Abstract, Vth International Congress of Nephrology, Mexico, 119 (1972).

10. W. A. Rightsel, T. Okamura, T. Inagami, J. A. Pitcock,, Y. Takii, B. Brooks, P. Brown, and E. E. Muirhead, Juxtaglomerular cells grown as monolayer cell culture contain renin, angiotensin I-converting enzyme, and angiotensins I and II/III, Circ. Res., 50(6):822-829 (1982).

11. R. Re, J. T. Fallon, V. Dzau, S. C. Quay, and E. Haber, Renin synthesis by canine aortic smooth muscle cells in culture, Life Sci., 30:99-106 (1982).

BRADYKININ COMPETITIVE ANTAGONISTS FOR CLASSICAL KININ SYSTEMS

John M. Stewart and Raymond J. Vavrek

Department of Biochemistry, University of Colorado School of Medicine, Denver, Colorado 80262

SUMMARY

The substitution of D-phenylalanine for proline at position 7 of bradykinin (BK) converts BK into a specific antagonist. Additional modifications of the nonapeptide structure, especially the inclusion of β-2-thienylalanine residues (Thi) for phenylalanine at positions 5 and 8, increase antagonist potency in the classic smooth muscle (isolated rat uterus and guinea pig ileum) and rat blood pressure kinin assays. [$Thi^{5,8}$,$DPhe^7$]-BK had a pA_2 value of 6.5 for inhibition of the BK response on rat uterus, and 6.3 on guinea pig ileum. Addition of Lys-Lys- or a D-Arg- residue to the N-terminal of $D-Phe^7$-substituted antagonists decreases uterine agonist activity, but does not affect inhibitory potency on the ileum. Addition of a D-proline residue in place of proline in position 3 of D-Arg- extended antagonists produces specific uterine inhibitors which show no antagonism on the ileum. The $D-Phe^7$-analogs did not inhibit smooth muscle responses to substance-P or angiotensin-II, and the antagonism of kinin responses was competitive.

INTRODUCTION

Studies of the role(s) of the nonapeptide BK (Arg-Pro-Pro-Gly-Phe-Ser-Pro-Phe-Arg) in mammalian physiology have been severely restricted by the lack of specific inhibitors of its physiological and pharmacological activities. In spite of more than two decades of investigation,[1,2] no specific sequence-related antagonists of the classical biological activities of BK on smooth muscle and blood pressure have been described. The antagonism of BK activity reported for heptyl amides of single amino acids[3] and of C-terminal tripeptide fragments of BK[4] was not specific for BK; these compounds also inhibited myotropic action of other agonists.

In a reassessment of the effects of substituents in position 7 of BK, brought about by the unexpectedly high agonist activity of [Aib^7]-BK,[5] the proline residue at position 7 of BK was replaced by several D-aliphatic and aromatic amino acid residues. The first antagonist was found among these analogs.

METHODS

Peptides were synthesized by the solid phase method on a Beckman 990 synthesizer and were purified by countercurent distribution. Purity of the synthetic peptides was assured by this layer chromatography and electrophoresis, and amino acid compositions and molecular weights were determined by quantitative amino acid anlysis. The analogs were assayed for myotropic activity on the isolated rat uterus and guinea pig ileum, and for their ability to lower blood pressure in the anesthesized rat, as previously described.[5,6] In the blood pressure assay, peptides were injected by both the iv (jugular vein) and ia (carotid artery) routes in order to estimate destruction in the pulmonary circulation. Abbreviations: Hyp = 4-hydroxy-proline, Δ-Pro = 3,4-dehydro-proline, Aib = α-amino-isobutyryl, CDF = p-chloro-D-phenylalanine, DNAL = β-(2-naphthyl)-D-alanine, MDY = O-Methyl-D-tyrosine, DPhg = D-phenylglycine, DhPhe = D-homophenyla-lanine.

RESULTS AND DISCUSSION

Table 1 lists the BK analogs having a single substitution,in position seven, that were synthesized and assayed for agonist and antagonist activity in this study. Only the Aib analog and two analogs with L-proline derivatives at position 7 (dehydro-Pro and hydroxy-Pro) showed significant smooth muscle agonist activity. [D-Ala^7]-BK and [D-Val^7]-BK showed weak agonist activity on the rat uterus but were devoid of BK-like activity on the guinea pig ileum.

DPhe^7 -BK also had weak BK-like agonist activity on the rat uterus and on rat blood pressure (1-4% agonist potency relative to BK), with moderate resistance to enzymatic breakdown in the rat pulmonary circulation,[6] but showed antagonism of the response of the guinea pig ileum to BK. This is the first observation of specific antagonism of a classical BK-response on smooth muscle caused by a sequence-related analog of BK. Determination of the inhibitor potency by means of pA$_2$ calculations of Schild[7] on the ileum preparation indicated a moderate level of antagonism of BK, pA$_2$ = 5.0. The pA$_2$ value represents the negative logarithm of the molar concentration of antagonist necessary to reduce the response of a double ED$_{50}$ dose of BK to the response of an ED$_{50}$ dose, where the ED$_{50}$ dose causes a half maximal contraction of the tissue.

Substitution of the proline residue in position 7 of BK with other D-aliphatic amino acid residues produced BK analogs with very weak agonist activity on the uterus, and no BK-like activity on ileum. Insertion of D-amino acid residues with large hydrophobic side chains or D-homo-phenylalanine or D-phenylglycine at position 7 gave analogs with little or no BK-like agonist effect on the smooth muscle preparations. The analog with D-histidine at position 7 had low agonist potency on uterus and none on ileum.

Selective further modification of [DPhe^7]-BK gave antagonists with greater potency and breadth of action (See Table 2). Replacement of the two phenylalanine residues at positions 5 and 8 of BK by the isosteric thienylalanine residue has been shown to increase the agonist potency of BK up to 10-fold.[8] Since the increased potency of this analog was thought to be due to increased receptor affinity,[9] this modification was tried with the antagonist. Replacement of the two phenylalanine residues in [D-Phe^7]-BK with thienylalanine increased the potency of the antagonist by

TABLE 1. Activities of Bradykinin Analogs with D-Aliphatic and
D-Aromatic Substitutions at Position 7

RESIDUE at 7	BIOLOGICAL ACTIVITIES		
	RUT	GPI	RBP-IA
Proline	100	100	100
Glycine	0.2	0.07	0.6
Alanine	1	1	-
Histidine	-	0.1	-
Hydroxyproline	2	3	-
Δ-Proline	25	12	-
des-Proline	0	0	-
Sarcosine	-	13	-
α-Aminoisobutyric	55	418	32
D-Proline	1.5	-	-
D-Alanine	0.3	0	0.03
D-Valine	5	0	0.3
D-Phenylalanine	1	AMTAGONIST	-
p-Chloro-D-Phe	7	0.2	1
D-Naphthylalanine	0.9	0.08	-
O-Methyl-D-tyrosine	AG	0	-
D-Tryptophan	4	0	-
D-Phenylglycine	0	AG	-
D-Homophenylalanine	-	AG	-
D-Tyrosine	0.2	0	-

RUT = isolated rat uterus; GPI = isolated guinea pig ileum; RBP-IA =
rat blood pressure, intracarotid injection.

For other abbreviations, see text.

TABLE 2. Bradykinin Inhibition by [D-PHE^7]-BK Analogs[a]

ANALOG	RUT	GPI
Bradykinin	AG (100%)	AG (100%)
[DPhe^7]-BK	AG (1%)	5.0
[Thi^{5,8}]-BK	AG (1000%)	AG (200%)
[Thi^{5,8}, DPhe^7]-BK	6.5	6.3
Lys-Lys-BK	35	–
DArg-BK	AG (143%)	AG (103%)
Lys-Lys-[DPhe^7]-BK	AG (0.3%)	5.1
DArg-[DPhe^7]-BK	AG (0.14%)	5.0
DArg-[Thi^{5,8}, DPhe^7]-BK	5.5	6.1
Lys-Lys-[Thi^{5,8}, DPhe^7]-BK	6.0	5.3
[DPro^3]-BK	AG (0.01%)	AG (0.02%)
[DPro^3-DPhe^7]-BK	0	0
[DPro^3, Thi^{5,8},DPhe^7]-BK	0	0
DArg-[DPro^3,DPhe^7]-BK	4.6	0
DArg-[DPro^3,Thi^{5,8},DPhe^7]-BK	5.2	0

[a] Data are given as pA$_2$ values according to Schild[7] or as agonist potency (AG) relative to BK = 100%. Thi = β-(2-thienyl)-L-alanine.

an order of magnitude on the ileum preparation (pA$_2$ = 6.2), and produced the first antagonist of the response of rat uterus to BK (pA$_2$ = 6.5) (the pD$_2$ of BK on the uterus is 7.9 and on the ileum is 7.5). [Thi^{5,8},DPhe^7]-BK is the most potent antagonist of BK smooth muscle activity we have at this time.

The resistance of N-terminal-extended BK analogs to kininase degradation, especially those with Lys-Lys-extentions,[10] suggested that long-acting antagonists of BK activity might be obtained by modifying the [D-Phe^7]-BK inhibitors with a Lys-Lys-extension. Additionally, our observations (Vavrek and Stewart, unpublished) that a D-Arg residue added to the N-terminal of BK agonists tends to increase uterine potency without affecting ileum activity prompted the synthesis of D-Arg-extended [D-Phe^7]-BK analogs as possible tissue specific inhibitors.

N-Terminal extension of [D-Phe[7]]-BK with Lys-Lys- or with the D-Arg residue reduced agonist potency in the uterus assay but had no effect on the antagonism seen in the ileum assay. Similarly, the inhibitory effect of [Thi[5,8],DPhe[7]]-BK was diminished on the uterus with the addition of either Lys-Lys- or D-Arg to the N-terminal. In the ileum assay addition of D-Arg to the very potent [Thi[5,8],DPhe[7]]-BK antagonist had little effect on inhibitory potency.

Odys reported that [D-Pro[3]]-BK showed significantly higher receptor binding in bovine myometrium membrane preparations than would be predicted by its low (<0.01%) smooth muscle potency.[9] Since high biological receptor binding coupled with low intrinsic activity are necessary conditions for competitive inhibitors, D-proline was incorporated into position 3 of our BK antagonists. This modification totally eliminated the agonist and antagonist activity of [DPhe[7]]-BK and [Thi[5,8],DPhe[7]]-BK in the smooth muscle assays. However, when a D-proline residue was introduced into position 3 of the D-Arg-extended analogs of these two inhibitors, a unique selectivity in the smooth muscle assays toward inhibition of the BK response on the uterus was found. The D-Arg extended antagonists containing D-proline in position 3 showed no agonist or antagonist activity on the guinea pig ileum preparation.

To determine whether DPhe[7]-containing sequence-related BK analogs were specific antagonists for BK-like activity, tests were made of the ability of these peptides to inhibit the myotropic activity of BK and two BK homologs of physiological importance, Met-Lys-BK and kallidin (Lys-BK), along with angiotensin-II(ANG) and substance P (SP) on guinea pig ileum (See Table 3). In each case the BK-related antagonists inhibited the action of BK-related kinins, but had no effect on ANG or SP. This kinin-specificity was also observed when DArg-[Thi[5,8],DPhe[7]]-BK was found to inhibit the activity of BK, Met-Lys-BK and Lys-BK, but not that of ANG, on the rat uterus. In the smooth muscle work, the antagonists produced parallel shifts of dose-response curves, indicating competitive antagonism.

The in vivo effects of three of our antagonists on blood pressure in the anesthesized rat[6] were determined. When DArg-[DPhe[7]]-BK, [Thi[5,8],DPhe[7]]-BK or DArg-[Thi[5,8],DPhe[7]]-BK were infused at a rate of 25ug/min, the response to a 25mm depressor dose (ED25mm) of BK was decreased from 25mm to 10mm. The blood pressure effect of BK returned to

TABLE 3. Specificity of [DPhe[7]]-BK Antagonists in Smooth Muscle Assays

ANALOG	RAT UTERUS				GUINEA PIG ILEUM				
	BK	KAL	MKBK	ANG	BK	KAL	MKBK	ANG	SP
[DPhe[7]]-BK	(AG)	–	–	–	5.0	5.6	6.0	No	No
DArg-[DPhe[7]]-BK	(AG)	–	–	–	5.6	6.0	6.3	No	No
[Thi[5,8],DPhe[7]]-BK	6.5	–	–	–	6.3	6.4	5.2	No	No
DArg-[Thi[5,8],DPhe[7]]-BK	5.5	5.5	5.8	No	6.1	6.7	6.4	No	No

Results are given as pA$_2$ values.[7] KAL = Kallidin; MKBK = Met-Lys-BK. Other abbreviations are given in the text.

normal within 5 minutes of terminating the antagonist infusion. The antagonists also showed inhibition when a mixture of BK and an antagonist was injected as a bolus by either the iv or ia route.

CONCLUSIONS

For the first time, a single residue modification of the BK sequence has produced an analog with BK antagonist activity. Substitution of the proline at position 7 of BK with D-phenylalanine is the key modification necessary for converting BK-agonists into BK antagonists. Antagonist potency can be increased significantly by additional modification of [DPhe^7]-BK by replacing phenylalanines at positions 5 and 8 with thienylalanine and making further modifications. The antagonists are specific for BK-like agonists in the classic in vitro smooth muscle assays. These antagonists also inhibit the in vivo rat blood pressure lowering effect of BK in a reversible manner.

ACKNOWLEDGEMENTS

This work was supported by grant HL-26284 from the NHLBI-NIH. The authors wish to thank Constance Young for performing the bioassays and Virginia Sweeney for the amino acid analyses.

REFERENCES

1. E. Schroeder, Structure-activity relationships of kinins, in: Handbook of Experimental Pharmacology, Vol. XXV, ed. by E. G. Erdos, Springer-Verlag, pp. 324-350, (1970).
2. J. M. Stewart, Chemistry and biologic activity of peptides related to bradykinin, in: Handbook of Experimental Pharmacology, Vol. XXV Supplement, ed. by E. G. Erdos, Springer-Verlag, pp. 227-272, (1979).
3. A. Gecse, E. Zsilinszky, and L. Szekeres, Bradykinin antagonism, Adv. Exptl. Med. Biol., 70:5-13, (1976).
4. G. Claeson, J. Fareed, C. Larsson, G. Kindel, S. Arielly, R. Simonsson, H. L. Messmole, and J. U. Balis, Inhibition of the contractile action of bradykinin on isolated smooth muscle preparations by derivatives of low molecular weight peptides, Adv. Exptl. Biol. Med., 120B:691-713, (1979).
5. R. J. Vavrek and J. M. Stewart, Bradykinin analogs containing α-aminoisobutyric acid (Aib), Peptides, 1:231-235, (1980).
6. J. Roblero, J. W. Ryan, and J. M. Stewart, Assay of kinins by their effects on blood pressure, Res. Commun. Pathol. Pharmacol., 6: 207-212, (1973).
7. H. O. Schild, pA, a new scale for the measurement of drug antagonism, Br. J. Pharmacol., 2:189, (1947).
8. F. W. Dunn and J. M. Stewart, Analogs of bradykinin containing β-2-thienyl-L-alanine, J. Med. Chem., 14:779-781, (1971).
9. C. E. Odya, T. L. Goodfriend, and C. Pena, Bradykinin receptor-like binding studied with iodinated analogs, Biochem. Pharmacol., 29: 175-185, (1980).
10. E. Schroeder, Synthese und biologische aktivitat bradykininwirksamer undeca-, dodeca- und tridecapeptide, Experientia, 21:271-276, (1965).

542

SMOOTH MUSCLE SELECTIVITY IN BRADYKININ ANALOGS WITH MULTIPLE D-AMINO

ACID SUBSTITUTIONS

Raymond J. Vavrek and John M. Stewart

Department of Biochemistry, University of Colorado School of
Medicine, Denver, Colorado 80262

SUMMARY

Two novel analogs of bradykinin (BK), [DAla^7]-BK and DArg-BK,
exhibited a dissociation of smooth muscle activities toward higher
potency on the uterus than on the ileum, in spite of increased metabolic
stability to pulmonary enzymatic breakdown in the rat blood pressure assay.
Analogs having a combination of the substitution of D-alanine in position
7 with a D-aromatic amino acid residue in position 6 show even greater
uterus specificity. The addition of a D-arginine residue to the N-terminal
greatly enhances this selectivity. Relative to BK, these poly-substituted
analogs are up to 17 times as potent on the uterus as on the ileum. Still
greater uterus selectivity is found among analogs in which glycine re-
places the serine residue at position 6 and a D-hydrophobic amino acid
residue (such as D-phenylalanine or D-p-chloro-phenylalanine) is present
in position 7. These [Gly^6, D-Hydrophobic^7]-BK analogs are 20-40 times
as potent on uterus as on ileum. [Gly^6,DPhe^7]-BK is the most uterus-
selective analog described. In contrast, [Aib^7]-BK is quite ileum-
selective, having a uterus/ileum potency ratio of 0.1.

This study represents an approach to engineering tissue selectivity
into BK analogs by modification of several residues in the BK sequence.

INTRODUCTION

The pharmacological potencies of bradykinin (BK) (Arg-Pro-Pro-Gly-
Phe-Ser-Pro-Phe-Arg) analogs in the guinea pig ileum assay generally
correspond to their resistance to pulmonary enzymatic breakdown as
determined in the anesthetized rat.[1] Results on the isolated rat uterus
(RUT) generally show less correlation with the pulmonary breakdown values.
These differences in potencies in the two smooth muscle assays is thought
to be due to the presence of kininases in ileum, while uterus is
relatively free of such enzymes. In analogs with little or no pulmonary
destruction in the rat blood pressure (RBP) assay relative to BK it is
rate to see high uterus potency coupled with low ileum potency; the reverse is usually the rule.

We reported earlier that the substitution of an α-amino-isobutyric acid (Aib) residue for proline at position 7 in BK produced the most potent 7-position analog of BK yet described.[2] [Aib[7]]-BK was shown to be 4 times as potent as BK on the ileum, and 5 times as potent on the rat blood pressure after iv administration. Its destruction in the pulmonary circulation was about half that of BK, which might explain some, but not all, of the increased potency in the ileum assay. This observation with the Aib-substituted analog prompted an examination of the effect of various D- and L-aliphatic and aromatic substituents at position 7 on biological activity, both singly and in combination with modifications at position 6. The α-aminoisobutyric residue is symmetrical; there are no D- and L-forms. For this reason, it is not clear if a D-amino acid residue at position 7 might be compatible with high BK-like potency; the Aib residue might be combining with the receptors in either its D-like or L-like conformation. Earlier, [DPro[7]]-BK had been shown to have extremely low biological activity.

METHODS

All peptides were synthesized by the solid phase method on an automatic Beckman 990 synthesizer, cleaved from the solid support with anhydrous HF, and purified by countercurent distribution. Peptides were analyzed for purity and composition, and their biological activities were determined as previously described.[2]

RESULTS AND DISCUSSION

The bioassay results obtained for 9 mono-substituted and 14 di- and tri-substituted BK analogs are listed in Table 1. The ratios of the potencies of the analogs, relative to BK, in the uterus and ileum assays are given at (RUT/GPI). This ratio is used as an indication of the tissue selectivity of the various analogs. In the table the RUT/GPI ratio for BK is arbitrarily designated as 1.0, so that all ratios are relative to that of BK. The uterus is normally more sensitive to BK ($pD_2=7.9$) than is the ileum ($pD_2=7.5$) in our assays.

Analogs with single D-amino acid (i.e., D-phenylalanine, p-chloro-D-phenylalanine, D-tryptophan) substitutions for serine in position 6 were remarkably potent in the BK assay systems, in spite of both a change in amino acid configuration at that position, and hence a significant change in overall backbone conformation, and an increase in hydrophobic character and side chain bulk. This group of analogs exhibited moderate resistance to enzymatic destruction in the rat pulmonary circulation, and a reasonably constant ratio of uterus to ileum potency (RUT/GPI=0.3-0.6).

Neither the D-alanine nor D-valine substitution for proline at position 7 of BK gave analogs with the high potency on the ileum and iv rat blood pressure seen with [Aib[7]]-BK. On the contrary, both were totally inactive in the ileum assay at doses up to 1000 times that of BK; in the rat blood pressure assay they had very low agonist potency, although they showed excellent resistance to pulmonary degradation. As noted earlier[2] D-amino acid substitutions at the Pro[7]-Phe[8] bond of BK, which is the primary site of cleavage of BK by angiotensin converting enzyme in the lung, would be expected to confer pulmonary stability on the molecule. Substitution of a glycine residue in position 7, which would allow a great deal of backbone flexibility compared with the structurally constrained proline residue, gave an analog with low BK-like potencies in all the assays and little resistance to pulmonary degradation.

Table 1. Bioassay Data for Bradykinin Analogs Containing Substitutions in Positions 6 and 7.

ANALOG	RUT	GPI	RUT/GPI	RBP-IA	RBP-IV	% D
BK	100	100	1.0	100	100	99
[Gly^6]–BK	29	61	0.5	–	–	–
[DPhe^6]–BK	6	13	0.5	0.2	8	35
[CDF^6]–BK	52	159	0.3	14	336	26
[DTrp^6]–BK	29	47	0.6	3	60	44
[Gly^7]–BK	0.2	0.07	2.9	0.6	0.7	95
[Aib^7]–BK	53	418	0.1	32	530	49
[DAla^7]–BK	0.3	0	*	0.03	2	0
[DVal^7]–BK	5	0	*	0.3	6	0
[Gly^6,Aib^7]–BK	2	4	0.5	0.3	6	0
[DPhe^6,DAla^7]–BK	11	6	1.8	0.6	18	0
[CDF^6,DAla^7]–BK	111	120	0.9	57	1151	77
[DTrp^6,DAla^7]–BK	31	18	1.7	2	52	45
[Gly^6,DVal^7]–BK	6	0.2	30.0	–	–	–
[DPhe^6,DVal^7]–BK	1	0	*	0[a]	0[a]	–
[CDF^6,DVal^7]– BK	1	0	*	0.9	14	35
[Gly^6,DPhe^7]–BK	31	0.8	38.8	2	22	20
[Gly^6,CDF^6]–BK	117	5	23.4	73	349	79
[CDF^6, DPhe^7]–BK	0.3	0.01	30.0	0	0	–
[CDF^6, CDF^7]–BK	0.2	0.2	1.0	0[b]	0[b]	–
DArg–BK	143	103	1.4	66	218	92
DArg–[DPhe^6,DAla^7]–BK	12	0.7	17.1	0.06	3	0
DArg–[DTrp^6, DAla^7]–BK	15	3	5.0	3	76	54
DArg–[CDF^6,DAla^7]–BK	153	51	3.0	12	340	8

a. Gave a pressor, followed by a depressor, response.
b. Gave a pressor response.
Aib=α-aminoisobutyric acid; CDF=p-chloro-D-Phe; % D=percent destruction on passage through rat pulmonary circulation.

In the rat pulmonary circulation Lys-Lys-BK exhibits total resistance to enzymatic breakdown. An added D-arginine residue does not confer similar total resistance to degradation in the pulmonary circulation, but it does reduce the pulmonary degradation to 92%, in contrast to the 99% destruction of BK; this increased stability is reflected in the high iv potency on blood pressure. The increased stability is not reflected in smooth muscle activities. This analog is equipotent with BK on ileum, but shows a 40% increase in rat uterus potency. This result suggests that addition to this basic residue to the N-terminus of the peptide may enhance its affinity for uterus receptors.

The combination of a D-aromatic residue in position 6 with D-alanine or D-valine in position 7 gives analogs with inconsistent activities and potencies. With D-alanine in position 7 a CDF residue at position 6 produces a very potent BK-like agonist, with very high iv potency (more than 10 times that of BK) on the blood pressure. Neither a D-phenylalanine nor a D-tryptophan residue in position 6 produces the same remarkable potency, but both these analogs show enhanced potency on the uterus as compared with the ileum. And while [DPhe^6,DAla^7]-BK retains the high resistance to pulmonary breakdown of [DAla^7]-BK, [DTrp^6,DAla^7]-BK resembles [DTrp^6]-BK more closely in pulmonary breakdown as well as in potency on uterus and blood pressure.

With D-valine in position 7, addition of D-phenylalanine or p-chloro-D-phenylalanine in position 6 did not alter the potencies seen with [DVal^7]-BK itself. [DPhe^6,DVal^7]-BK produced an anomalous blood pressure response, however. An immediate pressor response, possibly due to increased release of catecholamines, was followed by a rapid reflex depressor response. One other analog, [CDF^{6,7}]-BK produced a pressor response in the rat.

The three BK analogs with glycine in position 6 and D-aromatic amino acid residues (DVal, DPhe, CDF), in position 7 exhibited the greatest separation of smooth muscle potencies observed so far. [Gly^6,DPhe^7]-BK, with less than 1% of BK agonist potency on the ileum, was almost 40 times as potent on the uterus.

Addition of D-arginine to the N-terminus of the three DAla^7-analogs did decrease potency on the ileum, but did not increase potency on the uterus, so that the overall selectivity toward the uterus was less than 10-fold in this group.

CONCLUSIONS

The ability described here to design BK analogs with high selectivity for one tissue suggests that the receptors in these two smooth muscles may belong to different classes. Heretofore it had been thought that the uterus and ileum receptors had essentially the same hormone structural specificities. These results suggest that configurational flexibility is tolerated to a greater degree at the biological receptors in the rat uterus than by those in the guinea pig ileum, especially when a glycine residue is inserted for serine in the BK sequence at position 6. This in itself does not necessarily indicate separate receptor classes in the two smooth muscle preparations. The effect could be due to several factors, including access to the receptor site, resistance to non-specific enzymatic breakdown in the tissues, or binding to adjacent non-specific hydrophobic sites in proximity to the receptor. Given the high ileum selectivity of [Aib^7]-BK, we now have analogs whose potencies on these two smooth muscles differ by a factor of 400. Receptor binding studies with tissue-specific BK analogs, such as the studies carried out by Odya on bovine uterine myometrium membranes[3,4] and by Snyder and Manning on guinea pig ileum membrane particles[5,6], will be useful in determining whether separate BK receptor classes exist in separate tissues.

546

ACKNOWLEDGEMENTS

This work was supported by Grant HL-26284 from the NHLBI-NIH. The authors thank Constance Young for performing the bioassays and Virginia Sweeney for the amino acid analyses.

REFERENCES

1. J. Roblero, J. W. Ryan, and J. M. Stewart, Assay of kinins by their effects on blood pressure, Res. Commun. Pathol. Pharmacol. 6: 207-212, (1973).
2. R. J. Vavrek and J. M. Stewart, Bradykinin analogs containing α-aminoisobutyric acid (Aib), Peptides 1:231-235, (1980).
3. C. E. Odya, T. L. Goodfriend, and C. Pena, Bradykinin receptor-like binding studied with iodinated analogs, Biochem. Pharmacol. 29: 175-185, (1980).
4. M. J. Frederick, R. J. Vavrek, J. M. Stewart, and C. E. Odya, Further studies of myometrial bradykinin receptor-like binding, Biochem. Pharmacol. 33:2887-2892, (1984).
5. R. B. Innis, D. C. Manning, J. M. Stewart, and S. H. Snyder, (H3)Bradykinin receptor binding in mammalian tissue membranes, Proc. Natl. Acad. Sci. USA 78:2630-2634, (1981).
6. D. C. Manning, R. J. Vavrek, J. M. Stewart, and S. H. Snyder, Multiple bradykinin receptor binding sites with picomolar affinities (submitted for publication).

KININS, RECEPTORS, ANTAGONISTS

Domenico Regoli

Department of Physiology and Pharmacology, Medical School
University of Sherbrooke, Sherbrooke, Canada, J1H 5N4

SUMMARY

1. Kinins are potent myotropic agents acting on a variety of smooth muscle preparations: isolated arteries, veins, intestines, tracheae, urinary bladders, uteri, etc. In these tissues, kinins activate at least two different receptor types, B_1 and B_2.

2. B_1 and B_2 receptors for kinins have been identified by measuring the order of potency of agonists and the affinities of specific and competitive antagonists. Results of pharmacological studies have been confirmed by several investigators using binding assays with labelled bradykinin (BK) or desArg^{9}BK.

3. Antagonists for kinins active on B_1 and B_2 receptors have been identified. Anti-B_1 antagonists are specific, competitive and fairly potent: anti-B_2 antagonists have been identified among compounds primarily developed as anti-tachykinins: these compounds are non-specific, non-competitive and rather weak. They however may provide interesting new pharmacological tools, active against both kinins and tachykinins, two groups of endogenous peptides involved in the inflammatory process.

4. The type (direct, indirect) and the site (endothelial cell, smooth muscle fiber, autonomic nerve endings) of action of kinins in isolated vessels have been investigated. The results of various studies indicate that kinins do not act on the sympathetic nerve terminals of isolated organs in contrast with other peptides. Kinins do not promote the release of histamine or of 5-hydroxy-tryptamine from isolated arteries and veins.

5. Kinins are equally active in the presence and absence of indomethacin (an inhibitor of cyclooxygenase) or of BW 755C (an inhibitor of lipoxygenase) in some organs, while the actions of kinins on other organs are reduced to a variable extent by these inhibitors. In general, B_1 receptor systems do not depend on the ctivation of arachidonic acid, while B_2 receptor systems do: activation of the arachidonic acid cascade may be a feature of B_2 receptors.

6. Stimulant effects of kinins on arterial or venous vessels are independent on the endothelium, while the relaxant effect on the dog cartoid

artery occurs only in vessels with intact endothelium. The mechanism of action of kinins and tachykinins appears to be different from that of acetylcholine, since the peptides effects are not influenced by BW 755C and ETYA, two inhibitors of lipooxygenase that reduce significantly the effect of acetylcholine.

INTRODUCTION

The active products of the kallikrein-kinin system (bradykinin, kallidin and some of their metabolites) have been shown to be active, as stimulants or inhibitors, in a variety of organs containing smooth muscles. The existence of such effects has allowed us to apply to the study of kinin receptors, a classical pharmacological approach that was elaborated and successfully used in the field of biologically active amines such as catecholamines,[1] histamine[2] and other peptides, such as angiotensin.[3] The approach consists in attempting to correlate changes of kinins chemical structure with those in biological activities, using a series of compounds acting as agonists and modified in such a way as to distinguish, within the peptide molecules, the chemical groups involved in the binding of kinins to receptors from those primarily implicated in the receptors activation. Such an analysis generally provides useful indication for the design of antagonists. The availability of agonists and antagonists permit the utilization of the two fundamental criteria for receptor characterization, namely the determination of the order of potency of agonists and the measurement of the affinity of competitive antagonists. The existence of specific receptors for any endogenous agent is however not sufficient to determine whether this agent acts directly on the effector cells to produce changes of smooth muscle tone or if it acts indirectly, on a non-muscular cell type, to release another myotropic endogenous agent. In this study, useful indication has been obtained on the localization of tissue receptors and on the mechanism of action of kinin peptides in some isolated vessels.

METHODS

A variety of isolated organs, from various species (Table 1) have been isolated and used, according to the procedures and techniques described in several publications from our laboratory.[4-7] For all technical details the reader is therefore referred to these publications. Various peptides

Table 1.

Tissue	Preparation	Effect	Sensitivity
ARTERIES	Rabbit aorta	contraction	+
	Dog carotid artery	relaxation	++++
VEINS	Rabbit mesenteric vein	contraction	++
	Rabbit jugular vein	contraction	++
	Dog saphenous vein	relaxation	+++
INTESTINE	Guinea pig ileum	contraction	+++
	Rat duodenum	relaxation	++
TRACHEA	Guinea pig trachea	relaxation	+++
		contraction	+
URINARY BLADDER	Hamster urinary bladder	contraction	++
	Dog urinary bladder	contraction	++
UTERUS	Rat uterus	contraction	+++

+ up to 10^{-7}M   ++ up to 10^{-8}M   +++ up to 10^{-9}M   ++++ up to 10^{-10}M

related to bradykinin (BK), or to kallidin (K) and to their fragments desArg^{9}BK and desArg^{10}K have been investigated. Details of the chemical features of these peptides have been published.[8,9]

RESULTS

Kinins produce contraction or relaxation of various isolated organs (Table 1), containing smooth muscle fibers. These include segments or strips of vessels (arteries, veins), intestines, tracheae, urinary bladders and uteri. The sensitivity of these preparations to kinins show large variations and threshold concentrations of bradykinin active on these preparations vary from 10^{-7} to 10^{-10} M.

Are such differences to be attributed to the existence of different receptor types? Experiments, designed to answer this question, were performed on isolated vessels, the rabbit aorta (R.A.), the rabbit jugular vein (R.J.V.) and the dog carotid artery (D.C.A.), using as agonists: a) the natural kinins, BK, K and Met-Lys-BK, b) BK and K metabolites originated from the action of carboxypeptidase (desArg^{9}BK and desArg^{10}K) or of carboxy-dipeptidases (desPhe^8, desArg^{9}BK and desPhe^9, desArg^{10}K), and c) synthetic analogues such as [Tyr(Me)^8]-BK.

As shown by the results summarized in Table 2, the relative activities of the various compounds can be separated into two patterns: in the R.A., the metabolites desArg^{9}BK and desArg^{10}K are more active than the kinins: in fact, BK has only 8% of relative activity, compared to its metabolites desArg^{9}BK and the synthetic compound [Tyr(Me)^8]-BK is almost inactive. In the other two preparations, the most active compounds are BK, [Tyr(Me)^8]-BK and K, while the fragments are very weak agonists. These results support the existence of two different receptor types for which we have proposed the denomination of B$_1$ (R.A.) and B$_2$ (R.J.V., D.C.A.).[10]

This suggestion was substantiated by the results obtained with antagonists, and summarized in Table 3.

Antagonists against the actions of kinins on B$_1$ receptors were identified by preparing and testing a series of 8 analogues of desArg^{9}BK in which the natural residues were replaced one by one with L-Ala. Six of the eight compounds did not exert any antagonism, [Ala^7]-desArg^9-BK was a partial

Table 2. Biological Activities of Kinins, and Some Metabolites

COMPOUND	PREPARATION		
	R.A.	R.J.V.	D.C.A.
Bradykinin (BK	8*	100	100
Lys-BK (K)	95	150	64
Met-Lys BK	98	50	40
desArg^{9}BK	100	0.01	0.01
desArg^{10}K	2100	1	3.8
desPhe^8,desArg^{9}BK	0.1	<0.01	<0.01
desPhe^9,des-Arg^{10}K	0.1	0.01	0.05
[Tyr(Me)^8]-BK	0.1	140	100

* Relative activity.

Table 3. Abbreviated Structures and Biological Activities of Analogues of desArg^{9}BK

Compound	Biological activity on the rabbit aorta			
	α^E	pD_2	pA_2	$pA_2 - pA_{10}$
desArg^{9}BK	1.0	7.29	-	-
[Ala^2]-desArg^{9}BK	1.0	5.86	-	-
[Ala^3]-desArg^{9}BK	-	4.74	-	-
[Ala^4]-desArg^{9}BK	-	4.45	-	-
[Ala^7]-desArg^{9}BK	0.6	5.64	(+)	-
[Ala^8]-desArg^{9}BK	-	4.78	(+)	-
[Leu^8]-desArg^{9}BK	0	0	7.27	1.00
[Leu^9]-desArg^{10}K	0	0	8.37	1.00

$+_E$ indicates that the compound has a weak antagonistic activity.
α^E: intrinsic activity.
pD_2, pA_2: apparent affinities of agonists and antagonists.

agonist and [Ala^8]-desArg^{9}BK was a weak antagonist. Further modifications in position 8 of desArg^{9}BK (results obtained with a large series of compounds have been presented and discussed in reference 10, brought to the obtention of the potent, specific and competitive antagonists, [Leu^8]-desArg^{9}BK and [Leu^9]-desArg^{10}K. The first antagonist shows a pA_2 of 7.27 and an affinity for the B$_1$ receptors similar to that of desArg^{9}BK (pD_2 7.79): the second compound is approximately 20 times more active.

When tested on various preparations (Table 4), the two compounds are active in preparations possessing B$_1$ receptors, while they are completely inactive in preparations that have receptors of the B$_2$ type.

In order to develop an antagonist that will eliminate the action of kinins on B$_2$ receptors, the complete series of L-Ala analogues of BK was prepared and tested. As shown by the results of Table 5, the nine compounds were all active on the DCA, eight of them were full agonists and they did not provide any useful indication as to the localization of the active site of bradykinin.

Table 4. Affinities (pA_2) of Kinin Antagonists on Various Preparations

Antagonist	Rabbit aorta	Rabbit jugular vein	Dog carotid artery
[Leu^8]-desArg^{9}BK	7.27 (1.0)	inactive	inactive
[Leu^9]-desArg^{10}K	8.37 (1.10)	inactive	inactive
	Rabbit mesenteric vein	Cat ileum	Rat uterus
[Leu^8]-desArg^{9}BK	7.20 (0.98)	inactive	inactive
[Leu^9]-desArg^{10}K	8.15	inactive	inactive

In parenthesis: $pA_2 - pA_{10}$

Table 5. Activities of L-Ala Analogues of Bradykinin (BK)

Compound	Biological activity (dog carotid artery)		
	α^E	pD_2	R.A.
BK	1.0	8.64	100
[Ala^1]-BK	1.0	5.97	0.2
[Ala^2]-BK	1.0	6.33	0.5
[Ala^3]-BK	1.0	8.34	50.0
[Ala^4]-BK	1.0	6.78	1.4
[Ala^5]-BK	-	4.40	>0.01
[Ala^6]-BK	1.0	6.49	0.7
[Ala^7]-BK	1.0	6.16	0.3
[Ala^8]-BK	1.0	5.40	0.06
[Ala^9]-BK	1.0	5.38	0.06

α^E, pD_2: as in Table 3.
R.A.: relative activity.

Following these experiments, a large number of bradykinin analogues containing one or two substitutions in various positions, particularly in positions 5 and 8, were prepared and tested, but no one showed antagonistic activity: the results of these experiments have been described and discussed in reference 10.

Recently, during a testing of a series of tachykinin antagonists,[11] some of these compounds were found to exert a weak antagonistic effect against bradykinin, in preparations containing B_2 receptors. The results of a few experiments, presented in Table 6, indicate that the two tachykinin antagonists are inactive on the rabbit aorta and one of them [pro^2, trp^{7,9,10}]-SP is active on both the rabbit jugular vein and the dog carotid artery while the other is active only on the vein.

These preliminary results need to be confirmed. Despite their non-specificity and non-competitivity, these compounds present some interest and are promising in that they could be developed further to give large

Table 6. Bradykinin Antagonists (pA_2)

Compound	Preparation		
	Rabbit aorta	Dog carotid artery	Rabbit jugular vein
[Leu^8]-desArg^{9}BK	7.27	inactive	inactive
[pro^2,trp^{7,9,10}]-SP	inactive	5.70	5.20
[pro^4,trp^{7,9},pNO$_2$Phe^8]-SP (4-11)	inactive	inactive	5.43

spectrum antagonists, active against BK, SP and possibly other peptides (for instance bombesin).[12] The multiple actions of such antagonists could be of some utility in physiopathology, for instance for blocking kinins and tachykinins in inflammatory tissues.

Side and Mechanism of Action of Kinins

Further experiments were performed in isolated vessels to determine the specificity of kinin actions and to establish whether these peptides act directly or by the intermediate of other endogenous agents. Previous reports[13,14] have shown that, contrary to angiotensin and substance P, bradykinin and desArg[9]BK did not potentiate the effects of electrical stimulation in the rat vas deferens[13] and in the guinea pig ileum.[14] In the same preparations, BK did not show any inhibitory effect, in contrast with opioid peptides and somatostatin. These findings suggest that kinins do not exert presynaptic facilitatory or inhibitory actions in isolated vessels: it is however possible that, in other preparations, kinins modulate presynaptic transmitter release indirectly by increasing the local production of prostaglandins.[15]

Experiments with antagonists, including atropine, propranolol, phentolamine, support the above conclusion. Moreover, the negative results observed with mepyramine, cimetidine and methysergide indicate that kinins may not act through the release of histamine or of 5-hydroxy-tryptamine in arterial and venous isolated vessels. In other systems, for instance in the rat isolated mast cells, BK and desArg[9]BK promote the release of histamine, although they are less active than substance P (unpublished results from the author and its coworkers, Ph. Devillier, A. Renoux and J. P. Giroud, Medical School, Cochin-Port Royal, Paris).

Experiments were also performed to exclude the contribution of prostaglandins and leukotrienes in the myotropic effects of bradykinin of the two isolated vessels. It is known (see reference 10) that BK promotes the release of prostaglandins and possibly leukotrienes from various organs, particularly preparations containing receptors of the B_2 type, as shown by the data summarized in Table 7. Indomethacin and BW 755C were however inactive against the effect of BK in several isolated vessels, including the rabbit jugular vein and the dog carotid artery.

Table 7. Bradykinin and the Arachidonic Acid Metabolites

Preparation	Effect	Indo-methacin	BW 755C	Receptor
Rabbit aorta	C	0	0	B_1
Rabbit jugular vein	C	0	0	B_2
Dog carotid artery	R	0	0	B_2
Rabbit mesenteric vein	C	0	0	B_1
Guinea pig ileum	C	+	0	B_2
Guinea pig trachea	R	+	+	B_2
Hamster urinary bladder		+	0	B_2
Human fibroblasts*				
(protein formation) (19)	BK	+	?	B_2
(incorporation of ^{3}H thymidine)	desArg^{9}BK	0	?	B_1

R: relaxation   C: contraction

0: inhibitors are inactive

+: inhibitors reduce the effect of BK

In these tissues, the relaxant action of bradykinin was found to be dependent on endothelium, confirming the reports by other investigators[16,17] and by ourself.[18]

As shown in Fig. 1,, endothelium is required only for the relaxant effect of BK in the dog carotid artery. The stimulant actions of the kinins on the rabbit aorta, the rabbit jugular and mesenteric veins are as good in the absence as in the presence of endothelium, no matter whether they are mediated by B_2 receptors (the rabbit jugular vein) or B_1 receptors (the rabbit aorta and mesenteric vein).

What is the mechanism kof this endothelium-mediated relaxant effect of BK in some isolated arterial vessels? Kinins, as well as substance P, appear to relax the isolated arterial vessels by a mechanism which is different from that of acetylcholine, since this agent is significantly less active in the presence of inhibitors of the lipooxygenase (BW 755C and ETYA) while BK and SP are not influenced (Table 8).

In other preparations, for instance in the gunea pig trachea, the cyclooxygenase and lipoosygenase inhibitors reduce the effects of the two peptides. As shown in Table 8, the three agents (BK, Ach, SP) are potent stimulants of the guinea pig trachea. The effect of bradykinin is reduced in the presence of both the cyclooxygenase (indomethacin (INDO)) and lipooxygenase (BW 755C and ETYA) inhibitors, while that of acetylcholine is only influenced (reduced) by BW 755C and ETYA (eicosatetrainoic acid),

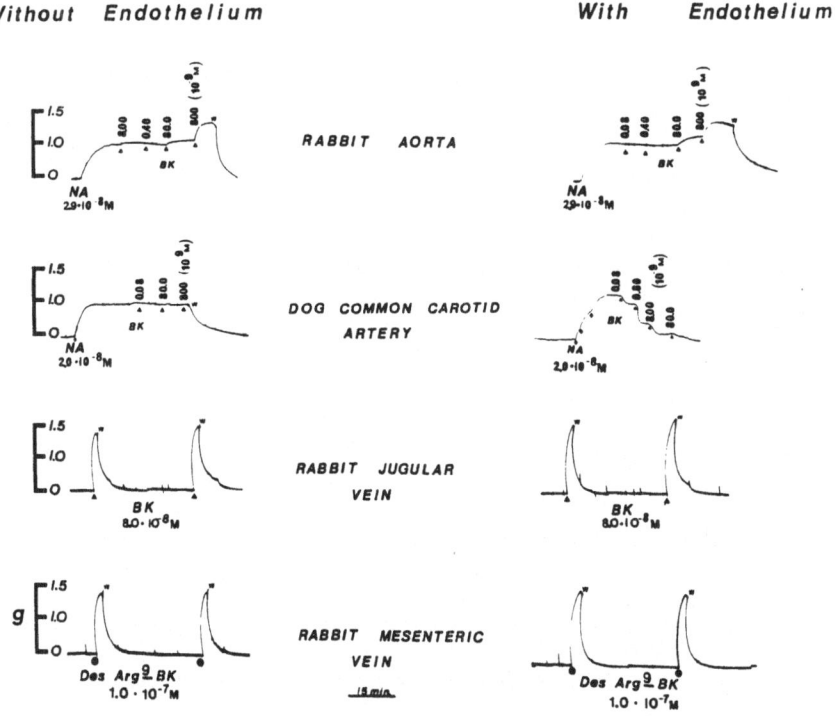

Fig. 1.   Effects of bradykinin (BK) on four isolated vessels in the presence and absence of endothelium. The two arteries were contracted with noradrenaline (NA) in order to quantify the relaxant effect of BK. Abscissa: time. Ordinate: tension in grams (g).

Table 8. Inhibitors of Arachidonic Acid. How They Influence the Effects
of Bradykinin (BK), Acetylcholine (Ach), and Substance P (SP)
in Two Preparations

Tissue	Agent/Effect		Control	Indo $(3\cdot10^{-5})$	BW 755C $(4\cdot10^{-5})$	ETYA $(3\cdot10^{-5})$
Dog carotid artery	BK $(8 \cdot 10^{-9}M)$	R	23 ± 5	25 ± 3	21 ± 4	24 ± 4
	Ach $(7 \cdot 10^{-8}M)$	R	34 ± 3	36 ± 2	25 ± 2**	27 ± 2**
	SP $(6.6 \cdot 10^{-9}M)$	R	23 ± 2	22 ± 2	19 ± 2	18 ± 3
Guinea pig trachea	BK $(8 \cdot 10^{-7}M)$	R	15 ± 2	0***	0***	0***
	Ach $(2 \cdot 10^{-7}M)$	C	27 ± 3	25 ± 2	0***	12 ± 3***
	SP $(7 \cdot 10^{-8}M)$	C	25 ± 2	39 ± 2***	21 ± 3	19 ± 3

Values are mm of relaxation (R) or of contraction (C)

** p <0.01   *** p <0.001

similar to what has been observed in the dog carotid artery. The myotropic
effect of SP is potentiated by indomethacin. These results suggest that
BK may promote the release of both prostaglandins and leukotrienes in the
guinea pig trachea, while acetylcholine and substance P interfere in some
way with the activities of lipooxygenase (the first) and of cyclooxygenase
(the second).

It is concluded that:

1. Kinins and related peptides exert direct, indirect and possibly gap-
junction mediated effects (Fig. 2), by acting on receptors localized
in the effector cell (as in Fig. 2-B), or by promoting the release of
other endogenous agents, such as prostaglandins, leukotrienes or histamine from another cell to activate the effector cell (as in Fig. 2-
A), or by activating a non-effector cell that however makes close
contact (gap-junctions) with the effector cell (as in Fig. 2-C).

2. Kinin receptors are of the two types, B_1, presumably localized in smooth
muscle membranes and B_2, localized in various tissue structures.
Further studies and the discovery and development of specific B_2 antagonists are needed to establish whether B_2 receptors, localized in various
cells, constitute an unique entity.

INDIRECT SIGNALING BY SECRETED CHEMICALS

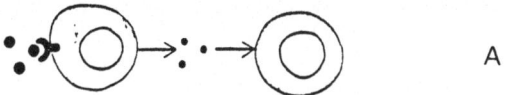

A

DIRECT SIGNALING BY PLASMA-MEMBRANE-BOUND MOLECULES

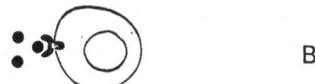

B

DIRECT SIGNALING VIA GAP JUNCTIONS

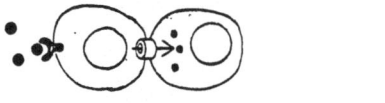

C

Fig. 2.

ACKNOWLEDGEMENTS

The author wishes to express his gratitude to Mrs. Cécile Théberge for the secretarial work. This work was performed with the financial support of the Medical Research Council of Canada (M.R.C.C.) and the Quebec Heart Foundation. The author is a Career Investigator of the M.R.C.C.

REFERENCES

1. H. O. Schild, Receptor classification with special reference to β-adrenergic receptors, in: "Drug Receptors," H. P. Rang, ed., University Park Press (1973).
2. A. S. F. Ash and H. O. Schild, Receptors mediating some actions of histamine, Brit. J. Pharmacol., 27:427-439 (1966).
3. D. Regoli, Receptors for angiotensin. A critical analysis, Can. J. Physiol. Pharmacol., 57:129-139 (1979).
4. D. Regoli, J. Barabé, and W. K. Park, Receptors for bradykinin in rabbit aortae, Can. J. Physiol. Pharmacol., 55:855-867 (1977).
5. J. Barabé, F. Marceau, B. Thériault, J.-N. Drouin, and D. Regoli, Cardiovascular actions of kinins in the rabbit, Can. J. Physiol. Pharmacol., 57:78-91 (1979).
6. R. Couture, P. Gaudreau, S. St-Pierre, and D. Regoli, The dog common carotid artery: A sensitive bioassay for studying vasodilator effects of substance P and of kinins, Can. J. Physiol. Pharmacol., 58:1234-1244 (1980).
7. J. Mizrahi, R. Couture, S. Caranikas, and D. Regoli, Pharmacological effects of peptides on tracheal smooth muscle, Pharmacology, 25:39-50 (1982).
8. W. K. Park, S. St-Pierre, J. Barabé, and D. REgoli, Synthesis of peptides by the solid-phase method. III. Bradykinin: Fragments and analogs, Can. J. Biochem., 56:92-100 (1978).
9. S. St-Pierre, P. Gaudreau, J.-N. Drouin, D. REgoli, and S. Lemaire, Synthesis of peptides by the solid-phase method. IV. Des-Arg[9]-bradykinin and analogs, Can. J. Biochem., 57:1084-1089 (1979).
10. D. Regoli and J. Barabé, Pharmacology of bradykinin and related kinins, Pharmacol. Rev., 32:1-46 (1980).

11. D. Regoli, E. Escher, and J. Mizrahi, Mini-Review. Substance P: Structure-activity studies and the development of antagonists, Pharmacology, 28:301-320 (1984).

12. J. Mizrahi, S. Dion, P. D'Orléans-Juste, and D. Regoli, Bombesin: Activities on smooth muscle and antagonism, Eur. J. Pharmacol., (Submitted).

13. D. Regoli, Peptide receptors on autonomic effectors: How should they be classified?, in: "Trends in Autonomic Pharmacology. Vol. 2," S. Kalsner, ed., urban and Schwarzenberg, München (1981).

14. D. Regoli, Neurohumoral regulation of precapillary vessels. The kallikrein-kinin system, J. Cardiovasc. Pharmacol., 6(Suppl. 2):S401-S413 (1984).

15. A. Nasjletti and K. U. Malik, Relationships between the kallikrein-kinin and prostaglandin systems, Life Sci., 25:99-110 (1979).

16. R. F. Furchgott, The requirement for endothelial cells in the relaxation of arteries by acetylcholine and some other vasodilators, TIPS, 3:173-175 (1981).

17. B. M. Altura and N. Chand, Bradykinin-induced relaxation of renal and pulmonary arteries is dependent upon intact endothelial cells, Brit. J. Pharmacol., 74:10-11 (1981).

18. D. Regoli, J. Mizrahi, P. D'Orléans-Juste, and S. Caranikas, Effects of kinins on isolated blood vessels. Role of endothelium, Can. J. Physiol. Pharmacol., 60:1580-1583 (1982).

19. R. H. Goldstein and M. Wall, Activation of protein formation and cell division by bradykinin and des-Arg[9]-bradykinin, J. Biol. Chem., 259:9263-9268 (1984).

EFFECTS OF KININS ON THE ISOLATED PERFUSED RAT KIDNEY AND EVIDENCE FOR THE

PRESENCE OF RENAL B_1 RECEPTORS*

Jorge A. Guimarães, Maria Aparecida R. Vieira,
Elizabeth Eich and Thomas Maack

Department of Biochemistry-ICB, UFRJ, Rio de Janeiro,
Brazil and Department of Physiology, Cornell University
Medical College, New York

SUMMARY

The kinins, particularly lysyl-bradykinin (LBK), have a bimodal effect
on the vasculature of isolated rat kidney. The vasorelaxant but not the
vasoconstrictor effect of LBK seems to be mediated by prostaglandins. The
vasoconstrictor action of LBK can be blocked by $(L-Leu)^8-des-Arg^9-BK$
indicating that the rat kidney vasculature has B_1 kinin-receptor which
mediates the effects of kinins and/or their C-terminal metabolites.

INTRODUCTION

Kinins appear to act on two different receptors recently characterized
and named B_1 and B_2 receptors by Regoli and Barabe.[1] The well known
vasocilating action of kinins[2] among other related effects such as hypotension and relaxation of large arteries and the contraction of smooth
muscles, have all been considered as a B_2 type-mediated response. This
type of receptor only recognizes the intact kinin molecule. Contrarily,
kinin-B_1 receptor, which recognizes the kinin fragments des-Arg^9-bradykinin
and des-Arg^{10}-lysyl-bradykinin, mediates the contraction of aorta and of
other large arteries.[3] Thus the existence of these receptors in the
kidney could explain some of the conflicting results found by different
authors concerning the renal vascular and hemodynamic actions of kinins.
It was then our purpose to test the direct effect of kinins in the
isolated perfused rat kidney and elucidate their mechanism of action on
renal vasculature.

METHODS

Isolated rat kidneys from Wistar rats (250-300 g) were perfused as
described by Maack[4] in a closed circuit system, with 60 ml of Krebs-
Henseleit bicarbonate buffer - 7.5% BSA, flucose and aminoacids. The
perfusate was gassed with 95% $O-5\%$ CO_2 at 37°C, pH 7.4. The initial
effective perfusion pressure was 90-100 mmHg.

---

*Work supported by grants from CNPq, FINEP, CEPG (UFRJ), Brazil and
N.I.H., AM 14241

Under control conditions, kidneys perfused in this manner maintain a constant renal vascular resistance for 90-120 min of perfusion. Isolated kidneys were allowed to stabilize for 20 min before experiments were started. After the stabilization period, two control clearance periods of 10 min each were performed. At the end the last control period, samples (0.1 to 1.0 ml) of the peptides and other test substances were added to the perfusate. Perfusion pressure (PP) and flow (RRF) were then continuously monitored. Results were expreseed in variations of the renal vascular resistance (RVR = PP/RPF). The peptides, bradykinin (BK), lysylbradykinin (LBK) and des-Arg^9-BK (DABK) (Sigma Chemical Co.) were diluted in the perfusion medium and added at the beginning of the experimental period as a single dosis. The B$_1$ kinin-receptor antagonist (1-Leu^8)-des-Arg^9-BK (LDABK) (Sigma Chemical Co.) was added to the perfusion medium 5 minutes before the addition of the agonists LBK or DABK.

RESULTS

Table 1 summarizes the effects of kinins and related peptides on renal vascular resistance (RVR) of the isolated perfused rat kidney (IPRK). Bradykinin (BK) and lysyl-bradykinin (LBK) added to the perfusate as a bolus at a final concentration of 0.07 uM induced a significant lowering of RVR which last for 5-7 minutes. At the first minute, this vasodilating effect was even more pronounced with LBK (data not shown) but with both kinins it was transient, being completely reversed after 10 minutes of perfusion.

In the kidneys perfused with BK, no further changes on RVR were seen up to the 20 min of perfusion. Contrarily, LBK after the 10th min of perfusion, consistently gave a rebound effect characterized by a significant increase on RVR. The variation of RVR induced by LBK on both the first (vasodilator) and second (vasoconstrictor) phase led to changes in the perfusion pressure while renal perfusion flow remained almost unchanged. The results also show that the vasodilator but not the vasoconstrictor effect of LBK was blocked by 5 uM indomethacin, thus suggesting that only the transient vasorelaxant effect of the decapeptide on IPRK is mediated by prostaglandins. These data also suggest that LBK may have a direct effect on the kidney vasculature.

Inasmuch as the kinins effects on the vascular bed of several tissue preparations may depend on distinct receptors,[1] we also studied the actions of a kinin fragment des-Arg^9-BK(DABK) and of the kinin-B$_1$ receptor antagonist (L-Leu)^8-des-Arg^9-BK(LDABK) on IPRK. DABK by itself had no vasodilating effect on the kidney. However, as shown in the Table DABK significantly increased RVR. This vasoconstrictor effect of DABK was not blocked by 0.2 - 20 ug/ml of BW-755C, an inhibitor of both pathways of arachidonic acid metabolism[5] (results not shown). As the results with DABK suggested the presence of B$_1$-receptor in the IPRK, the antagonist of this receptor (LDABK) was tested. As shown in the Table, LDABK strongly blocked the vasoconstrictor effect of DABK. The antagonist also inhibited the vasoconstrictor effect of LBK, while its vasorelaxant action, if anything, was even larger in the presence of the antagonist.

DISCUSSION

The present results demonstrate that in the perfused rat kidney BK and LBK induce different effects on renal vasculature. The kinins added to the perfusate cause a vasodilating effect leading to a lowering of RVR

Table 1. Effects of bradykinin, lysyl-bradykinin and kinin-fragments on the renal vascular resistance (RVR) of isolated perfused rat kidney

Test substances		Effect on RVR		
Kinins and fragments	Other substances	Experimental period (minutes)		
		5	10	20
BK (0.07 uM, n = 7)	–	0.93±0.02*	0.98±0.02	1.02±0.02
LBK (0.07 uM, n = 5)	–	0.94±0.02*	1.04±0.02	1.17±0.05**
LBK (0.07 uM)	Indomethacin (5 uM, n = 6)	0.98±0.01	1.04±0.01	1.13±0.03*
DABK (20 ug, n = 4)	–	1.02±0.005	1.04±0.005	1.06±0.05
DABK (20 ug)	LDABK (100 ug, n = 6)	1.04±0.015	1.07±0.018	1.07±0.018
LBK (0.07 uM)	LDABK (200 ug, n = 5)	0.89±0.037**	0.93±0.030*	0.94±0.027*

Values given are mean±SEM
*p<0.05 and **p<0.01 vs RVR of control period taken as 1.0.

which was markedly significant at the first minute of perfusion. While BK showed only vasodilation lasting for about 5 minutes, LBK induced both vasodilation (more pronounced but of shorter duration) and a rebound effect with a vasoconstrictor phase leading to a significant increase on RVR. It seems then possible to postulate that the transience of kinin vasodilating response as well as the bimodal effect of LBK may account for the conflicting results concerning the actions of kinins in the renal vasculature and its mediation by prostaglandins.[6,7] Moreoever, the vaso-constrictor effect induced by LBK is unrelated to the mediation by cyclo-oxygenase and/or lipoxygenase products.

The existence of two different types of kinin receptors as found in the vascular tissues such as the rabbit aorta[3] also implies different responses from the preparation. As proposed by Regoli and Barabé,[1] if the B_1 receptor is involved one would expect a higher effect of LBK than with BK because of the presence of an additional positive charge at the N-terminal lysine. It would be also possible that both kinin fragments Des-Arg[9]-BK and Des-Arg[10]-LBK could be agonists for the vasoconstriction of renal vasculature. Accordingly, when the former peptide was tested a dose- and time-dependent increase in RVR was found. The effect of Des-Arg[10]-LBK was not investigated in this work, but such fragment could be expected to be produced after the direct action of kininase I[8] on LBK. From this decapeptide DABK could also be formed upon the sequential action of a kinin-converting aminopeptidase[9] and kininase I.

As recently reported[10] a vasoconstrictor effect of BK on isolated rat kidney was seen when the organ was perfused with BK in presence of captopril, the potent inhibitor of angiotensin-converting enzyme.[11] This finding strongly suggests that the inhibition of kininase II would favor the action of kidney kininase I thus producing des-Arg^9-BK, which is no longer substrate for kininase II being however agonist of B_1-receptor. Our results clearly indicate the presence of both types of receptors in the kidney accounting for the two types of responses by renal vasculature upon interaction with BK, LBK or their fragments. Thus kinin-induced vasocilation and vasoconstriction of this vasculature may result in inducing distinct physiological responses of the kidney hemodynamics.

REFERENCES

1. D. Regoli, and J. Barabe, Pharmacology of bradykinin and related kinins, Pharmacol. Rev., 32:1-46, (1980).
2. M. Rocha e Silva, Present trends in kinin research, Life Sci., 15:7-22, (1974).
3. D. Regoli, Pharmacology of bradykinin and related kinins, Adv. Exp. Med. Biol., 156A:569-584, (1983).
4. T. Maack, Physiological evaluation of the isolated perfused rat kidney, Am. J. Physiol., 238:F71-F78, (1980).
5. G. A. Higgs, R. J. Flower, and J. R. Vane, A new approach to anti-inflammatory drugs, Biochem. Pharmacology, 28:1959-1961, (1979).
6. A. Nasjletti, and K. U. Malik, Renal kinin-prostaglandin relationship: Implications for renal function, Kidney International, 19:860-868, (1981).
7. H. S. Margolius, The kallikrein-kinin system and the kidney, Ann. Rev. Physiol., 46:309-326, (1984).
8. E. G. Erdos, and H. Y. T. Yang, in: Handbook of Experimental Pharmacology, Vol. 26, E. G. Erdos (ed.), Berlin: Spring-Verlag, pp. 289-323, (1970).
9. K. B. Alves, C. M. W. Brandi, J. C. Souza-Pinto, and J. A. Guimarães, Kinin-converting aminopeptidase from human urine: further purification and characterization through kinetic and inhibitory studies, Int. J. Biochemistry, (in press).
10. J. P. Curtin, and L. A. Arbeit, The effect of bradykinin on the renal blood flow of the rat, Abstract IXth, International Congress of Nephrology, 447A, (1984).
11. M. A. Ondetti, B. Rubin, and D. W. Cushman, Design of specific inhibitors of angiotensin-converting enzyme: A new class of orally active antihypertensive agents, Science, 196:441-444, (1977).

^{3}H-BRADYKININ BINDING SITE LOCALIZATION IN GUINEA PIG URINARY SYSTEM

Donald C. Manning and Solomon H. Snyder

Department of Neuroscience, The Johns Hopkins University
School of Medicine, Baltimore, Maryland 21205

ABSTRACT

Bradykinin (BK) causes vasodilation and increases free water and
sodium excretion in the kidney and stimulates smooth muscle contraction
in the ureter and bladder. Several proposed sites of action for BK include
the renal medullary collecting duct, renal blood vessels and the ureter
and bladder smooth muscle. This study employs ^{3}H-BK autoradiography to
localize the sites of BK action. ^{3}H-BK binding sites in the kidney are
localized in the medullary interstitium where BK may produce prostaglandins
which mediate its blood flow, natriuretic and diuretic effects. ^{3}H-BK
binding sites in the ureter and bladder are localized in the lamina
propria below the basal epithelial layer and absent over the muscle layers
suggesting an indirect action on urinary tract smooth muscle.

INTRODUCTION

Bradykinin (BK), when injected into the renal artery, can stimulate
vasocilation and increase free water and sodium excretion.[1,2] This finding associated with the excretion of urinary kallikrein has prompted
many investigations into the location and function of the renal
kallikrein-kinin system. Kallikrein has been localized by biochemical[3]
and immunohistochemical[4,5] methods to the luminal and basolateral anti-
luminal membranes of cells of the distal nephron. Kininogen is also
present in the cells of the distal tubules and collecting ducts.[6]
Kininase II (Peptidyl-dipeptidase) activity appears to be mostly
localized to the proximal tubule[7] effectively preventing filtered kinins
from acting at distal sites in the nephron. BK's actions in the kidney
are at least partially linked to the production of prostaglandins including PGE_2, PGF_2 and PGI_2.[8] Indeed, kinins have been shown to release
prostaglandins from renal medullary interstial cells[9] and renal papillary
collecting tubule cells[10] in culture.

The successful localization of many components of the renal kinin
system has been met with questions and controversies as to the kinin
site(s) of action. So far it has been difficult to determine if the

principle site of action is directly on the collecting duct, the vasculature or at some other site with indirect prostaglandin mediated effects.

BK can effect other areas of the urinary tract as well causing smooth muscle contraction in the bladder[11] and ureter[13,14] and dilation of the bladder vascular bed.[12]

Saturable ^{3}H-BK binding sites with picomolar affinity and pharmacological properties consistent with relevant BK receptors can be identified in membrane preparations of the kidney, ureter and bladder.[15] This study employs ^{3}H-BK in vitro receptor autoradiography to localize these binding sites in the guinea pig urinary system.

METHODS

The autoradiographic localization of ^{3}H-BK receptor binding sites is accomplished by using a modified version of Young and Kuhar's coverslip method.[16] Guinea pigs are perfused through the heart with 500 ml of 0.1% formaldehyde in a mixture of equal parts phosophate buffered saline and 20% sucrose, pH 7.4. The tissues are removed, embedded in homogenized calf cerebral cortex and frozen on dry ice. Ten micron sections are cut in a cryostat at -12^0C, thaw mounted onto chrome alum-gelatin subbed microscope slides and stored frozen at -20^0C.

When ready for use, the slides are warmed to room temperature, incubated for 120 min at 4^0C in media containing 20 mM TES pH 6.8, 1 mM 1-10-phenanthroline, 0.2% bovine serum albumin (protease free), 1 mM dithiotheitol, 140 µg/ml bacitracin, 0.1 mM SQ20,881, 300 mM sucrose and 0.5 mM ^{3}H-BK (52 Ci/mmole). Blanks are incubated in the same media with the addition of 1 µM unlabeled BK or lysyl-BK.

After incubation the tissue sections are washed in 25 mM TES pH 6.8 and 10% sucrose for 20 min (2 x 10 min) at 4^0C then dried rapidly under cold, dry air, and apposed to either NTB-3 emulsion coated coverslips or LKB ultrafilm for 1-3 months. After exposure the coverslip/slide or ultrafilm are developed and the tissue stained with hematoxylin-eosin.

In the developed autoradiogram silver grains are localized over areas of radioactivity accumulation (mostly receptor bound as determined by comparison to blanks). These silver grains appear as white dots under darkfield illumination with the underlying tissue rendered invisible.

RESULTS

Saturable ^{3}H-BK binding sites have been localized by autoradiographic methods in guinea pig kidney ureter and urinary bladder. All localizations have been reproduced in triplicate in tissues from 3-4 separate animals.

Kidney

The kidney exhibits high levels of heterogeneously distributed ^{3}H-BK binding sites (Figure 1) which are almost exclusively restricted to the medulla with the highest density in the inner medulla (Figure 1B).

Essentially all of these sites represent saturable binding as determined by the lack of autoradiographic grains over sections incubated with a large excess of unlabelled BK (Figure 1C).

Closer analysis of the streaking grain pattern in the inner medulla reveals that the binding sites are restricted to the interstitial regions between the collecting ducts (labelled i in Figures 1D and E) and not over the ducts (between the arrows, labelled ct in Figures 1D and E). Sparse labelling is present in the cortex and absent over any identifiable blood vessels as well as proximal or distal convulted tubules and thick limbs of Henle's loop. At this level of fixation it is not possible to distinguish vasa recta or thin limbs of Henle's loop in the medullary interstitium.

Qualitatively similar grain reductions occur when sections are incubated with 20 nM BK, lysyl-BK and 200 nM methionyl-lysyl BK. No detectable reduction in grain density is observed with 1 µM DesArg^{9}BK.

Ureter

^{3}H-BK binding sites in the ureter are heavily localized over the immediate subepithelial region of the lamina propria with a decreasing gradient of concentration extending to the muscle layer (Figure 2B). No significant grain accumulation greater than background is present over the epithelial and smooth muscle (Figure 2D). The grain densities are reduced to background levels in sections incubated with excess unlabelled lysyl-BK.

Bladder

^{3}H-BK binding sites in the urinary bladder are heterogeneously distributed with high densities over the immediate subepithelial layer of the lamina propria, lower densities over widely dispersed mucosal blood vessels and approximately background levels over the muscle layers. As with the other areas of the urinary tract, incubation of tissue sections with excess unlabelled lysyl BK reduces grain density to background levels. Figure 3D emphasizes the sharp concentrated localization of binding sites just beneath the basal layer of transitional epithelium.

DISCUSSION

One of the major findings of this study is the autoradiographic localization of ^{3}H-BK binding sites in the renal mudullary interstitium suggesting that this area may be a major site of action for BK in the kidney. The absence of significant ^{3}H-BK binding over the distal tubule or renal blood vessels however does not preclude direct binding interactions there. Recently Tomita and Pisano[17] have published evidence for ^{3}H-BK binding interactions in cortical collecting tubule segments of isolated nephrons with an affinity of 12.9 nM. The assay in this study is designed to label binding sites with affinities higher than 1 nM. The low concentrations of ^{3}H-BK and the long wash time in this study allows ligand to dissociate off binding sites with affinities in the nanomolar range and therefore would not be significantly labelled in the autoradiograms. The selection against low affinity sites would also lower the possibility that the binding site distribution in the present study represents enzymes as one would not expect BK to exhibit affinities in

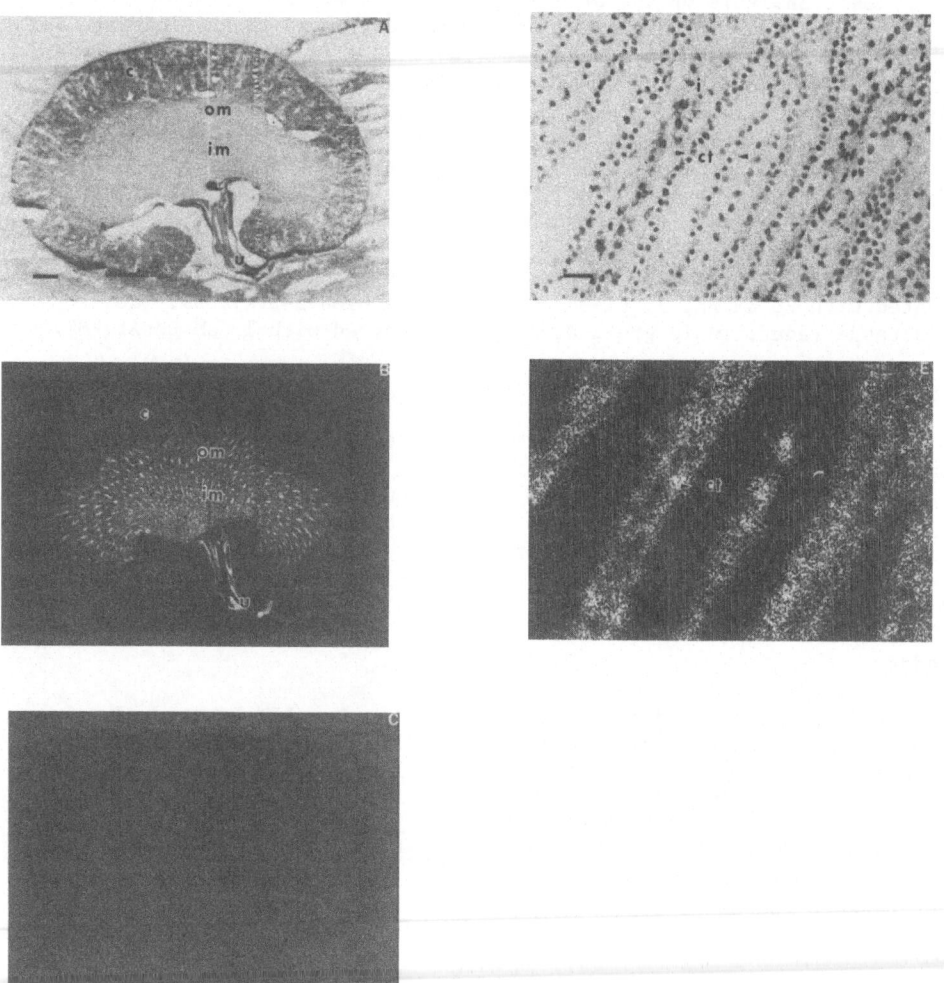

Figure 1.   Autoradiographic localization of ^{3}H-BK (0.5 nM) binding in
guinea pig kidney.   (A) Low power brightfield photomicrograph
(bar = 100 μM).   (B) Darkfield photomicrograph from LKB ultrafilm after exposure to tissue section in A.   Note the high
grain density representing ^{3}H-BK binding sites over the inner
medulla (im), outer medulla (om) and ureter (u) and the
relative absence of grains over the cortex (c).   (C) Darkfield
photomicrograph of Ultrafilm grain density after exposure to
kidney section incubated with ^{3}H-BK (0.5 nM) and 1 μM unlabelled
lysyl-BK.   (D) High power brightfield photomicrograph (bar =
5 μM) of renal inner medulla showing a field of collecting
tubules (ct) with peritubular limits indicated by arrows and
interstitium (i).   (E) High power darkfield photomicrograph
of tissue section field in D from overlying NTB-3 emulsion
coated coverslip.   Note the discrete localization of grains in
the interstitium and the relative lack of grains over the
collecting tubule (between arrows).

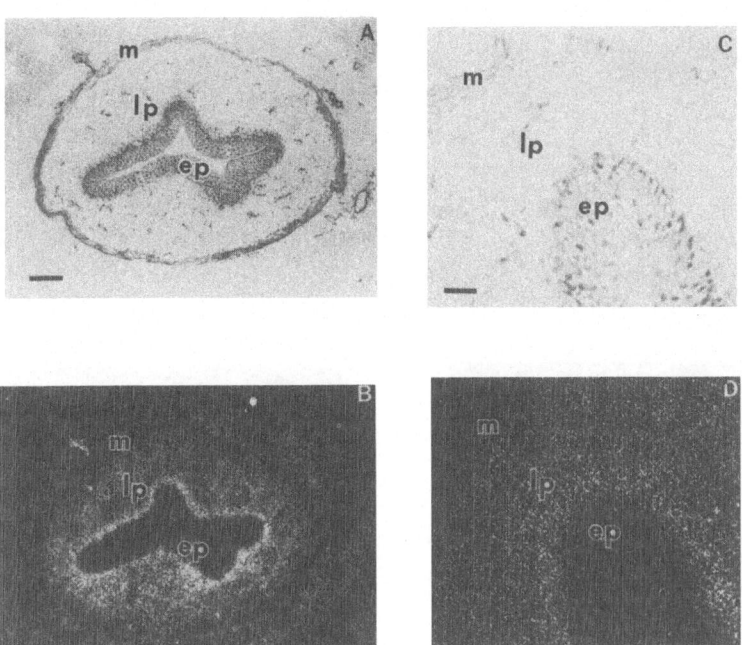

Figure 2. Autoradiographic localization of ^{3}H-BK (0.5 nM) binding in guinea pig ureter. (A) Low power brightfield, photomicrograph (bar = 100 μM) of ureter cross section. (B) Darkfield photomicrograph of NTB-3 emulsion coated coverslip overlying section in A. Note the high grain density over the lamina propria (lp) especially the subepithelial area and the relative lack of grains over the epithelium (ep) and muscle layer (M). (C) High power brightfield photomicrograph (bar = 25 μM) from A. (D) Darkfield photomicrograph of C emphasizing the sharp boundary of grain density in the lamina propria at the basal layer of the epithelium and the lack of grains over the muscle layers.

the subnanomolar range for enzymes. In addition SQ 20881 was used in the incubation cocktail to competitively inhibit angiotensin converting enzyme binding.

The ^{3}H-BK binding site distribution in the inner medulla could represent interactions with the thin limbs of the loop of Henle, vasa recta or interstitial cells, however unambiguous cellular localization is not possible with this technique. The renal medullary interstitial cell is the most likely site of kinin action of the ones listed here. These cells are known to contain large quantities of lipids and they have been shown to produce prostaglandins upon kinin stimulation.[9] Several investigators have localized kallikrein to the basal membrane of cells in the distal tubule[3,4] particularly the connecting tubule[5] in addition other studies have reported kallikrein in the renal venous effluent. These findings imply transfer of the enzyme through the interstitium and renal lymph[18] where kallikrein has been found in small but measurable quantities.[19] The localization of kallikrein and the presence of kininogen in collecting tubule cells[6] suggests possible generation and action of kinin within the institium and possible interaction with the binding sites identified here to produce prostaglandins which would mediate the vasodilatory, natiuretic and diuretic actions.

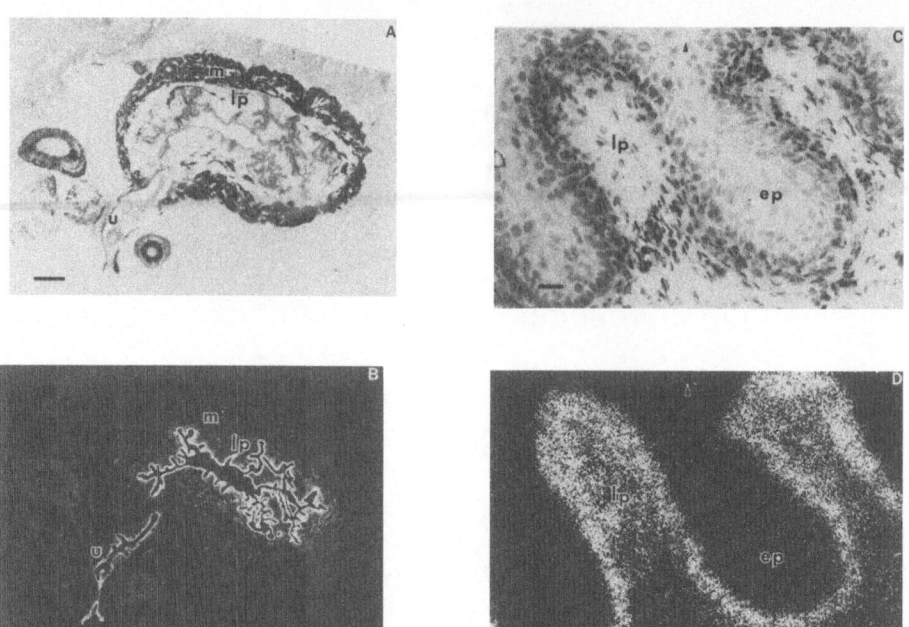

Figure 3. Autoradiographic localization of ^{3}H-BK (0.5 nM) binding in guinea pig urinary bladder. (A) Low power brightfield photomicrograph (bar = 1 mm). (B) Darkfield photomicrograph from LKB Ultrafilm after exposure to tissue section in A. Note the high grain density in the lamina propria (lp) especially in the immediate subepithelial area, following the epithelial foldings. Note also a lower grain density in the deeper areas of the lamina propria representing blood vessel binding. Binding is also present in the lamin propria of the ureter (u) but absent over the muscle layers (m). (C) High power brightfield photomicrograph (bar = 25 μM) at the lamina propria - epithelium junction. The arrow points in the direction of the bladder lumen. (D) Darkfield photomicrograph of section in C. Note the sharp boundary of grain density in the lamina propria at the basal border of the epithelium.

The immediate subepithelial localization of ^{3}H-BK binding sites in the ureter and bladder with an absence over the muscle layers is puzzling. The subepithelial lamina propria regions are rich in both capillaries[20] and nerves[21] suggesting that BK's action on smooth muscle may be indirect through capillary endothelium derived prostaglandins or neurons. Kinins may also mediate mucosal effects in the ureter and bladder not yet described. In the bladder however, the ^{3}H-BK labeling over intramural blood vessels is consistent with BK's ability to dilate this vascular bed.[12]

ACKNOWLEDGEMENTS

Supported by USPHS grants DA-00266 and NS-16375, RSA award DA-00074 to S.H. S. and a grant of the McKnight Foundation. We thank Nancy Bruce for manuscript preparation.

REFERENCES

1. M. A. Baraclough and I. H. Mills, Effect of bradykinin on renal function, Clin. Sci., 28:69-74, (1965).
2. M. Marin Grez, P. Cottone, and O. A. Carretero, Evidence for an involvement of kinins in regulation of sodium excretion, Am. J. Physiol., 223:797-796, (1972).
3. K. Yamada, W. W. Schulz, D. S. Page, and E. G. Erdos, Kallikrein and prekallikrein on the basolateral membrane of rat kidney tubules, Hypertension 3 (suppl II):II-59-II-64, (1981).
4. T. B. Orstavik, K. Nustad, P. Brandtzaeg, and J. V. Pierce, Cellular origin of urinary kallikreins, J. Histochem. Cytochem.,24:1037-1039, (1976).
5. C. D. Figueroa, I. Caorsi, J. Subiabre, and C. P. Vio, Immunoreactive kallikrein localization in the rat kidney, J. Histochem. Cytochem., 32:117-121, (1984).
6. D. Proud, M. Perkins, J. V. Pierce, K. N. Yates, P. F. Highet, P. L. Herring, M. M. Mangkonkonok, R. Bahu, F. Carone, and J. J. Pisano, Characterization and localization of human renal kininogen, J. Biol. Chem., 256:10634-10639, (1981).
7. P. E. Ward, E. G. Erodos, C. D. Gedney, R. M. Dowben, and R. C. Reynolds, Isolation of membrane bound renal enzymes that metabolize kinins and angiotensin, Biochem. J., 157:643-650, (1976).
8. A. Nasjletti, and K. U. Malik, The renal kallikrein-kinin and prostaglandin systems interaction, Ann. Rev. Physiol., 43:597-609, (1981).
9. R. M. Zusman and H. R. Keiser, Prostaglandin biosynthesis by rabbit renomedullary interstitial cells in tissue culture, J. Clin. Invest., 60:215-223, (1977).
10. F. C. Grenier, T. E. Rollins, and W. L. Smith, Kinin-induced prostaglandin synthesis by renal papillary collecting tubule cells in culture, Ann. J. Physiol., 241:F94-F104, (1981).
11. G. Falconier-Erspamer, L. Negri, and D. Piccinelli, The use of preparations of urinary bladder smooth muscle for bioassay of discrimination between polypeptides, Naunyn-Schmiedeberg's Arch. Pharm., 279:61-74, (1973).
12. S. Matsumura, N. Taira, and K. Hashimoto, The pharmacological behavior of the urinary bladder and its vasculature of the dog, Tohoku J. Exp. Med., 96:247-258, (1968).
13. M. Marin-Grez, G. Bonne, and F. Gross, Ureteral contractions induced by rat urine in vitro: Probable involvement of renal kallikrein, Experentia, 36:865-866, (1980).
14. P. Labay and S. Boyarsky, Bradykinin: Effect on ureteral peristalsis, Science, 151:78, (1966).
15. D. C. Manning, R. Vavrek, J. M. Stewart, and S. H. Snyder, Multiple bradykinin binding sites with picomolar affinities, In preparation.
16. W. S. Young and M. J. Kuhar, A new method for receptor autoradiography: [^{3}H]opioid receptors in rat brain, Brain Res., 179:255-270, (1979).
17. K. Tomita and J. J. Pisano, Binding of [^{3}H]bradykinin in isolated nephron segments of the rabbit, Am. J. Physiol., 246:F732-F737, (1984).
18. R. Garcia, G. Thibault and J. Genest, Lymphatic, renal and urinary kallikreins in the rat, Am. J. Physiol., 247:R29-R33, (1984).

19. D. Proud, S. Nakamura, F. A. Carone, P. L. Herring, M. Kawamura, T. Inagami, and J. J. Pisano, Kallikrein-kinin and renin angiotensin systems in rat renal lymph, Kidney Int., 25:880-885, (1984).
20. J. T. Velardo, Histology of the ureter, in: The ureter, 2nd ed., H. Bergman, (ed.), Springer-Verlag, pp. 13-15, (1981).
21. M. Aung-Khin, The innervation of the ureter, Invest. Urol., 10: 370-378, (1973).

ACTION AND METABOLISM OF DES(ARG)KININS IN MESENTERIC ARTERIES

Laurie Churchill, John C. McGiff and Patrick E. Ward

Department of Pharmacology, New York Medical College

Valhalla, New York 10595

SUMMARY

Kallidin and bradykinin can be hydrolyzed at their C-termini to produce des(Arg[10])kallidin and des(Arg[9])bradykinin respectively. These des(Arg)kinins, previously thought to be biologically inactive, are now known to have potent effects on B_1 receptors. Although stimulation of B_1 receptors has been reported to produce peripheral vasodepressor responses in certain experimental states, only constriction has been reported in isolated vessels (i.e., rabbit aorta, basilar artery, mesenteric vein). In the present study, we have investigated the biologic activity of des(Arg) kinins on a peripheral resistance vessel (rabbit mesenteric artery). We found that des(Arg)bradykinin relaxes mesenteric arteries, and that its potency relative to kallidin and bradykinin is consistent with the presence of B_1 receptors. Further, intact mesenteric arteries, and a plasma membrane fraction purified from these arteries, contained a carboxypeptidase activity which was capable of producing des(Arg)kinins from both kallidin and bradykinin. Thus, these data demonstrate that the vasculature has the enzymatic capacity to form B_1 kinins, and that stimulation of B_1 receptors in resistance vessels can be associated with peripheral vasodilation.

INTRODUCTION

Glandular and plasma kallikreins hydrolyze kininogen substrates to produce kallidin and bradykinin respectively[1]. Kinins cause peripheral arterial vasodilation, venule constriction, increased flow in capillary beds and increased vascular permeability. However, both peptides are rapidly inactivated by vascular and circulating angiotensin I converting enzyme (ACE; EC 3.4.15.1)[2,3], and are also hydrolyzed by plasma carboxypeptidase N (CPN; EC 3.4.17.3) to produce des(Arg)kinins[4,5]. Until recently, des(Arg)kinins were thought to be biologically inactive. However, Regoli and co-workers[6,7] have reported that these kinin metabolites demonstrate significant biologic activity, and are resistant to degradation by ACE.

Regoli and co-workers have identified and characterized two types of kinin receptors (B_1 and B_2) which differ with regard to order of potency of agonists, pA_2 values and susceptibility to blockade by specific antagonists[6-9]. Bradykinin is a potent and relatively specific B_2 agonist,

```
                              Am M                        C P
                               ↓                           ↓
  KALLIDIN:           LYS-ARG-PRO-PRO-GLY-PHE-SER-PRO-PHE-ARG
                                                          ↓
  BRADYKININ:             ARG-PRO-PRO-GLY-PHE-SER-PRO-PHE-ARG
                           ↓
  DES(ARG10)KALLIDIN:  LYS-ARG-PRO-PRO-GLY-PHE-SER-PRO-PHE

  DES(ARG9)BRADYKININ:    ARG-PRO-PRO-GLY-PHE-SER-PRO-PHE
```

Figure 1

while kallidin has both B_1 and B_2 agonist activity. Conversely, des(Arg[10]) kallidin and des(Arg[9]) bradykinin do not have any significant capacity to stimulate B_2 receptors. However, these peptides are 200 and 10 fold more potent, respectively, than bradykinin, in stimulating B_1 receptors. The effects of des(Arg) kinins can be blocked by specific B_1 antagonists including Leu[9]-des(Arg[10]) kallidin and Leu[8]-des(Arg[9]) bradykinin[10,11].

Stimulation of B_1 kinin receptors produces contractile responses in a number of vascular bioassay tissues including the rabbit mesenteric vein, basilar artery and aorta[7,10,12]. Tissue injury or certain experimental stress conditions have been shown to enhance B_1 receptor levels. Vessels containing B_1 receptors demonstrate increased sensitivity to des(Arg)kinins during incubation in vitro[13] and after lipopolysaccharide treatment in vivo [14]. Infusion of des(Arg[9]) bradykinin to these animals is associated with a vasodepressor response which is blocked by B_1 antagonists. These data indicate that although B_1 kinins are reported to produce constriction in isolated vasculature, a more general effect may be peripheral vasodilation.

The present study was carried out to investigate the effect of des(Arg) kinins on the vascular tone of peripheral resistance vessels. Further, studies were conducted to determine whether certain vascular enzymes such as Aminopeptidase M (AmM; EC 3.4.11.2)[15] and a carboxypeptidase (CP)[16] may be involved in the local metabolism of B_1 kinins (Figure 1).

METHODS

Superfusion Bioassay

Male, New Zealand white rabbits (2-3 kg) were anesthetized with Keto-set, Ace Promazine and Rompin, and were bleed from the abdominal aorta. The mesenteric artery was carefully removed and immediately placed in ice cold oxygenated Krebs. The vessel was cleaned of any adherent fat or connective tissue, and was cut into a spiral strip with care being taken not to rub the intimal surface or stretch the tissue. The strip was then suspended in a polypropylene chamber and was superfused with oxygenated Krebs solution (pH 7,4,37°C) at 10 ml/min. The tissue was attached to a Grass force transducer and the resting tension adjusted to one gram. After a one hour incubation period, the tissue was precontracted with phenylephrine (10 μM). Agents were given in bolus directly over the tissue. All results are shown as means ± standard error of the mean.

Vessel Subcellular Fractionation

Mesenteric arteries were obtained from the above animals and the vessels were subfractionated as previously described[15] to obtain a purified vascular plasma membrane (VPM) fraction.

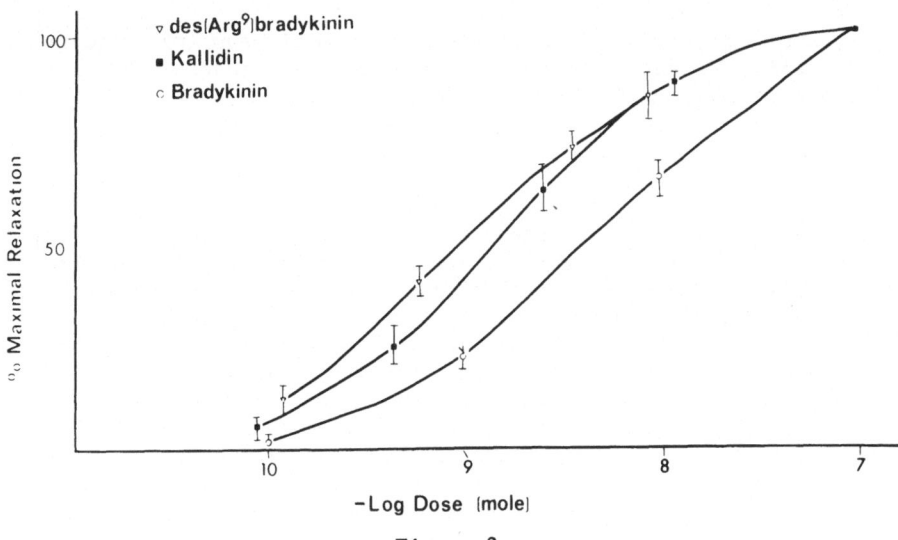

Figure 2

Peptide Metabolism

The presence of a CPN-like enzyme was determined using hippuryl-L-arginine (HLA) as substrate[16]. HLA (2 mM final concentration) was incubated in 50 μl of 100 mM Tris/HCl (pH 7.4) with 5 μl of VPM. The arginine product was measured qualitatively after separation via thin layer chromatography (TLC) on MN 300 cellulose plates[17]. Five μl aliquots were spotted at timed intervals and immediately dried. Plates were developed in butanol: acetic acid: water (4:1:5) and the products visualized by staining with 0.4% (w/v) ninhydrin in acetone[18].

Qualitative analysis of kallidin metabolism by VPM was also carried out by TLC as above. The incubation consisted of kallidin (0.5 mM final concentration) in 50 μl of 100 mM Tris/HCI (pH 7.0) with 1 mM captopril and 2.5 μl VPM. Enzyme inhibitors were preincubated for 30 minutes before addition of substrate.

RESULTS

Rabbit Mesenteric Artery Bioassay

As shown in Figure 2, des(Arg[9]) bradykinin, kallidin and bradykinin all produced dose dependent relaxation of the precontracted rabbit mesenteric artery (n=4). The dose response curves obtained show that des(Arg[9])-bradykinin and kallidin are significantly more potent than bradykinin in producing relaxation. The EC_{50}'s were 1.0 ± 0.2, 1.4 ± 0.2 and 5.1 ± 0.8 nmols for des(Arg) bradykinin, kallidin and bradykinin respectively.

Peptide Metabolism

When VPM from mesenteric arteries was incubated with the synthetic CPN substrate HLA, Arg was produced in a time dependent manner indicating the presence of a carboxypeptidase. Experiments were then carried out to determine if this activity could hydrolyze the carboxy terminal Arg from kallidin. Incubation of VPM with kallidin (in the presence of captopril) produced increasing concentrations of Lys and Arg with time, demonstrating the hydrolysis of kallidin at both the amino terminus to produce bradykinin, and at the carboxy terminus to produce des(Arg)kinins. Indeed, when this reaction was carried out in the presence of an AmM inhibitor (amastatin; 0.1 mM)[17], Lys production was completely inhibited whereas Arg production was not altered. Conversely, when a CPN inhibitor was added (MERGETPA; 0.1 mM)[4], the production of Arg was selectively inhibited.

DISCUSSION

The results of the present study show that des(Arg^9) bradykinin (B$_1$ agonist) and kallidin (B$_1$/B$_2$ agonist) are approximately five times more potent than bradykinin in producing relaxation of the rabbit mesenteric artery. This order of potency is consistent with the presence of B$_1$ receptors. If, in fact, the relaxation produced by des(Arg^9) bradykinin is due to B$_1$ stimulation, this is the first report of relaxation of an isolated vessel via B$_1$ receptors. To date, only contractions of isolated vessels has been reported, despite the fact that B$_1$ stimulation in LPS treated rabbits produces a significant vasodepressor response[14]. Nevertheless, further studies will be required using the more potent B$_1$ agonist des(Arg^{10})kallidin and specific B$_1$ antagonist before any final conclusions can be made.

The physiologic significance of B$_1$ kinins is probably related not only to the presence of receptors and the response elicited, but also to the presence of specific enzymes which can form and/or degrade des(Arg)kinins at or near vascular cell surface receptors. Bradykinin can be formed within the circulation by plasma kallikrein, and kallidin may be formed by circulating and/or vascular glandular kallikrein[19-21]. Therefore, both kallidin and bradykinin may be available in vivo for conversion to des (Arg)kinins by vascular peptidases. Our results show that a carboxypeptidase is present in vasculature and this data is consistent with the results of Ryan et al.[22] reporting CPN-like activity on the surface of vascular endothelial cells. Indeed, some of the B$_1$-like activity of kallidin could be due to local formation of des(Arg^{10})kallidin. Nevertheless, this possibility must remain speculative until dose response experiments can be carried out under conditions where the vascular CPN-like activity is inhibited.

In summary, the results of this study have demonstrated that the rabbit mesenteric artery has the capacity to convert kinins (B$_2$ agonists) into des(Arg)kinins (B$_1$ agonists) and that stimulation of B$_1$ receptors results in vascular relaxation. The possible significance of B$_1$ kinins to control of local blood flow and systemic blood pressure remain to be determined.

ACKNOWLEDGEMENTS

This work was supported by NIADDKD grant #1 RO1 28184.

REFERENCES

1. Erdos, E.G., ed.: Handbook of Experimental Pharmacology, Vol 25 (Suppl. I), Springer-Verlag, Heidelberg (1979).
2. Soffer, R.L.: Angiotensin converting enzyme and the regulation of vasoactive peptides. Ann. Rev. Biochem. 45: 73-94 (1976).
3. Erdos, E.G.: Kininases. In: Handbook of Experimental Pharmacology, ed. by E.G. Erdos. Springer-Verlag, Heidelberg. Vol. 25 (Suppl. I), pp. 427-487 (1979).
4. Plummer, T.H. and Ryan, T.J.: A potent mercapto-by-product analogue inhibitor for human carboxypeptidase N. Biochem. Biophys. Res. Commun.98: 448-454 (1981).

5. Levin, Y., Skidgel, R.A. and Erdos, E.G.: Isolation and characteri-
    zation of the submits of human plasma carboxypeptidase N (kininase
    I). Proc. Natl. Acad. Sci. U.S.A. 79: 4618-4622 (1982).
6. Regoli, D. and Barabe, J.: Pharmacology of bradykinin and related
    kinins. Pharmacol. Rev.32: 1-46 (1980).
7. Barabe, J., Marceau, F., Theriault, B., Drovin, J.N. and Regoli, D.:
    Cardiovascular actions of kinins in the rabbit. Can. J. Physiol.
    Pharmacol. 57: 78-91 (1979).
8. Gaudreau, P., Barabe, J., St.-Pierre, S. and Regoli, D.: Pharmacolog-
    ical studies of kinins in venous smooth muscles. Can. J. Physiol.
    Pharmacol. 59: 371-379 (1981).
9. Marceau, F., Lussier, A., Regoli, D. and Giroud, J.P.: Pharmacology
    of kinins: Their relevance to tissue injury and inflammation.
    Gen. Pharmacol. 14: 209-229 (1983).
10. Regoli, D., Barabe, J. and Park, W.K.: Receptors for bradykinin in
    rabbit aorta. Can. J. Physiol. Pharmacol. 55: 855-867 (1977).
11. Marceau, F., Barabe, J., St.-Pierre, S. and Regoli, D.: Kinin re-
    ceptors in experimental inflammation. Can. J. Physiol. Pharmacol.
    58: 536-542 (1980).
12. Whalley, E.T., Fritz, H. and Greiger, R.: Kinin receptors and angio-
    tensin converting enzyme in rabbit basilar arteries. Naunym-
    Schmiedeberg's Arch. Pharmacol. 324: 296-301 (1983).
13. Regoli, D., Marceau, F. and Barabe, J.: De novo formation of vascular
    receptors for bradykinin. Can. J. Physiol. Pharmacol. 56:
    674-677 (1978).
14. Regoli, D., Marceau, F. and Lavigne, J.: Induction of B_1-receptors
    for kinins in the rabbit by a bacterial lipopolysaccharide. Eur.
    J. Pharmacol. 71: 105-115 (1981).
15. Ward, P.E.: Immunoelectrophoretic analysis of vascular, membrane
    bound angiotensin I converting enzyme, aminopeptidase M, and
    dipeptidyl (amino) peptidase IV. Biochem. Pharmacol. 33:
    3183-3193 (1984).
16. Juillerat-Jeanneret, L., Roth, M. and Bargetizi, J.: Some properties
    of porcine carboxypeptidase N. Hoppe-Seyler's Z. Physiol. Chem.
    363: 51-58 (1982).
17. Palmieri, F.E., Petrelli, J.J. and Ward, P.E.: Vascular, plasma
    membrane aminopeptidase M: Metabolism of vasoactive peptides.
    Biochem. Pharmacol. (in press).
18. Toennies, G. and Kolb, J.J.: Techniques and reagents for paper
    chromatography. Anal. Chem. 23: 823-826 (1951).
19. Lawton, W.J., Proud, D., Frech, M.E., Pierce, J.V., Keiser, H.R. and
    Pisano, J.J.: Characterization and origin of immunoreactive
    glandular kallikrein in rat plasma. Biochem. Pharmacol. 30:
    1731-1737 (1981).
20. Scicli, A.G., Orstavik, T.B., Rabbito, S.F., Murray, R.D. and
    Carretero, O.A.: Blood kinins after sympathetic nerve stimulation
    of the rat submandibular gland. Hypertension. 5: (Suppl. I):
    I-101-I-106 (1983).
21. Nolly, H. and Lama, M.C.: Vascular kallikrein: a kallikrein-like
    enzyme present in vascular tissue of the rat. Clin. Sci. 63:
    249s-251s (1982).
22. Ryan, U.S. and Ryan, J.W.: Endothelial cells and inflammation.
    Clin. Lab. Med. 3: 577-599 (1983).

ACTIVATION BY BRADYKININ AND VASOACTIVE INTESTINAL PEPTIDE OF ADENYLATE

CYCLASE FROM IMMUNOLOGICALLY SENSITIZED LUNG MEMBRANES

Alison L. Gadd and Kanti Bhoola

Department of Pharmacology, Medical School, University of
Bristol, Bristol BS8 1TD, England

SUMMARY

Bradykinin receptors on normal lung membranes seem to be coupled to
adenylate cyclase. Stimulation of the enzyme from sensitized lung membranes by adrenaline and vasoactive intestinal peptide was markedly
reduced, whereas the ability of bradykinin and histamine to activate the
sensitized adenylate cyclase was unaffected. Additional experiments are
necessary in order to delineate the precise molecular events associated
with activation of each of the two presently known bradykinin receptor
types.

INTRODUCTION

Several peptides, including kallidin, bombesin, vasoactive intestinal
peptide (VIP) and substance P are believed to be released from or localized
in mammalian lung tissue. Kallidin (lysyl-bradykinin) is considered to be
formed after allergen-dependent degranulation of mast cells, through the
action of a tissue kallikrein on kininogen. VIP, bombesin and substance P
appear to be associated with neural elements in lung tissue. Both bradykinin[1] and VIP[2] increase cyclic AMP levels in lung slices and tracheal
rings respectively. We therefore designed experiments to examine whether
these regulatory peptides simulate known bioactive amines and activate the
adenylate cyclase of normal lung membranes; in addition, we compared their
efficacy on the enzyme in immunologically sensitized (IgE/IgG) membranes.

METHODS

Extrinsic or allergic bronchial asthma is caused by an immediate
hypersensitivity reaction to allergens, and is primarily mediated by IgE
antibodies.[3] Sensitized guinea-pigs are often used to study such reactions
even though the main homocytotropic antibody produced is IgG. However,
induction of both IgE and IgG antibodies occurs when guinea-pigs are
immunized in a specific manner.[4] Male guinea-pigs (250-350g) were therefore sensitized by an intraperitoneal injection of 1 µg ovalbumin and 100
mg aluminium hydroxide in 2 ml saline (0.9% w/v). Control animals were
sham injected with adjuvant. After a seven week interval the guinea-pigs
were killed by cervical dislocation. Confirmation of sensitization was

obtained in experiments on the isolated ileum of the animals injected with ovalbumin (Schultz-Dale reaction). Subsequently IgE/IgG antibodies were identified by passive cutaneous anaphylaxis[5] in the serum of sensitized guinea-pigs. The two groups can be readily differentiated since IgE antibodies exhibit a longer sensitization latency and have a greater affinity for their mast cell and basophil receptors. Both antibodies (IgE and IgG) were absent in the sera of control animals.

Lungs of control and sensitized animals were perfused with ice-cold saline (0.9%), homogenized and a plasma membrane fraction (1600g x 10 min) prepared for measurement of adenylate cyclase.[6]

RESULTS

Recently we reported that basal adenylate cyclase activity was markedly increased in the lung membranes of guinea-pigs in whom circulating IgE and IgG antibodies were identified (Fig. 1).[7] Receptor-adenylate cyclase coupling involves the interaction of three components: a receptor, a guanine nucleotide regulatory protein and a catalytic unit (Fig. 2). Guanosine triphosphate (GTP) is necessary for receptor-mediated activation of adenylate cyclase.[8] The increase in basal activity noted in the lung membranes of guinea-pigs with circulating IgG/IgE antibodies appeared to be due to a 10-fold increase in the potency of GTP for the sensitized enzyme (Fig. 3). Furthermore, a significant reduction was observed in the activation of the sensitized cyclase by the β-adrenoceptor agonists, adrenaline (Fig. 4), isoprenaline and salbutamol.

Of the four regulatory peptides tested, bradykinin (10^{-7} - 10^{-11} M), bombesin (10^{-7} - 10^{-11} M) and VIP (10^{-5} - 10^{-9} M) produced a dose-related increase in the activity of lung membrane adenylate cyclase, whereas substance P (10^{-4} - 10^{-8} M) was ineffective. Even though bradykinin and bombesin were more potent in activating the enzyme, a greater maximal stimulation was observed with VIP (Fig. 5). Next, we examined the ability of bradykinin and VIP to stimulate the enzyme in sensitized (IgE/IgG) lung membranes. When compared with control membranes, stimulation by VIP was significantly reduced (P <0.01), with an approximately 10-fold loss of efficacy (Fig. 6). In contrast, no alteration was evident in the bradykinin (Fig. 7) or forskolin (Fig. 8) activation of adenylate cyclase from sensitized lung membranes.

DISCUSSION

Our results suggest that bradykinin receptors on lung membranes are linked to adenylate cyclase. Structure-activity relationships[9] and the recently developed antagonist[10] indicate the existence of two kinin receptor populations. The question therefore arises as to the precise molecular mechanisms involved in mediating the cellular actions of kinins and whether kinin receptors are directly coupled in addition to adenylate cyclase to other known second messenger systems (calcium ionophore and chloride cotransporter;[11] hydrolysis of phosphoinositids and activation of guanylate cyclase).

Immunological sensitization of lung membranes resulting in the formation of IgE/IgG antibodies selectively altered the receptor coupled activation of adenylate cyclase. Whereas stimulation of the enzyme by bradykinin or histamine was unaffected, activ4tion by adrenaline or VIP was reduced significantly. Activation of the catalytic unit through the N protein (see Fig. 2) by sodium fluoride or forskolin was unaffected in the sensitized membranes. Therefore, the molecular lesion in the IgE sensitized

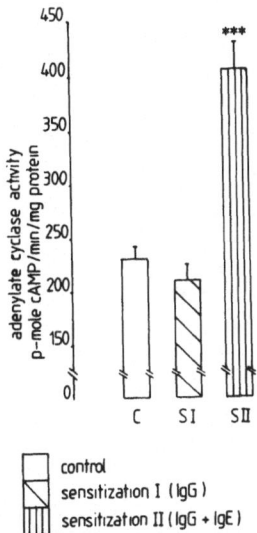

Fig. 1. Effect of immunological sensitization on the basal activity of
lung membrane adenylate cyclase. ☐ – control; ▧ – sensitization
I (IgG); ▥ – sensitization II (IgGE + IgG). Results are mean ±
S.E.M. of 8 experiments performed in triplicate. *** p < 0.001.

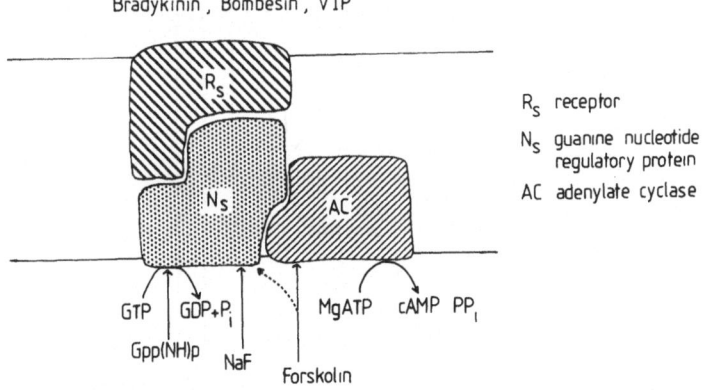

Fig. 2. Schematic diagram of receptor-adenylate cyclase coupling.

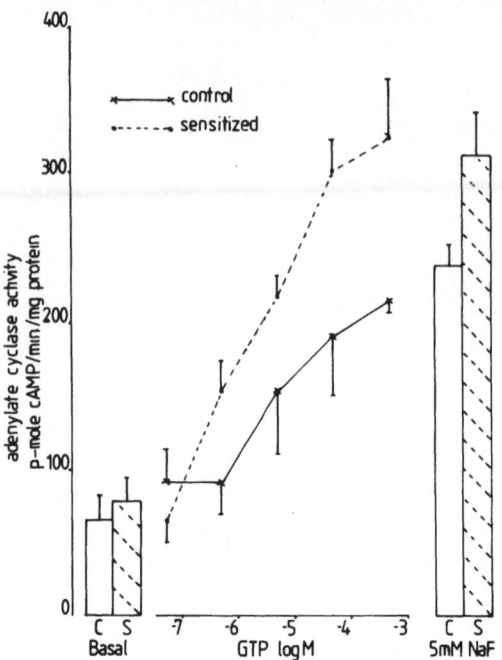

Fig. 3. Effect of GTP on adenylate cyclase of control and sensitized (IgE/IgG) lung membranes. ☐ - control x———x; ▨ - sensitized o-----o; NaF: Sodium fluoride. Results are mean ± 1 S.E.M. of 3 experiments performed in triplicate.

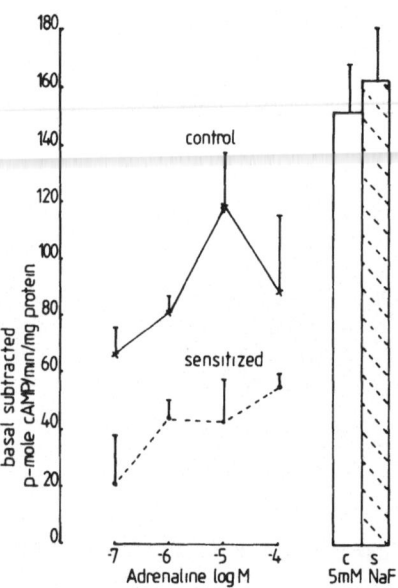

Fig. 4. Effect of adrenaline on adenylate cyclase of control and sensitized (IgE/IgG) lung membranes. ☐ - control x———x; ▨ - sensitized o-----o;NaF: Sodium fluoride. Results are mean ± 1 S.E.M. of 5 experiments performed in triplicate.

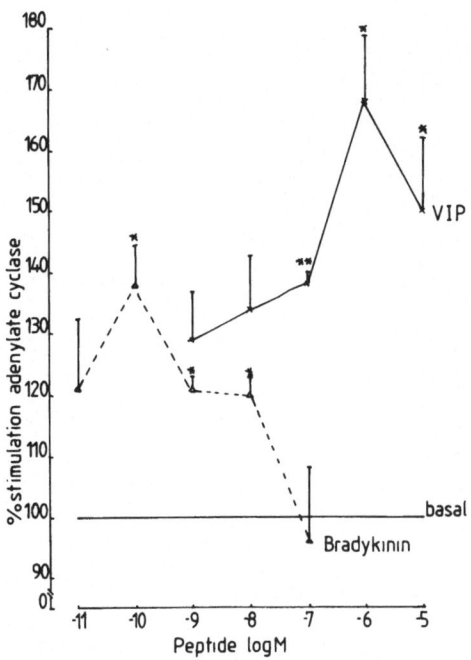

Fig. 5. Effect of bradykinin and VIP on adenylate cyclase of lung membranes.
Δ-----Δ Bradykinin; x———x VIP. Results are mean ± 1 S.E.M. of
3 experiments performed in triplicate. * p < 0.05; ** p < 0.01.

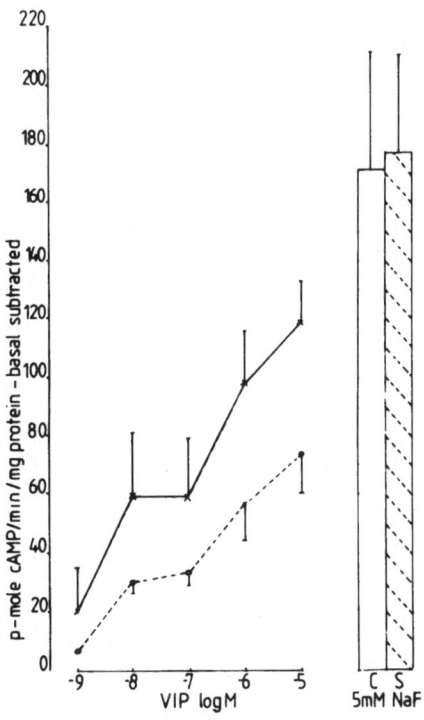

Fig. 6. Action of VIP on control and sensitized (IgE + IgG) adenylate
cyclase of lung membranes. □ - control x———x; ▨ - sensitized
o-----o; NaF: Sodium fluoride. Results are mean ± 1 S.E.[3]. of 3
experiments performed in triplicate.

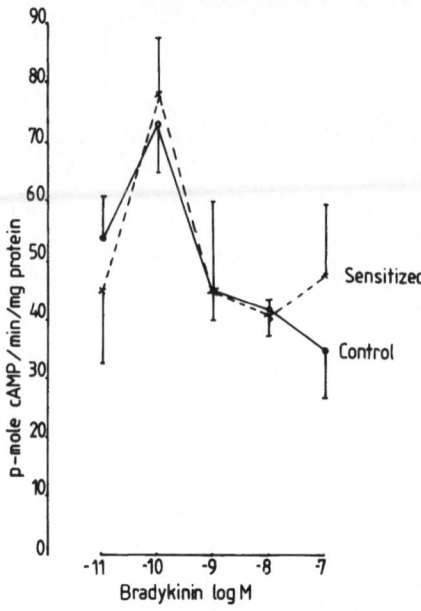

Fig. 7. Action of bradykinin on control and sensitized (IgE + IgG) adenylate cyclase of lung membranes. ☐ – control x———x; ⊠ – sensitized o-----o. Results are mean ± 1 S.E.M. of 3 experiments performed in triplicate.

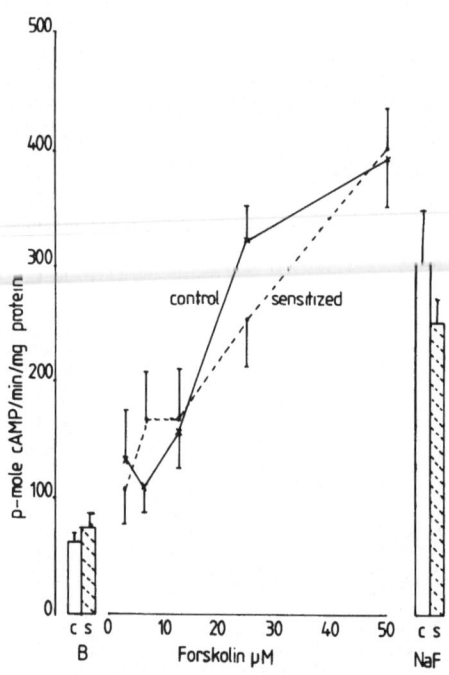

Fig. 8. Effect of forskolin on control and sensitized (IgE + IgG) adenylate cyclase of lung membranes. ☐ – control x———x; ⊠ – sensitized o-----o. Results are mean ± 1 S.E.M. of 3 experiments
performed in triplicate.

adenylate cyclase may reside at the coupling site between the receptor and N protein rather than in a reduction of receptor numbers.

ACKNOWLEDGEMENTS

Alison Gadd was a NAPP Scholar (Cambridge Science Park, Cambridge, England).

REFERENCES

1. J. Stoner, V. C. Maganiello, and M. Vaughan, Effect of bradykinin and indomethacin on cyclic GMP and cyclic AMP in lung slices, Proc. Nat. Acad. Sci. USA, 70:3830-3833 (1973).
2. E. K. Frandsen, G. A. Krishna, and S. I. Said, Vasoactive intestinal polypeptide promotes cyclic 3'5'-monophosphate accumulation in guinea-pig trachea, Br. J. Pharmac., 62:367-369 (1978).
3. K. Ishizaka, Cellular events in the IgE antibody response, Advan. Immunol., 23:1-75 (1976).
4. P. Andersson, Antigen-induced bronchial anaphylaxis in actively sensitized guinea-pigs, Allergy, 35:65-71 (1980).
5. N. Watanabe and Z. Ovary, Antigen and antibody detection by in vivo methods: A re-evaluation of passive cutaneous anaphylactic reactions, J. Immun. Methods, 14:381-390 (1977).
6. B. L. Brown, J. D. M. Albano, R. P. Ekins, A. M. Sgherzi, and W. Tampion, A simple and sensitive saturation assay method for the measurement of adenosine 3',5'-cyclic monophosphate, Biochem. J., 121:561-562 (1971).
7. K. D. Bhoola, A. L. Gadd, and J. Maguire, Does immunological sensitization alter the activity of lung adenylate cyclase, Br. J. Pharmac., 80:605P (1983).
8. M. Rodbell, The role of hormone receptors and GTP-regulatory proteins in membrane transduction, Nature, 284:17-22 (1980).
9. D. Regoli, Kinins, receptors, antagonists, in: "Kinins-84," (1984).
10. J. M. Stewart and R. J. Vavrek, Bradykinin competitive antagonists for classical kinin systems, in: "Kinins-84," (1984).
11. A. W. Cuthbert, P. V. Haluska, H. S. Margolius, and J. A. Spayne, Mediators of the secretory response to kinins, Br. J. Pharmac., 82: 597-607 (1984).